# ENVIRONMENTAL EMERGENCIES

WARD

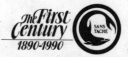

ENVIRONMENTAL EMERGENCIES

# ENVIRONMENTAL EMERGENCIES

## Charles E. Stewart, M.D., F.A.C.E.P.

Director of Research and Education
Spectrum Emergency Care, Inc.
Colorado Springs, Colorado
and
Medical Director, At-Large
Synergon
St. Louis, Missouri

With illustrations by Cynthia Suchovsky

**WILLIAMS & WILKINS**
Baltimore • Hong Kong • London • Sydney

*Editor:* Laurel Craven
*Associate Editor:* Carol Eckhart
*Copy Editor:* Janis Oppelt
*Designer:* Dan Pfisterer
*Illustration Planner:* Lorraine Wrzosek
*Production Coordinator:* Barbara J. Felton

Copyright © 1990
Williams & Wilkins
428 East Preston Street
Baltimore, Maryland 21202, U.S.A.

Accurate indications, adverse reactions, and dosage schedules for
drugs are provided in this book, but it is possible that they may
change. The reader is urged to review the package information data of the
manufacturers of the medications mentioned.

*Printed in the United States of America*

**Library of Congress Cataloging-in-Publication Data**

Stewart, Charles E. (Charles Edward), 1947–
     Environmental emergencies / Charles E. Stewart.
          p.     cm.
     Includes index.
     ISBN 0-683-07932-8
     1. Medical emergencies.   2. Wounds and injuries.   I. Title.
     [DNLM:  1. Emergencies.   2. Wounds and Injuries.     WO 700 S849e]
     RC86.7.S75     1989
     616.02′5—dc20
     DNLM/DLC
     for Library of Congress                                          89-8902
                                                                              CIP

90  91  92  93  94
1  2  3  4  5  6  7  8  9  10

# Preface

## EARTH, AIR, FIRE, AND WATER

The ancients expressed their awe of the forces of nature that surrounded them and deified the forces that shook, baked, froze, and pelted them. Thunder and lightning were the gods of laughter and/or wrath. Sprites dwelled in trees and brooks. The seasons and the days changed due to the mystical forces of these primitive deities. Daily existence depended on the benevolence of the gods of nature and it is natural that the awe was expressed in worship.

As we became more civilized, we started to tame our personal environment. Despite the vagaries of climate and geography, humankind has spread over the earth. Humans thrive on virtually all parts of the earth (both land and water) and can survive both below and above it. Given sufficient energy and commitment, we can live in relative comfort anywhere on the face of the earth, and even off of it.

Perhaps because of our increasing ability to control our personal environment, we are now challenging nature in our play. Daily, more humans migrate to more hostile climates and rugged lands just "for the fun of it." In urban areas, runners, cyclists, and other athletes attempt to extend their personal performance envelopes in all seasons.

Unfortunately, in our urbanization and dependence upon technology, we have lost much of our ancestors' lore and skills of survival in the wilderness and under hazardous conditions. More importantly, we often fail to realize that Mother Nature's rules are inviolate and do not discriminate by color, income, or even species. Skilled professionals skirt disaster when they ignore or deny these rules. For those who are unskilled in wilderness lore, gambling with Mother Nature may have a tragic outcome.

As our transportation skills improve, the ravages of the wilderness may also be brought closer to the urban community. In some cases, as distances diminish, the disease process may not be recognized until the victim is far from the environment from which it was acquired. Such patients may sorely tax the abilities of physicians unaccustomed to environmentally induced ailments.

As we move from the roads and urban environments into the trailhead, we expect the medical professions to follow, protect, rescue, and heal us. The medical profession is not always well prepared to do this. The emergency services may be asked to search for and rescue patients in formidable areas or weather. The local emergency service often simply does not have the training, skills, or equipment to effect these rescues or searches. Even more importantly, once the victim has been rescued and brought to the medical facility, the physicians may not have experience or training in management of the disease or trauma in question.

Until recently only a few medical practitioners had addressed the problems engendered by the environment. In many cases military or naval physicians with extensive experience and hard data were ignored by their civilian colleagues. One or two physicians in each region would be considered "expert" in the management of near-drowning, heat-induced illnesses, snake and arthropod envenomation, cold-related injuries, and hypothermia. Unfortunately those considered to be experts often have had little experience in the management of environmental emergencies in their field of expertise. At times, the intrepid physician who had accompanied a "trek" or who had a hobby of a certain disease or skill would be considered the expert. With little exception, therapy was based on anecdotal accounts, unfounded opinion, or "series" of only a few patients. Lore and conjecture abounded, but few "facts" were subjected to controlled evaluation. (To give due credit, some of these avocationally oriented physicians were so appalled by the lack of information about "their" topic that they became focal points for research efforts and teams. Likewise, some environmentally related diseases are so rare in the general population that few physicians will ever see these maladies.)

It was easily noted that the "experienced" source physicians were not the practitioners who provided primary or emergency care to the patient. A radiologist or radiation physicist would be appointed as a hospital's "radiation emergency officer," with absolutely no *field* experience in emergency management of a traumatized, contaminated victim. Surgeons who saw three or four patients with chemical burns per year would give "astute" advice on "antidote therapies" to the emergency physicians managing such patients. True hazards to medical staff and emergency medical service (EMS) providers were generally ignored in the management of these chemical injuries. Plastic surgeons who could not explain the difference between AC and DC current pontificated on electrical injuries. Cardiologists who were accustomed to overloaded hearts would dehydrate young healthy patients with high altitude pulmonary edema, oblivious to the differences in the two diseases.

Lay people and the lay press were often no better. "Weather experts" would talk of wind-chill factors as absolute temperatures, and responsible journalists ignored the plight of the elderly hypothermic or hyperthermic patient. Road races and/or bicycle races were planned without adequate water supplies or in conditions of extreme heat or humidity. Medical support for these events was often lacking or inadequate. Sports coaches would advocate water-deprivation and wind-sprint "toughening" in 90+ (F) temperature and humidity conditions for summer football training. Otherwise responsible leaders would proceed on late summer mountain treks without appropriate survival skills and gear for all members of the party. Three Mile Island was crafted into a disaster, yet no significant injuries were attributable to radiation exposure.

Fortunately, many of these abuses, oversights, and ill-founded opinions are fading, to be replaced with facts rather than fancy. Lore and conjecture are being replaced with abundant research in the mechanics, pathology, and treatment of wilderness-related emergencies. Multiple groups of both lay and medical providers now have training programs in wilderness emergencies. Those who plan athletic events require an appropriate supply of water and medical support, and there are cancellation plans for conceivable contingencies.

Three concurrent events have changed the medical community's lack of interest and knowledge about wilderness emergencies: the development of the specialty of Emergency Medicine; the migration of the physicians themselves to the trailhead for their recreation; and the "malpractice crisis" experienced by all physicians.

The development of a specialty that prides itself on its ability to treat anyone who can walk, crawl, or often enough, who must be carried through the doors of the emergency department has been a landmark in the treatment of environmental emergencies. In the search for their own "turf" in a specialty that crosses the conventional specialty boundaries, emergency physicians have discovered the lack of knowledge and ongoing research in environmental emergencies. A review of the literature from the 1960s and 70s and a cursory comparison with the 1980s shows an abundance of new research and papers about problems that have been with us since ancient times. Indeed, most of the newer texts and research on environmental emergencies have been edited and written by physicians in emergency medicine. The old anecdotes and opinions are questioned by this new breed of physicians. These same stalwart physicians deliberately developed a style of practice that allows them to journey to the outback for long periods of time. When these physicians are faced with problems in the wilderness, they seek or develop the solutions to these problems. As members of rescue parties, disaster aid teams, and wilderness outing staffs, these physicians want answers rather than "opinions." This desire sparks research activities.

The care of patients who have environmentally provoked problems has also been advanced by the malpractice crisis. A physician who holds himself/herself out as a consultant physician is now held to a nationwide standard of care. With the knowledge that the plaintiff's attorney will bring a true expert on frostbite, snake envenomation, or heat-induced illness to the trial arena, it is difficult to accept ill-founded advice or dogma. All physicians, regardless of specialty, are less likely to rely on lore, anecdote, or gut feelings to treat patients. Advice will be sought, and responses such as, "We do it that way here," will be avoided.

The author's personal quest for and contemplation of the beauty of nature has led him and his family directly into an arena where Mother Nature rules instantly and quite personally. This text represents the quest for answers to questions encountered both trailside and bedside. It also reflects hours in the treatment of patients in wilderness settings and in repairing the ravages of those who have unsuccessfully argued with Mother Nature.

Unfortunately, many questions in medicine are answered with new questions, and environmental emergencies are no exception. Multiple areas of needed research have been identified in this text. It is a fond hope that along with the new questions some answers will be found.

# Acknowledgments

Special mention must be made to Michael Clifford, MD, J. Theodore Youngberg, MD, Keith Conover, MD, and Michael Robinette, MD, who made substantial contributions to the chapters on altitude-related emergencies, venomous land animals, wilderness emergencies, and diving emergencies, respectively. Their abundant contributions, advice, and commentary made these chapters possible. In some cases, they provided the expertise to combine literary research with hard field experiences.

Kenneth Phillips, PAC, proofread, edited, and offered jibes and commentary about many chapters. His constant reminder that the military had "done this" is evident in the multiple military sources found. His additional experience under hostile fire and hostile weather provided yet another view.

Cindy Suchovsky graciously contributed the illustrations. Explaining the concepts to be illustrated necessitated organization and simplification. Her embellishments of the concepts greatly enhance this text. She not only was a joy as a collaborator, but became a friend in the process.

Authors often put their family "on hold" while writing, but this manuscript became a family effort. Carol, Robin, and Tracy listened and watched and read many times over. This book would have been impossible without the efforts of my wife, Carol, who read and edited every word. Her wit and clarity of speech are reflected throughout the text. Her patience with a husband oblivious to all surroundings was extraordinary. Her "just one more pass" (trail, hill, stream, or mile as the case may be . . . ) philosophy to the wilderness provided more stimuli to master yet another survival skill.

Passing the lore and the crafts to our two children helped me simplify many a difficult concept. Our daughters, Robin and Tracy, gleefully pointed out poisonous mushrooms and bugs, taste tested every water purification method listed, and learned to appreciate the simple beauties of a mountain moonrise in the preparation. Lugging camera and notepad into the fields, mountains, and deserts, they became skilled in observation at an early age. Faced with a wife and two young daughters who all wanted to see the other side of the mountain, the author perforce capitulated, despite mere personal frailty. Younger days and earlier hikes provided insights about altitude illnesses and hypothermia in childhood and tested the mettle of parents who were determined not to give up the outback.

Distinctive mention must be made of the United States Army, which unwittingly provided the early impetus for the book by frequently exposing the author's frame to the elements, during his years of service. Although the author is profoundly a civilian in outlook, commanders through the ages have braved not only hostile fire, but hostile weather. It was truly amazing to note how many times the "wheel" of any specific topic of wilderness medicine had been previously "invented" by a military or naval physician.

A special note of thanks should also be given to Betsy Mueth (Spectrum/Synergon) and Carol Eckhart and Barbara Felton (Williams & Wilkins), who helped research, edit, and publish this manuscript. In the process, they became not only tutors but friends.

Finally, thanks to Zenith Data Systems.

The author's Z-183 allowed him to concentrate on the message, not the mechanics. It, alas, did not survive the task, suffering a fall from a height 2 months before completion of the manuscript. Sadly mourned, it has been replaced with a SuperSport.

# Contents

# CHAPTER 1

# The Spectrum of Heat Illness

## INTRODUCTION

In the United States, it is estimated that over 4000 people die each year from heatstroke, most of them elderly.[1] Exceptionally high rates of severe illness occur and many people succumb during periods of sustained hot weather (heat waves).[2] Military recruits and athletes who are undergoing rigorous training and conditioning under hot and humid environmental conditions are particularly susceptible to heatstroke. These statistics may represent only the tip of the iceberg, with other deaths due to the effects of the heat misdiagnosed as the result of coronary or cerebral vascular disease. Other patients with marginal capacity to handle the increased stress of a hot summer day will succumb from the original disease, causing "excess" deaths from the cardiovascular or cerebrovascular diseases. During a heat wave, the deaths from cardiovascular disease may increase to 10 times the normal death rate.[3]

Though heat illnesses are eminently preventable, thousands of people continue to suffer from them each year. Physicians have recognized the problem for over 2000 years: The Old Testament mentions heatstroke following physical exercise in the hot fields.[4,5] In addition to heat-induced annihilation of a Roman army in 24 B.C., there were 11,000 deaths in Peking during a heat wave in 1743.[6,7] Mass casualties in the 1959, 1960, and 1980 pilgrimages to Mecca totaled in the thousands.[8]

In this chapter, the spectrum of heat illness is discussed and patients in need of urgent care from heat illnesses are identified. Each form of heat illness is in turn reviewed, focusing on the common causes and risk factors, prompt diagnosis, and emergency management.

## HEAT CONTROL MECHANISMS

Humans run. The rest of the animal world does not have that capability to the same degree that humans do. The cheetah can run faster, and the antelope can spring quicker, but humans can run longer. A human being in good condition can literally run a horse, a deer, or an antelope to death in a 24-hour period. Apache war parties on foot could, and frequently did, outdistance mounted pursuers in the West of the 1800s. Indeed, some paleoanthropologists feel that humans have evolved their shape and even possibly their intelligence because of the adaptations needed to hunt by relentlessly running down prey.[9]

Human beings evolved in a hot dry plain/savannah environment, such as the Africa of a few million years ago. The adaptations to this hot climate and our style of life include a cardiovascular system designed to support long distance running and a heat exchange system to support the increased heat loads of prolonged exertion. The development of a relatively hairless skin, abundant sweat glands, and an enduring cardiovascular system is a combination unrivaled throughout the animal world.

Heat production mechanisms include basal

**Table 1.1.**
**Spectrum of Heat Illness**

| |
|---|
| Failure of Thermoregulation |
| Heatstroke |
| Thermoregulation Maintained |
| Heat exhaustion<br>Heat syncope<br>Heat edema<br>Heat cramps |

metabolism and active energy metabolism, generated by exercise. Body temperature represents a balance between heat loss and heat production. When the heat loss reflex mechanisms are overwhelmed, heat illness results. (See Table 1.1.)

## Heat Loss Mechanisms

In humans, the heat loss mechanisms are evaporation, conduction, convection (a form of conduction), radiation, and, to a lesser degree, respiratory transpiration. (See Table 1.2.)

### EVAPORATION

"Horses sweat. Men perspire. Ladies glow." The old adage to remind a "lady" of the proper vocabulary terms was wrong. Men and women **sweat**, and, in comparison, horses only glow. A horse that is sweating is in stress and needs

**Table 1.2.**
**Heat Gain and Loss Mechanisms**

| |
|---|
| Heat Loss Mechanisms |
| Evaporation<br>Conduction<br>Convection<br>Radiation<br>Transpiration |
| Heat Gain Mechanisms |
| Metabolism<br>  Basal<br>  Exercise<br>Conduction<br>Convection<br>Radiation |

special care—cooled down slowly and walked until dry. A sweating, exhausted human with adequate water supply is in good shape and only needs to sit down and cool off. A result of this is that the human being can tolerate heat stresses that will kill other animals.

Evaporation of perspiration is a major source of heat loss in the human being. The average human dissipates about 1 kilocalorie (kcal) of heat for each 1.7 cc of sweat, when the sweat is completely vaporized (580 kcal per liter). Maximal sweating is between 1.5 and 2.5 liters per hour. At least 20% drips from the body, but if the remainder was evaporated, the body would shed about 900 to 1400 kcal an hour.

When sweat rolls off the body instead of evaporating, little additional heat is lost. The theoretical maximum heat loss is not reached in areas of high humidity as the evaporation of water vapor is slowed when the ambient humidity increases and the surrounding air becomes saturated with water vapor. The usual heat loss attained in most climactic conditions is about 600 kcal. If exercise and basal rates of heat production exceed that rate, the body starts to gain heat.

When sweat does not evaporate, inadequate cooling prompts increased sweating. The body water is lost, at least initially, almost entirely from the circulating blood volume.[10] If the water is not replaced, the resulting dehydration adds to the strain on the cardiovascular system. Older individuals and infants have reduced sweat gland activity and a lesser circulatory response to heat.

If the individual is unable to sweat for any reason, the core temperature will rapidly rise with heat exposure because the individual has lost the most effective defense mechanism available. The ability to work in hot climates declines remarkably at about 5 to 8% dehydration weight loss, precisely as the ability to sweat starts to diminish.

It is interesting to note that during the Six-day War of 1967, Egyptian troops, following practices of strict water rationing inherited from their Russian advisors, sustained over 20,000 casualties from heatstroke! During the same time, Israeli troops with abundant field water supplies and command-enforced water policies had minimal heat casualties.[11] It is thought that dehydration was a major contributor to this phenomenal heat casualty rate. As a result of this tragedy, Russian units now have mandatory liberal water rationing policies enforced by the commanders during battle.[12]

With acclimation to the heat, the rate of sweating is increased, sodium excretion in the sweat is decreased, and both blood volume and cardiac output are increased. The degree of acclimation appears to be proportional to the imposed heat stress.

## TRANSPIRATION

The loss of heat through exhaled water vapor is called transpiration. Transpiration cools, even if the surrounding temperature is greater than the temperature in the body. As noted earlier, transpiration is an important mechanism of heat loss in furred animals such as dogs and explains the animal's panting on hot (dog) days. Transpiration is only a minor source of heat loss in human beings, however. In humans, less than 5% of excess heat is usually lost through warming tidal air. A panting human may increase the heat loss via the lungs, but there is also the danger that respiratory alkalosis may occur as the $PaCO_2$ is lowered.

## CONDUCTION

Conduction is loss or gain of heat through direct contact of the body with a cooler surface or medium such as water. Obviously, conduction does not cool the body if the ambient temperature is greater than the body temperature. Indeed, in desert climates, where surface temperatures of 70°C (160°F) are not uncommon, heat can be gained through the feet from the hot ground. Conduction losses are quite important in *HYPO*thermia, but in the discussion of heat-related illnesses, conduction losses may be safely neglected.

## CONVECTION

Convection is loss or gain of heat through contact with moving air surrounding the body. The thin layer of air surrounding the body is cooled or warmed by the body's temperature. As the wind or motion strips away this layer, it must be cooled or warmed again. On cool windy days, heat loss may be markedly increased by convection. Again, convection will

not cool the body when the air temperature is greater than about 33°C (92°F); indeed, the body may gain heat from hot air that is in contact with the body.

## RADIATION

Radiation is gain or loss of heat through energy emission from the skin surface. Radiation will not cool when the surrounding temperatures are greater than the temperature of the radiating body. Heat will be gained from areas that are warmer than the body, and depending upon the location, heat may be gained and lost at the same time (for example, stand partly in the sun and in the shadow on a cool day). During a sunny day, the bright sun will transfer about 150 kcal per hour to the human body. The cutaneous vasodilation reflexes will raise skin temperature in hot weather, thereby facilitating heat loss by radiation.

## Heat Production Mechanisms

Within the body, there are two major sources of heat production—basal metabolism and active energy or volitional exercise metabolism. (See Table 1.2.)

## BASAL METABOLISM

Basal metabolism produces an average of 65 to 85 kcal per hour at normal body temperatures. In patients who have a fever or who are modestly hyperthermic, basal metabolism increases at about 13% for every degree Centigrade rise in temperature.

## VOLITIONAL EXERCISE

Energy metabolism produces heat from exercise ranging from 300 kcal per hour for moderate work to 1000 kcal per hour for strenuous exercise. Seizures, combative behavior, and straining at restraints can all qualify as strenuous exercise. (See Fig. 1.1.)

Strenuous exertion can markedly raise the body temperature. Elite marathoners, for example, are able to generate heat at 15 to 18 times the basal metabolic rate and sustain this intensity for more than 2 hours. If no heat were lost externally, the core temperature of these athletes would increase by 1°C

| Activity | Heat Production (Kcal/Hr) |
|---|---|
| Rest (seated) | 90 |
| Walking leisurely | 120 |
| Walking (2 MPH) | 180 |
| Housework | 240 |
| Bicycling at 8 MPH | 300 |
| Walking (2 MPH) | 300 |
| Vigorous exercise | 400 |
| Shoveling snow | 400 |
| Running (5 MPH) | 550 |
| Running ( )6 MPH) | 700 |

**Figure 1.1.** Body heat production (70-kilogram men).

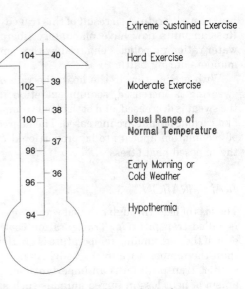

**Figure 1.2.** Range of normal rectal temperature.

every 5 minutes. In 1945, Assmussen and Boje showed that during extreme physical exertion deep muscle temperature rose to 41.1°C (106°F).[13] Later, in 11 young unacclimated males that were exercising in hot air for 1 hour, blood temperatures as high as 41.6°C (107°F) were measured by Rowell and his associates.[14] Rectal temperatures in normal, physically conditioned men performing strenuous exercise may rise to 42°C (107.6°F).[15] (See Fig. 1.2.)

Of particular interest are the many biochemical changes that accompany strenuous exercise. Severe acidosis, decreased renal function, rhabdomyolysis, decreased liver function, and increased enzymes are all found following strenuous exercise.[16] It is thought that some of these changes may be due to a localized hypoxia from the overuse.

## ACCLIMATION TO HEAT

If a heat-acclimated athlete were compared (during vigorous exercise) to a similar athlete who is not acclimated to heat, one would note that the unacclimated athlete has a higher heart rate and rectal temperature. The unacclimated athlete has a faster depletion of glycogen, lower plasma volume, higher concentration of sodium and potassium in sweat, and a lower rate of sweating. The unacclimated runner will have a greater susceptibility to heat illness and a greater perceived exertion and fatigue level. This acclimation process takes place over a 2- to 3-week process and involves both short term and long-term

changes to protect the athlete from the effects of the heat.

## Short-Term Acclimation

The human body acutely responds to heat stress by altering the magnitude of contribution of each of the heat loss and production mechanisms. As the body temperature rises, the hypothalamic thermoregulatory center is stimulated by the sensory input from the peripheral thermoreceptors and central blood temperature receptors.[17] As a result of this stimulation, the compensatory cooling mechanisms are initiated. First, the shivering response is inhibited. Secondly, increased sweating is initiated. Finally, cutaneous vasodilation commences.

The concomitant response to all of these reflexes is a mandatory increase in cardiac output. In the face of the cutaneous vasodilation, there is increased cutaneous circulation (the erythematous skin "blush" seen with heat exposure). This increased blood flow to the skin will result in increased heat transfer from the core and increased heat losses due to radiation and convection if the ambient temperature is favorable. (See Fig. 1.3.)

This diversion of cardiac output is why even trained athletes experience fatigue quicker in hot climates. The increased loss of water and electrolytes caused by profuse sweating

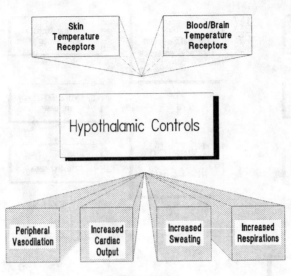

**Figure 1.3.**

can rapidly cause dehydration and compound the fatigue.

## Long-Term Acclimation

Acclimation to heat is a physiological process by which an individual becomes even more able to tolerate the effects of the heat and more efficient in disposing of excess heat loads. By this process, profound adaptations take place that involve the cardiovascular, endocrine, and exocrine systems. (See Fig. 1.4.)

Obviously, the degree of acclimation must be qualified by the amount and degree of stress. The Pittsburgh steel worker toiling next to his furnace has a different level of heat stress than a secretary answering a phone in an office without air conditioning. A significant level of acclimation is achieved by brief exposure to daily heat stress for 10 to 20 days, but full acclimatization may require up to 2 months to achieve.[18-20] This partial acclimation may be achieved by exposure to dry air at 49°C (120°F) for 90 to 120 minutes per day. Shorter periods of exposure to humid air may achieve the same results.

## Physiological Changes of Adaptation

Four major physiological changes occur to allow long-term management of this increased heat load.

### ENHANCEMENT OF METABOLIC EFFICIENCY

Skeletal muscle glycogen stores and the total number of mitochrondria increase in both cardiac and skeletal muscle. The net effect is to make more use of efficient aerobic metabolism rather than the less efficient anaerobic metabolism. This means that more adenosine triphosphate (ATP) is produced with less energy wasted (hence, less heat produced).

### ENHANCEMENT OF SWEATING

Both the quality and quantity of sweat produced is more efficient after acclimatization. The maximum sweating rate increases from 1.5 liters per hour in the unacclimatized person to from 2.5 to 3 liters per hour in acclimatized people. The acclimatized person will enhance dissipation of heat by evaporative cooling.

In acclimatized individuals, sweating is initiated at a lower core temperature than in the unacclimatized. This, of course, means that the acclimatized person will start the most efficient cooling process at an earlier set point.

### ENHANCEMENT OF MYOCARDIAL EFFICIENCY

In the acclimatized person, the myocardial efficiency is improved. There is an increase

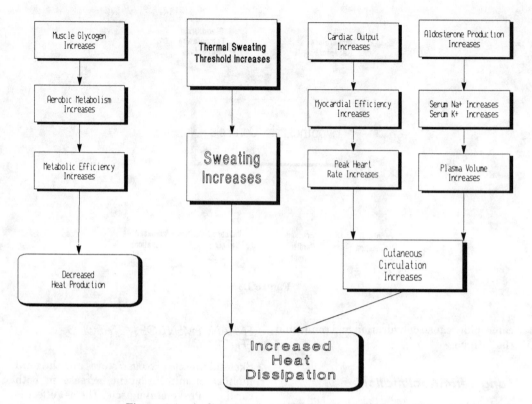

**Figure 1.4.**  Acclimatization to heat (10 days to 2 months).

in both cardiac output and stroke volume but a decrease in peak heart rate.[21,22] The net effect is to increase the ability of the circulation to dump heat to the environment through the vasodilated cutaneous circulation. These responses may not occur if the patient is taking drugs with myocardial depressant functions or if the myocardial reserves are marginal.

## SODIUM AND POTASSIUM CONSERVATION

In the least trained persons, the sweat chloride levels are as high as 40 to 50 mEq/L, producing the possibility of a profound sodium loss.[7] In heat-acclimatized persons, the concentration of sodium chloride in the sweat may decrease to as little as 2 to 5 mEq/L. This concentration will increase somewhat as the quantity of sweat increases, even in the acclimatized individual. Trained (conditioned and acclimatized) individuals also produce a more dilute urine, again reducing the amount of sodium loss.

Sodium conservation by the kidneys and sweat glands occurs when aldosterone secretion is increased during acclimation. Sodium retention also appears to increase the plasma and extracellular volumes, allowing more evaporative heat losses before dehydration occurs.[7,23-25]

Less conditioned individuals seem to be less heat tolerant and take longer to acclimatize to work in the heat. Football, jogging, and armed forces training programs have many people who are pushed to or beyond their limit of tolerance for physical activity and have high associated rates of heat injury.

One detriment of the effects of acclimatization appears to be a potassium depletion as a result of sweat and urinary losses that are mediated by increased aldosterone effects as noted above. Military recruits who are undergoing intense physical exertion in hot weather may have an average deficit of 500 or more mEq of potassium.[26] The potassium deficit is apparently corrected by poorly defined mechanisms as the person becomes more fully acclimated.

## THE SPECTRUM OF HEAT EMERGENCIES

The clinical picture of heat illnesses is a spectrum ranging from the deep coma and fatalities of heatstroke to the faints of heat syncope or the pains of heat cramps. In this continuum, heat dissipation reflexes may or may not be lost, depending upon the severity of the disease. (See Table 1.1.)

## Epidemiology

As was noted, humans are unique in their ability to shed excess heat and maintain composure, occupation, and existence. When that unique heat loss system is overwhelmed, heat illness will surely result. Whether by intent or inadvertently, we regularly place ourselves in positions of heat stress and suffer the inevitable consequences. Each year, 4000 or more people die in the United States from heatstroke. Eighty percent are over the age of 50, but there is appreciable mortality in young people. Heatstroke is the second leading cause of death among athletes in this country, ranking directly behind head and spinal injuries.[20] Other high-risk groups include the chronically ill or bedfast, the mentally ill, those taking antipsychotic or anticholinergic drugs, those who work under high heat loads, and alcoholics.[27]

No single, identified pattern consistently provokes heatstroke, although most *epidemics* have occurred when the temperature exceeds 32°C (90°F) with relative humidity above 50% for 2 or more days. However, factors such as conditioning, medications, underlying disease, or previous history of heatstroke play a predictive role in identifying patients at highest risk.

The prevalence of the more minor heat illnesses is unknown and, quite possibly, unknowable. Certainly every exercising athlete at one time or another has suffered heat cramps and may have felt lightheaded and dizzy after severe exercise in the heat.

## Etiology

Why some people develop heat illnesses and others do not is not yet known, but the operating factors of high temperature, increased metabolic oxygen demands, and relative hypoxia seem to define the damaging factors. Even the healthiest of persons can experience heat illness under the right circumstances.

## HOW HOT IS TOO HOT

Some authors theorize that there is a set maximum core temperature beyond which heat illness is inevitable. Strangely, difficulty arises in defining exactly when body temperature is "too high." As previously noted, athletes in good shape have measured core temperatures of 41°C (106°F) and beyond. Gilat and co-workers studied the change of rectal temperatures in eight highly acclimatized Israeli soldiers while carrying loads of 35 kilograms during a desert march. Five of the eight had rectal temperatures ranging from 41.5 to 42.4°C (106.7 to 108.3°F) upon completion of the march.[28]

Obviously, some authorities would consider these temperatures to be "heatstroke," yet these athletes required no therapy other than oral replenishment of water and electrolytes. The athletes also suffered no worse central nervous system effects than euphoria when the march was finished.

Other authors have noted this tolerance of markedly elevated core temperatures and redefine heat stroke by adding a time exposure factor or an upward shift of the temperature "set point."[29] The cause of heatstroke in apparently similar patients is unknown.

One hypothesis that may put all of the parts together is as follows. Cellular metabolism increases about 13% for each centigrade degree rise in temperature. At 40.5°C (105°F), the cellular metabolism is 50% above normal. As the core temperature rises, if the oxygen supply does not keep pace with the intracellular needs, the cells will become hypoxic and begin to die. In a conditioned athlete, the heat is dissipated well, and the heart and cardiovascular system can provide for the cardiovascular load of the heat dissipation, supply necessary oxygen and metabolic substrates and meet the circulation needs of the exercise. In the poorly conditioned, chronically ill, dehydrated, or the very young, the cardiovascular system is not able to provide for the needs of both circulation and cooling. As the temperature rises, even in the fit and conditioned, at some point, the cardiovascular system is unable to both provide adequate circulation and continue cooling efforts. The result is multisystem breakdown with diffuse cellular death. The cellular breakdown appears to be responsible for some of the delayed morbidity in those patients who survive the emergent phase.

## Predisposing Factors

As noted, man is superbly adapted to a hot climate, with the ability to shed large amounts of excess heat efficiently. If the exogenous burden of heat is too great, if endogenous production is too large, or if other factors supravene, then our ability to deal with excess heat will fail. If the exposure is too great, all will have failure of heat regulation; if it is marginal, only a few individuals will experience the failure of the heat elimination processes. A discussion of the factors that predispose to cooling system breakdown follow.

### EXOGENOUS HEAT GAIN FROM THE CLIMATE

Severe climactic conditions, particularly those with high humidity without wind, predispose to heatstroke. These severe conditions may be due to a generalized climactic change or to the change in a small local environment (a "microclimate").

Generalized climactic changes (heat waves)—such as the 1980 heat wave in Kansas City, Missouri, where for the months of June and July, the high for the day went below 32°C (90°F) just twice and for 17 days in a row it was above 37.7°C (100°F)—are well known to predispose to heatstroke in epidemic proportions. Indeed, during that heat wave 1 out of every 1000 people died or were hospitalized from heat-related illnesses.

Less well appreciated are the effects of a microclimate on individuals. Incarceration in "The Black Hole of Calcutta," working in mines and around furnaces or boilers and other similar unusual circumstances, are associated with markedly increased incidence of heatstroke and other heat illnesses. These hot and often humid microclimates provide abundant heat gain and little opportunity for heat losses.

Deaths have also been reported from saunas, steam rooms, whirlpool baths, and hot tubs. It has been thought that the resulting severe hyperthermia has been induced by the rapid conduction of heat by the water. The hyperthermia may be aggrevated by the peripheral vasodilation, erect posture, and alcohol ingestion that may often accompany the use of hot tubs and saunas. Indeed, some of our "hot tub drownings" may actually have been heat stress related.

Another special microclimate is the unprotected hot car. Temperatures in automobiles left exposed in the sun can reach up to 60°C (140°F). The message is obvious for parents leaving children in an exposed vehicle.

The effect of the microclimate has been shown to markedly influence risks of heat illness for those who have other risk factors, particularly if the patient is unable to remove him- or herself from the microclimate. Investigators from the Centers for Disease Control (CDC) studied risk factors for both fatal and non-fatal heatstroke during the 1980 heat wave. The factors identified as decreasing the risk of classic heatstroke in this study included spending time in air conditioning, among shrubbery or trees, or on lower floors of buildings.[27,30] All of these factors were shown to favorably influence the microclimate surrounding the patient.

There is a strong, inverse relationship between daily hours of home air conditioning and classic heat illnesses. The value of air conditioning was suggested by the reduction of summer deaths in nursing homes in California after air conditioning became widespread.[31] Indeed, during the 1980 heat wave, the CDC estimated the risk of dying from heatstroke to be 49 times greater for those persons without home air conditioning than those with 24-hour-a-day air conditioning. The same investigators found that spending time in air conditioned places also decreased the risk of heatstroke during a heat wave.

### INCREASED ENDOGENOUS HEAT PRODUCTION

Any factor that increases the amount of heat that is produced to a point beyond the capacity of the body to eliminate it will eventually produce heat illnesses. The most common factor that increases heat production is, of course, increased exercise.

## Exercise

Extremes of exercise under hot environmental conditions may lead to heatstroke or other heat illness even in normal persons. As noted previously, rectal temperature rises are common in extremes of exercise. Misconceptions—such as avoidance of water during exercise, wearing heat-retaining clothing, and pushing people to the limits of tolerance—all contribute to the increased incidence of heatstroke among athletes. In the 1980 CDC heatstroke study mentioned above, reduction of activity markedly reduced the risk of heatstroke.

It should be noted again that seizures, delirium tremens, combative behavior, and straining at restraints all qualify as extremes of exercise. Although not customarily listed as exercise, vigorous muscular contractions in these activities may produce just as much heat as the marathon runner's exercise. It is partly for these reasons that the alcoholic may be at higher risk of heat injury than his nonalcoholic peers.

Core body heat gains of 1 degree centigrade per 5 minutes are possible with strenuous exercise if the microclimate precludes heat losses. This situation may be found in some boiler areas, foundries, and mines. The heat stroke incidence for these areas is significantly higher than similar areas where no exercise is required.

## Febrile Illness

Any patient with a febrile illness has a greater chance of developing a heat illness during hot humid weather. Compared to peers, the febrile patient has an increased metabolic rate that produces an even greater heat burden. Often this heat burden may be combined with the effects of the illnesses, such as vomiting or diarrhea, which may lead to dehydration, pulmonary dysfunction that may decrease oxygen intake, or dermatitis that prevents effective sweating.

## Drugs

Drugs, such as cocaine, phencyclidine (PCP), and lysergic acid diethylamide (LSD), that cause a hyperactive state and increase the body's metabolic rate may predispose the patient to development of heatstroke. Needless to say, it does not matter whether the drug causes the hyperactivity by direct action such as strychnine or by indirect central nervous system (CNS) effects such as PCP.

Tricyclic antidepressants and amphetamines can also boost heat production by both stimulating the hypothalmus and increasing muscle activity. Several reports have implicated amphetamines in the pathogenesis of hyperthermia in association with massive rhabdomyolysis. The threshold of damage may be easily surpassed when one is under the influence of a drug that blunts the recognition of fatigue and increases the motor activity. (See Table 1.3.)

Withdrawal from alcohol, opiates, and barbituates or other drugs with subsequent

**Table 1.3.**
**Drugs That Predispose to Heatstroke**

Anticholinergics[58]
  Atropine
  Scopolamine
  Benztropine mesylate
  Belladonna and synthetic alkaloids
  Antihistamines[59]
Phenothiazines[60,61]
Butyrophenones
Tricyclic antidepressants
  Amitriptyline (Elavil)
  Imipramine (Norpramin)
  Nortriptyline (Tofranil)
  Protriptyline (Vivactil)
Monoamine-oxidase inhibitors
  Isocarboxazid (Marplan)
  Nialamide (Niamid)
  Phenelzine (Nardil)
  Tranylcypromine sulfate (Parnate)
Glutethimide
Lysergic acid diethylamide (LSD)
Phencyclidine (PCP)
Lithium
Diuretics
Sympathomimetics[62]
  Amphetamines
  Epinephrine
  Ephedrine
  Levarterenol
Anesthetic Agents
  Nitrous oxide
  Succinylcholine
  Ethyl chloride
  Halothane
  Ether
Alcohol

hyperactive withdrawal states will likewise increase the endogenous production of heat by increased muscle activity. Lithium carbonate may also increase muscle activity.

## IMPAIRMENT OF HEAT DISSIPATION

### Clothing

Heat-retaining clothing will cause the effective absence of sweating as a cooling force by complete inhibition of evaporation, in the most extreme case. If the athlete is exercising heavily in rubber "sweat suits" to lose weight, heat production may be massive, and heat losses minimal. Fatal heatstroke has occurred in men exercising in plastic sweat suits, even when the temperature is as low as 26.6°C (80°F). Physical exercise in these and other occlusive garments can cause a body temperature rise of as much as 5°C (9°F) per hour. Firemen and emergency medical technicians on rescue duty in multilayer protective garments attending to fire or chemical rescue have also had episodes of heatstroke with even shorter exposures. The psychotic, dressed in inappropriate multilayered clothing, may be in a similar situation.

### Obesity

Overweight people are less heat tolerant than people of normal weight. During strenuous exercise, they are at a much higher risk for heat illness. It is not apparent whether the obesity or the accompanying lack of physical condition is the problem. Certainly, fat is an insulator and decreases heat loss to the environment. The obese person may also be unable to attain the cardiovascular output necessary for effective cooling due to lack of conditioning.

### Dehydration

Dehydration blunts the response to heat stress in at least two ways. First, the depleted blood volume means that there is less fluid that can be lost as sweat before terminal reflexes decrease perspiration. Secondly, the lower blood volume means that the cardiovascular system can less easily afford to shunt blood to the periphery to dump heat by radiation.

Progressive dehydration may occur during a long run or other prolonged vigorous exercise, even though the athlete drinks during the exercise. Hot, exercising athletes simply do not adequately rehydrate themselves voluntarily. Thirst is not a reliable indicator of dehydration; athletes, workers, and soldiers must be taught to "overdrink."

The Israeli Defense Forces consider water replacement so important in prevention of heat stroke that a commander is courtmartialed if water replacements are not ensured for every member of his command. The Israelis consider 1 liter per hour to be a minimum for each soldier. They further note that the water should be cooled and flavored for best palatability. The commanders have been instructed to check the urine concentration on every exposed soldier at midday.[32]

### Age

The elderly are at a high risk of developing heat illnesses under otherwise tolerable conditions. A possible cause for the decrease in heat tolerance among active elderly persons is a lessening of sweat production. Underlying cardiac pathology, use of multiple drugs, general frailty, and poor physical conditioning all may contribute to the increased incidence of heatstroke in the elderly. The neglected, debilitated nursing home resident may not be able to ambulate to obtain water and suffer severe dehydration as a consequence.

Children are also more susceptible than adults to climatic heat waves. Heat intolerance in children exercising in hot areas is attributable to greater surface area to mass ratios, lower sweating rates, and greater metabolic heat production.[30] Hyperthermia during extreme hot weather is particularly likely to develop in children with diarrhea, respiratory tract infections, or neurologic illness.[33]

### Chronic Disabling Diseases

Chronic disabling diseases of virtually any form will increase the risk of heatstroke. Important among these diseases are diabetes, malnutrition, and disorders that impair the sweating responses.

### Heart Disease

Since cardiac output must be increased to adapt to increases in heat exposure, people with cardiac disease are at increased risk of developing heatstroke. Likewise, those persons taking drugs that limit the cardiovascular responses will suffer more from heat exposure. (See section on drugs below.) In the presence of cardiovascular disease, heat stress that would be normally tolerated may rapidly precipitate heatstroke.

## Drugs

Many cases of drug-induced heat stress have been reported in the literature. (See Table 1.3.) Though the true incidence of the relationship is unknown, it is thought to be high because of the large numbers of patients who suffer from exposure to heat stress while taking these medications.[34]

There are five major mechanisms by which drugs may affect the ability to dissipate heat to control the body temperature:

1. Depression of the thermoregulatory center of the anterior hypothalamus can affect the control of the body temperature "set point" probably through interference with or by depletion of dopamine (phenothiazines are prime examples of drugs with this effect).[35]
2. Anticholinergic agents can block the sweating response and affect the body's ability to maintain normal body temperature by inhibition of sweating. (Atropine, tricyclic antidepressants, and a large group of other medications have some effects here.)[36]
3. Any drug that causes cutaneous vasoconstriction will markedly decrease the body's ability to lose heat. These medications include the sympathomimetics such as norepinephrine or pseudophrine.
4. Diuretics may cause relative dehydration by decreasing total body water stores. If the patient is dehydrated, sweating may be diminished or abolished, and cardiovascular responses to heat are markedly hampered.
5. If the cardiovascular responses to heat stress are blocked, the body is less able to tolerate increased heat. If beta blockers or calcium channel blockers are prescribed, the diminished cardiovascular response to stress puts the patient at greater risk from heat stress.

Phenothiazines deserve particular note as etiologic agents of heatstroke, because they have multiple effects and are associated with high incidences of heatstroke. In one series of 51 psychotic patients with heatstroke, 48 were taking antipsychotic agents.[37] The CDC study on the effects of the 1980 heat wave in St. Louis likewise noted a large increase in the mortality rates among psychiatric patients taking major tranquilizers.[27]

During low ambient temperatures, the phenothiazines will impair the body's response to cold and abolish shivering. During heat stress, the phenothiazines depress the anterior hypothalamus and prevent or slow down the onset of sweating. The thermal changes produced by chlorpromazine are transient, indicating that the drug, in therapeutic doses, causes a temporary biochemical impairment of the function of the hypothalmus.[38] In addition to a suppressive effect upon temperature regulation, phenothiazines exert anticholinergic effects peripherally, including reduction of sweating.

Additionally, confusion in diagnosis may be found with the onset of the neuroleptic malignant syndrome that has been associated with the high-potency antipsychotic drugs, such as haloperidol or fluphenazine.[39] The neuroleptic malignant syndrome is characterized by muscular rigidity, altered consciousness, autonomic instability, and high temperatures. It should be considered in anyone taking antipsychotic drugs, whether or not there is environmental heat stresses. The syndrome is not associated with high environmental temperatures and core body temperatures above 41°C (106°F) have not been reported.

Alcohol also deserves a particular note as multiple investigators have noted an increased risk for alcoholics.[27] The 1980 CDC risk factors study found that a history of alcoholism was significantly associated with heatstroke death with a relative risk of about 15 times the normal populations risks. This may be due to inhibition of the secretion of antidiuretic hormone or due to some other aspect of the syndrome of alcoholism. The risk does not appear to be directly related to the amount of alcohol intake.

## Prior Heatstroke

Current evidence suggests that those persons who have had a prior history of heatstroke are at an increased risk of another attack. The feeling is that the genetic or physiologic predisposition of the person is the reason for this increased incidence and not some damage induced by the prior heatstroke.

### Fatigue and Lack of Sleep

U. S. Army evaluations have noted that fatigue and lack of sleep are associated with increases in heatstroke and other heat illnesses. This has been corroborated with pilgrims to Mecca in Saudia Arabia.[8]

## MINOR HEAT EMERGENCIES

If the rate of heat gain exceeds the heat loss by only a small amount, the heat loss mechanisms may not be overwhelmed but may not completely protect the patient. This leads to a minor heat emergency.

### Heat Edema

```
    Characteristics of Heat Edema
  Self-limited
  Usually limited to lower extremities
  Usually asymptomatic
      (shoes may fit too tightly)
  Treatment:
      Reassurance
      Elevation
      ? Support hose
      ?? Diuretics
```

Swelling of the feet and ankles is often reported during the summer months. This heat edema is worse during the first few days of heat exposure and is often asymptomatic (except the shoes are "too tight"), worryng the physician more than the patient. The presence of edema tends to raise the spectre of congestive heart failure, (CHF) thrombophlebitis, cirrhosis, and other dreaded diseases. Many such individuals have no underlying disease (e.g., heart disease, hepatic or renal disease) to explain the abnormality. The edema is usually minimal, is not accompanied by any significant impairment in function, and often resolves after several days of acclimatization. It is presumed that cutaneous and muscular vasodilatation, combined with venous stasis leads to a vascular leak and accumulation of interstitial fluid in the lower extremities. The most important reason to be aware of this clinical syndrome is to prevent overly vigorous treatment in patients with this problem. For heat edema, brief diagnostic evaluation is in order, but invasive diagnostic or therapeutic intervention is clearly inappropriate for this self-limited disease. A characteristic history and otherwise normal examination is usually all the diagnostic work-up requires. In questionable cases, a chest x-ray may be taken to ensure that underlying CHF is not missed. Therapy consists of reassurance, elevation, and use of support hose. There are no studies to support or refute the use of mild diuretics if the edema is bothersome. Certainly, if diuretics are administered, strict attention should be paid to fluid status, and dehydration must be prevented. Accurate and detailed assessment of this problem's pathophysiology has not been established (and may not be needed) as the problem resolves without any therapy.

### Heat Cramps

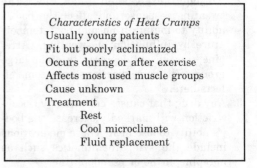

```
    Characteristics of Heat Cramps
  Usually young patients
  Fit but poorly acclimatized
  Occurs during or after exercise
  Affects most used muscle groups
  Cause unknown
  Treatment
      Rest
      Cool microclimate
      Fluid replacement
```

Heat cramps are painful, involuntary spasms of major muscles used in intense exercise. They usually occur in unacclimated persons and are more common after profuse sweating. Body temperature is usually normal with heat cramps; other minor heat syndromes may accompany the heat cramps. Fortunately, heat cramps are limited both in duration and morbidity.

The cause of any cramp is usually not clear, and heat-related cramps are no exception. Heat cramps are common in hot weather and are believed to be from the sodium and water losses described above. The cramps are presumably due to a rapid change in the extracellular osmolality. Other factors, such as alkalosis that decreases the ionized calcium or diuresis that causes a loss of magnesium or calcium, may play a role.

Massage and stretching will help to alleviate the pain and may allow the athlete to resume competition. Muscle cramps also can be treated with simple oral fluid replacement. In severe cases, intravenous fluid replacement and judicious doses of diazepam may be useful. Magnesium sulfate and calcium chloride have been considered, but there is no study to refute or support their use.

Prevention of heat cramps is best done by maintaining adequate hydration.

## Heat Syncope

> *Characteristics of Heat Syncope*
> Self-limited
> Probably vasovagal in origin
> Exacerbated by parade posture
> Exacerbated by dehydration
> Treatment:
>     Postural adaptation
>     Raise legs
>     Oral fluids
>     ? Intravenous rehydration

The next increment in the severity of heat-induced illnesses is syncope in those exposed to, and unaccustomed to, the increased ambient heat. Peripheral pooling of blood in the lower extremities can cause any person to "faint" with prolonged standing or use of a "tilt table." This physiologic aberration of the vasomotor control is exacerbated in high temperatures by the normal heat loss mechanism of peripheral vasodilatation. Volume loss secondary to the sweating further exacerbates inadequate blood return to the central circulation. The summation of these mechanisms appears to be similar to a vasovagal syncope. The soldier or bandsman in a parade on a sweltering Memorial Day is an ideal candidate for this form of heat illness.

Most patients with this syndrome can be treated with postural adaptation alone. The patient should receive oral fluids and be encouraged to avoid prolonged standing. If at all possible, the individual who has suffered a heat-related syncope should be removed from the hot environment.

If many people in a group start to suffer from heat exhaustion or syncope, the group should recognize that the necessary conditions for production of heatstroke are present and reduce the activity accordingly.

Patients should be instructed about the cause of the syncope and how to prevent repeated episodes. An appreciable amount of venous circulation can be maintained with minimal knee bending or "isometric" maneuvers when at the "attention" position. Support hose may also help to prevent venous pooling.

If these maneuvers fail, or if the patient is not in the parade type activities, they should be encouraged to assume a horizontal or head between the knees position whenever they recognize the symptoms of this postural syncope.

## Heat Exhaustion

> *Characteristics of Heat Exhaustion*
> Ill-defined precursor of heatstroke
> Mild dehydration often noted
> Postural hypotension noted
> Mild mental status changes
> Slightly elevated temperature
>     (to 40°C (104°F))
> Treatment
>     Rapid cooling
>     Remove from heat exposure
>     IV rehydration with 1 liter normal saline
> SUSPECT HEATSTROKE
> Limit activity of companions

Heat exhaustion is an ill-defined illness intermediate between the previously mentioned syndromes and the morbidity and mortality of frank heatstroke. The syndrome is characterized by minor changes in mental status, hyperventilation, dizziness, nausea, headache, and temperature elevation. Dehydration and postural hypotension are common. Individuals with heat exhaustion sweat freely and may complain of chills. The body temperature is generally between 39°C (102.2°F) and 40°C (104°F). The skin is usually cool and moist with piloerection.

Water deficiency is believed to be a contributing factor in heat exhaustion. During extreme environmental heat stress, a 1 liter per hour water loss is not uncommon; this loss may increase to between 1.5 to 2 liters per hour. With sweat containing between 20 and 50 mEq of sodium chloride, both sodium and water are rapidly depleted. This combined electrolyte and volume deficiency can contribute to a deficit in peripheral and cerebral perfusion.

The condition is easily treated with oral fluids such as pedilyte and Gatoraide. Severe cases with nausea may require intravenous rehydration. External cooling is helpful and either evaporation or ice may be used.

Some authorities feel that heat exhaustion is a mild form of heatstroke and should be treated vigorously. If multiple people in an area start to have symptoms of heat exhaustion, suspicions for heatstroke should be markedly raised. Coaches, trainers, or group leaders should decrease or postpone training and increase water and rest breaks.

## HEATSTROKE

| Clinical Characteristics of Heatstroke | | |
| --- | --- | --- |
| | Classic | Exertional |
| Age group affected | Older/very young | Young/fit |
| Occur in epidemics | Yes (heat waves) | Yes (group athletics) |
| Predisposing illness | Yes | No |
| Prevailing weather | Heat wave | Variable |
| Sweating | Often absent | Often present |
| Acid/base changes | Respiratory alkalosis | Metabolic acidosis/respiratory alkalosis |
| Rhabdomyolysis | Uncommon | Common |
| Acute renal failure | Rare | Common |
| DIC | Rare | Common |
| CPK elevation | Mild | Marked |
| Major organ system | CNS | Renal/muscle/hematologic |
| Lactate | Usually low | Usually high |

### Diagnosis

Heatstroke occurs when the body heat loss mechanisms are either overwhelmed or are insufficient to meet environmental demands. Typically it has been taught that a "classic triad" of heatstroke—coma, hot dry skin, and a temperature greater than 41°C (106°F)—was needed for the diagnosis of heatstroke. This classic triad leads to substantial underdiagnosis. *The diagnosis of heatstroke must be suspected whenever alteration or loss of consciousness (including bizzarre behaviour) occurs under any possible condition of heat load.*

It is important to note that an elevated body temperature is neither the sole criterion of the syndrome, nor needed for a diagnosis. There are several studies in the literature of body temperatures as high as 42°C (108°F) in athletes engaged in vigorous activity, and in cancer patients treated with hyperthermia techniques without clinical symptoms. Likewise, a patient may have been cooled by bystanders or emergency response teams and no longer has a temperature greater than 41°C (106°F) upon arrival to an emergency department.

It is also important to note that patients with heatstroke may be either anhidrotic or moist and sweaty. Sweating does not rule out heatstroke, especially in young healthy adults.

In milder cases of heatstroke, the patient may have regained consciousness prior to being seen by the emergency physician so that none of the features of the "classic triad" are met. The patient may have only mild confusion or altered behavior that passes a cursory inspection.

In these milder cases of heat stroke, the patient is often diagnosed as having heat exhaustion. Without laboratory and electrocardiographic confirmation that no damage existed, it is difficult to separate mild cases of heat stroke from heat exhaustion.

Any patient with an exposure to heat stress and with an alteration of consciousness should be evaluated immediately as a possible heatstroke patient. Core temperature should be taken rectally, preferably with a continuously reading thermometer. Any hyperthermia should be immediately treated and the patient investigated for multiple system involvement. The diagnosis of heatstroke calls for a high index of suspicion and mandates rapid action, before all of the "facts" may be available.

## Heatstroke Variants

There appears to be two distinct major variants of heatstroke: classic heatstroke and exertional heatstroke. In some cases, the symptoms, signs, and clinical milieu may overlap.

### CLASSIC HEATSTROKE

Classic heatstroke presents with hyperpyrexia, coma, and hot dry skin. Clinical descriptions of classical heatstroke are based on observations made about clusters of cases during heat waves. The population at risk appears to be the aged and chronically ill. A smaller subset of cases may be found in those taking major tranquilizers and/or alcohol or in the very young. A point to be strongly emphasized in the etiology of this form of heatstroke is that the temperature and humidity are often high and have been at sustained highs for night and day for several days. (See Table 1.4.) Because the heat wave will affect an entire city or area, classic heatstroke frequently occurs in epidemics.

The elderly patient, after being subjected to this heat stress for several days, may become dehydrated and then start to show symptoms of confusion, delirium, or lethargy. The elderly patients, living alone or left unattended in a nursing home or with no one to care for them, initially may not be recog-

**Table 1.4.**
**Risk Factors for CLASSIC Heatstroke**

Daily hours of home air conditioning (inverse)
Ability to care for self (inverse)
Reduction in physical activity during heat
  (inverse)
History of alcoholism
Use of a drug from list below:
  Antipsychotics
  Anticholinergics
  Tricyclics
  Major tranquilizers[27]

**Table 1.5.**
**Risk Factors for Exertional Heatstroke**

Fit, young athletes
Overweight
Unacclimatized
Unusual exertion
High humidity
High temperature
Heavy clothing or uniform
Dehydration (usually mild)
Lack of sleep
Recent use of alcohol

nized as ill. After 2 to 3 days of unrelieved heat stress, the elderly may lapse into a coma. If still unattended, they may die and later be found in bed.

### EXERTIONAL HEATSTROKE

Exertional heatstroke is typically seen in fit, young, unacclimatized athletes who are exercising in the heat. It usually presents as an acute derangement of mental function. Incoherent speech, confusion, delirium, seizures, decerebrate posturing, transient hemiplegia, and frank coma may all be presenting symptoms. Initial symptoms may go unnoticed, with the victim feeling increasingly hot and noting dizziness or a decrease in concentration. Many athletes are familiar with these symptoms but think that they are the normal result of exertion. Other early neurologic warning signs include irritability, confusion, agitation, or incoherent speech. These young, healthy patients also may have no prodrome or warning symptoms before collapse. (See Table 1.5.)

Since sporting events are frequently sites of intense competition and consequent exertion, many simultaneous cases of exertional heatstroke may be seen in summer runs, football practices, and similar sporting events.

Patients with heatstroke of either variety will have tachycardia due to the shunting of blood through dilated skin vessels. Hyperventilation likewise is universal with rates up to 60 per minute. This hyperventilation may cause a respiratory alkalosis that leads to hypercapnea and frank tetany. Vomiting and diarrhea are commonly found with heatstroke. (See box for a comparison of the features of both types of heatstroke.)

| Precautions to Prevent Heatstroke in Hot Climates | |
| Wet Bulb Globe Temperature Index | Precautions |
| --- | --- |
| Under 18°C (65°F) | No precautions are needed. Observe those athletes who lose over 3% of body weight. |
| 18.8–23.3°C (66–74°F) | Insist that unlimited amounts of water be given. Flavored or iced water is preferable. Coaches or rare officials should ensure that .5 to 1 liter of water per hour is consumed. Moderate risk of heat injury exists. |
| 23.3–27.7°C (74–82°F) | Any person who is susceptible to heat or humidity probably should not run in races. Coaches must ensure adequate water consumption of 1 to 2 liters per hour. Water should be cooled and flavored. High risk of heat injury exists. |
| 27.7°C (Over 82°F) | Work/rest cycles of 30 minutes/30 minutes for all work. Alter practice schedule and conduct practice in shorts. Practice at 6 A.M. is preferable. Races and competitive athletic events should probably be rescheduled. Severe risk of heat injury exists. |

## Complications

### HYPOTENSION

Hypotension and shock are also early manifestations of heatstroke. The mechanism of the hypotension is complex and probably due to three or four factors that simultaneously combine to present a multifactoral but ubiquitous picture of hypotension and shock.

### Hypovolemia

Hypovolemia is often present. With the rapid loss of fluid (2 to 3 liters per hour) found in the unconditioned unacclimatized person, large volume losses may rapidly occur. The Israeli experiences with exertional heatstroke suggest that the rapid infusion of 1 to 2 liters of Ringer's lactate or normal saline will be helpful. Needless to say, in the patient with cardiac failure or underlying cardiac disease, volume overload must be avoided.

### Peripheral Vasodilation

Peripheral vasodilation with the subsequent peripheral pooling of blood is both a mechanism of heat reduction and a source of hypotension. The shunting of blood first leads to a tachycardia as noted above. After the heart is unable to further compensate for the apparent decrease in blood volume, a high output failure intervenes with subsequent hypotension. This hyperdynamic state resembles that seen with sepsis. At least one study has noted that older patients who have

had symptoms for less than 6 hours have had a hyperdynamic state (high output cardiac failure), while the patients with symptoms for more than 12 hours have had a hypodynamic state (low output cardiac failure).[40] The author of that article feels that the spectrum of circulatory responses to heatstroke is more a function of the patient's cardiac reserves than age alone. Younger patients with exertional heatstroke do not usually have low output heart failure.

### Cardiac Dysfunction

Cardiac dysfunction is a major component of the hypotension of heatstroke. Myocardial infarction (MI) and heart failure are repeatedly reported from heatstroke. Vascular obstruction is usually not the cause of the MI. Though the mechanisms involved in the genesis of myocardial infarctions with heatstroke are not completely understood, some authorities feel that the basis for the infarction is hypoxia caused by the increased oxygen demands from the increased work load and the temperature-related metabolic requirements.

### Disseminated Intravascular Coagulation

Disseminated intravascular coagulation (DIC) is often found in the patient with heatstroke and subsequent bleeding can contribute to the hypotension. Evidence for disseminated intravascular coagulation in heatstroke is supported by the findings of increased levels of fibrin split products, hypofibrinonemia, thrombocytopenia, and prolonged prothrombin times.[41,42]

Proposed mechanisms of the bleeding disorders found with heatstroke include:

1. Hepatic necrosis with impairment of the clotting factors. Beard and Hickton in 1982 noted that there was a generalized fall in coagulation factors known to be produced in the liver, together with evidence of hepatic damage, even in moderate cases of heatstroke.[42] These investigators attributed the coagulation disorders to a failure of hepatic synthesis.
2. Tissue damage with subsequent release of thromboplastic substances that cause intravascular thrombosis (consumption coagulopathy). Low levels of factors II, VII, V, and X suggest that tissue damage may act as a trigger mechanism for DIC leading to a consumption coagulopathy that proceeds through the extrinsic clotting system pathway.
3. Vascular damage with subsequent increased capillary permeability.
4. Thrombocytopenia.

It should be emphasized that any or all of the mechanisms proposed may be operative in each case of heatstroke that is complicated by bleeding disorders. Patients with bleeding disorders differ from nonbleeders in that they appear to have higher rectal temperatures, more significant hypotension, higher incidence of shock, and a higher mortality rate.[43]

### RESPIRATORY

Pulmonary edema, caused by both cardiac dysfunction and intravascular coagulopathy is common in heatstroke. This pulmonary edema leads to tachypnea, further hypoxemia, and hypercapnea. Circulatory failure has also been attributed to an increase in the pulmonary vascular resistance.[44] Pulmonary edema with wedge pressures of 25 to 40 mm of mercury ranges have been reported, and autopsy results confirm the pulmonary edema. Because of these findings, cautions about fluid administration are often noted in the literature.[45,46] Other recent investigators have found low pulmonary artery wedge pressures and feel that there is no evidence for left ven-

tricular failure.[40] These authors did administer all fluid replacements and challenges (mean fluid administration of $5,719 \pm 568$ ml) with careful monitoring of serial pulmonary artery wedge pressures. Again, these studies were in older patients.

### RENAL

Aberrations in renal function are quite common in heatstroke and probably reflect the hypovolemia and hypoperfusion associated with the syndrome. Unless it is transient, acute tubular necrosis may require dialysis for treatment. Both red and white blood cells and protein are found in the urine. The urine may contain ketones and casts of white blood cells, hyaline, and granular nature. The specific gravity is usually low because of the kidney's decreased ability to concentrate the urine. The urine is sometimes "machine oil" in nature, concentrated and colored with blood and myoglobin from muscle destruction if rhabdomyolysis is present.

The necessity for dialysis does not carry the ominous prognosis of chronic renal failure. Most patients will eventually recover normal or near normal renal function.

### HEPATIC FUNCTION

The liver is also commonly injured in heatstroke. Hepatocellular necrosis can produce marked liver enzyme and bilirubin elevations and impair the synthesis of clotting factors. These hepatocellular enzymes reflect liver cell death, which may be corroborated on biopsy or postmortem examination. The liver is frequently enlarged and tender on examination. Frank jaundice may occur from the cell destruction and concomitant liver failure. These abnormalities, especially common in the exertional form of heatstroke, usually peak about 48 to 72 hours after the insult. A SGOT (AST) level above 1000 international units will bode for a poor outcome.

### MUSCULOSKELETAL

Rhabdomyolysis leading to myoglobinuria is often reported and may be a significant factor in producing renal failure. Both degeneration of muscle and the increased metabolic requirements in the face of cardiovascular collapse combine to produce a profound lactic acidosis. Although conventionally taught that rhabdomyolysis is seen commonly only in exertional heatstroke, patients with classic heatstroke and rhabdomyolysis have been reported to be common in recent literature.[47]

## NEUROLOGIC

As has been mentioned before, a disturbance of the central nervous system is necessary for the diagnosis of heatstroke. Confusion, irrational behavior, ataxia, or a sudden alteration or loss of consciousness are characteristic disturbances. Convulsions are common during the course of heatstroke and may be expected to occur in as many as one third of cases.[48] Seizures that occur early, before or during cooling, carry little prognostic import, but can increase metabolic oxygen consumption. Seizures that occur after cooling reflect either the effects of damage to the brain parenchyma, thrombosis, or hemorrhage. As such, the prognosis of the patient with a late convulsion is poor. Ischemic cord lesions, diffuse brain damage, hemiplegia, and long-term ataxia have all been described as late complications of heatstroke. Prolonged coma after restoration of a normal body temperature is indicative of a poor prognosis.

## Laboratory Findings

*Cooling of the heatstroke victim takes precedence over ALL lab, x-ray, and ECG procedures. Critical treatment must not be delayed in those who have heatstroke.*

## ELECTROCARDIOGRAM FINDINGS

Electrocardiograms (ECGs) may show some conduction changes or nonspecific ST segment changes. Frequently, changes of myocardial ischemia are reported. Although ischemic changes may be noted on an ECG, structural lesions that would compromise cardiac flow are only rarely found. One can hypothesize that a generalized increase in tissue oxygen consumption versus supply is mirrored by these findings of cardiac ischemia.

## CLOTTING STUDIES

As noted previously, clotting studies are routinely abnormal during heatstroke with frank disseminated intravascular coagulation being frequently found. Clotting disturbances may be found with decreased platelets, decreased prothrombin (PT), and decreased fibrinogen. These disorders may be the result of direct thermal damage to the hepatic cells and enzyme and are exacerbated by the multiorgan failure that ensues.

## ELECTROLYTES

Hypokalemia, hypophosphatemia, and hypocalcemia are found in heatstroke with the specific etiology in each case not yet fully understood. Certainly, a deficit in total body potassium due to obligatory sweating losses is expected. Muscle breakdown may cause the rapid rise of serum potassium. If hyperkalemia is found, it must be managed urgently as it is a serious complication. Early dialysis is probably the treatment of choice, although Kayexalate enemas, insulin, and glucose infusions are recommended by some authors. Serum sodium measurements often range from 120 to 150 mEq. Hypocalcemia is most common on the second or third day following heatstroke. It is thought to be due to deposition of calcium on areas where muscle breakdown has occurred. Tetany is unusual unless bicarbonate excess has been iatrogenically induced.

## BLOOD SUGAR

Khogali noted that 70% of his patients had an abnormally high blood sugar. In the majority of these patients, there was no prior history of diabetes.[8] Prior investigators have also noted that high serum glucose measurements were common in nondiabetic heatstroke patients.[49] Only 30% of these patients will have sugar in the urine.

## ARTERIAL BLOOD GASES

Metabolic abnormalities in classic heatstroke patients commonly include a moderate hypokalemia and a mild respiratory alkalosis. Lactic acidosis is relatively uncommon and is an ominous finding.

In exertional heatstroke, metabolic acidosis is common and often severe enough to need treatment. The metabolic acidosis appears to be increased lactic acid levels due to a combination of acute hypoxemia, shock, and increased metabolic demand. Respiratory alkalosis is also commonly found in conjunction with the metabolic acidosis either compensating or as part of a complex combination of metabolic acidosis and respiratory alkalosis.[47]

A possible explanation for the metabolic changes that have been seen is that the patient exposed to high heat stresses will first start to hyperventilate and develop respiratory alkalosis. If the heat exposure outstrips the ability to compensate, increased tissue oxygen consumption and relative hypoxia will follow. Lactic acid will then be produced and metabolic acidosis ensues.

## HEPATIC FUNCTION TESTS

With the liver and muscle damage noted, the SGOT, lactate dehydrogenase (LDH), and creatinine phosphokinase (CPK) are markedly elevated on admission.

## HEMATOLOGIC CHANGES

Increased numbers of hypersegmented polymorphoneucleocytes in the peripheral blood are often found in patients with heatstroke.[50] The etiology of the nuclear white cell changes is not clear. Spherocytosis is reported in patients with heatstroke and is thought to account for a shortened red cell life span noted in heatstroke.[51] Spherocytosis has also been reported together with increased fragility, red cell budding, and fragmentation in red blood cells heated for 15 minutes in vitro to 50°C (122°F), but the clinical applicability of this study may be questioned.[52]

## Therapy

Although the mainstay of therapy in the heatstroke victim is rapid core body cooling, good emergency practice dictates that life support ABCs take precedence over all other types of therapy. This axiom is particularly true because of the hypermetabolic state of heatstroke, with accelerated oxygen consumption for all tissues. The margin of safety in airway management is reduced by this increased oxygen consumption. Pulmonary edema and hypoxemia are also commonly found in heatstroke, and myocardial infarction is not uncommon.

Intubation should be considered early in the course of treatment since coma, convulsions, and vomiting are all common. Oxygen should always be administered at the highest available concentrations through an endotracheal tube or a nonrebreathing mask.

An intravenous line must be started, and half normal saline or normal saline is probably the fluid of choice. In the patient with pulmonary edema or myocardial dysfunction, central venous pressure or preferably a Swan-Ganz catheter is indicated for monitoring fluid status. A Swan-Ganz catheter is likewise frequently indicated in the elderly patient with borderline cardiovascular function and heatstroke.

Rhythm monitoring is routinely indicated since these patients have myocardial ischemia and dysrhythmias and may have frank infarction.

A urinary catheter will allow monitoring of urine output and osmolarity.

A temperature probe should be inserted in either the rectum or the esophagus. Glass thermometers are dangerous in seizing, delirious, or obtunded patients. Ordinary clinical electronic thermometers may be unable to measure temperatures above 42°C (107.6°F).

## COOLING

The primary therapy of heatstroke is cooling of the patient. The patient should be removed from the heat, immediately if possible. The clothing should be removed, and core body cooling should be instituted. The temperature should be reduced to 39°C as quickly as possible. The more rapid the cooling, the lower the mortality that has been observed, particularly in exertional heatstroke. Some cooling modalities that have been used are shown in Table 1.6.

**Table 1.6.**
**Common Cooling Methods**

Ice packs
Large Fans (with or without water mist)
Cold water immersion
Peritoneal lavage
Rectal lavage
Gastric lavage
Cardiopulmonary bypass

## Traditional Methods

Ice water soaks, immersion in iced baths, ice to groin, neck, and axilla and cooling blankets have been used by multiple centers as cooling modalities. Sheets or towels that have been soaked in ice water are an easy method to use. The patient should have all clothes removed and then be covered with towels or sheets. The towels should then be soaked in ice water and ice chips. The sheets or towels keep the ice water in contact with the skin and prevent the ice from running on the floor. A large fan will accelerate the cooling rate. The sheets or towels should be changed frequently and kept cold. Body massage may aid circulation and prevent the reflex vasoconstriction. This method can be managed by any emergency department, requires no special equipment, and provides rapid cooling with little risk.

Immersing the victim in cold water tubs has not been proven to be more effective and may make monitoring more difficult, although it has been enthusiastically recommended by some. Management of a seizing, incontinent, vomiting, obtunded patient with an endotracheal tube, multiple intravenous lines, catheter and rhythm monitoring in a tub of ice water is unpleasant and difficult. If a dysrhythmia supervenes, defibrillation can be hazardous or fruitless until precious minutes are wasted drying the patient.

## Evaporative Method

Recent investigators have abandoned ice water cooling in favor of the more theoretically sound method of evaporative cooling.[53,54] Evaporation of water involves the removal of 540 kcal per kilogram of water evaporated, while melting of ice to water involves the removal of only 80 kcal per kilogram. This means that evaporation of water from the skin will cool the patient up to four times more quickly than an ice water bath. The skin temperature is kept at 30 to 32°C (86°F to 89.6°F) to enhance vasodilation and increase heat flow. Shivering is much less prevalent.

Current methods of evaporative cooling include the use of a body cooling unit (BCU) that sprays 15°C water about the patient suspended in a net hammock. High speed fans ensure the most rapid evaporation possible. Although not found in most U. S. emergency departments, the effects of the BCU can be emulated with fans and mist sprayers. Evaporative cooling will work only if the patient has been completely undressed and is not covered with sheets or towels.

This method of cooling presupposes a dry microclimate to allow evaporation to take place. If the patient is not in an air conditioned area or an area of low relative humidity, the needed evaporation will not take place. Evaporative cooling also presupposes an intact circulation to take cooled blood from the skin to the core. If the patient is in shock, evaporative cooling will most likely not be as effective as ice water cooling.

## Other Cooling Methods

Other methods of cooling either require special equipment, special training, or have large risks. There are no studies available that have tested the efficacy of these methods against the more commonly employed methods. Numerous anecdotal reports describe the use of one or more of these methods in groups of one or two patients.

- Peritoneal lavage with iced Ringer's lactate or dialysate solution provides faster core cooling but requires both special training and equipment. It has the theoretical advantage of cooling the liver preferentially, which may decrease the hepatic complications often associated with heatstroke.
- Cardiopulmonary bypass provides rapid core cooling but requires preparation and specially trained teams and should be reserved for patients in whom standard therapy proves ineffective. Cardiopulmonary bypass carries with it the risk of bleeding in the face of the frequent bleeding disorders associated with heatstroke.
- Ice water enemas and ice water gastric lavage may cause water intoxication and may be detrimental to physician-nurse relations. They also contribute little to cooling in comparison to the vast skin surface areas.
- Chilled air or oxygen administration is frequently difficult to arrange as most hospitals do not have this equipment readily available. It likewise contributes little to cooling in comparison to other more common methods.

## HYPOTHERMIA

After reaching 39°C (102.2°F) current practice dictates that the cooling measures should be modified or slowed to avoid deep overshoot into the hypothermic range. There is some controversy that carefully monitored cooling of the patient into the hypothermic range may allow for better recovery of stressed and hypoxic neurons. This thought awaits a good controlled study.

## ADJUNCTIVE THERAPY

Aspirin will not control the temperature of the heatstroke victim and may aggravate the clotting disorders and should not be used.

Shivering while the patient is being cooled is a frequent problem. The shivering will cause an increase in oxygen consumption and will also increase the metabolic heat production. Valium (diazepam) 5 to 10 mg intravenously will abolish the shivering reflexes. Diazepam also has significant anticonvulsant properties and does not significantly potentiate hypotension. It can cause respiratory depression and appropriate airway maintenance equipment should be ready if the patient has not already been intubated.

Thorazine (chlorpromazine) (10 to 25 mg given very slowly intravenously) has also been recomended if the patient starts to shiver during cooling. Although chlorpromazine can affect the normal thermoregulatory mechanisms, and has been implicated in the cause of heatstroke, after the onset of the heatstroke, there is no contraindication to its use on this basis. Chlorpromazine has the additional beneficial effect of increasing peripheral vasodilation and thus promoting heat exchange. It should be noted that the phenothiazines can potentiate hypotension, cause arrhythmias, and lower the seizure threshold. For these reasons, the phenothiazines should be used both cautiously and then only if the patient starts to shiver. Diazepam appears to be a better choice in this regard.

Alcohol baths should not be used because of risk of topical absorption or inhalation of the alcohols and subsequent toxic blood levels. Children are particularly susceptible to this toxic absorption.

Dantrolene has been proposed as a treatment for heatstroke, extrapolating from its efficacy in patients with malignant hypothermia.[55,56] Dantrolene, a hydantoin derivative, is the current treatment of choice for malignant hypothermia. Its mechanism appears to be a calcium-release inhibition in the skeletal muscle's sarcoplasmic reticulum. The drug does not seem to have significant cardiovascular effects when given in doses of up to 10 mg per kg by intravenous infusion. The usual starting dose for therapy is 1 mg per kg. The major side effects appear to be muscle weakness and nausea and are manifest by about 2.5 mg per kg. There are no controlled studies about its use, and further investigation is needed before advocating its use in heatstroke.

## HYPOTENSION

Hypotension is often an early manifestation of heatstroke as has been noted previously. Particularly in exertional heatstroke, large volume deficits are common and should be rapidly corrected. The Israeli army advocates the immediate use of at least 2 liters of Ringer's lactate in all suspected cases of heatstroke, even on the battlefield. The amount of fluids and rate of administration should be based upon hemodynamic parameter, level of consciousness, and urine output to determine the adequacy of resuscitation. Major fluid shifts can occur in those patients with acute rhabdomyolysis.

Fluid administration during treatment of classic heatstroke patients should be conservative. The elderly patient with marginal cardiovascular status may easily be given excessive fluids with subsequent volume overload.

Many authors note that the next step in the treatment of hypotension associated with heatstroke should be continuing the cooling process. Certainly with the classic form of cooling with ice or iced cloths, a degree of peripheral vasodilation is induced, and the increased peripheral resistance may relieve the hypotension. This would be expected to be most effective in the patients with a hyperdynamic state and high output cardiac failure, rather than those with hypotension from pump failure.

Alpha sympathomimetic drugs, such as epinephrine or norepinephrine should be avoided as they impair heat dissipation by induction of peripheral vasoconstriction. Use of either dopamine or isoproterenol has been advocated and makes better physiologic sense.

The splanchnic vasodilation of small doses of dopamine may aid cooling. There is no large study that addresses its use in patients with heatstroke.

Bicarbonate should be given for significant acidosis, but metabolic acidosis is often found in conjunction with a significant respiratory alkalosis. The dose of bicarbonate given should be addressed after results of arterial blood gases are available.

## Further Treatment

### CENTRAL NERVOUS SYSTEM (CNS) ABNORMALITIES

As noted before, depression of the level of consciousness is an essential component of the diagnosis of heatstroke. It is important to carefully evaluate the patient for the presence of cerebral edema. If cerebral edema is found, mannitol 0.5 to 1 gm/kg and dexamethasone 10 mg IV may both be indicated, although these drugs remain controversial. If a focal neurologic lesion is noted, the patient should have a computerized tomographic scan to rule out the presence of correctable neurosurgical lesion.

Seizures should be treated with intravenous diazepam (Valium) or barbiturates in conventional doses. Some authors advocate early treatment of patients with prophylactic doses of diazepam to prevent seizures prior to their occurrence. Phenytoin has been recommended but may also precipitate dysrhythmias and hypotension.

### RENAL FUNCTION

The kidneys are severely affected by heatstroke but usually these changes are reversible. Victims of heatstroke routinely will have elevated BUN and creatinine levels and almost always have abnormalities of the urine. The management most frequently reported to decrease the effects of the heatstroke is the early and vigorous use of mannitol in 0.25 gm/kg dosages. Urine flow should be maintained at rates of 50 to 75 ml/hr. Alkalinization of the urine should also be considered. Hyperkalemia may occur in patients with renal failure or rhabdomyolysis and may require emergency dialysis.

### GASTROINTESTINAL FUNCTION

Nasogastric aspiration is routinely required to prevent regurgitation of stomach contents. Ileus is a frequent component of the heatstroke syndrome. Gastric bleeding is also frequently reported and will be recognized earlier with the nasogatric (NG) tube in place. If gastrointestinal GT bleeding occurs, it should be treated with cimetidine 300 mg IV q 6 hours.

## Prognosis

The high morbidity and mortality of heatstroke stands in stark contrast to that of profound hypothermia, where the prognosis is not generally related to the depth of temperature but rather to underlying diseases. The overall prognosis of heatstroke depends upon the body habitus, the functional reserve capacities, intercurrent chronic diseases, and delay in institution of cooling.

In general, there are three major prognostic groups found in heatstroke:

1. The first group consists of those who have had a prolonged period of coma, delayed seizures, coagulation abnormalities, acute tubular necrosis, and profound hypotension. Few of these patients awaken from coma and mortality is quite high. Hypotension that does not respond to fluids or cooling is particularly ominous. The levels to which the SGOT, SGPT, and LDH are elevated is of prognostic significance with early high elevations being poor prognostic indicators.
2. The second group consists of those patients who have regained consciousness within 4 to 10 hours. The hepatic and renal pathology reaches a peak within 3 to 5 days and then subsides. Some of these patients have transient or permanent neurologic sequellae. Ataxia and cerebellar pathology is particularly common. These patients often have long-lasting deficits in thermoregulation.
3. The third group has only transient unconsciousness, rarely lasting greater than 3 hours. Hepatic and renal pathology is limited in scope. There is a rapid recovery.

Poor prognostic signs for all patients with

heatstroke include a core temperature greater than 41.1°C (106°F), particularly if prolonged; SGOT greater than 1000 in the first 24 hours; prolonged duration of coma; hypotension that does not respond to cooling and fluid repletion; and either renal failure or hyperkalemia. Patients with classic heatstroke who have serum lactate of greater than 3 mmol/L within the first 24 hours, who are dependent upon pressor agents or who develop a complication of an underlying disease, will also do poorly.

Common causes of death in these patients include irreversible CNS damage; irreversible bleeding diathesis; hyperkalemia; renal failure; hepatic failure; and late sepsis.

## Differential Diagnosis

Heatstroke is a diagnosis of exclusion, but treatment is begun well before other diagnoses are considered. The patient with heatstroke will respond to treatment and begin to improve. If they do not improve, other possibilities in the differential diagnosis are considered based upon history, initial blood work, early clinical course, and occasionally lumbar puncture.

Purely clinical grounds are sometimes not accurate, but measurement of SGOT, LDH, and SGPT may show the early elevations associated with heatstroke. Although these elevations are not pathognomonic, they may help in confirming presumed cases of heatstroke. In any case, treatment of the elevated temperature and the ABCs takes priority over all other diagnostic tests. (See Table 1.7.)

**Table 1.7.**
**Diseases That May Mimic Heatstroke[8]**

Cerebral hemorrhage
Encephalitis
Hypothalamic hemorrhage
Infectious hepatitis
Malaria
Malignant hyperthermia
Meningitis
Tetanus
Thyroid storm
Typhus
Typhoid fever

## Prevention

### WET BULB GLOBE TEMPERATURE (WBGT) INDEX

Heatstroke becomes more likely when humidity and temperature are both high. This may be predicted by the use of the WBGT index. The effects of humidity and radiant heat are added to the dry air temperature to predict the heat stress. The dry air temperature is measured with a shaded regular thermometer. A thermometer enclosed in a wet wick (wet-bulb) measures the effects of humidity on the temperature and accounts for 70% of the reading. The radiant effects of the sun are estimated by the use of a thermometer enclosed in a 6-inch hollow black sphere. (See Fig. 1.5.)

The WBGT is available from all weather stations and most television and radio stations during periods of high heat stress. It may be calculated by:

$$\text{WBGT} = .7 \text{ (wet bulb temp)}$$
$$+ .2 \text{ (black globe temp)}$$
$$+ .1 \text{ (dry bulb temp)}$$

The dry bulb temperature alone is generally considered to be a poor indicator of heat stress since it neglects the effects of radiant heat, air movement, and humidity. Of these, humidity appears to have the greatest effect, since high humidity precludes effective evaporation.

If a means for assessing the WBGT is not readily available, an alternative equation may be employed using the dry air temperature and the water vapor pressure:

$$\text{WBGT} = (0.567 \, T_{db}) + (0.393 \, P_a) + 3.94$$

$$\text{Where } T_{db} = \text{dry bulb temperature}$$
$$P_a = \text{water vapor pressure}$$

These environmental variables should be readily available from local weather or radio stations.

If the WBGT index is above 32°C (90°F) in the hottest 2-hour part of the day, physical training and strenuous exercise should be suspended. See box for further details. The American College of Sports Medicine recommends that if the WBGT is above 28°C

$$\text{WBGT Index} = 0.7 \text{ WB} + 0.2 \text{ BG} + 0.1 \text{ DB}$$

## Example

```
Black Globe Temperature 120 *.2 = 24
Wet Bulb Temperature      80 *.7 = 56
Dry Bulb Temperature     100 *.1 = 10
```

90 WBGT Index

**Figure 1.5.** Wet bulb-globe temperature index.

(82°F) consideration should be given to postponing or rescheduling races and similar activities.

## ACCLIMATION

---

*Safe Heat Acclimation for Athletes*

Complete heat adaptation takes as long as 3 weeks.

Train either early morning or late evening for the first week's workouts.

Gradually schedule workouts closer to midday.

On particularly hot days, resume interval training in early morning or later in the evening. (See WBGT temperature guidelines.)

Ensure appropriate fluids at all times

  Drink cold fluids if at all possible.

  Drink 6 to 8 ounces of fluids every 10 to 15 minutes (Remember that thirst is a poor guide to acute dehydration)

  Electrolyte replacement solutions are optional but should have no more than 120 mmol/L concentration of all electrolytes.

---

Acclimation to the heat can be achieved in about 2 weeks for those who must exercise in hot and humid ambient temperatures. Prior physical conditioning is an important part of acclimation. In practical terms, the more fit the athlete and the less effort that it takes to maintain a given pace, the fewer problems the athlete will have with the heat.

The principle of acclimation is gradual increase to tolerance of physical activity during periods of heat and humidity. The runner should start with 15 to 20 minutes of training during the warmest hours of the day. It is important for the trainer or athlete to assess progress honestly. If the runner looks or feels tired and depleted at the end of a 20-minute run, "pushing" will achieve only an injured or ill athlete. At the end of 2 days with no ill effects, the runner should increase the duration to 35 or 40 minutes for 2 to 4 more days. If this remains satisfactory, then the duration can be increased to 1 hour.

The athlete should monitor heart rate and weight during the training process. If the heart rate does not decline during and after the workout, adaptation is not progressing satisfactorily. If the athlete notes a daily weight loss of more than 2 pounds (1 kilogram), dehydration is a distinct possibility. Extra water should be consumed, even more than dictated by thirst. Remember that the athlete working in the heat does not have adequate thirst to prevent dehydration.

## FLUID INTAKE—GENERAL

It is especially important to maintain adequate fluid intake. Thirst is a poor indicator of dehydration, and there is no signal for salt depletion. Cool, mildly flavored water is tolerated better than warm brackish water. A good indication of adequate fluid intake is clear urine. Salt tablets and salted beverages are of questionable benefit. Salt intake with meals may be increased. Do not advise those patients at risk to markedly increase their fluid intake if they have heart, kidney, or liver disease.

## INFANTS AND CHILDREN

Children should not be bundled and should not be left in cars or hot buildings. Children with a febrile illness, vomiting, diarrhea, or an upper respiratory tract infection should be promptly treated for these illnesses. For a given level of dehydration, children have a greater increase in core temperature than do adults.[57] If possible, these patients should be provided with air conditioning. Abundant fluids, fans, and antipyretics are alternatives, but the patient should be carefully monitored.

## OTHER HIGH-RISK PERSONS

During high ambient temperatures, those people at high risk should avoid the heat as much as possible and should reduce activity as much as possible. No one at risk should sleep in direct sunlight.

CDC studies showed that increased survival resulted from increasing time in air conditioned places and use of fans. Those patients who do not have home air conditioners should be advised to window shop in air conditioned malls for at least 1 to 2 hours during the hottest part of the day. Certainly, those who live on the top floors of multilevel apartment buildings should realize that increased heat stress is associated with this location.

Physicians should advise family members or friends to check on "loners" frequently during the day with at least one personal visit, daily. The elderly person living alone should be encouraged to adopt a social activity in an air conditioned place on a daily basis. Physicians should see patients on diuretics, anticholinergics (to include tricyclics), calcium blockers, beta blockers, phenothiazines, and cardiac medications on a more frequent basis during the summer months. Medications should be carefully titrated to effect, with a decrease of doses during hot weather if possible.

## ALCOHOL AND PSYCHOTROPIC MEDICATIONS

Alcoholics and patients who are taking psychotropic drugs are particularly susceptible to heatstroke. Education of family, friends, and patients to the preventative measures outlined is essential for psychiatric and alcoholic patients. Physicians who prescribe these psychotropic medications or care for alcoholics should be aware of the patient's social situation and counsel the patient and supporting persons well about the increased dangers of heatstroke while taking the psychotropic drugs. Physicians and nurses who prescribe or administer psychotropics may wish to decrease the doses to the lowest level compatible with the patient's pathology during a heat wave. Alcohol consumption in alcoholics should be limited during heat waves but not completely withdrawn. For those who do abruptly decrease their alcohol consumption during a heat wave, prompt treatment of impending delirium tremens may be lifesaving.

## TRAINING AND COMPETITION IN THE HEAT

Organizers of athletic events should be cautious of regional weather variations in scheduling for competition. Races should be organized to avoid the hottest parts of the day and, preferably, the hottest months of the year. Summer events should be scheduled before 8:00 A.M. (ideally) or in the evening after 6:00 P.M. to avoid the additional stresses of solar radiation.

Sweat suits and water "rationing" should be condemned. Coaches should keep water in the players, not on the field.

Athletes doing moderate to heavy work in the heat must sweat and may lose from 3 to 5 liters of water per hour. Depending upon environmental and work conditions, he or she may require up to 16 liters of water to drink per day. The loss of 3 liters of water is equal to about 2% of the body weight. Between 2 to 6% dehydration, the athlete's performance is impaired, both physically and mentally. Beyond 7% dehydration, the body will no longer tolerate sweating or cutaneous vasodilation and these mechanisms of heat control are lost.

During a training session, run, or race, the athlete should drink 6 to 8 ounces of water or some kind of fluid every 20 minutes. Athletes who drink anything—water, sugar water, sports drinks, or whatever—show fewer symptoms of heat stress. Cooled drinks may or may not lower core temperature, but they are more palatable and make the athlete feel better. After training, have the athletes end the training session with a long celebratory drink of at least 10 to 20 ounces of water.

There is no good evidence that one "sport drink" is better than another or even better than water for short training sessions. Glucose repletion may be a cogent factor for recommending sugar containing solutions for training sessions, runs, or races longer than 90 minutes.

For those who need to increase fitness and are not currently in good physical condition, fitness training should be done when the air is cooler, before 9 A.M. and after 6 P.M. Even then, humidity may mandate a reduction in the pace or duration of fitness training.

## SUMMARY

The diagnosis of heatstroke should be considered in all patients with an alteration of consciousness and an elevated temperature. Heatstroke is particularly common in elderly urban dwellers who have been taking phenothiazines and have an altered cardiovascular system.

The syndrome carries a high morbidity and mortality and needs emergent treatment. Rapid cooling with iced towels or water mist and fans is the treatment of choice. Hypotension, seizures, disseminated intravascular coagulation deficits, and oliguria are all common complications of this disorder.

Prevention of the heat illness syndromes is, of course, the best of all possible environmental medicines.

## References

1. Ellis FP. Mortality from heat illness and heat aggravated illness in the United States. Environ Res 1972;5:1–58.
2. Impact assessment: US social and economic effects of the great 1980 heat wave and drought. Environmental Data and Information Service, National Oceanographic and Atmospheric Administration, Sept 7, 1980, p 12.
3. Centers for Disease Control. Heatstroke-United States 1980. MMWR 1981;30(23)277–279.
4. II Kings 4:18–20.
5. Judith 8:2–3.
6. Stine RJ. Heat illnesses. JACEP 1979;8(4):154.
7. Knochel JP. Environmental heat illness: an eclectic review. Arch Int Med 1974;133:841–864.
8. Khogali M. Epidemiology of heat illnesses during the Makkah pilgrimages in Saudi Arabia. Int J Epidem 1983;12(3):267–273.
9. Johanson J, Lucy E.: The beginnings of humankind. New York: Simon and Schuster, 1980.
10. Dept of The Army. TB MED 507. United States Printing Office, 1978.
11. Mcgough S, Bunker C. DASG-HCO Subject: report of visit to Israeli Defense Forces (IDF)— Tel Aviv, Israel, 4–15 June 1976. Department of the Army, Surgeon General.
12. Hubbard RW. A brief analysis of Soviet hot weather operations doctrine. USARIEM Briefing Material, 1979.
13. Assmussen E, Boje O. Body temperature and capacity for work. Acta Physiol Scand 1945; 10;475–482.
14. Rowell LB, Brengelmann GL, Blackmon JR, et al. Splanchnic blood flow and metabolism in heat stressed man. J Appl Physiol 1968;24:475–484.
15. Gilat T, Shibolet S, Sohar E. Mechanism of heat stroke. J Trop Med Hyg 1963;66:204–212.
16. Demos MA, Gitin EL. Acute exertional rhabdomyolysis. Arch Int Med 1974;133:233–239.
17. Stine RJ. Heat illness. JACEP 1979;8:154–160.
18. Smith LH Jr. Heat stroke. West J Med 1974; 121:305–312.
19. Gottschalk PG, Thomas JE. Heat Stroke. Mayo Clin Proc 1966;41:470–482.
20. Knochel JP. Dog days and Siriasis: how to kill a football player. JAMA 1975;233(6):513.
21. Bonner RM, Harrison MH, Hall CJ, et al. Effect of heat acclimatization on intravascular responses to acute heat stress in man. J Appl Physiol 1976;41:708–713.
22. Finberg JPM, Berlyne GM. Modification of renin and aldosterone response to heat by acclimatization in man. J Appl Physiol 1977;42:554–558.
23. Conn JW. Aldosteronism in man: some clinical and climatological aspects. Part 1. JAMA 1963;183:775–781.
24. Bonner RM, Harrison MH, Hall CJ, et al. Effect of heat acclimatization on intravascular responses to acute heat stress in man. J Appl Physiol 1976;41:708–713.
25. Finberg JPM, Berlyne GM. Modification of renin and aldosterone response to heat by acclimatization in man. J Appl Physiol 1977;42:554–558.
26. Knochel JP, Dotin LN, Hamburger RJ. Pathophysiology of intense physical conditioning in a hot climate. I. Mechanisms of potassium depletion. J Clin Invest 1972;51:242–255.
27. Kilbourne EM, Choi K, Jones TS, et al. Risk factors for heatstroke: a case-control study. JAMA 1982;247(24):3332–3336.
28. Gilat T, Shibolet S, Sohar E. Mechanism of heat stroke. J. Tropi Med Hyg 1963;66:204–212.
29. Attia M, Khogali M, El-Khatib G, et al. Heat stroke: an upward shift of temperature regulation set point at an elevated body tempera-

ture. Int Arch Occup Environ Healt 1983;53:9–17.

30. Jones TS, Liang AP, Kilbourne EM, et al. Morbidity and mortality associated with the July 1980 heat wave in St. Louis and Kansas City, Mo. JAMA 1982;247(24):3327–3331.

31. Ellis FP. Mortality from heat illness and heat aggravated illness in the United States. Environmental Research 1972;5:1–58.

32. Hubbard RW. An analysis of current doctrine in use (USA vs IDF) for the prevention and treatment of heat casualties resulting from operations in the heat. Commanding Officers Conference 4th MAW/MARTC 2–4 October, 1978.

33. Cardullo HM. Sustained summer heat and fever in infants. J. Pediatr 1949;35:24–42.

34. Stadnyk AN, Glezos JD. Drug induced heat stroke. Can Med Assoc J 1983;128:957–959.

35. Forester D. Fatal drug-induced heat stroke. JACEP 1978;7(6);243–244.

36. Cullumbinde H, Miles J. The effect of atropine on men exposed to warm environments. Q J Exp Physiol 1956;41:162–176.

37. Bark NM. The prevention and treatment of heatstroke in psychiatric patients. Hosp Community Psychiatry 1982;33(6):474–476.

38. Ayd FJ Jr. Fatal hyperpyrexia during chlorpromazine therapy. J Clin Exp Psychopathology 1956;17:189–192.

39. Caroff SN. The neuroleptic malignant syndrome. J. Clin Psych 1980;41:79–83.

40. Sprung CL. Heat stroke in the elderly. Chest 1979;75(3):362–366.

41. Mustafa KY, Khogali M, Gumaa KA, and Abu Al-Nasr NM. Disseminated intravascular coagulation among heat stroke cases. In Khogali M, Hales J, editors: Heat stroke and temperature regulation. Sydney, Academy Press, 1983:109–117.

42. Beard ME, Hickton CM. Hemostasis in heat stroke. Br J Hemotology 1982;52:269–274.

43. Mustafa KY, Omer O, Khogali M, et al. Blood coagulation and fibrinolysis in heat stroke. Br J. Hematology 1985;61:517–523.

44. O'Donnell TF Jr, Clowes GHA Jr. The circulatory abnormalities of heatstroke. N Engl J Med 1972;287:734–737.

45. Malamud N, Haymaker W, Custer RP. Heat stroke: a clinico-pathologic study of 125 fatal cases. Milit Surg 1946,99.397–449.

46. Shibolet S, Coll R, Gilat T, et al. Heatstroke: its clinical picture and mechanism in 36 cases. Q J Med 1967;36:525–548.

47. Sprung CL, Portocarrero CJ, Fernaine AV, Weinburg PF. The metabolic and respiratory alterations of heat stroke. Arch Int Med 1980;140:665–669.

48. Gauss H, Meyer KA: Heat stroke: Report of 158 cases from Cook County Hospital. Am J Med Sci 1917;154:554–564.

49. Green WL. A 65 year old woman with heat stroke. Am J Med 1967;43:117–119.

50. Navari RM, Sheehy TW, McLean BK, Sutton FD. The peripheral blood smear in heat stroke: an aid to diagnosis. Alabama J Med Sci 1983;20(2):137–140.

51. Halden ER, Jones F, Sutherland DA, et al. Hematologic studies in heat stroke: the anemia of heat stroke with emphasis on a hemolytic component. Am J Med 1955;19:141–142.

52. Ham TH, Sayre RW, Dunn RF, et al. Physical properties of red cells as related to effects in vivo. II. Effect of thermal treatment of rigidity of red cells, stroma, and the sickle cell. Blood 1968;32:826–871.

53. Weiner JS, Khogali M. A physiological body cooling unit for treatment of heat stroke. Lancet 1980;2:507–509.

54. Graham BS, Lichtenstein MJ, Hinson JM, Theil GB. Non-exertional heatstroke: physiologic management and cooling in 14 patients. Arch Int Med 1986;146:87–90.

55. Lydiatt JS, Hill GE. Treatment of heat stroke with dantrolene [Letter]. JAMA 1981;246(1):41–42.

56. Paasuke RT. Drugs, heat stroke, and dantrolene. Can Med Assoc J 1984;130:341–343.

57. Bar-Or O. Climate and the exercising child: a review. Int J Sports Med. 1980;1:53–65.

58. Adams BE, Manoguerra AS, Lilja GP, Long RS, Ruiz E. Heat stroke associated with medications having anticholinergic effects. Minn Med 1977:60;103–106.

59. Litman RE. Heatstroke in parkinsonism. AMA Arch Int Med 1952;89:562–567.

60. Zelman S, Guillan R. Heat stroke in phenothiazine treated patients: a report of three fatalities. Am J Psychiatry 1970;126:1787–1790.

61. Greenblatt DJ, Greenblatt GR. Chlorpromazine and hyperpyrexia: a reminder that this drug affects the mechanisms which regulate body temperature. Clin Pediatr (Phila) 1973; 12:504–505.

62. Litman RE. Heat sensitivity due to autonomic drugs JAMA 1952;149:635–636.

# CHAPTER 2

# Burns

## Part 1
## Thermal Burns

### INTRODUCTION

Among the environmental injuries sustained by man, by far the most common are burns. The National Consumer Commission has estimated that there are at least 2 million individuals in the United States alone that are burned each year. Of these patients, some 100,000 will require hospitalization, and about 20,000 will die.[1] Burns are not only common, they are abundantly lethal. The emergency provider may find caring for the burned patient stressful, frightening, and even repugnant. Thermal burns are perhaps the most devastating injury suffered by an individual.

The skin separates us from our environment. It provides the bulk of cooling for the stress of heat, regulates the egress of bodily fluids, and prevents outside agents and bacteria from entering the body. The skin is the largest organ in the body. It also provides us with much of our concept of the beauty of a person. When the skin is broached by a burn, we lose some or all of these factors to a degree depending upon the extent of the burn. While a minor burn requires little treatment, a 20% full thickness burn is an injury equivalent to having both legs crushed.[2] In this chapter, the effects of thermal, chemical, and electri-cal injuries will be discussed and management plans for each injury developed.

### DEMOGRAPHICS

Children are more likely to suffer a thermal injury than adults. Children are active, curious, and unaware and uninformed, a combination of traits that can result in many burns. Indeed, children under six have more burns than any other age group.[3] Children are most frequently victims of scald burns, while adults are most frequently burned with inflammable liquids. Males are more frequently burned than females. Structural fires account for 45% of burn-related deaths, primarily due to inhalation injuries.

Survival of the burn patient is dependent upon the amount and depth of the burn, on the age of the patient, and upon other associated injuries. Predicting the mortality risk for a given patient helps in deciding where to transport the patient, assigning the appropriate level of care, and comparing different therapies. There are multiple formulas for calculation of the expected mortality.[4-7]

### TYPES OF BURNS

Burns are classified by the agent that causes them. Common categories are thermal, electric, radiant, and chemical. Additionally, thermal burns are categorized according to their causes such as flame, flash, scald, and

**Table 2.1.**
**Etiology and Distribution of Burns**

Distribution of Etiology of Burns in 143 Patients[39]

| Source | Percent |
|---|---|
| Flash | 15% |
| Flame | 29% |
| Scald | 33% |
| Contact | 5% |
| Chemical | 7% |
| Electrical | 7% |
| Unknown | 4% |

Distribution of nonfatal burns

| Source | Percent |
|---|---|
| Contact with hot objects | 24% |
| Scalds | 21% |
| Explosions | 10% |
| Ignition of fabric | 12% |
| Welding and soldering | 4% |
| Trying to extinguish house fire | 11% |
| Electrical short circuits | 1% |
| Gasoline related | 1% |
| Motor vehicles | 10% |
| Other | 6% |

contact burns. Radiant burns are discussed in the sections on radiation and sunburn. (see Table 2.1)

## Pathophysiology of Thermal Burns

Burns are caused by the transfer of energy to the skin at a faster rate than the body or skin can dissipate it. The depth of a burn depends upon the temperature and duration of the heat applied, and the ability of the tissues to dissipate the transferred energy. The rate of heat transfer is more critical than the total amount of heat transferred.

In scald burns, the magnitude of injury is dependent upon the specific heat from the liquid, which is the amount of heat needed to raise a liter of liquid a degree centigrade. A higher specific heat means that the liquid's capacity to store and release heat is higher. Water has a higher specific heat than most substances found in nature. This means that the heat stored in small quantities of hot water is sufficient to cause thermal injuries. The maximum temperature that liquid water can attain at sea level is, of course, 100°C (212°F).

Other liquids, such as tar, sulfur, or molten metals, can attain higher temperatures. Unfortunately, sulfur and tar also have higher specific heats than water does; thus, the burns from these two substances can cause severe burns during scalds. Likewise, steam temperatures can be elevated far above the boiling point of water, resulting in severe burns.

The length of time during which the liquid contacts the skin is another important determinant. At temperatures above 70°C (158°F), the contact time for hot water to cause complete necrosis of the epidermis is less than 2 seconds. It is fortunate that water is not particularly viscous and streams to the floor unless impeded by clothing. In immersion scalds, the duration of contact between the hot liquid and skin is considerably longer than when the water flows onto the skin, thus increasing the severity of the injury.

It is obvious that if the liquid solidifies upon contact, is hotter than water, or ignites other materials, the burn will be more severe. An obvious example is the severity of the molten metal burn where the liquid is hotter than water.[8] Because it solidifies upon contact, it also has a much longer contact time.

## VASCULAR CHANGES IN BURNED SKIN

Almost immediately after the burn, the vessels in the area adjacent to the burn are altered. At first, an intense vasoconstriction is caused by the release of numerous vasoactive substances from the injured cells.

After a few hours, the vessels dilate from the release of kinins from the damaged mast cells in the area. During the vasodilation, the capillaries become more permeable, with subsequent extravasation of plasma into the burned wound.

Ischemia from the initial vasoconstriction and subsequent microthrombus formation may extend the area of the burn. The ischemia may be present to a depth as much as three to seven times greater than the area of the cells directly damaged by the heat. Because of this ischemia, final determination of the depth of the burn may be delayed as long as 5 days.

Many authorities recognize three concentric layers of vascular changes due to the effects of the burn and subsequent ischemia.[9]

The center of the burn is often called the *zone of coagulation* and represents the area of direct destruction of the cells by the heat.[10] Within this area, all blood vessels are thrombosed. As the intensity of the heat or the length of the exposure increases, this zone of coagulation will extend deeper and wider.

Surrounding the zone of coagulation is a *zone of stasis*. In this area, there is vasoconstriction and some microvascular thrombosis. In the zone of stasis, some blood vessels will remain patent even though blood flow is reduced overall. It is in this zone that injury is potentially reversible or may be converted into a wider zone of coagulation with subsequent cell death. Circulation can be restored to this area with prompt proper treatment in many cases.

Surrounding the area of vascular stasis is an area of minimal damage, the *zone of hyperemia*. The bright red color that blanches on pressure is noted at the margin of all burn wounds and, in the most minimal cases, may comprise the entire wound.

## WATER AND HEAT LOSSES

In addition to the direct reactions to a thermal burn, burns that destroy the epidermis will permit increased insensible water losses of up to 15 times normal. As the water evaporates, body heat is lost with the possibility of hypothermia ensuing. These heat and water losses can be considerable when the patient is evacuated by helicopter due to the increase in air flow around the patient. The results of heat and water losses must be considered in the treatment plans. There is an enormous increase in caloric requirements to balance the metabolic expenditure consequences of these losses.

## INFECTION POTENTIAL

Following a severe skin burn from any source, the skin undergoes coagulation necrosis and becomes a superb growth medium for bacteria. Because the local blood supply is also compromised in the burned tissues, the local defense mechanisms may be inadequate. The degree and consequences of the resultant bacterial invasion will vary directly with the severity of the wound and are modified by the subsequent therapy. This bacterial invasion is one of the most frequent fatal complications of a serious burn and should not be underestimated.

## ASSESSMENT OF THE BURN

The assessment of burn injury involves two major factors: the depth and extent of the damage. These two factors help to determine the capacity for regeneration, the potential for bacterial invasion, and other complications. Included in the initial assessment of the burn should be the assessment of the potentially exacerbating factors such as age, prior medical history, allergies, and current medications.

### Initial History

Obtain the history of the injury from the patient, relatives, or emergency response crew. Remember that although the burn may ultimately be fatal, if the patient has survived the initial insult, the burn wound itself is not likely to be the IMMEDIATE threat to life.[11] Gas explosions, propane explosions, or other explosive injuries may cause substantial associated injuries. Confinement in an enclosed car or a room may be associated with pulmonary injuries from inhalation of toxic gases. The patient may have been involved in an accident that preceded the burn or may have leaped to escape being more severely burned. There may be penetrating injuries from associated blast effects, electrical injuries, or myriad other situations. These potentially life-threatening injuries may take precedence over the burn wound management and should be dealt with as necessary.

The history should include any associated illnesses such as diabetes, hypertension, metabolic disorders, or cardiac and pulmonary diseases. It is important to find out any allergies and current drug therapy. The patient's age should be noted at this time. Remember that burns occurring at the extremes of age will be associated with the highest morbidity and mortality.

### Depth of the Burn

The depth of a burn provides the initial clue to the severity of the injury, but it may not be possible to accurately determine the depth

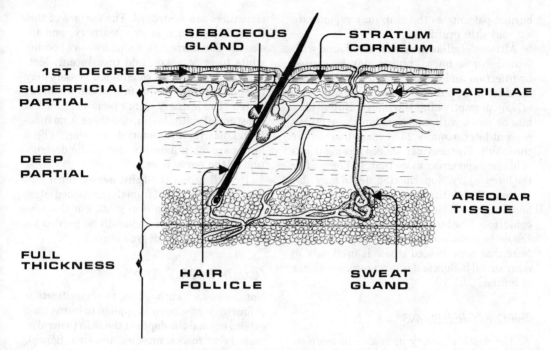

**Figure 2.1.** Depth of burn.

of a burn until debridement has been performed. What initially appears to be a second degree burn may evolve into a third degree burn by infection or vascular changes from other burn injuries. Determination of the depth of burn is most important in establishing wound care priorities. (See Fig. 2.1.)

## FIRST DEGREE BURNS

A first degree burn affects only the epidermis. It results in vasodilation and congestion of the dermal vessels. The resultant erythema will blanch upon pressure. There is no bullae formation, and the wound is quite painful. Premature cell death often results in desquamation or peeling a few days after the burn. Healing is not accompanied by scarring or discoloration. There is no substantial clinical significance to this injury in the otherwise healthy adult, unless a great extent of the body is involved. Needless to say, these burns are quite painful.

## SECOND DEGREE BURNS

A second degree burn involves a portion of the dermis and produces an epidermolysis. The resultant edema and fluid exudate yields

bullae formation, a hallmark of the second degree injury.

By definition, the full thickness dermis is not destroyed in a second degree burn, and the epidermis can reconstitute over a period of time without significant scarring or contracture formation. Since nerve fibers in the skin are often spared, these burns are exquisitely painful.

The intact blisters maintain a sterile waterproof covering of the wound, and healing occurs by continued growth of the remaining basal cells. Underlying the blister formation may be an erythematous or waxy base, depending upon the depth of the burn. Once a blister is broken, a weeping wound will result. There is then a concomitant increase in evaporative water and heat losses and exposure of naked nerve fibers.

Deep second degree burns occur when the damage is extensive, but the deeper structures retain viable skin elements. This is most often true in deep burns of the back, palms, and soles. At times, the only remaining elements may be very deep in the dermis, such as sweat glands and hair follicles. This burn may develop the same eschar as the third degree burn. It is important to recognize these deeper second degree burns in extensively burned patients as the skin may regenerate without skin grafting.

Although bullae are classically found with second degree burns, bullae may be caused by infection and by superheated steam. Bullae due to second degree burns develop relatively promptly after the injury. Bullae may also be noted with infection, but these bullae present later, usually 24 or more hours after the insult. The provider should be suspicious of blisters appearing more than 16 hours after the burn injury. Superheated steam may also cause bullae as the heat causes water to boil and vapor to form between the dermis and epidermis. The burns from *superheated* steam should be considered third degree at all times. Note that superheated steam is used only in commercial boilers and is not a common source of injury.

### THIRD DEGREE BURNS

As the depth of injury increases in more severe burns, all epidermal and supporting structures are destroyed. The surface of this third degree burn is dry, leathery, and inelastic. The burned skin surface may become white to gray, waxy, and translucent. Mottling and superficial coagulated vessels may be seen through the surface of the resultant eschar. The leathery eschar permits rapid and substantial water losses, and there is no functional barrier to bacterial invasion. These burns are often painless, due to the destruction of the nerve fibers.

By definition, the third degree burn will not regenerate except from the unburned edges of the skin or from a skin graft. For this reason, surgical intervention will be needed for all but small third degree burns.

### FOURTH DEGREE BURNS

Not used by all authorities, the classification of fourth degree burn is applied to burns that extend beyond the depth of the skin to involve underlying fascia, muscles, tendons, nerves, periosteum, and vessels. Occasionally, even

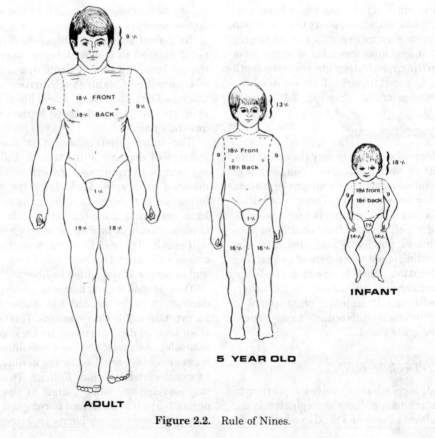

**Figure 2.2.** Rule of Nines.

bone may be involved. This burn classification is most often used with electrical injuries, but severe charring of extremities may also be termed fourth degree lesions. The natural history of this wound is the same as a third degree burn with the added deeper destruction and dysfunction. There is no difference in the initial treatment of a third degree burn and a fourth degree burn.

## Extent of the Burn Surface

Unfortunately for burn surgeons, the human frame is not a right cylinder. If this were so, calculation of the burned surface area would be simple, and a determination of the percentage of burned surface area would be easy. Since our frame is irregular, and varies in its irregularity with age and sex, determination of the fraction of burned surface area is not simple. Because of the complexity, multiple schemes have evolved for the estimation of the total burned surface area (TBSA).

### RULE OF NINES

The rule of nines apportions a 9% segment to each of eleven major body surfaces and the

remaining 1% is apportioned to the groin. (see Fig. 2.2.) This scheme is for the adult human. For children, a greater percentage is assigned to the head and a lesser percentage to the lower extremities.

### LUND AND BROWDER CHART

Since the proportions of surface areas of the younger patients will vary with age, schemes to approximate the burn surface area will fail unless these variations are taken into account. The most accurate method of determining the extent of the burn is the Lund and Browder chart, which accounts for changes in the sizes of body parts that occur with growth.[12] These calculations can be quite time consuming, and the rule of nines is more frequently used in field emergency services (though less accurate for the pediatric population). (See Fig. 2.3.)

### RULE OF PALMS

The rule of palms is convenient for measurement of small burn surfaces. The palm of the patient's hand is roughly 1% of the patient's total body surface area. Estimation of the

| Age vs. Area | | | | | | | | | |
|---|---|---|---|---|---|---|---|---|---|
| Area | Birth 1 yr. | 1-4 yr. | 5-9 yr. | 10-14 yr. | 15 yr. | Adult | 2° | 3° | Total |
| Head | 19 | 17 | 13 | 11 | 9 | 7 | | | |
| Neck | 2 | 2 | 2 | 2 | 2 | 2 | | | |
| Ant. Trunk | 13 | 13 | 13 | 13 | 13 | 13 | | | |
| Post. Trunk | | | | | | | | | |
| R. Buttock | $2^1/_2$ | $2^1/_2$ | $2^1/_2$ | $2^1/_2$ | $2^1/_2$ | $2^1/_2$ | | | |
| L. Buttock | $2^1/_2$ | $2^1/_2$ | $2^1/_2$ | $2^1/_2$ | $2^1/_2$ | $2^1/_2$ | | | |
| Genitalia | 1 | 1 | 1 | 1 | 1 | 1 | | | |
| R. U. Arm | 4 | 4 | 4 | 4 | 4 | 4 | | | |
| L. U. Arm | 4 | 4 | 4 | 4 | 4 | 4 | | | |
| R. L. Arm | 3 | 3 | 3 | 3 | 3 | 3 | | | |
| L. L. Arm | 3 | 3 | 3 | 3 | 3 | 3 | | | |
| R. Hand | $2^1/_2$ | $2^1/_2$ | $2^1/_2$ | $2^1/_2$ | $2^1/_2$ | $2^1/_2$ | | | |
| L. Hand | $2^1/_2$ | $2^1/_2$ | $2^1/_2$ | $2^1/_2$ | $2^1/_2$ | $2^1/_2$ | | | |
| R. Thigh | $5^1/_2$ | $6^1/_2$ | 8 | $8^1/_2$ | 9 | $9^1/_2$ | | | |
| L. Thigh | $5^1/_2$ | $6^1/_2$ | 8 | $8^1/_2$ | 9 | $9^1/_2$ | | | |
| R. Leg | 5 | 5 | $5^1/_2$ | 6 | $6^1/_2$ | 7 | | | |
| L. Leg | 5 | 5 | $5^1/_2$ | 6 | $6^1/_2$ | 7 | | | |
| R. Foot | $3^1/_2$ | $3^1/_2$ | $3^1/_2$ | $3^1/_2$ | $3^1/_2$ | $3^1/_2$ | | | |
| L. Foot | $3^1/_2$ | $3^1/_2$ | $3^1/_2$ | $3^1/_2$ | $3^1/_2$ | $3^1/_2$ | | | |
| | | | | | | | | Total | |

**Figure 2.3.** Lund and Browder chart. By permission of *Surgery, Gynecology & Obstetrics*.

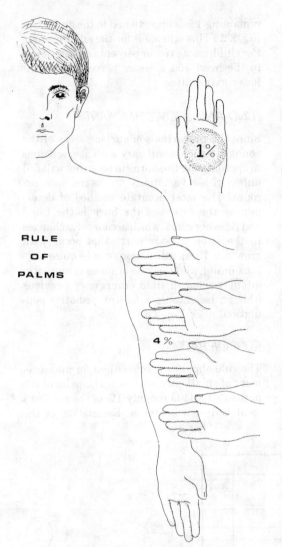

RULE
OF
PALMS

**Figure 2.4.** Rule of palms.

number of palms for a small burn will give a rough approximation of the burned surface area. This method is not accurate for large burned surfaces. (See Fig. 2.4.)

## Classification of Burns

The American Burn Association guidelines are useful in determination of the overall severity of a burn. Those burns that involve inhalation injuries or are caused by electricity are significantly more dangerous than thermal burns are alone.[13] Extensive burns and burns that involve areas that are difficult to treat or are associated with high rates of infection are also more dangerous.

Finally, those burns in patients at the extremes of age or those patients with extremes of risk due to preexisting disease will have more mortality or morbidity associated with the injury.[14] Those preexisting diseases that increase the risk of a major burn include (but are not limited to) major cardiovascular or respiratory diseases, hepatic and renal diseases, insulin dependent diabetes, alcoholism, severe psychiatric illness, and head injuries with unconsciousness. Patients with sickle cell disease should also be considered to be in this category because they frequently will develop a sickle cell crisis in response to major burns.

---

*Major Burn Injuries*
Second degree burns greater than 25% TBSA in adults
Second degree burns greater than 20% TBSA in children
Third degree burns greater than 10% TBSA
Burns of hands, face, eyes, ears, feet, or perineum
All inhalation injuries
Electrical burns
Burns complicated by fractures or other trauma
Burns in poor risk patients

*Moderate Uncomplicated Burn Injuries*
Second degree burns greater than 15% TBSA in adults
Second degree burns greater than 10% TBSA in children
Third degree burns greater than 2% TBSA that do not involve ears, eyes, face, hands, feet, or perineum

*Minor Burn Injuries*
Second degree burns less than 15% TBSA in adults
Second degree burns less than 10% TBSA in children
Third degree burns that are less than 2% and do not involve any of the critical areas

---

## CARE OF THE BURN PATIENT AT THE INJURY SCENE

Prior to initiation of medical care, the patient should be extricated from the source of heat if necessary and the sources of heat removed from the body. Under no circumstances should the emergency care provider enter burning buildings without proper protective equipment that includes self-contained breathing apparatus. The rescuer who succumbs to smoke, toxic gases, or flames has helped no one and becomes a casualty that needs to be extricated himself. The approach to the chemically contaminated victim should also occur after thorough preparation and donning of proper protective equipment for the agents involved.

Smoldering or burning clothing should be extinguished and then cut away. Failure to remove burning clothing, followed by application of high-flow oxygen, is unnecessarily hazardous to both patient and medical staff. It is wise to always remove all of the clothes of a burn victim to ensure that no embers or smoldering sections remain to be transported in the vehicle. Chemically contaminated garments should be removed and the victim washed with copious amounts of water (with only a few exceptions). Needless to say, washing of the victim should be done at a decontamination station, not in the vehicle.

Burns may be inflicted in children as a form of abuse. Contact burns with matches, cigarettes, irons, or hot metal appliances, and scald burns are common forms of this type of child abuse. If the history seems inconsistent with the trauma noted, or if the parent's concern seems inconsistent with the potential injuries of a child, the physician should be alerted to the possibility of child abuse. Frequent locations of nonaccidental burn trauma include the backs of the hands, legs, buttocks, and feet.[15,16]

If the transport time to the hospital is less than 15 minutes, the burn patient may be covered with a sheet (sterile if possible) and transported without further delay. If the transport time exceeds 30 minutes, at least one large bore line of Ringer's lactate should be started in any available site. Use of intravenous lines through burned tissue should be avoided if at all possible. If the transport time is less than 30 minutes and greater than 15 minutes, local protocols should be consulted. For severe burns, associated injuries, inhalation injuries, and patients with associated preexisting diseases, air transport directly from the site to a specialized burn center may be indicated.

If communications are available from the site to the receiving emergency department,

the receiving emergency department should be notified so that appropriate arrangements can be made. Only the information that is used to classify the severity of the burned patient should be communicated to the hospital via radio (e.g., depth of burn, percentage of burned skin, location of the injuries, age of the patient, presence of inhalation or electrical injuries, and significant other illnesses).[17]

Moist soaks or ice applications are often recommended to relieve the pain of a superficial burn. If the patient has more than a single extremity burned, the patient should not have cold water or ice applied. If the burn is third degree, the patient also does not need the application of ice or cold water. It is, unfortunately, entirely too common that a patient is brought to the emergency department by inexperienced EMTs or well meaning friends who have applied ice water to the burns and have the patient sitting in a pool of cold water on the cot. With an immersion of this sort, it is easy to imagine (and document) the rapid development of hypothermia. The patient with a burn does not need the additional stress of hypothermia and its associated problems.

## Field Considerations (Long Transport Times)

If transport of the patient is delayed due to weather, unavailability of transport, distance, terrain, or any other factor, airway support and fluid status should be monitored carefully and corrected as needed. Any of the fluid resuscitation "burn budgets" may be used as described below.

In this long transport mode, if intravenous fluids are not available for any reason, oral fluid replacements may be required. The decision to give oral fluids in this situation should not be made lightly, since about 30% of patients with a burn of 20% or more of the body surface area will develop an adynamic ileus. The complications of an adynamic ileus and administration of oral fluids are patent. Obviously, if contraindications to the administration of oral fluids exist (such as abdominal trauma, facial trauma, or unconsciousness), oral fluids should not be given. The practitioner with a severely burned patient beyond the roadhead or in very inclement weather has a practical and therapeutic dilemma in prevention of burn shock.

Treatment of the patient's burned surface areas in the field during the first 48 hours should be limited to a gentle cleansing with diluted povidone-iodine solution or a diluted solution of baby shampoo or mild dish soap. Needless to say, water used to cleanse burns should be properly treated as described in the chapter on water purification. Grease-based ointments and salves should not be used. Water-soluble antibiotic creams such as Silvadine may be used if available. These dressings should be changed every 12 to 24 hours. Burn dressings should be fabricated from the cleanest cloths available, if no sterile dressings are at hand.

Nonmentholated shaving cream may suffice as a burn dressing to keep the eschar moist and prevent increased fluid losses. Shaving creams are easy to cleanse from the burn and may have a minimal antibacterial action. It should be emphasized that this is not an approved or advertised use of these products and is offered as a field expedient only.

During long transports, care should be taken to keep burned extremities elevated so that excessive edema formation does not occur. Circumferential extremity burns should be treated as outlined below to prevent limb ischemia. Circumferential chest injuries may also necessitate an escharotomy prior to or during an extended transport to prevent respiratory embarrassment.

## EMERGENCY DEPARTMENT MANAGEMENT OF BURNS

Once the patient has arrived in the emergency department, definitive management of the burn begins. It should be remembered that for the patient with an extensive burn, this is only the beginning of a definitive treatment program that may last for years. The emergency physician's goal is to give the maximum chance for survival of both body and burned surfaces for the patient with a severe burn. This may mean that the emergency physician's appropriate role is that of stabilization and referral rather than definitive therapy. Burn care has advanced tremendously over the past 20 years through the joint efforts of cognizant emergency providers and burn researchers in specialized burn units. The average hospital, quite simply, does not have the resources or training for management of the severely burned patient.

## Appraisal of the Burn

Upon arrival of the patient, the physician needs to reassess the basics: Airway, Breathing, and Circulation (ABC). Airway swelling, respiratory distress, and signs of potential inhalation injury should be sought and corrected immediately.

Although impairment of circulation is not usually a problem in the early and uncomplicated burned patient, burned patients have frequently sustained additional trauma in the process of exiting the burning area or as a consequence of the burn. These additional problems should be sought aggressively by the emergency physician. As the formation of local edema in the burn progresses, hypovolemia (burn shock) becomes likely and must be corrected. Locally impaired circulation by circumferential burns of extremities is also likely and must be corrected.

## Inhalation Injuries

Postburn lung dysfunction is a major cause of mortality in the burned patient. Of the 84 people who died in the 1980 MGM Grand Hotel fire in Las Vegas, 79 died of smoke inhalation.[18] Increasing use of plastics and other materials that liberate noxious fumes when ignited has increased the potential for inhalation injury. Objective criteria for diagnosis of inhalation injuries, such as fiberoptic bronchoscopy and Xenon lung scans, have shown such injuries in up to one third of all burn victims.[19,20] These problems should not be underestimated. Patients with a burn and an inhalation injury have twice the mortality of patients with only a burn.

The emergency physician should anticipate the presence of a pulmonary or respiratory injury due to the inhalation of smoke and other products of combustion. In cases with upper airway damage, rapid intubation may literally be lifesaving. For further diagnostic and therapeutic information about this complex problem, please refer to the section on inhalation injuries at the end of this chapter.

## Burn Shock

Following a severe burn, adult patients may lose up to 10 to 15 liters of fluid due to increased capillary permeability at the burn site and to a lesser degree throughout the body. This isotonic fluid and protein leak from the intravascular compartment to the cellular interstitium with the greatest losses occurring during the first 8 to 12 hours.[21-24] If untreated, this transfer of fluid may cause hypovolemic shock.

Fluid resuscitation "budgets" developed over the past two decades have virtually eliminated death due to burn shock. In fact, burn edema due to increased capillary permeability and overzealous fluid administration is now the most common complication of a burn.[25]

Fluid resuscitation becomes critical in adults who have sustained more than 15% burns of their body surfaces and in children or elderly patients with 10% or more body surface burns. The goals of fluid resuscitation are to maintain cardiovascular hemodynamics, prevent renal and pulmonary complications, and to correct acid/base abnormalities.

## CALCULATING FLUID REPLACEMENTS

In 1942, Harkins and associates devised a formula for calculating the fluid and electrolyte requirements of severely burned patients.[26] Our concepts of the fluid and electrolyte replacements needed in the burned patient have been derived from suggestions by many investigators since that time. The author has had the most experience with the modified Brooke Burn Unit and the Parkland formulae, but all of the formulas appear to be based upon relatively sound principles.[27,28] (See Table 2.2.) Children will require more precise fluid replacement than adults for similar burns.[29]

Because the most drastic fluid shifts occur in the first 8 to 12 hours after the burn, most formulas advocate replacing half of the first 24 hours calculated fluid requirements during the first 8 to 12 hours. When calculating the replacement, be certain to consider the time of the burn, not the time of arrival of the patient in the emergency department. On the other hand, care must be taken not to overwhelm the patient's cardiovascular system with massive fluid administration rates if the patient arrives late in the course of the burn. Judgment becomes critical when the patient arrives 4 to 6 hours after a severe burn and has not had adequate fluid resuscitation. Unfortunately, this is a common situation during transport of a burn from the outback, such as occurs with brush or forest fires.

In general, use the formula recommended by the local burn center. Although good results have been obtained with all formulas and budgets, the local burn team may be more familiar with a different formula.[30] Since they are going to be responsible for the care of this patient for an extended time, it is thoughtful to find out, in advance, the burn center's preferences to make their task easier. This admonition applies to both field and hospital EMS providers.

**Table 2.2.**
**Burn Resuscitation Formulas in the First 24 Hours**

| Investigator | Electrolyte | Colloid | Water |
|---|---|---|---|
| Evans | 1 cc/kg/% burn | 1 cc/kg/% burn | $D_5W$ 2000 cc |
| Brooke Burn Unit | 1.5 cc/kg/% burn | 0.5 cc/kg/% burn | $D_5W$ 2000 cc |
| (Revision 1979) | 2–3 cc/kg/% burn | Lactated Ringer's | |
| Baxter | 4 cc/kg/% burn | Lactated Ringer's | |
| Monafo | Hypertonic lactated saline | | |
| | To maintain urine at 30 cc/hr | | |
| | (About 2 cc/kg/% burn) | | |

## MONITORING THE STATE OF HYDRATION

All of the burn formulas and budgets are merely guidelines and a rigid application of formulas will ignore the variability of both burn and patient. The burn fluid replacement formulas frequently result in over- or under-hydration at the extremes of weight and burn size. Do not rely on a single parameter to judge the efficacy of fluid replacement. Look for a combination of the following factors:

Clear sensorium
Extremity capillary filling and warmth of
    extremities
Vital signs normal or near normal
Decreasing hematocrit
Adequate urine output
    30 to 50 cc/hr in adults
    0.5 to 1 cc/kg/hr in children

Hematocrit, blood pressure, and pulse have significant limitations as indicators of shock in the burned patient. The blood pressure in children and young adults is often stable until late in the clinical picture of shock. With the increased metabolic rates associated with thermal trauma, a pulse in excess of 100 is often found and is compatible with adequate fluid resuscitation.

Hematocrits of 55 to 60% are common in the first 24 hours after serious burn injuries, even with adequate fluid administration. Decreasing hematocrits are to be expected with adequate fluid resuscitation but may also be a hallmark of occult bleeding. If the patient apparently requires fluid far in excess of the burn budget, a vigorous search for occult bleeding is indicated.

Central venous pressure lines may also not show the patient's fluid status in the patient with extensive burns. This is particularly true in the case of fluid overload. A more reliable indicator of fluid status is the pulmonary wedge pressure (Swan-Ganz catheter).

### Circumferential Burns

In severe burns of the extremities, especially those with circumferential or total involvement, it is imperative to establish the adequacy of perfusion. Marked edema from the deep dermal and third degree burn within the confines of inelastic eschar or the rigid fascial compartments of the extremity can limit the arterial supply and the venous outflow. The resultant tissue hypoxia can cause muscle necrosis that results in further swelling and further decrease in blood supply.

The appropriate preventative measures include early removal of rings and jewelry and elevation of the limbs. If the extremity appears cyanotic distal to the injury or capillary filling time is increased despite these measures, escharotomy should be considered. Doppler flow detectors also may be used to assess small vessel blood flow. If the patient has weak or absent distal peripheral pulses or progressive neurological signs (such as paresthesias or deep tissue pain), escharotomy is indicated.

The escharotomy should be made in both the mid medial and the mid lateral line of the limb and carried down to the ends of the fingers or to unburned skin. The incisions should be carried across involved joints and should be incised only to the depth that allows the cut edges of the eschar to separate. As the eschar has had the cutaneous nerve endings destroyed, there is no need for anesthesia.

Thoracic escharotomy may be required to prevent respiratory decompensation in the patient with circumferential chest burns. The incisions for thoracic escharotomy are in the midaxillary lines, across the costal margins, and along the clavicles. These incisions should be considered in all patients with a circumferential chest injury, particularly if combined evaluation and transport time from injury to evaluation at a burn center is greater than 60 minutes.

Fasciotomy may become necessary in the following situations:

A high-voltage injury with deep tissue
    damage
Associated skeletal or crush injuries
Thermal injuries that extend to the fascia
    (fourth degree injuries)

A tissue pressure of greater than 30 mm Hg, obtained by inserting a needle into the tissues and attempting to infuse saline or by attaching a manometer, is indicative of impending vascular compromise. When in doubt, perform a fasciotomy or escharotomy rather than risk a subsequent amputation.

## Care of the Burn Wound

Care of the burn wound should be directed towards four principles:

1. Prevention of infection
2. Decrease of burn fluid losses
3. Relief of pain
4. Salvage of all viable burn tissue

It should be emphasized that the best coverage for tissue is skin. Although acceptable artificial substitutes are now available, there is still nothing better than the "real thing." If bullae are present, these skin coverings should be preserved if at all possible. All cleansing and debridement should be directed to ensure maximum salvage of tissue in the burned patient.

### CLEANSING THE WOUND

Before cleansing the burn, soak off charred clothing with sterile saline, and clip any hair within about 2 inches about the burn. Gently cleanse the burn with mild soap and water, debriding it of all foreign particulate matter and charred tissue. The process is easier if the affected area is immersed in warm saline or water.[31] The use of a Hubbard or similar immersion tank is ideal for treatment of larger burns, but washing under running tap water will suffice for smaller burns.

The question of whether or not to debride intact bullae remains controversial. The blister provides a sterile biological dressing and should be left intact unless it is extremely large or inhibits motion. If the blisters are ruptured, hemorrhagic, or purulent, they should be debrided.

The burns caused by tar, sulfur, or clinging materials such as plastics should be immersed in cold water to rapidly cool the substance to room temperature. If this has not been done at the scene by the EMS providers, it should be done upon arrival at the emergency department, but the injury will be predictably worse. Total body immersion and subsequent hypothermia should be avoided.

Mechanical debridement of these substances can cause considerable tissue damage and pain. These clinging substances cause burns that are often deep second degree, leaving only the hair follicles to generate new skin growth. Pulling the clinging material off potentially removes the hair follicles as well. The best methods of tar removal include application of either a petroleum-based substance such as Vaseline or a Neosporin ointment or a polyoxyethylene sorbitan-based compound such as Neosporin cream or Medasol.[32-37] A proposed and unvalidated field expedient treatment for tar burns is mayonnaise.[38] If all of the tar is not immediately removed, the wound should be dressed with the petroleum-based ointment, and the dressings changed every 6 hours.

Sulfur, molten plastics, and molten metals should also be rapidly cooled until they are at body temperature. Molten metals will not be dissolved by any of these methods, but the application of petroleum-containing substances may also create an emollient surface between the cast and the underlying skin.

### USE OF ANTIBIOTIC CREAMS

There are a number of ways to manage a burn once it has been cleansed. For the early care of a burn, little wound coverage is needed. Dry sheets (sterile if at all possible) will prevent air exposure to the burned tissues and will decrease pain. If something "must" be applied to the wound, a water-soluble base is mandatory. Do not use petroleum-based ointments, unless the burn is due to sulfur or tar.

For smaller burns, treated as an outpatient, studies show that any of a variety of medications are appropriate. These medications include povidone-iodine, silver sulfdiazine, Furacin, or Sulfmylon. For the larger burn, an appropriate first choice is silver sulfdiazine, but the preferences of the local burn center should be determined before treatment. Some authorities do not wish to have any topical medications applied until they have evaluated the patient themselves.

## Adjunctive Therapies

### NASOGASTRIC SUCTION

Nasogastric suction using a Salem sump or similar tube should be initiated early in the emergency department. Many patients with a burn of greater than 25% TBSA will develop an ileus in the first 24 to 48 hours that will often last for several days. If the patient has nausea, distention, or vomiting with lesser burns, a nasogastric tube will often help.

Curling's ulcer (burn stress ulcers) will often be prevented by instillation of cimetidine (Tagamet) or other $H_2$ blockers or antacids instilled into the nasogastric tube.

## ANTIBIOTICS

In the early postburn period, antibiotics are rarely indicated. The burn unit physician should be consulted prior to use of any antibiotics. The single exception to this is the patient who has been on antibiotics for an antecedent illness. These patients should be continued on their antibiotics.

## TETANUS IMMUNIZATION

The burn injury is considered a high risk wound for tetanus. If the patient has had a tetanus immunization within 5 years, no further therapy is needed. If the patient's last tetanus immunization is greater than 5 years ago, then a tetanus booster of 0.5 cc of an age-appropriate toxoid should be given. If the patient has never had a full series of tetanus immunizations, then the patient should receive hyperimmune tetanus antitoxin and the tetanus immunization series initiated.

## PAIN MEDICATION

Patients with extensive severe burns often experience little pain. Paradoxically, more minor burns are much more painful, as the cutaneous nerve endings are damaged but not destroyed. Burn patients with partial thickness injuries will experience environmental aggravation of the injury and will benefit by simply covering the burn with a sheet.

Although there is an overwhelming tendency to use narcotics for the burn patient early in the course of the burn, it is often unwise. Most assuredly, if narcotics are used, small frequent intravenous doses should be employed. There are no contraindications to the intravenous route, and it provides rapid action, assured uptake, and easy control. If the patient becomes hypovolemic for any reason, narcotics injected intramuscularly or

---

*The "FIRE DRILL"*

1. Remove all clothing. "Undress to assess." Extinguish all smoldering clothing. Remove all chemicals.
2. Ensure that the airway is intact and start the patient on 100% oxygen by face mask. Assume that an inhalation injury exists until you prove otherwise.
3. Estimate the severity of the burn. Ascertain the depth and extent of the burn. Seek associated illnesses, injuries, and potentially complicating past medical illnesses. Ensure that allergies and current medications are recorded.
4. Ensure that circulation is intact and stays that way to all tissues. Evaluate circumferential burns for distal perfusion adequacy.
5. Calculate fluid requirements and ensure that replacement is underway if needed. If not at a burn unit, and the patient has a moderate or severe burn, ensure that the patient is appropriately transferred.
6. Ensure that baseline laboratory data is obtained. This usually includes:
   Complete blood count
   Prothrombin time/partial thromboplastin time
   Electrolytes
   Carbon monoxide level
   Blood sugar
   Blood urea nitrogen and creatinine
   Chest x-ray
   Blood gases
   ?? Type and cross blood if the patient has greater than 35% burn
   Obtain baseline weight if at all possible
   Other studies as clinically indicated

subcutaneously will not be absorbed until the circulatory status is restored. Anxiolytics, such as diazepam 5 to 10 mg intravenously, may be just as effective as narcotics in relief of pain.

If the burn patient becomes restless or agitated, check the oxygenation and then check the fluid replacement status. Anxiety and agitation are often early signs of hypovolemia and hypoxemia. To treat either of these conditions with narcotics is to invite disaster. Since both conditions are commonly found in association with severe burns, THE PATIENT MUST BE EVALUATED FOR HYPOXEMIA AND HYPOVOLEMIA BEFORE EACH DOSE OF PAIN MEDICATION.

## References

1. Trunkey DD. Transporting the critically burned patient. In: Wachtel TL, et al, eds. Current topics in burn care. Rockville MD: Aspen Publications, 1983:15–18.
2. Bassin R. Ambulatory treatment of burns. Hospital Physician 1977;8:20–23.
3. Demling RH. Burns. N Engl J Med 1985;313:1389–1398.
4. Zawacki BE, Azen SP, Imbus SH, Chang YT. Multifactoral probit analysis of mortality in burned patients. Ann Surg 1979;189:1.
5. Roi LD, Flora JD Jr, Davis TM, Wolfe RA. Two new burn severity indices. J Trauma 1983;23:1023.
6. Roi LD, Flora JD, Davis TM, et al. A severity grading chart for the burned patient. Ann Emerg Med 1981;10:161–163.
7. Tobiasen J, Hiebert JM, Edlich RF. The abbreviated burn severity index. Ann Emerg Med 1982;11:260–262.
8. Kahn AM, McCrady-Kahn VL. Molten metal burns. West J Med 1981;135:78–80.
9. Arturson MG. The pathophysiology of severe thermal injury. J Burn Care Rhabil 1985;6:129–146.
10. Zawacki BE. The natural history of reversible burn injury. Surg Gynecol Obstet 1974;139:867–872.
11. Bowen J. Emergency management of burns and pre-hospital treatment. Emergency Product News 1976;Sept/Oct:96–100.
12. Lund CC, Browder NC. The estimation of areas of burns. Surg Gynecol Obstet 1944;79:352–358.
13. Thompson PB, Herndon DN, Traber DL, Abston S. Effect on mortality of inhalation injury. J Trauma 1986;26:163–165.
14. Ostrow LB, Bongard FS, Sacks ST, et al. Burns in the elderly. Amer Fam Phys 1987;35:149–154.
15. Hobbs CJ. When are burns not accidental? Arch Dis Child 1986;61:357–361.
16. Lenoski EF, Hunter KA. Specific patterns of inflicted burn injuries. J Trauma 1977;17:842–846.
17. Bourne MK. Thermal burns: a comprehensive approach for prehospital care providers. JEMS 1987;May:42–47.
18. Crapo RO. Smoke inhalation injuries. JAMA 1981;246:1694.
19. Moylan JA, Chan CK. Inhalation injury—an increasing problem. Ann Surg 1978;188:34.
20. Cahalane M, Demling RH. Early respiratory abnormalities from smoke inhalation. JAMA 1984;251:771.
21. Demling RH. Fluid resuscitation after major burns. JAMA;250:1438.
22. Caravajal HF. A physiologic approach to fluid therapy in severely burned children. Surg Gynecol Obstet 1980;150:379.
23. Harms BA, Bodai BI, Kramer GC, et al. Microvascular fluid and protein flux in pulmonary and systemic circulations after thermal injury. Microvasc Res 1982;23:77.
24. Brouhard BH, Caravajal HF, Linares HA: Burn edema and protein leakage in the rat. I. Relationship of time of injury. Microvasc Res 1978;15:221.
25. Caravajal HF, Stewart CE. Emergency management of burn patients: the first few hours. Emerg Med Reports 1987;8:129–136.
26. Harkins HN, Lam RC, Romence H. Plasma therapy in severe burns. Surg Gynecol Obstet 1942;75:410–420.
27. Monafo WW, Halverson JD, Schechtman K. The role of concentrated sodium solutions in the resuscitation of patients with severe burns. Surgery 1984;95:129–134.
28. Rubin WD, Mani MM, Hiebert JM. Fluid resuscitation of the thermally injured patient. Clin Plas Surg 1986;13:9–20.
29. Merrell SW, Saffle JR, Sulliban JJ, et al. Fluid resuscitation in thermally injured children. Am J Surg 1986;152:664–669.
30. Pruitt BA. Fluid resuscusitation for extensively burned patients. 1981;21(supp):690–691.
31. Haynes BW Jr. Emergency department management of minor burns. Top Emerg Med 1981;3:35.
32. Stratta RJ, Saffle JR, Kravitz M, et al. Management of tar and asphalt injuries. Am J Surg 1983;146:766–769.
33. Bose B, Tredgett T. Treatment of hot tar burns. CMA J 1982;127:21–22.
34. Pruitt BA, Edlich RF. Treatment of bitumen burns [Letter]. Ann Emerg Med 1982;11:697.
35. Pruitt BA, Edlich RF. Treatment of bitumen burns. JAMA 1982;247:1565.

36. Ashbell TS, Crawford HH, Adamson JE, Horton CE. Tar and grease removal from injured parts. Plas Reconst Surg 1967;40:331.
37. Schiller WR. Tar burns in the southwest. Surg Gynecol Obstet 1983;157:38–39.
38. Shea PC, Fannon P. Mayonnaise and hot tar burns. J Med Assoc Ga 1981;70:659–670.
39. Edlich RF, Larkham N, O'Hanlan JT, et al. Modification of the American Burn Association injury severity grading system. JACEP 1978;7:226–228.

# Part 2
# Inhalation of Smoke and Toxic Gases

## INTRODUCTION

Inhalation injury is a vague term that encompasses a number of injuries from a variety of mechanisms. The lungs represent such a large surface area that they readily absorb toxic materials into the systemic circulation. In addition, the lung surface is necessary for life. Other organs can suffer substantial damage and maintain support until the organ recovers, but if the lung is severely damaged, treatment options are limited. If the lung is unable to function, life span is measured in moments.

The importance of this cannot be overstated. Between 8000 and 12,000 people die from fires in the United States each year. Over 60% of these victims have no burns and are thus presumed to have died from toxic gas inhalation. In North Dakota alone, of 28 work-related deaths in 1983, 5 were due to suffocation or inhalation of toxic gases.[1] Certainly, other states had an incidence of toxic gas inhalation similar to this.

It should be clearly noted that some of these toxins and gases talked about in this section are NOT due to burning material but are included as prime examples of toxic inhalations. Other gases are elaborated from pyrolysis on occasion but may also be found in industry or laboratories.

Over 100 chemical compounds or moieties have been identified from the burning of common materials. It is literally impossible to catalog each and every possible toxin that can be inhaled, and, indeed, the purpose of this text is not to serve as such a catalog. Instead, a general approach to the inhalation of toxic material is more appropriate for the student of environmental emergencies. Multiple handbooks, computer catalogs, and other references exist that document inhalation agents, specific tests to identify them, treatment, and, most importantly, proper protective gear to avoid them.

There are many variables to be considered when an exposure to a potential toxic agent occurs:

1. The type or types of gases (or particulates) involved
2. The duration of exposure
3. The concentration of the gas
4. The water solubility of the material
   If the agent is water soluble, it may be absorbed more easily. Less soluble and particulate materials tend to pass into the lower airways and alveoli.
5. The time lapse from exposure to proper treatment
   Usually, the diagnosis of a toxic inhalation is obvious. Occasionally, the emergency provider must have a high index of suspicion in order to make the diagnosis.
6. The underlying health of the subject
   Obviously, cardiovascular and respiratory illnesses may increase the lethality of a specific toxin. Other toxins may affect those who are very young or old or pregnant. Use of cigarettes, industrial exposures, and licit or illicit drugs may alter the effects of a toxin.

The airway and pulmonary problems that can occur from inhalation of noxious agents can be classified into five groups: displacement or consumption of the available oxygen, respiratory obstruction from thermal injury, pulmonary thermal injury, pulmonary damage from noxious fumes or particulates, and inhalation of cellular toxins such as carbon monoxide.

Another factor to be considered is that frequently in a fire—and occasionally in non-fire-related inhalation injuries—multiple factors, toxins, and sites of injury may be present. It is common, for example, for the fire to partly consume oxygen, elaborate carbon dioxide, cyanide, and soot and to produce superheated air. Needless to say, the injury resulting from breathing these mixtures is also a mixture of the "pure" varieties of inhalation injury.

## ENVIRONMENTAL HYPOXIA

Consumption of oxygen by a fire may decrease oxygen concentrations from 21% to 10% or lower.[2] This decrease results in simple hypoxia that is further aggravated by the impaired oxygen-carrying capacity and tissue injury caused by an inhalation injury.

Other gases may mechanically displace the oxygen from the local environment. Sewers, holds of ships, mines, pits, silos, and tanks are notorious for oxygen displacement by another gas. The most common gases are methane, ethane, propane, and butane. These gases are colorless and odorless. In industrial practice, mercaptans are added to produce the typical "gas" smell.

In general, symptoms of hypoxia are produced when the oxygen content falls to below 15% within an enclosed space. Unfortunately, if the oxygen is less than 6 to 8%, the first symptom may be collapse.

Self-contained breathing apparatus should be employed to examine any suspected area until the oxygen content of the local atmosphere can be verified.

## THERMAL UPPER RESPIRATORY INJURY

Thermal injury of the upper respiratory tract often causes laryngeal and supraglottic edema. Marked edema may accumulate within minutes to hours and may be worsened by overzealous fluid administration.[3] Upper airway obstruction may develop from this laryngospasm, laryngeal edema, accumulation of secretions, or extrinsic obstruction due to neck or facial burns. Injury below the vocal cords is seen in less than 5% of patient who present with moderate or severe surface burns.

It should be emphasized that the most common cause of death in the early phases of burn treatment is this *upper* respiratory tract injury. The extent of this injury and the level of respiratory tree involvement depend upon the specific inhaled gases, the length of exposure, and the environment of the exposure. (See Fig. 2.5). Emergency intubation or tracheostomy may be required to prevent rapid airway obstruction due to edema.

## THERMAL PULMONARY INJURY

Thermal injury of the lung itself is rare. Gases have a relatively low specific heat and, therefore, transfer of heat from the gas to the tissues occurs rapidly. As a hot gas passes through the respiratory tract, it converts the liquid water normally found in the oropharynx and upper respiratory tract into water vapor, losing much of its energy. Most often, this heat transfer, even of superheated gases, occurs in the supraglottic and laryngeal areas, hence the propensity of burns in this area. Inhalation of superheated steam is capable of producing a direct mucosal injury as far distal as the major bronchioles. The superheated water vapor has a much higher specific heat and is able to transfer more thermal energy to the distal lung.[4] It also loses little of its energy by vaporization of respiratory tract liquids. This may produce a true pulmonary parenchymal injury.

## TOXIC AIRWAY INJURY

Pulmonary parenchymal and tracheobronchial injuries may also result from toxic products of combustion or from inhalation of toxins. Most fires release a large number of toxic gases including acids, aldehydes, phosgene, chlorine, ammonia, hydrogen chloride, acroleins, nitrogen oxides, cyanide, and other toxic substances. While these products may irritate the upper airway, they often also inflict a primary lung damage. This lung damage may be manifested by mucosal and pulmonary edema, increased capillary permeability, and sloughing of the mucosal lining. Alveolar irritants may cause little irritation to the eyes, nose, or upper airway. The result may be a very insidious injury that presents hours after the exposure. Fatal bacterial pneumonia may complicate the pulmonary injury.

Other major complications of inhalation of these toxic products include bronchospasm, chemical pneumonitis, and the adult respiratory distress syndrome (ARDS).

## INHALATION OF TOXIC GASES

Toxic gases may be clinically indetectable because they may be both colorless and odorless. Tests to detect many gases may be difficult to perform, at site or in the hospital.

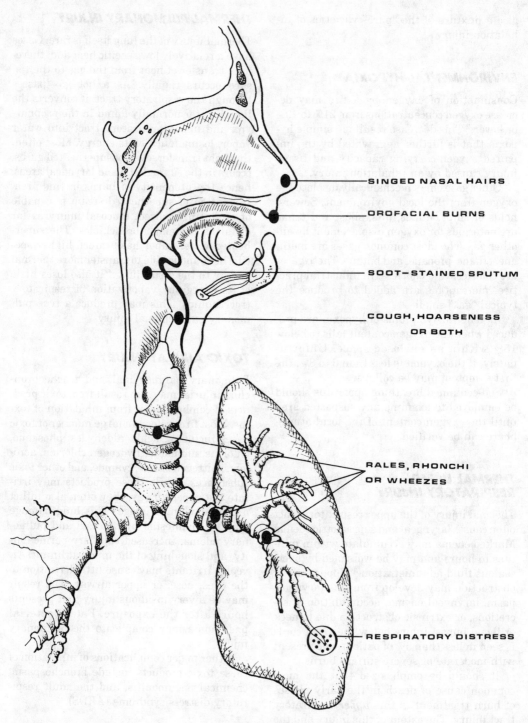

**SINGED NASAL HAIRS**

**OROFACIAL BURNS**

**SOOT-STAINED SPUTUM**

**COUGH, HOARSENESS OR BOTH**

**RALES, RHONCHI OR WHEEZES**

**RESPIRATORY DISTRESS**

**Figure 2.5.**

The result of inhalation of most gases is poorly studied, and there are few diagnostic studies that confirm an exposure after the gas has been eliminated. There are, of course, exceptions to this, such as carbon monoxide.

## Diagnosis of the Inhalation Injury

Diagnosis of the inhalation injury is of paramount importance. Effective early therapy is often lifesaving. Often, the injury is obvious with clinical signs including pharyngeal or laryngeal edema, wheezing, stridor, hoarseness, respiratory distress, and cough yielding carbonaceous sputum. More often, the clinician makes the diagnosis from the usual history and physical examination.

In the absence of obvious injury, the clinician must have a high index of suspicion and respond accordingly. Certain mechanisms of injury place the victim in an extremely high-risk category:

History of a fire in an enclosed area
Exposure to the smoke of synthetic materials, particularly the plastics
Loss of consciousness at any time during the fire
Inhalation of steam

Certainly, if the victim has been found with these high-risk categories, the clinician should seek an inhalation injury assiduously. Victims with these histories should be hospitalized and observed for at least 24 hours because of the possible development of delayed symptoms of inhalation injury. The on-scene emergency providers will often give the best historical information available about the mechanism of injury in these cases and should be questioned carefully.

### PHYSICAL FINDINGS

Once thought to be a clear-cut decision based upon common physical findings and historical data, the diagnosis of inhalation injuries is somewhat more complicated than previously presented. Facial burns, carbonaceous sputum, wheezing, and singed nasal hairs are often cited as classic hallmarks of inhalation injury.

Facial burns, carbonaceous sputum, wheezing, and singed nasal hairs are, unfortunately, not diagnostic. Facial burns portend a possible inhalation injury, but 86% of patients without an inhalation injury have some degree of facial burns. Also, the converse appears to be false, with only 50% of victims of inhalation injuries having facial burns.[5,6] Singed nasal hairs are an accurate indicator of pulmonary injury in only 13% of the patients. Only 50% of the burn victims with a proven inhalation injury had production of carbonaceous sputum or had wheezing.

### DIAGNOSTIC TESTS

Diagnostic tests that may yield better results include flexible fiberoptic bronchoscopy, standard pulmonary function testing, and xenon lung scans.

### Pulmonary Function Testing

Pulmonary function testing will show increased work of breathing, increased airway resistance, decreased lung compliance, and decreased flow rates in the presence of a pulmonary injury. Normal spirometry probably excludes a significant injury to the lower respiratory tract.[7] Unfortunately, these data are often not obtainable if the patient is unconscious or not cooperative. Arterial blood gases often show a normal pH and $PCO_2$ or a mild hypoxemia. An increased arterial-alveolar oxygen gradient may also be found. Measurement of carboxyhemoglobin is important and is a useful screening test for inhalation injuries.

### Fiberoptic Bronchoscopy

Fiberoptic bronchoscopy is easily performed in the emergency department and will detect edema, swelling, and obstruction readily. Endoscopic criteria used to diagnose the inhalation injury include mucosal erythema, hemorrhage, necrosis, ulcerations, and the presence of carbonaceous deposits. Fiberoptic bronchoscopy will not help in the diagnosis of the injury that is limited only to the lung parenchyma.

If the patient is identified by fiberoptic bronchoscopy or laryngoscopy as having burns of the upper airway, the patient needs to be rapidly intubated. The fiberoptic laryngoscope may be employed for this examination with an appropriate endotracheal tube in place over it for rapid emplacement. A fiberoptic laryngoscope may be useful in diagnosis of the pulmonary injury but is limited to only the proximal mainstem bronchi and trachea in its field of view.

### Xenon Lung Scan

Another test for determination of an inhalation injury is the xenon lung scan. Xenon[133] is an inert, insoluble gas that is injected intravenously. After injection, it normally is cleared by exhalation within 90 to 180 seconds after the first pass through the lungs. If the patient retains xenon in the lung, or has unequal clearing, the exam is abnormal and an inhalation injury is suspected. Unfortunately, prior lung disease such as asthma or bronchitis may cause a false positive result.

### Other Lab Tests

**Arterial Blood Gases.** Arterial blood gases may increase the index of suspicion of an inhalation injury but do not provide a diagnosis. A distinct advantage is that the arterial blood gases frequently return before all other laboratory examinations! If good $PaO_2$, $PCO_2$, and $O_2$ saturation are found in the presence of an obviously dyspneic or apneic patient, inhaled toxins such as carbon monoxide or cyanide should be suspected. The laboratory should measure the saturation and not calculate it for best results.

**Carboxyhemoglobin Level.** As noted below in the section on carbon monoxide (CO) poisoning, the CO level may correlate with symptoms, but absence does not rule out carbon monoxide poisoning or effects. Since carbon monoxide is elaborated in nearly all fires, carbon monoxide levels may be used as a screening test to increase suspicion of other inhaled toxins.

**Chest X-ray.** The chest x-ray should be obtained on all patients with a suspected inhalation injury. The chest x-ray may be normal for nearly 24 hours after the injury and, as such, is an unreliable screening tool. If positive, the pattern may be mixed, show an alveolar infiltrate, an interstitial infiltrate, or congestive heart failure. X-rays may show concomitant injuries such as fractured ribs or pneumothorax.

The burned patient with a potential inhalation injury should NEVER be sent to x-ray without a qualified attendant. Likewise, intubation should not be delayed by an x-ray performed merely to confirm the obvious.

**Soft Tissues of the Neck.** X-ray views of the soft tissues of the neck will rule out and document any suspect obstruction of the upper airway. The epiglottis and trachea should be visible on the lateral and anterior-posterior views respectively.

**Electrocardiogram.** Since hypoxia is such a frequent concomitant of most inhalation injuries, an electrocardiogram (ECG) is indicated both as a baseline and to assess hypoxic insults to the myocardium. If the ECG is abnormal, the patient should be monitored for any dysrhythmias. As always, if old records are available, old ECGs should be obtained for comparison.

**Urinalysis.** Although urinalysis may not seem like a test of the respiratory tree, the inhaled toxic gas may have systemic effects. The urine should be checked for hematuria and proteinuria. Proteinuria should suggest carbon monoxide, hydrogen sulfide, halogens, or carbon disulfide for example. Hematuria may suggest hydrogen sulfide, halogens, or carbon disulfide inhalation.

**Miscellaneous Laboratory Tests.** Ethanol levels should be obtained, particularly if the patient has any altered mental status. Cigarette smoking and alcohol consumption are commonly and tragically associated.

Cyanide levels are often unavailable or greatly delayed. Suspicion must guide the practitioner who does not have this laboratory exam available readily.

### Clinical Course

The progression of the inhalation injury is related to the extent and intensity of both the chemical and thermal components. In severe inhalation injuries, respiratory distress may begin within minutes to hours. In these cases, the problem is likely to be multifactorial in involvement. An inhaled gas does not necessarily produce a simple injury.

## Airway

Hypoxia and anoxia or direct toxic effects of rapidly acting toxins may incapacitate the patient within moments. Bronchospasm and alveolar damage may cause rapid deterioration and high mortalities in these patients.[3] Irritant effects may cause edema of the airway that may lead to respiratory obstruction. Absorbed acids, toxins, and irritants may cause an inflammatory response with release of histamine and other vasoactive substances or smooth muscle spasm.

Soots, tars, resins, epithelial debris, and necrotic tissue may act as a physical plug to small airways. Plugging from debris and spasm may lead to atelectasis, air trapping, or emphysematous areas. This plugging may also set the stage for recurrent pneumonia, empyema, abscesses, and all of the myriads of complications of the aspirated foreign body.

Pulmonary edema has been noted with some agents to develop between 8 and 36 hours. It occurs somewhat earlier with underlying pulmonary disease, congestive heart failure, or past history of myocardial ischemia. It may be precipitated by an iatrogenic fluid load. The chest x-ray lags about 4 to 12 hours.

This pulmonary edema of inhaled toxins responds poorly to the classic diuretic therapy. An early use of positive end expiratory pressure (PEEP) should be considered in these cases. The administration of fluids should be guided by pulmonary artery pressures if the patient develops pulmonary edema after an inhalation injury.

The last pulmonary complication to develop is often a bacterial bronchopneumonia that develops after the lung's defenses have been destroyed by the toxin.

## Cardiovascular

Cardiovascular collapse may result from the hypoxia or from the direct action of such toxins as freon. These toxins may precipitate arrhythmias, cardiac arrest, hypotension, conduction blocks, or pulmonary edema. The hypoxia may cause infarcts or ischemic ECG changes.

## Central Nervous System

Early general symptoms of toxic gas inhalation include restlessness, "intoxication," headache, dizziness, confusion, seizures, or coma. One question needs to be answered immediately: Are the symptoms due to the toxin or merely hypoxia? This question is best answered by removing the person from the offending agent and applying 100% oxygen. Always remember to include trauma, alcohol, and drugs (licit and illicit) in the differential.

## Hepatic and Renal Systems

Again: Is the damage noted due to the toxin or to hypoxia? The inhaled toxin may cause hepatic necrosis, such as is found with the hydrocarbons. Acute tubular necrosis may result from toxic effects elsewhere, such as from the rhabdomyolysis or hemolysis, that may be found with carbon monoxide and other inhaled toxins.

## Gastrointestinal Systems

Nausea and vomiting are very common symptoms that result from multiple types of inhaled toxins. The most prominent examples are the nausea and vomiting from carbon monoxide, or the salivation, urination, vomiting, and diarrhea seen with organophosphates.

## Skin and Musculoskeletal Systems

The skin should be checked for the usual cyanosis, cherry red color, brownish tinge. The inhaled toxin may lead to necrosis, ulcers, or frank burns on exposed skin.

The musculoskeletal system may suffer from the effects of the toxin, such as rhabdomyolysis from carbon monoxide or from the positioning in long duration coma.

## **Treatment**

### COMBINED THERMAL AND INHALATION INJURY

Effective treatment of the inhalation injury depends first upon an accurate initial diagnosis and early recognition of complications. The appropriate airway treatment principles for both prehospital and emergency department care alike are:

1. Ensure and protect an adequate airway.

2. Correct hypoxia and potential CO and hydrocyanic acid (HCN) toxicity.
3. Clear airway debris and secretions.

The victim of an inhalation injury who is alert, awake, and conversant needs no airway protection but should be placed on 100% oxygen pending CO levels. The patient with stridor or severe dyspnea should be intubated rapidly, placed on 100% oxygen by endotracheal tube, and considered for bedside bronchoscopy. The patient who is unconcious following exposure to smoke should be rapidly intubated to protect the airway.

Any patient with "classic" findings of an inhalation injury deserves confirmatory flexible fiberoptic bronchoscopy and pulmonary function testing if the patient is capable of cooperation. To intubate, by rote, the patient with "classic" hallmarks of inhalation injury, but who is in no respiratory distress, phonating well, and with normal pulmonary functions, is inappropriate. To deny intubation because of the lack of classic symptoms and signs when signs of respiratory distress develop or when pulmonary function testing is markedly abnormal is also inappropriate. If the patient has an alteration of consciousness or loss of the gag reflex, intubation is indicated for airway protection.

Although the nasal route is preferred for intubation in the literature, this is not a clearcut decision in the patient with an inhalation injury. An adult flexible fiberoptic bronchoscope requires an 8 mm tube orifice in order to pass. Mucous plugging, soot, and debris in the airway may require repeat bronchoscopy for pulmonary toilet. The oral route will allow placement of a larger tube and subsequent repeat bronchoscopy through the tube.

Later treatment includes prompt recognition and treatment of bacterial infections and reversal of ventilation-perfusion abnormalities. In many cases, these occur during the more prolonged hospital stays and are well covered in the many definitive texts upon the management of burns.

Although once advocated, tracheostomy is no longer recommended. Emergent tracheostomy has no advantage over intubation and is fraught with many more complications, particularly when performed through burned skin. For facial trauma, severe respiratory distress, or massive facial burns, cricothyrotomy is preferred as the surgical airway of choice.

Once the patient has been intubated, humidified oxygen at high flows should be maintained. As noted earlier, carbon monoxide toxicity is an integral part of smoke inhalation and is best treated in the short term by administration of high-flow oxygen. Patients with chronic lung disease are not exempt from this treatment. Although hypoxia may be providing the stimulus for their respiratory drive, the dangers of the potential inhalation injury far outweigh the danger of giving oxygen at high flow to these patients. The clinician should be alert to the respiratory rate and status in any case.

Frequent pulmonary toilet, humidified oxygen, postural drainage, coughing, and encouragement of deep breathing all aid in clearing the airway of debris and secretions. Frequent airway suctioning is often needed to remove this debris. Occasionally, repeat fiberoptic or rigid bronchoscopy is useful to remove debris. As noted previously, escharotomy of chest and abdominal burns may be required for circumferential burns.

Prophylactic antibiotics are not used since studies have shown that overgrowth of resistant organisms usually results. Prospective studies indicated that steroids are not beneficial and are associated with a significant increase in mortality even when used briefly.

## IRRITANT GAS EXPOSURE

Treatment for exposure to irritant gases is mainly supportive, since few specific antidotes exist. Since so many delayed symptoms may appear, all patients with toxic gas exposure should be hospitalized for observation for 24 hours.

Airway support and oxygenation should be promptly instituted. Humidified oxygen at high flows should be given to all patients as soon as practicable. Airway support should include intervention to prevent upper airway compromise as indicated.

As cardiac toxicity and arrhythmias are common, cardiac monitoring should be instituted promptly.

If the patient has bronchospasm or wheezing, a trial of nebulized aerosol bronchodilators such as albuterol, terbutaline, or Bronchosol is indicated. Aminophylline intravenously may also be used to treat bronchospasm. Pulmonary edema from toxic gas exposure frequently does not resolve with diuretics. Positive pressure breathing such as PEEP and intubation are often required.

---

*Treatment of Irritant Gas Injuries*
Tracheobronchitis
  Humidification with cool mist (100% oxygen at first)
Bronchospasm
  **Epinephrine**
  Adults 0.3 ml 1:1000 Q20 minutes X 3 PRN
  Children 0.01 cc/kg Q20 min X 3 PRN
  **Aminophylline**
  6 mg/kg bolus over 20 minutes IV
  0.9 mg/kg/hr maintenance
  **Aerosol Therapy**
  Bronchosol or terbutaline in usual doses
Conjunctivitis and Corneal Defects
  Irrigation with saline
  Fluorescein stain for corneal abrasions
  Ophthalmologic referral
Chemical Skin Burns
  Treat as described in section on chemical burns
Pulmonary Edema
  Intubation
  Supplemental humidified oxygen
  Positive end expiratory pressure if $PaO_2$ is less than 50 despite supplemental oxygen
  Swan-Ganz catheter monitoring for blood volume and fluid resuscitation
  Antibiotics only when infection is documented
  Steroids are controversial

---

# DESCRIPTION OF SPECIFIC TOXIC GASES

## Carbon Monoxide

Carbon monoxide poisoning has been with humans since they brought fire into their caves. Today, carbon monoxide poisoning is the single largest cause of death by poisoning in the United States.[9] Bernard in the 1850s first described the hypoxic effects of the gas.

## ETIOLOGY

Carbon monoxide poisoning is frequent in burned patients and is thought to be a common cause of death in those trapped in fires. Fires that occur in a closed space environment are subject to incomplete combustion with subsequent carbon monoxide production. Motor vehicles can produce exhaust CO concentrations from 0.05 to 7%. The average automobile can produce a near lethal level of carbon monoxide in a single car garage in in under 10 minutes. Blast furnaces, propane fork lifts, and methylene chloride paint strippers are also causative agents in CO poisoning.[10,11]

## PHYSIOLOGICAL EFFECTS OF CARBON MONOXIDE

One major toxic property of carbon monoxide results from its propensity to combine with hemoglobin and form carboxyhemoglobin (COHb). Since carbon monoxide has an affinity for hemoglobin that is 210 to 250 times that of oxygen, even low levels of CO will produce significant accumulations of COHb. This now ineffective hemoglobin reduces the body's oxygen-carrying capacity proportionately. Carbon monoxide also binds to proteins in the extravascular spaces, particularly myoglobin. This is the classic model that was taught in most medical schools and emergency training programs until recently.

Unfortunately, symptoms appear not to be due just to the combination with hemoglobin and the subsequent hypoxia. Two additional effects seem to worsen the overall presentation of carbon monoxide toxicity.

COHb shifts the dissociation curve to the left, reducing the oxygen delivery to the tissues even in the face of tissue hypoxia.

Carbon monoxide also impairs oxygen usage in tissues by interference with the cytochrome oxidase systems. That means that it not only affects oxygen delivery but blocks oxygen utilization in the cells. Tissues of highest metabolic rates appear to be most susceptible to effects of this binding. This is consistent with the observation that relatively low CO levels may be far more damaging than a shorter, high level exposure resulting in the same COHb levels.[12]

Fortunately for the victims of CO poisoning, the oxygen displacement caused by CO is reversible. Carbon monoxide is reversibly bound to the various heme pigments and enzymes and readily dissociates from them under certain defined circumstances. This binding is competitive with oxygen and increasing the presence of oxygen will increase the dissociation of the carbon monoxide.

Occasionally, after a CO victim has been treated with 100% oxygen at one atmosphere, it has been observed that there is a rebound in the COHb level, and it goes up again after the oxygen is stopped. This shows that CO is more slowly removed from tissues than from blood.

If the patient is removed from the source of carbon monoxide and treated with carbon monoxide-free room air, it takes about 5 hours to rid one half of the carbon monoxide. Administration of 100% oxygen shortens the half-life of the COHb complex to 40 minutes. Administration of hyperbaric oxygen at three atmospheric pressures cuts this half-life to 23 minutes. These figures are widely quoted, and somewhat arbitrary, since they can vary dramatically from individual to individual.

## CLINICAL PICTURE

Although many authors have felt that the blood level of carbon monoxide correlates closely with the symptoms of carbon monoxide poisonings, newer evidence shows that chronic lower levels may cause more damage than was formerly appreciated. The acute symptoms correlate poorly with the blood COHb levels.[13,14] In the words of one investigator who treated over 400 cases, the neurologic symptoms and the COHb levels correlated like "a buckshot graph."[15] In fact, dogs have been deliberately poisoned with long-term administration of CO and have then undergone complete exchange transfusion with little improvement.

Although the entire organism is affected by carbon monoxide poisoning, the heart and nervous system are the most sensitive to hypoxia and, hence, account for the major toxic manifestations. The extent of these manifestations depends upon a total COHb concentration, duration of exposure, activity, and the underlying state of the organism. The manifestations of acute carbon monoxide poisoning include headache, dizziness, nausea, vomiting, drowsiness, tachypnea, chest pain, pallor, confusion, irritability, irrational behavior, and loss of consciousness.

When the acute carbon monoxyhemoglobin level is below 10%, few people have symptoms. In patients with coronary artery disease or in young children or infants, these lower concentrations of carbon monoxide may cause symptoms. Infants have a higher susceptibility to carbon monoxide because of their increased ventilatory rates. Pregnancy poses an even higher risk to the fetus.[16] If the exposure is over a longer period of time, there will be more symptomatology at lower levels.

At a carbon monoxyhemoglobin level of 10 to 20%, the patient will usually have a headache, nausea, and vomiting. The patient may also have some ataxia, loss of short-term memory, and loss of manual dexterity.

More severe headache weakness, dizziness, dimness of vision, nausea, and vomiting appear with blood levels of 20 to 30% of carbon monoxide. These are intensified with activity and are often accompanied by tachycardia, tachypnea, and syncope.

At 30%, the victim often becomes confused and lethargic. Frequently, ECG tracings will show some depression of the ST segment. At about 30% carbon monoxyhemoglobin, increasingly confused victims may be unable to extricate themselves from the situation, even if consciousness is maintained.

When the COHb level rises to between 40 and 60%, the patient becomes comatose. Levels over 60% are usually fatal.

### Neurological Complications

The expected neurological complications of severe hypoxia are found with exposure to carbon monoxide.[17] Coma, decerebrate rigidity, seizures, dysphasia, absent-mindedness, and generalized loss of cognitive and psychomotor abilities are all noted.[18] CO toxicity in children, particularly, appears to affect the neurologic system. This may be due to their increased metabolic rate and subsequent increased ventilation.[19] The degree and rate of recovery from the neurological symptoms is variable and clinical improvement may not be seen for 3 to 6 weeks after the injury.

Blindness, both temporary and permanent, visual field defects, and retinal hemorrhages have been documented with CO poisoning. If retinal hemorrhages are found in the presence of headache, nausea, dizziness, seizures, or unexplained coma, carbon monoxide should be suspected as an etiology. Delayed neurological sequelae are found in 10% of admitted patients with carbon monoxide poisoning.[20] There is some evidence that hyperbaric oxygen therapy may lower this incidence.[18]

## Cardiac Complications

The ECG may be the most sensitive measure of myocardial damage from carbon monoxide. The electrocardiographic changes range from acute dysrhythmias, ST segment and T wave abnormalities, intraventricular block, and myocardial ischemia to the signs of frank infarction. In patients with preexisting cardiovascular disease, carbon monoxide poisoning can precipitate an acute myocardial infarction.

## Muscle Complications

Rhabdomyolysis with subsequent myoglobinuria has been frequently described in patients with carbon monoxide poisoning. An unconscious patient should be carefully evaluated for soft tissue swelling, urine myoglobin, and signs of peripheral ischemia. CPK will be elevated markedly by muscle necrosis.

## Skin Complications

Erythema, edema, blisters, and bullae are all noted in carbon monoxide toxicity and have been mistaken for burns or trauma in the unconscious patient. The "classic" cherry red color is rarely found in the living patient.

## DIAGNOSIS

Carbon monoxide is a particularly insidious threat when an unsuspected source releases the gas among sleeping persons. Tightly sealed tents, cooking fires used for heating, and tired climbers have proven to be a fatal combination on multiple occasions. Mountain cabins or camping trailers with poorly serviced heating units may be deadly to hunters. When two or more people develop nausea and a headache while in a closed cabin or tent, carbon monoxide poisoning should be suspected

and all should be rapidly moved to the outdoors. The physician should be particularly alert for a family or group who has developed nausea, headache, or vomiting several nights in a row.

Routine arterial blood gases are not helpful in the diagnosis of carbon monoxide poisoning. The $PaO_2$ reflects the dissolved oxygen concentration rather than the hemoglobin saturation and is, therefore, usually normal. A relatively normal $PaO_2$ with a low $PaCO_2$ may suggest hyperventilation to compensate for the tissue hypoxia. The most reliable means of detection is a carbon monoxide oximeter. An older colorimetric assay is useful but not as accurate.

It should be reemphasized that carbon monoxide levels in the blood stream is not a definitive index of the toxic effect if the patient has received 100% oxygen en route to the hospital. COHb in the blood is cleared in about 80 minutes with 100% oxygen and the level may be only modestly elevated after a prolonged transport to the hospital. The tissue CO levels may take longer to change and are not reflected by blood CO measurements. Consequently, treatment decisions should be governed by signs and symptoms of CNS dysfunction rather than blood levels.

## Prehospital Emergency Therapy

As in all toxic exposures, the first priority of therapy in the treatment of the patient is to ensure that the rescuer does not become a victim. The rescuer should not enter burning buildings without proper protective equipment! In the case of a nonfire situation as would be found with a defective heater or furnace, the exposure time to the rescuer should be limited to the minimum necessary to ensure that all are removed from danger.

The prehospital and emergent treatment of suspected carbon monoxide poisoning includes increasing the inspired $FiO_2$ and the alveolar ventilation. The administration of 100% oxygen is routinely used and is safe, convenient, and inexpensive.

The patient should receive oxygen by a tight-fitting rubber mask, similar to an aviator's mask, if possible. A simple face mask, even with high flows of oxygen, simply does not deliver 100% oxygen. A nonrebreathing mask with reservoir will suffice for prehospital and emergent therapy but is less efficacious than the tight-fitting mask.[21]

## TRANSPORT DECISIONS

Patients with known or strongly suspected carbon monoxide poisoning may be better served by diversion to a hospital with a hyperbaric chamber.[18,22] Oxygen should be provided during the air transport by a tight-fitting face mask. Such patients require cardiac monitoring and intravenous access.

## Hospital Treatment

The treatment of carbon monoxide poisoning in the hospital is identical to the prehospital environment. Indeed, the emergency department cannot give any better therapy for **known or highly suspected** carbon monoxide poisoning than intubation and ventilation with 100% oxygen. Needless to say, this therapy can be given by a qualified paramedic in an ambulance en route to a hyperbaric chamber. Treatment of seizures, acidosis, and dysrhythmias again follows standard protocols and medications carried in paramedic-equipped transport. The diagnostic expertise of the emergency physician will be invaluable in the patient where the diagnosis is unknown at onset.

Hyperbaric oxygen is the ultimate form of increasing the $FiO_2$. Guidelines for hyperbaric therapy vary. No one questions the efficacy of hyperbaric oxygenation when the CO level is above 40% or when accompanied by coma, seizures, or alteration of consciousness. No one questions that the asymptomatic patient with CO levels of less than 10% requires little therapy other than oxygen by face mask. It is in the intermediately affected patient that the controversy exists.

In making the decision to treat with hyperbaric oxygen, several items need to be weighed carefully:

The COHb level does not always reflect the true severity of the illness since tissue levels cannot be measured.

Patients with chronic exposures can be severely poisoned while demonstrating only modest levels of COHb.

Chronic sequelae have been noted at relatively low levels of measured COHb.

Transport time to the nearest hyperbaric

chamber may equal clearance times for the CO from the system.

Monoplace hyperbaric chambers do not allow access to the patient to treat associated injuries.

Hyperbaric oxygen is a relatively expensive form of therapy, but has few complications and little contraindication.[23] The major problem with this form of therapy is accessibility of the chamber. The ideal situation is found in the multiplace chamber, where an assistant can accompany the patient.

The use of steroids to reduce cerebral edema in poisoning by carbon monoxide is unsubstantiated.[24]

## HYPERBARIC OXYGEN CRITERIA

A conservative set of criteria for the use of hyperbaric oxygen are as follows:

1. Patients with alteration of consciousness should be treated with hyperbaric oxygenation. If there is any difficulty in determination of a change in the level of consciousness, psychometric testing should be employed. History of an alteration of consciousness at the scene but normal consciousness at the emergency department should be treated with hyperbaric oxygenation.
2. Patients with evidence of hypoxic ECG changes or dysrhythmias should be treated with hyperbaric oxygenation. Most authorities would argue that chest pain, seizures, and dysrhythmias are indications, not contraindications, for HBO.
3. Patients with greater than 25% CO levels should be treated regardless of symptoms.

An important consideration is the sound clinical judgment of the examiner. If the patient appears ill despite the "numbers," then hyperbaric oxygenation is properly ordered by the clinician. It should be noted that at least one lawsuit has inferred negligence for failing to use hyperbaric oxygenation in a case of carbon monoxide poisoning.[25]

## Cyanide Poisoning

Cyanide is usually thought of in the solid forms but those patients suffering from severe smoke inhalation syndromes also have been found to have elevated cyanide levels.[26]

Those patients with high cyanide levels also appear to be the same group of patients with elevated carbon monoxide levels. As a product of combustion, it is commonly mixed with isocyanates, which are intense respiratory irritants.

Cyanide is found in the burning fumes of x-ray film, wool, silk, nylon, paper, urethanes, and some plastics. It is also found in laboratories, photographic studios, and blast furnaces and is used as a fumigation agent. Precious metal extraction and electroplating are done with cyanide compounds. Potassium cyanide crystals are used as a poison for animals and are favorite agents of both homicide and suicide. Cyanide is employed as a war gas by the Warsaw Pact countries.

Cyanide appears to act by inhibition of the cytochrome oxidase system and subsequent interruption of the aerobic cellular metabolism. This leads to a profound lactic acidosis as the body attempts to use the less efficient anaerobic metabolism. Subsequent central nervous system (CNS), respiratory, and myocardial depression complicate the picture. The dose at which 50% of the exposed people will die ($LD_{50}$) is 0.5 mg/kg for hydrogen cyanide. The military incorrectly calls cyanide a "blood agent," implying that the action is in the blood when it is, in fact, a tissue toxin.

Diagnosis is difficult without a history of cyanide exposure. There is no readily available assay that can be done in "real time" to confirm the poisoning while trying to treat an acutely poisoned patient. Before any cyanide level is correlated with clinical appearance, the elapsed time since the exposure and since the specimen was obtained must be considered. The "Lee-Jones" test may be performed on gastric aspirate but is not useful in inhalation injuries.

**Lee Jones Test**

Add crystal FeSO4 to 5 to 10 cc of gastric contents.

Add 4 to 5 drops of 20% NaOH.

Boil and allow to cool.

Add 8 to 10 drops of 10% HCL.

Positive for cyanide is a greenish blue color.

Salicylates will turn greenish blue and then purple.

Arterial blood gases will often show a metabolic acidosis with normal oxygenation and calculated hemoglobin saturation. Venous gases have the same pattern, because the oxygen is not used up! Venous blood often looks arterial in color. The measured arterial oxygen saturation will be decreased, while the calculated saturation is normal.[27]

This picture of an abnormal hemoglobin and less than adequate saturation is found commonly in only four poisons. The toxidrome includes cyanide, carbon monoxide, hydrogen sulfide, and methemoglobin. Methemoglobin and COHb are easily measured. Hydrogen sulfide and cyanide are treated in a similar manner. Cyanide levels should be obtained in all cases.

## SYMPTOMS

The symptoms are relatively nonspecific. It is not the surely lethal agent of the thrillers, however. Early symptoms may include dryness and burning of the throat and air hunger. In small doses, headache, confusion, anxiety, dizziness, nausea, palpitations, tachycardia, tachypnea, and combativeness may all be found. In large doses, bradycardia, bradypnea, coma, gasping respirations, apnea, and death may all be common manifestations. The examiner should be suspicious if the patient has had an abrupt collapse without apparent cause that does not respond well to oxygen administration. An audible gasp is thought to be characteristic of extreme exposure to HCN.

Cyanide exposure may be diagnosed by history of probable exposure and an odor of bitter almonds but only 50% of people can detect this smell of cyanide. An elevated anion gap metabolic acidosis may exist but is not diagnostic.

## TREATMENT

The mainstays of treatment are oxygen and ventilation. Therapy beyond the basics is controversial and includes the classic Lilly cyanide kit, hyperbaric oxygenation, and massive doses of vitamin $B_{12}$. Contaminated clothing must be removed and the skin washed. If cyanide was ingested, gastric lavage should be done. Activated charcoal will not adsorb cyanide.

### Lilly Cyanide Kit

Proposed in the 1930s by Chen and colleagues, intentional production of methemoglobin is used to compete with cyanide for sites on the cytochrome oxidase system.[28] Methemoglobinemia is produced by inhalation of amyl nitrite and then intravenous administration of sodium nitrite. About 30% methemoglobinemia is considered optimum, and the levels should be kept below 40%. After the methemoglobin has relieved the symptoms, the cyanide is converted to thiocynate by the use of sodium thiosulfate. The thiocynate ion then allows renal excretion. A high tissue oxygen markedly potentiates the effects of this treatment.

Therapy with nitrites is not innocuous and the doses given to an adult can cause a fatal methemoglobinemia in children. In those with mixed gas exposure, induction of methemoglobinema may induce tissue hypoxia. Too rapid administration of the sodium nitrite may cause vasodilation and hypotension. If methylene blue is given, all of the cyanide bound to the methemoglobin will be released with a relapse of symptoms. Instructions are on the cyanide kits and should be followed explicitly.

### Hyperbaric Oxygenation

Hyperbaric oxygenation may be the ideal adjunct to both hydroxycobalamin and nitrite therapies. Hyperbaric oxygenation will mitigate concern about the methemoglobinemia formed by nitrite administration since the dissolved oxygen in the tissues and blood stream can support the metabolic requirements. The oxygen may act competitively to displace cyanide from the cytochrome oxidase.[29] In the case of a mixed gas inhalation, carbon monoxide will be effectively displaced from hemoglobin and will allow higher levels of nitrite to be used. Hyperbaric oxygen therapy should not be used to replace the chemical treatments, however, due to the deleterious effects of delay in institution of the treatment in most cases.

### Hydroxycobalamin (Vitamin B₁₂ₐ)

Hydroxycobalamin has been used to prevent cyanide toxicity from prolonged administration of sodium nitroprusside as well as in the acute treatment of cyanide poisoning.[30,31] This agent reacts directly with the cyanide and does not act on the hemoglobin. B$_{12}$ appears to be a preferable antidote for patients with another concurrent gas exposure such as carbon monoxide. There is limited use in the United States to date, but more than 15 years of experience are documented in the French literature.[32] Hydroxycobalamin is essentially devoid of complications but is not currently available in the United States.

Another antidote available in Europe is dicobalt-EDTA, sold as Kelocyanor.[33] This agent chelates cyanide as the cobalticyanide. It does cause a significant hypertension and may cause dysrhythmias if no cyanide is present. Kelocyanor and hydroxycobalamin may be given together for additive effect.[34] Dicobalt-EDTA is thought to act more quickly than the nitrites method.

### Ammonia

Ammonia is a colorless gas most often used in fertilizers but also frequently employed in the production of plastics, cyanides, nitrates, and nitriles and in explosives manufacture. In the household, it can be manufactured by mixing ammonia solution and bleach (sodium hypochlorite). It may be produced by combustion of wool, silk, nylon, and melamine.

Ammonia is highly water soluble and affects the eyes and upper airway with chemical burns, pneumonitis, and airway edema. Inhalation causes a direct caustic and necrotizing action on the pulmonary parenchyma. Conjunctivitis and lacrimation are noted at low levels and may cause temporary blindness. At concentrations greater than 1500 parts per million, laryngospasm may be induced with subsequent respiratory arrest.

Chest examination at the time of admission may be a prognostic factor. Patients with abnormal examinations generally have a more protracted and more complicated hospital course.

Emergent treatment is removal of the patient from the exposure. The patient should be started on 100% high-flow oxygen. Therapy is supportive. Airway control in the face of laryngeal and glottic edema may be difficult.

### Hydrogen Sulfide

Hydrogen sulfide is an extremely toxic, colorless gas that smells of rotten eggs. In high concentrations, it causes paralysis of the olfactory nerve, and the smell may not be apparent. It is a common respiratory irritant and asphyxiant with exposures found in sewer and oil workers, metal smelters, and tanning hides. It is produced by burning of wool and hides, from petroleum products, vulcanization of rubber products, and some fertilizers. Deaths from hydrogen sulfide have been reported in people who work with decaying organic material, such as fish, sewage, and manure.

The toxicity of hydrogen sulfide approaches that of cyanide. It is an irritant to both eyes and respiratory tract with tearing and coughing early in the exposure. The CNS symptoms are tremors, convulsions, and coma. A common picture is a sudden collapse, with clothes smelling of rotten eggs.[35] Respiratory tract edema and pulmonary edema are indicative of a large exposure.

Hydrogen sulfide acts quickly enough that rescuers without self-contained breathing apparatus frequently also succumb. Rapid removal of the victim from the contaminated environment is essential. High-flow oxygen, with assisted ventilations if required, should be started in all exposed victims. The victim's skin should be irrigated and contaminated clothes removed.

Hydrogen sulfide causes reversible inhibition of the cytochrome oxidase system, with effects that are similar to those of cyanide. Methemoglobin generation is thought to hasten the formation of sulfmethemoglobin and subsequent excretion, but this site of action is somewhat controversial. Rapid improvement has been noted when amyl nitrite and sodium nitrite were administered to hydrogen sulfide poisoned patients.[36,37] A logical treatment plan is use of the Lilly cyanide kit without use of the thiosulfate.

Hyperbaric oxygen may be helpful in the treatment of this toxin.[38,39] The role of hyperbaric oxygen therapy, however, has not been confirmed by experimental data.

### Carbon Disulfide ($CS_2$)

Carbon disulfide is a volatile liquid used as a disinfectant, fumigant, oil solvent, and grease remover. Chronic exposure to $CS_2$ results in permanent peripheral and neurological damage with optic and peripheral neuropathy and possible Parkinson's syndrome.

The inhalation of carbon disulfide results in CNS stimulation followed by respiratory and CNS depression. It is thought that carbon disulfide has a mechanism of toxicity that is similar to hydrogen sulfide. This would indicate that production of methemoglobin might enhance the metabolism of this drug.

### Chlorine

Chlorine is a greenish-yellow gas, somewhat heavier than air with a pungent odor. It is involved in more industrial accidents than any other gas. Chlorine is used in water purification, bleaching and manufacture of bleach, as a reagent in the production of plastics, and other chemicals. A principle war gas of World War I, chlorine was the cause of many allied casualties in that war. Bleach, when mixed with an acid such as vinegar, will produce chlorine gas.[40]

Chlorine is a local irritant that can cause bronchitis, pulmonary edema, and cutaneous and respiratory burns. High concentrations of chlorine gas will produce chemical skin burns. Major injuries will almost always have a pulmonary component, however.

Chemical burns from chlorine are treated as an acid burn. Minor injuries should receive symptomatic therapy. Eye irritation should be treated with a minimum of 1 liter of saline irrigation and ophthalmologic referral. Treatment of pulmonary edema is symptomatic with humidified oxygen, bronchodilators and consideration of PEEP. Both epinephrine and aminophylline were used without problems in a recommendation based upon review of the literature and experience with 100 casualties in an exposure.[41] There is little recent experimental work on chlorine poisoning. Use of steroids and prophylactic antibiotics is controversial.

### Phosgene ($COCl_2$) and Hydrogen Chloride ($HCl$)

These two gases are similar, and phosgene decomposes to HCl and CO. They are colorless and somewhat heavier than air. In the pure form, they are reputed to have the smell of new mown hay, but this would be absent in the fire situation. Unfortunately, pyrolysis of plastics, polyvinylchlorides, and chlorinated hydrocarbons produce these gases in modern house fires. Use of carbon tetrachloride fire extinguishers may produce phosgene.

Phosgene was used as a war gas in World War I and was responsible for over 60 to 80% of the inhalation injury deaths of that war. It is a relatively slow-acting agent and may have lengthy exposure with subsequent alveolar damage. This slow action is thought to be due to a poor water solubility.

It causes vasoconstriction of the pulmonary venous circulation, which increases the risk of pulmonary edema. The pulmonary edema of phosgene gas exposure has been associated with severe fluid sequestration in the lungs and may require fluid replacement.[42] Field care consists of decontamination and high-flow oxygen. Skin surfaces and eyes should be copiously irrigated after exposure. The patient who has been exposed to phosgene must be hospitalized for observation. Meticulous pulmonary care is needed for treatment of victims.

## Arsine

Arsine is a colorless, relatively nonirritating gas with an odor like garlic. It is produced when acids are mixed with arsenic containing metals or ores. Most commonly, exposure to arsine is found in the semiconductor industries but may also be found in the smelting and refining industries. Hobbies that involve acid flux solder, plumbers, and lead plating also produce arsine gas. Arsine may also be generated by the combustion of fossil fuels.

Arsine gas binds with the sulfhydryl group in hemoglobin, causing hemolysis and producing methemoglobinemia. The resultant hemoglobinuria may cause renal failure. A characteristic triad is seen 24 to 48 hours after exposures:[43]

Abdominal pain
Methemoglobinuria
Jaundice

Malaise, headache, dizziness, confusion, nausea, and vomiting are also common with this gas.

Exchange transfusion is used to remove the hemoglobin-fixed arsine. The hemoglobin-arsine moiety does not dialyze.

## Nitrogen Dioxide

Nitrogen dioxide exposure is seen in farmers and other agricultural workers. Nitrogen-rich plants and fertilizers are oxidized to nitrogen dioxide in silos and other storage areas. Blasting, arc welding, the production of explosives, and burning of dynamite may produce nitrogen dioxide. The reduction of organic material by nitric acid will also produce this reddish gas.

Nitrogen dioxide may produce an acute picture that ranges from mild dyspnea to frank pulmonary edema, depending upon the severity of exposure. Three to four weeks after large exposures, the patient may develop bronchiolitis fibrosa obliterans. This phase of exposure is frequently fatal, but progression may be arrested by steroids.

## Metal Fume Fever

A metal fume is a suspension of microscopic oxidized particles of the metal, ranging in size from 0.02 to 0.25 microns. Most commonly, exposures are seen after welding or smelting brass, copper, tin, magnesium, or nickel. Smelting cadmium, cobalt, manganese, or chromium may also cause this disease. A similar picture is seen with exposure to hot polymers in "polymer fume fever."

The symptoms are those of influenza with the sudden onset of thirst, fever, chills, myalgias, nausea, vomiting, and headache. A completely characteristic course is complete resolution of the symptoms over the weekend (24 to 48 hours). Much less commonly found are airway and lung parenchymal injury and acute renal injury. With chronic exposure, a long-lasting tracheobronchitis or pneumonitis may be found. Serum or urinary heavy metal levels do not appear to correlate with symptoms.

The pathogenesis is uncertain. The most commonly accepted theory is an allergically mediated complex, but other theories propose direct toxic effects, an endotoxin-like effect, and anaphylaxis.[44]

Treatment is removal from the source. Therapy is supportive with bed rest, analgesics, and fever control for symptomatic relief. Milk is often recommended to relieve the nausea and vomiting associated with metal fume fever.

## SUMMARY

The prudent emergency provider will recognize that the diagnosis of a specific toxic gas inhalation is difficult. It depends upon historical data, "toxidromes," and a high index of suspicion. The variability of possible gas composition and effects and of the body's response to these agents make the identification of the agent difficult, if not impossible. If a significant toxic gas inhalation is suspected, an aggressive response with airway support and high-flow oxygenation should be instituted. Hyperbaric oxygenation therapy should be considered if a specific gas is identified or highly suspected, and this gas is responsive to HBO. Once these therapies have been instituted, identification of the gas may be attempted, and the need for subsequent intervention evaluated.

## References

1. Primary analysis of injury events reported in North Dakota, 1985–1987. North Dakota Injury Surveillance System. North Dakota State Department of Health, July 1987.
2. Cohen MA, Guzzardi LJ. Inhalation of products of combustion. Ann Emerg Med 1983;12:628–632.
3. Robinson L, Miller RH. Smoke inhalation injuries. Am J Otolaryngol 1986;7:375–380.
4. Moritz AR, Henriquez FC, McLean R. The effects of inhaled heat on the air passages and lungs: an experimental investigation. AM J Pathol 1945;21:311–331.
5. Moylan JA, Alexander LG. Diagnosis and treatment of inhalation injury. World J Surg 1978;2:185.
6. Moylan JA. Smoke inhalation and burn injury. Surg Clin North Am 1980;60:1533.
7. Whitener DR, Whitener LM, Robertons KJ, et al. Pulmonary function measurements in patients with thermal injury and smoke inhalation. Am Rev Resp Disease 1980;122:731.
8. Peters WJ. Inhalation injury caused by the products of combustion. Can Med Assoc J 1981;125:249.
9. U. S. Public Health Service. Vital Statistics of the United States. Government Printing Office, 1976.
10. Horowitz Z. Carboxyhemoglobinemia caused by inhalation of methylene chloride. Am J Emerg Med 1986;4:48–51.
11. Sturmann K, Mofenson H, Caraccio T. Methylene chloride inhalation: an unusual form of drug abuse. Ann Emerg Med 1985;14:903–905.
12. Kindwall EP. Carbon monoxide poisoning. In: Hamilton RW, Peirce EC, eds. Hyperbaric oxygen in emergency medical care. Bethesda, MD: Undersea Medical Society, 1983.
13. Mofenson HC, Caraccio TR, Brody GM. Carbon monoxide poisoning Am J Emerg Med 1984;3:254–261.
14. Olson KR. Carbon monoxide poisoning: mechanisms, presentation, and controversies in management. J Emerg Med 1984;1:233–243.
15. Kindwall EP. Carbon monoxide poisoning. In: Hamilton RW, Peirce EC, eds. Hyperbaric oxygen in emergency medical care. Bethesda, MD: Undersea Medical Society, 1983.
16. Margulies JL. Acute carbon monoxide poisoning during the pregnancy. Am J Emerg Med 1986;4:516–519.
17. Eltorai IM, Strauss MB, Hart GB, Montroy RE. Carbon monoxide neural toxicity with report of a clinical case. Arizona Med 1984;16:729–734.
18. Myers RAM, Linberg SE, Cowley RA. Carbon monoxide poisoning: the injury and its treatment. JACEP 1970;8:479–484.
19. Crocker PJ, Walker JS. Pediatric carbon monoxide toxicity. J Emerg Med 1985;3:443–448.
20. Choi IS. Delayed neurologic sequellae in carbon monoxide intoxication. Arch Neurol 1983;40:433–435.
21. Kindwall EP. Hyperbaric treatment of carbon monoxide poisoning. Ann Emerg Med 1985;14:1233–1234.
22. Haddad LM. Carbon monoxide poisoning: to transfer or not to transfer? [Letter]. Ann Emerg Med 1986;15:1375.
23. Norkool DM, Kirkpatrick JN. Treatment of acute carbon monoxide poisoning with hyperbaric oxygen: A review of 115 cases. Ann Emerg Med 1985;14:1168–1171.
24. Crocker PJ. Carbon monoxide poisoning: the clinical entity and its treatment. Military Med 1984;149:257.
25. Kindwall EP. Hyperbaric treatment of carbon monoxide poisoning [Editorial]. Ann Emerg Med 1985;14:1233–1234.
26. Clark CJ, Campbell D, Reid WH. Blood carboxyhaemoglobin and cyanide levels in fire survivors. Lancet 1981;1:1332–1335.
27. Hall AH, Rumack BH. Clinical toxicology of cyanide. Ann Emerg Med 1986;15:1067–1074.
28. Chen KK, Rose CL, Clowes GHA. Methylene blue, nitrites, and sodium thiosulfate against cyanide poisoning. Proc Exp Biol Med 1933;31:250–252.
29. Kindwall EP. Carbon monoxide and cyanide poisoning. In: Davis JC, Hunt TK, eds. Hyperbaric Oxygen Therapy. Bethesda MD: Undersea Medical Society, 1977:177–190.
30. Cottrell JE, Casthely P, Brodie JD, et al. Pre-

vention of nitroprusside-induced cyanide toxicity with hydroxycobalamin. N Engl J Med 1978;298:809–811.

31. Graham DL, Laman D, Theodore J, Robin ED. Acute cyanide poisoning complicated by lactic acidosis and pulmonary edema. Arch Intern Med 1977;137:1051–1055.

32. Jouglard J, Fagot G, Deguigne B, et al. L'intoxication cyanhydrique aigue et son traitement d'urgence. Marseille Medicale 1971;9:571–575.

33. Vogel SN, Sultan TR, Ten Eyck RP. Cyanide poisoning. Clin Toxicol 1981;18:367–383.

34. Bismuth C, Cantineau JP, Pontal P, et al. Priorite de l'oxygenation dans l'intoxication cyanhydrique. J Toxicol Med 1984;4:107–121.

35. Hoidal CR, Hall AK, Robinson MD, et al. Hydrogen sulfide poisoning from toxic inhalations of roofing asphalt fumes. Ann Emerg Med 1986;15:826–830.

36. Stine RJ, Slosberg B, Beacham BE. Hydrogen sulfide intoxication: a case report and discussion of treatment. Ann Intern Med 1976;85:756–758.

37. Peters JW. Hydrogen sulfide poisoning in a hospital setting. JAMA 1981;246:1588–1589.

38. Whitcraft DD, Bailey TD, Hart GB. Hydrogen sulfide poisoning treated with hyperbaric oxygen. J Emerg Med 1985;3:23–25.

39. Smilkstein MJ, Bronstein AC, Pickett HM, et al. Hyperbaric oxygen therapy for severe hydrogen sulfide poisoning. J Emerg Med 1985;3:27–30.

40. Jones FL. Chlorine poisoning from mixing household cleaners. JAMA 1972;222:1312.

41. Hedges JR, Morrisey WL. Acute chlorine gas exposure. JACEP 1979;8:59–63.

42. Everett ED, Overholt EL. Phosgene poisoning. JAMA 1968;205:103–105.

43. Fowler BA, Weissberg JB. Arsine poisoning. N Engl J Med 1974;291:1171–1174.

44. Mueller EJ, Seger DL. Metal fume fever-a review. J Emerg Med 1985;2:271–274.

# Part 3
# Caustic Skin Burns

## INTRODUCTION

Chemicals that "burn" present a special problem to both the therapist and the patient. Unlike a thermal burn, chemicals continue to burn until they are removed or inactivated. If the removal is delayed by as little as 3 minutes, the severity of the burn may be markedly increased.

Chemical skin burns most often occur in the workplace and in most cases, the chemical that caused the burn is well known. There are more than 25,000 chemicals, however, that can burn the skin or mucous membranes.[1]

Both acids and alkalies are widely used as major raw materials and for cleaning, curing, extracting, and preserving products. Sodium, ammonium, lithium, potassium, barium, and calcium hydroxides are used in industrial processes. The most commonly used industrial acids include sulfuric, nitric, acetic, hydrochloric, formic, picric, tungstic, tannic, sulfosalicylic, trichloroacetic, and cresylic. Chromic and hydrofluoric acids are widely used in the microinstrument and microelectronics industries. Sulfuric acid and nitric acid are used in the steel industry for casting iron and steel and removing slag wastes. Many military personnel and employees in the defense industry are exposed to uncommon and extremely potent compounds. Hospital and reference laboratory workers may also have exposure to uncommon and powerful agents.

Hobbyists are exposed to an increasing variety of agents, and these chemicals are causing more varied skin burns. The number of hobby-related cases will undoubtedly rise as more people become involved in more complex hobbies.

Skin burns from household chemicals may be caused by contact with phenols (deodorants, sanitizers, disinfectants), sulfuric acid (toilet bowl cleaners), sodium hypochlorite (bleaches), and lye (drain cleaners and paint removers).

Caustics may be used as a form of revenge or punishment in some subcultures. Self-abusive individuals may apply these substances for a variety of reasons.

Although any of the caustic agents mentioned earlier (and thousands not mentioned) can cause a skin burn, multiple series show that lye and sulfuric acid account for the majority of chemical injuries. In certain areas, hydrofluoric acid is commonly used and may be the most popular causative agent. In military training areas, the most common agent encountered is white phosphorus, which is uncommonly encountered in civilian life.[2,3]

## PATHOPHYSIOLOGY

Chemical agents usually produce actions different than thermal burns. The chemical reaction may be an oxidizing or reduction reaction or may be a protoplasmic poison, desiccant, vesicant, or a corrosive.

The amount of tissue destruction is determined by the extent and nature of the exposed surface, the concentration of the agent, the duration of exposure to the agent, and the nature of the agent. With some chemicals, the injury is deceptively mild on first appraisal, with only a mild discoloration or blanching of the skin. Over the ensuing 24 to 36 hours, the damage may progress to an extensive necrosis of the skin and underlying structures with substantial systemic effects. In contrast, other agents produce a tough leathery eschar or a liquification necrosis soon after contact with the skin.

Unlike the thermal burn, the chemical agent will continue to "burn" until the substance is inactivated or removed from the area or until the substance exhausts its capacity to damage the protoplasm. The capacity for tissue destruction varies from agent to agent. The damage caused by a chemical burn may be more severe than that caused by a thermal burn because the agent rapidly and deeply penetrates through the skin.[4] The chemical agent may have systemic side effects that incapacitate.

Also unlike the thermal burn, the chemical agent penetrates clothing, skin folds, and surface body openings. Tympanic membrane perforations and parotid fistulas are seen with facial lye burns. Marjolin's malignant scar ulcerations appear to be more common with chemical agents than with thermal burns.[5]

## ALKALI BURNS

The initial reaction of an alkali is a saponification reaction (soap formation) with subsequent liquification necrosis of the body fats. As these organic complexes penetrate further into the tissues, they carry the unattached alkali ions with them and continue to destroy. This penetration also limits the contact with water on the skin surfaces.

A strong alkali instilled or spilled into the eye produces an immediate opacification of the cornea and coagulation of the proteins of the sclera or cornea. The pH of the anterior chamber rises within 2 to 3 minutes, causing damage to the iris, lens, and ciliary body. This may lead to an irreversible loss of vision within 3 minutes. While the eye is the most sensitive tissue of the body, the other tissues sustain progressive destruction until all of the alkali is removed or consumed.

Among the common alkalies, ammonium hydroxide has the fastest rate of skin penetration followed in order by sodium hydroxide, potassium hydroxide, lithium hydroxide, strontium hydroxide, barium hydroxide, tetraethylammonium hydroxide, calcium hydroxide, and magnesium hydroxide.[6] Collagenase may be elaborated by some cells with further increase in the speed of skin and tissue penetration.

## ACID BURNS

In general, the acid burn is not as serious as the alkali burn but is far more fulminant. Acids are water soluble and easily penetrate into the subcutaneous tissues. The tissues coagulate soon after contact and a tough leathery eschar forms, limiting further spread of the agents. Some acids, such as fuming nitric or sulfuric, act as desiccants and create an even more impenetrable eschar. (See Table 2.3.) The exothermic reactions of the desiccant acids can cause thermal injury and exacerbate the chemical burn.

## IMMEDIATE THERAPY

The cornerstone of chemical burn therapy is removal of the noxious substance. Irrigation of the burn with large volumes of water under low pressure dilutes the toxic agent and washes it out of the tissues. "The solution to chemical pollution is dilution." Irrigation should be with low pressure and high volumes because the chemical may be splashed onto the patient or the medical team that is treating the patient.

Table 2.3.
**Eschar Appearance with Certain Acid Burns**

| Acid | Appearance of Eschar |
| --- | --- |
| Sulfuric | Green black to dark brown |
| Nitric | Yellow eschar and tissue staining |
| Hydrochloric | Yellow-brown eschar and tissue stains |
| Trichloracetic | Whitish with a soft slough |
| Hydrofluoric | Grayish to brown eschar |

---

*Management guidelines for chemical burns*
1. **Evaluate ABCs.**
2. **Start decontamination.**
   a. Ensure medical personnel are protected.
   b. Remove all clothing (undress to access and assess).
   c. Wipe away or debride all solid chemical particles.
   d. Inspect hair, nails, and web spaces for collections of the chemical.
   e. Remove caked compounds with green soap solution (liquid soap and 10% isopropyl alcohol).
3. **Obtain history.**
   a. Type and concentration of chemical
   b. Nature and duration of exposure
   c. Concomitant traumatic injuries
   d. Preexisting medical illnesses
   e. Tetanus immunization and allergies
4. **Start treatment with specific antidotes if applicable.**
5. **Identify hospitalization criteria.**
6. **Check effectiveness of irrigation.**
   Use pH paper; if the pH is not neutral, continue irrigating for an additional hour.
7. **Arrange follow-up and consultation**
   Follow-up checks at 24 hours, 72 hours, and 7 days.
**Do not use a closed dressing on a chemical burn!**

---

To further limit the damage to the tissue, and reduce penetration, particulate matter should be debrided from the wound before or during the irrigation. The patient's clothing and protective garments must be removed to prevent further injury to the patient and possible injury to the medical team.

The severity of the chemical injury is directly proportional to the length of time that the substance remains on the skin. If removal of the substance is delayed, tissue damage is greater. Studies of acid and alkali burns have shown the contrast between the effects of early and late irrigation. When the irrigation was initiated within 1 minute after contact, the burn was substantially less severe than when the irrigation was delayed for 3 minutes.[7] When the irrigation was delayed for 15 minutes in acid burns, the tissue pH was not altered by lavage. Likewise, when irrigation was delayed for 1 hour in alkali burns, the tissue pH remained alkaline.

Good experimental studies show that irrigation of tissues for at least 1 hour is needed to reverse tissue pH changes due to alkali chemical injuries.[7] Some studies suggested that severe alkali burns should be irrigated for 8 to 24 hours.[8] An appropriate regimen for this extended hydrotherapy is 2 hours of shower alternated with 2 hours of rest.[9] If an alkali burn has a soapy feeling or if the tissue pH has not returned to normal, irrigation must be continued.

Burns of the eye may be treated with continuous irrigation through a Morgan irrigating contact lens. An alternative is a small-bore soft catheter fixed in the palpebral sulcus or the IV tubing held by an attendant.

Neutralization of the chemical with a weak acid or base opposite is not recommended for at least two reasons:

1. Irrigation should not be delayed while waiting for a specific antidote—immediate irrigation provides the best removal of the agent.
2. Neutralization may produce an exothermic reaction with the heat of the reaction causing further damage. As early as 1927, the dangers of neutralization of chemical injuries were recognized.[10]

Specific antidotes exist for certain chemical agents and are listed in Table 2.4. As noted previously, nonspecific neutralization is generally a waste of time.

## SELECTED SPECIFIC AGENTS
### Hydrofluoric Acid Burns

Hydrofluoric acid is used in the glass and semiconductor industries as an etching agent, in the plastic industries in production of various plastic materials, and in the nuclear industries as a solvent for uranium. Many rust removal agents contain hydrofluoric acid. Most hydrofluoric acid burns appear to come from either the semiconductor or the glass injuries.

Hydrofluoric acid is very damaging to tissues even at low concentrations. The fluoride ion causes a liquefaction necrosis of the skin and subcutaneous tissues. The salts formed by this destruction are soluble and will permeate through the tissues with continued destruction.[11] Because the salts continue to be bioactive, the fluoride ions must be inactivated. Calcium and magnesium ions will form

**Table 2.4.**
**Summary of Treatment Measures for
Specific Chemical Burns**

Irrigation with water

Chromic acid
Cantharides
Lyes and alkalies
Potassium hydroxide
Sodium hydroxide
Ammonium hydroxide
Barium hydroxide
Calcium hydroxide
Sulfosalicylic acid
Acetic acid
Cresylic acid
Potassium permanganate
Dimethyl sulfoxide (DMSO)
Sodium hypochlorites
Phenol
Hydrofluoric acid
Dichromate salts
Tungstic acid
Picric Acid
Trichloracetic acid
Formic acid
Gasoline

Calcium salts irrigation or injection

Hydrofluoric acid

Cover burn with oil

Sodium metal
Lithium metal
Potassium metal
Mustard gas

Cover with water

Phosphorus metal

Special measures for certain chemicals

Sodium, potassium, and lithium metals: pieces
    must be excised
Phenol: polyethylene glycol wipes
White phosphorus: copper sulfate irrigation
Alkyl mercury agents: debride and remove
    vesicle fluid

insoluble salts with the fluoride ions.[12] All
other salts are soluble and dissociate completely, allowing the continued diffusion of
ions into the tissues.

Immediately after the exposure, the area
should be flooded with copious amounts of

water at low pressures. After the area has
been flooded with water for 30 minutes, the
remaining fluoride ions can be fixed in insoluble salts with the application of magnesium oxide topical ointments, calcium chloride, or calcium gluconate solutions. Some
authorities also recommend the use of qua-
ternary ammonia compounds such as Hib-
clens or Zephiran. These ammonia compounds have a dubious effect upon fluoride
skin poisoning.[13]

The initial presentation is usually pain at
the site of the exposure. Local erythema and
edema may be present. The pain is uniformly
described as excruciating, particularly after
exposure to solutions of greater than 20%
concentration. Also, the pain is described often
as deep, throbbing, or burning. Regional nerve
blocks may be required for relief.

As the injury progresses, erythema and
edema progress to blanching. Bullae denote
a more severe burn that requires aggressive
treatment. A grossly necrotic area may develop with a subsequent tissue slough and
slowly healing lesion. In severe cases, bone
injury may be manifest and severe decalcification may be noted. Hydrofluoric acid burns
have caused systemic hydrofluorosis with
subsequent death.[14–16]

If there is evidence of skin damage, even
including erythema, the skin has been pen-
etrated by fluoride ions, and these must be
inactivated. The area should be copiously
flushed with running water while materials
and further preparations are in progress. All
bullae and vesicles should be aspirated to remove fluoride-containing fluids. Care must
be taken not to spill the aspirate on any other
part of the skin. The lesions must then be
debrided.

After debridement of the lesions, 10 percent calcium gluconate is injected into the
burn to further bind the fluoride ions. About
0.5 ml of solution should be injected intra-
dermally for every square centimeter of tissue damage. The injection is extended about
0.5 centimeters into the margins of the burn
to bind ions that may have already migrated
there. To ease the pain of injection, use a 27-
or 30-gauge needle and slowly infiltrate the
area. The calcium gluconate injection is usually effective in relieving the pain of the burn.
(See Fig. 2.6.) Unfortunately, the volume of
the calcium chloride is limited to only 0.5 cc
per injection. This severely restricts the

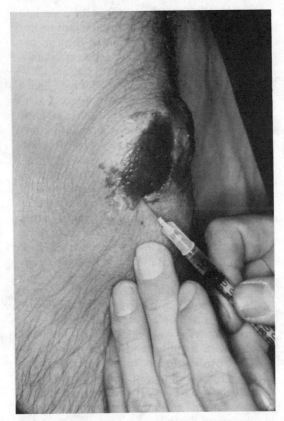

**Figure 2.6.** Injection of 0.5 cc per square centimeter of 10% calcium gluconate solution into the eschar and surrounding tissues in a hydrofluoric acid burn. The patient experienced complete relief of pain from the injection.

amount of calcium that can be injected therapeutically at 1 sitting. Recurrence of the pain is an indication of further fluoride ion migration and another injection is needed.

After the injection of calcium, the area may be covered with either calcium or magnesium oxide dressings. Magnesium oxide dressings are less expensive and easier to obtain but not as effective as calcium-based dressings.[17] Calcium chloride soaks may also be used. Some authors recommend 2.5% calcium gluconate in a gel vehicle, but further clinical trials are indicated before advocating this more costly therapy.[18] It must be inspected frequently to determine if there is any further damage. Recurrence of pain is an indication for reinspection and reinjection. A fluoride burn should always be reinspected at 24-hour in-

tervals, no matter how small or innocuous it seems.

Hydrofluoric acid can rapidly penetrate the nail bed and destroy the underlying nail bed and matrix. Infiltration of calcium ions into the subungual spaces is extremely painful and may cause vascular compromise in the restrictive space between nail and nail bed. When ungual areas are involved in a hydrofluoric acid burn, the affected nail must usually be excised under regional anesthesia. Removal of the nail will allow regeneration after the injury.

In serious fluoride burns of extremities, give intraarterial infusions of calcium chloride or calcium gluconate over a period of 4 hours.[19] If the patient has no pain relief or has recurrence of the pain, a second intraarterial injection is used. Intraarterial injection of calcium may eliminate the need to remove the nails in digital injuries.

Treatments that have been proposed in the past include steroids, systemic steroids, and early surgical excision of the lesion. Steroids have not shown any beneficial effects, and surgical therapy may be unnecessarily mutilating.

Skin burns with hydrofluoric acid are rarely associated with significant systemic absorbtion of fluoride ions. The fluoride ion can cause decalcification of bone and systemic hypocalcemia as a result of the formation of the poorly soluble calcium fluoride complexes. This precipitous drop in serum calcium has been implicated in fluoride-induced sudden death.[20] The mechanism of death is usually intractable ventricular fibrillation, but this dysrhythmia does not respond to intravenous calcium. Other authors feel that the leak of potassium from fluoride-damaged cells has caused a fatal hyperkalemia. This hyperkalemia is mediated by calcium-dependent channels and has been blocked in dogs by quinidine. There are no reported trials of quinidine in fluoride toxic humans with hyperkalemia, hypocalcemia, and ventricular dysrhythmias, but in view of the poor response to extant therapies, quinidine may be appropriate in these selected patients.[21,22]

If there is any evidence of systemic fluorosis or the possibility of inhalation injury, the patient should be admitted to the hospital and observed for at least 24 hours. In these patients, monitoring of liver function studies, renal function studies, electrolytes, and serial serum calcium levels is indicated.[23]

### Elemental Sodium, Potassium, and Lithium Burns

Sodium, potassium, and, to a lesser extent, lithium will spontaneously ignite when in contact with water, including water vapor in the air or on the skin. Using water to irrigate these burns will only intensify the combustion effects. When these metals combine with water, sodium, potassium, and lithium hyroxide are formed. These are, of course, among the strongest of alkalies and capable of causing severe caustic burns.

To extinguish these burning metals, the oxygen and water must be removed from the area. A class D fire extinguisher or sand may be used to smother the fire. After the fire is extinguished, the area should be covered with oil, such as mineral oil or cooking oil, to isolate the metal from water. Small metal pieces should be removed by debridement to fresh tissue. Embedded pieces must be removed surgically. Following debridement, and ensuring that **all** pieces are removed, the area must be irrigated with water, using the same techniques as for an alkali burn.

### Other Metals

Water is generally contraindicated for extinguishing burning metal fragments because of the hydroxides and hydrogen gases that are produced when water is added to hot metals. Particularly injurious are burning fragments of elemental magnesium, which produces magnesium oxide. If the pieces of magnesium are not removed, the small ulcers that form will slowly enlarge and become extensive lesions. After these fragments of burning metal are removed, the resultant wounds must be treated as alkali burns.

### PHOSPHORUS BURNS

White phosphorus is a waxy translucent substance that ignites spontaneously on contact with air. It is usually preserved under water and becomes a liquid at 44°C. White phosphorus is used in the construction of military weapons and fireworks and is a component in insecticides and rodent poisons.

Following an explosion of a white phosphorus munition, flaming droplets of white phosphorus are flung widely about and dense clouds of white smoke with a typical "garlic-like" smell are produced. The flaming pieces of phosphorus cause primarily thermal tissue damage but may also cause high-speed projectile injuries.[24] The smoke is made by the oxidation of phosphorus to phosphoric acid, which can damage the lungs as well as the skin. Some "tracer" bullets have white phosphorus as a major component. This may lead to absorption of retained phosphorus fragments after either an explosion of a phosphorus-based shell or after a bullet wound with a tracer bullet.

Phosphorus is highly fat soluble and is easily absorbed from phosphorus particles driven into the subcutaneous lipid tissues or from the gastrointestinal tract if ingested. The two most common systemic effects are hepatotoxicity and renal damage, but changes in blood phosphorus and calcium levels are also noted. ECG changes with prolongation of the QT interval, ST segment depression, T-wave changes, and bradycardia are also noted. Sudden death has been reported in patients with reversed calcium-phosphorus ratios but is fortunately rare.[25] Monitoring for electrocardiographic abnormalities and changes in serum calcium and phosphorus is appropriate for patients with significant wounds. In cases where systemic absorption is suspected, BUN, creatinine, serum phosphorus, and liver enzymes should be assessed frequently.

Flaming white phosphorus is extinguished by immersing the pieces in water. Surface particles and particles embedded in clothing should be promptly removed. During transport, the EMTs should cover the burned areas with moistened cloths to prevent further burning.

The wound should then be washed with a 1 percent copper sulfate solution. The copper sulfate solution combines with the phosphorus to form copper phosphate, which can be readily identified as black particles.[3] These black pieces can be easily debrided. If the particles are not debrided, they will be absorbed and systemic effects will ensue.[26]

Once debridement is completed, then no further copper sulfate solution is needed. The copper sulfate solution should not be used for a prolonged period, because of the risk of systemic copper poisoning. Systemic copper poisoning can be manifested by vomiting, diarrhea, oliguria, intravascular hemolysis, hematuria, hepatic necrosis, and cardiovascular collapse. The hemolysis is thought to be due to copper's inhibition of the erythrocyte hexose monophosphate shunt. This results in a hemolysis similar to that found in G6PD deficiency disease.

To minimize copper absorption, the wound may be irrigated with a solution of 5 percent sodium bicarbonate and 3 percent copper sulfate suspended in 1 percent hydroxyethyl cellulose.[27] Wet dressings of copper sulfate in any form should never be applied to the wound. Following debridement, the wound should be irrigated with copious amounts of water to remove the copper salts.

Metabolic derangements have been noted with white phosphorus injuries. Hypocalcemia, hyperphosphatemia, and ECG abnormalities are all noted.[28] The electrocardiographic abnormalities include prolongation of the QT interval, bradycardia, and nonspecific ST-T wave changes.

## Phenol Burns

Phenol is an aromatic acid alcohol that is a highly reactive and corrosive contact poison. The phenols have been used as bactericidal agents and are used in industry as bases for plastics and organic polymers. In the form of creosote, it is also used as a preservative for wood.

Phenols were first used as antiseptics by Lister in 1867, and their effects on tissues have been well studied.[29] In either the vapor or the liquid, phenol is rapidly absorbed through the skin surfaces. Phenol vapors are easily absorbed by the lungs. If the skin absorption is significant, the exposure may result in toxic effects on the cardiovascular and central nervous systems. These can include:

Central nervous system depression
Hypotension
Intravascular hemolysis
Pulmonary edema
Shock
Death

The most common manifestation of sys-temic phenol poisoning is a profound fulminant central nervous system depression with coma, hypothermia, loss of vasomotor tone, and respiratory arrest. In many cases, loss of consciousness may be noted within 30 minutes of skin contact. Cardiopulmonary collapse freqently accompanies this CNS presentation and is due to the cardiac depressant effects of phenol. In animal studies, as little as 0.625 mg/kg of phenol has caused death.[30,31]

Phenol skin burns are characterized by initial pain, followed by numbness as the nerve endings are anesthetized.[32] The skin then blanches and an eschar forms over the burned area during a period of hours. Phenols in strong concentrations rapidly produce a whitish slough, which turns to a greenish-black or copper-colored eschar. Formation of coagulation necrosis of the dermis will delay the absorption, but this delay is only temporary.

Treatment must be initated immediately. Before washing a contaminated area, remove any liquid on the skin. Swabs, gauze pads, or even clothing is acceptable for this. If polyethylene glycol is not available, glycerol may aid in the removal. Removal of the liquid should not wait until these materials are available.

Water irrigation is not recommended by some authorities. In severe phenol burns, the necrotic tissues may act as a temporary barrier that does not allow penetration of the water into the deeper layers of the injury. The water may also dilute the phenol and allow more rapid penetration into the skin. Nevertheless, if there is no ready access to specific solutes of phenol, immediate irrigation with water is probably better than allowing the substance to remain upon the skin.

Although water irrigation is effective for phenol burn, wiping the skin with undiluted polyethylene glycol 300 or 400 will dissolve and remove the phenols more quickly than water alone. Alcohols and glycerol would also be effective in removal of the phenols. Polyethylene glycol solutions are not irritating to the tissues and may safely be used to irrigate facial burns and eye injuries.

## Alcohol Burns

Isopropyl alcohol is a commonly used disinfectant in hospital settings and is used for cleaning in home and industry. In infants and small children, it can be associated with skin burns. The mechanism of action is thought to be deesterification of the skin.[33] The degree of burn is related to the concentration of the alcohol, the duration of the exposure, and the condition of the skin to which the alcohol has been applied. Premature infants are at most risk. Burns occur most often in areas of pressure and where the alcohol can pool, such as about the diapers.[34]

## Burns From Lime and Cement

Lime (calcium oxide) in the presence of water is converted to calcium hydroxide, a strong alkali with a pH as high as 12.9.[35] Perspiration and skin moisture are sufficient to initiate this reaction. Portland cement is composed of lime, magnesium and other metal oxides, and sand. Portland cement, hence, has the same potential to damage skin as lime. In premixed cement, the reaction with water is already underway, and the wet cement can produce third-degree alkali burns in as little as 2 hours of contact time.[36]

The professional cement worker is well aware of this potential for skin burns, but the amateur is not. Most injuries are, expectedly, in amateurs. The worker usually sustains ankle (boot cuff) injuries as the wet cement collects inside the shoes, or knee injuries as he kneels in the wet cement without protection.[37] (See Fig. 2.7.) The resultant burn is often serious, because it is not appreciated at once and the material is often allowed to remain in contact with the skin for a prolonged period of time.

Initial treatment of lime or cement spilled on the skin consists of brushing away the particulate matter and then irrigating with copious amounts of water. Wet cement burns should be flushed with copious amounts of water. The lesions should be treated as alkali burns.

Some EMS texts wrongly recommend only half of the treatment, e.g., brushing away the particulate matter. The remaining fine dust can be activated by the insensible perspiration and will cause an alkali burn. Irrigation with water is an integral part of the treatment of lime burns.[9]

To avoid the injuries, the danger of prolonged skin contact with wet cement or dry lime should be noted to all workers, printed

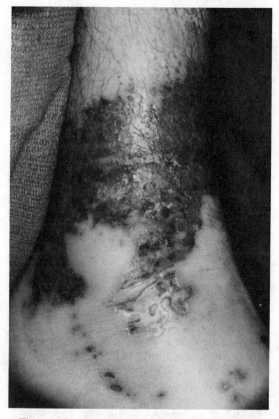

**Figure 2.7.** Appearance on the third postburn day of a "boot-cuff" burn from wet cement in an amateur laying a cement garage floor. The patient wore open-topped boots with an estimated contact time of 4 hours.

as a warning on the sacks, and disseminated to all health care providers. Watertight boots and gloves should be worn at all times when handling cement or lime. Boots should be tucked under the trousers so that cuff pockets of cement cannot form. Workers kneeling on wet cement should have a dry board or other protection against the wet cement.

## Gasoline Burns (Chemical)

Gasoline is a complex mixture of aromatic hydrocarbons, cycloalkanes, and alkanes. The hydrocarbons appear to be a major toxic agent in skin exposures. Constant contact with gasoline can result in a chemical burn in as little as 1 hour. The skin surface resembles a scald, and the burn is most often a second degree injury that heals without scarring.[38] The injury seems to be caused by the solvent effects of gasoline on the skin fats.

Exposure to gasoline may be complicated by the leading agents that are used to improve the performance characteristics. Significant lead absorption and subsequent neurological damage may ensue from gasoline exposure. Tetraethyl lead is more toxic than elemental lead in this regard.

Common complications from the contact effects of gasoline and other light petroleum products such as kerosene include toxic effects from inhalation and ingestion. In addition to the skin burn, the patient often may have serious multisystem effects, including organ system failure.

### Hydrocarbon toxicities
  Neurological disorders
  Pulmonary injuries
  Cardiovascular abnormalities
  Gastrointestinal disturbances
  Renal failure
  Hepatic failure

Inhalation or absorption of gasoline produces symptoms similar to those of ethanol intoxication, including ataxia, mental confusion, and slurred speech. High concentrations of gasoline vapors may lead to coma and death.[39] Once far more common, the gasoline "sniffer" is much less frequently found.

Cardiovascular complications include sudden death when inhalation is followed by strenuous exercise or stressful situations. Spontaneous and severe cardiac arrhythmias are the mechanism of death in these cases. Catecholamine release appears to increase the toxic potential of the petroleum distillate.

Gasoline absorption has produced renal damage to include glomerulonephritis and renal tubular acidosis. The hydrocarbon hepatitis is secondary to vascular endothelial damage and is usually a reversible lesion without long-term sequelae.

Initial treatment of the gasoline immersion burn is to remove the clothing and cleanse the skin surfaces. Further emergent treatment of a petroleum distillate burn should include low pressure irrigation with water for at least 1 hour. The patient should be admitted to the hospital and observed for at least 24 hours. A monitored bed is appropriate for these patients. Serum lead levels should be obtained and treatment initiated if the lead level is greater than 30 to 40 nanograms per 100 ml. Dimercaprol (British Anti-Lewisite)

**Table 2.5.**
**Indications for Hospitalization of Patients With Chemical Burns**

High-risk patients (concurrent illnesses)
Burns of hand, foot, face, eye, or perineum
Burns of greater than 15% of total body surface
Deep burns (deep second or third degree burns)
Burns with substances that have systemic
  toxicity

and calcium EDTA followed by penacillamine therapy for 15 to 20 days has proved efficacious in these cases.[40]

## SUMMARY

Fortunately, the chemical burn usually involves only a small part of the patient's surface area. In most cases, these burns can be managed on an outpatient basis.

Patients who require hospitalization include those with burns from chemicals that have long-term or distant effects such as gasoline, phenol, or hydrofluoric acid. Admission is also required when the burn involves a critical area or a large surface, and, of course, when the patient has a concurrent severe illness. (See Table 2.5.)

As a rule, most chemical injuries can be managed by copious irrigation with large quantities of water. This measure serves to both dilute and remove the agent. For elemental lithium, sodium, and potassium metals, the particles must be removed before irrigation. Special antidotes should be used, if available, in appropriate cases.

### References

1. Jelenko C III. Chemicals that "burn." J Trauma 1974;14:65–72.
2. Leonard LG, Scheulen JJ, Munster AM. Chemical burns: effect of prompt first aid. Trauma 1982;22:420–423.
3. Currerri PW, Asch MJ, Pruitt BA. The treatment of chemical burns: specialized diagnostic, therapeutic and prognostic considerations. J Trauma 1970;10:634–642.
4. Rodheaver GT, Herbert JM, Edlich RF. Initial treatment of chemical, skin, and eye burns. Compr Ther 1982;8:37–43.
5. Wolfort FG, DeMeester T, Knorr N, et al. Surgical management of cutaneous lye burns. Surg Gynecol Obstet 1970::873–876.
6. Kunkel DB. Burning issues: acids and alka-

lies. II. Skin and eye exposures. Emerg Med 1984;:165–172.

7. Bromberg BE, Sang IC, Walden RH. Hydrotherapy of chemical burns. Plast Reconstr Surg 1965;35:85.

8. Gruber RP, Laub DR, Vistnes LM. The effect of hydrotherapy on the clinical course and pH of experimental cutaneous chemical burns. Plast Reconstr Surg 1975;55:200.

9. Stewart CE. Chemical skin burns. Amer Fam Phys 1985;31:151–157.

10. Davidson EC. The treatment of alkali and acid burns. Ann Surg 1927;85:481.

11. Shewmake SW, Anderson BG: Hydrofluoric acid burns: a report of a case and review of the literature. Arch Dermatol 1979;115:593–596.

12. Carney SA, Hall M, Lawrence JC, Ricketts CR. Rationale of the treatment of hydrofluoric acid burns. Brit J Ind Med 1974;31:317–321.

13. Trevino MA, Herrmann GH, Sprout WL. Treatment of severe hydrofluoric acid exposures. J Occup Med 1983;25:861–863.

14. Mayer TG, Gross PL. Fatal systemic flourosis due to hydrofluoric acid burns. Ann Emerg Med 1985;14:149–153.

15. Tepperman PB. Fatality due to acute systemic fluoride poisoning following a hydrofluoric acid skin burn. J Occup Med 1980;22:691–692.

16. Burke WJ, Hoegg UR, Phillips RE. Systemic fluoride poisoning resulting from a fluoride skin burn. J Occup Med 1973;15:39–41.

17. Iverson RE, Laub DR. Hydrofluoric acid burn. Surg Forum 1970;21:517–519.

18. Milner JE. The office treatment of minor chemical skin burns. Cutis 1982;29:285–288.

19. Vance MV, Curry SC, Kunkel DB, et al. Digital hydrofluoric acid burns: treatment with intraarterial calcium infusion. Ann Emerg Med 1986;15:890–896.

20. Mayer TG, Gross PL. Fatal systemic fluorosis due to hydrofluoric acid burns. Ann Emerg Med 1985;14:149–153.

21. McIvor ME. Delayed fatal hyperkalemia in a patient with acute fluoride intoxication. Ann Emerg Med 1987;16:1165–1167.

22. Cummings CC, McIvor ME. Fluoride-induced hyperkalemia: the role of Ca2+ dependent K+ channels. Amer J Emerg Med 1988;6:1–3.

23. Trevino MA, Herrmann GH, Sprout WL. Treatment of severe hydrofluoric acid exposures. J Occup Med 1983;25:861–863.

24. Konjoyan TR. White phosphorus burns: case report and literature review. Mil Med 1983; 148:881–884.

25. Bowen TE, Whelen TH, Nilson TG. Sudden deaths after phosphorus burns: experimental observations of hypocalcemia, hyperphosphatemia, and electrocardiographic abnormalities following induction of a standardized white phosphorus burn. Ann Surg 1970;174:779–784.

26. Dempsy WS. Combat injuries of the lower extremities. Clin Plast Surg 1975;2:585–614.

27. Ben-Hur N, Appelbaum J. Biochemistry, histopathology and treatment of phosphorus burns. Isr J Med Sci 1973;9:40–48.

28. Bowen TE, Whelen TJ Jr, Nelson TG. Sudden death after phosphorus burns: experimental observations of hypocalcemia, hyperphosphatemia and electrocardiographic abnormalities following production of a standard white phosphorus burn. Ann Surg 1971;174:779–784.

29. Roberts HL. Chloracetic acids: a biochemical study. Ann Surg 1926;49:245–247.

30. Conning DM, Haynes MJ. The dermal toxicity of phenol: an investigation of the most effective first-aid measures. Brit J Ind Med 1970;27:155.

31. Brown VKH, Box VL, Simpson BJ. Decontamination procedures for skin exposed to phenolic substances Arch Environ Health 1975;20:1.

32. Abraham AJ. A case of carbolic acid gangrene of the thumb. Br J Plast Surg 1972;25:282–284.

33. Hodgkinson DJ, Irons GB, Williams TJ. Chemical burns and skin preparation solutions. Surg Gynecol Obstet 1978;147:534–536.

34. Schick JB, Milstein JM. Burn hazard of isopropyl alcohol in the neonate. Pediatrics 1981;68(4):587–588

35. Peters WJ. Alkali burns from wet cement. Can Med Assoc J 1984;130:902–903.

36. Rowe W, Williams GH. Severe reaction to cement. Arch Environ Health 1963;7:709–711.

37. Fisher AA. Cement burns resulting in necrotic ulcers due to kneeling on wet cement. Cutis 1979;23:272–274.

38. Hunter GA. Chemical burns of the skin after contact with petrol. Br J Plast Surg 1968; 21:337–341.

39. Poklis A, Burkett CD. Gasoline sniffing: a review. Clinical Toxicol 1977;11:35.

40. Simpson LA, Cruse CW. Gasoline immersion injury. Plast Reconstruct Surg 1981;67:54–57.

# CHAPTER 3

# Frostbite and Cold Injuries

## INTRODUCTION

Local cold injuries can occur both above and below freezing temperatures and inflict permanent disability and disfigurement to those who suffer. Frostbite is thought to be rare in civilian practice, and perhaps **major** cold injury is an uncommon disease in the civilian population of temperate climates.[1] There are no available statistics that document the multitudes of minor cold injuries that occur during colder weather as these injuries are not often reported and may never be seen by a physician. Military physicians maintain a close accounting of severe cold injuries during major campaigns, and the Surgeon General feels that this is a potentially major debilitating factor in any winter or mountain encounter. In the recent Falklands campaign, for example, cold injuries accounted for 9% of total casualties.[2] Indeed, the efforts of military surgeons have substantially contributed to both past and present treatment of cold injuries. One of the more famous military accounts governed the treatment of cold injuries for over a century:

> During the retreat of Napoleon's Grande Armee' from Moscow in 1812–1813, Baron Dominique Jean Larey was the Army Surgeon-General. He had ample opportunity to observe the ill effects of frostbite on his soldier-patients. He repeatedly saw the development of wet gangrene with massive tissue loss and frequent death. His eloquent advice was followed for over a century:[3]

*"When some external part of the body is caught by cold, instead of submitting the part to heat, which provides gangrene, it is necessary to rub the affected part with substances containing very little caloric. . . . For it is well known that the effect of caloric on an organized part that is almost deprived of life is marked by an acceleration of fermentation and putrefaction."*

What Baron Larey observed was the effect of a freeze-thaw-freeze cycle as his patients froze on the march, then thawed in front of a roaring fire and resumed march the next day. This cycle produced massive tissue loss from the initial freeze injury and the addition of a secondary burn injury with subsequent re-freezing. This experience has been repeated by the British in the trenches of World War I, Hitler in Moscow and the U.S. in Korea with similar catastrophic results.

The human peripheral circulation has a dense system of capillary loops that are able to markedly increase and decrease blood flow through the extremities. The cutaneous vascular tone is controlled by direct local effects as well as both central and peripheral reflexes due to heating and cooling. With heat stress, the cutaneous blood flow may increase from the normal 200 to 500 ml per minute to a maximum of 3000 ml per minute. With cold stress, this cutaneous blood flow may decrease to only 20 to 50 ml per minute for the entire skin surface. This decrease in peripheral blood flow causes a decrease in total body heat losses but at the expense of the peripheral circulation.

When the extremity is cooled to about 15°C, peripheral vasoconstriction is at a maximum, and blood flow to the tissues is minimal. If cooling is continued to about 10°C, a cold-induced vasodilation (the "hunting reflex of Lewis") is initiated.[4] This reflex is a periodic vasodilation with an associated increase in blood flow and hence heat transfer. This periodic vasodilation will continue in a cycle every 5 to 10 minutes and provides some protection from the hypoxic and thermal effects of the maximal vasoconstriction induced by the cold.

This reflex is more marked in those who have had long-standing and ancestral exposures to cold, such as Alaskan natives, and may be increased by prolonged and repeated exposure to the cold. Humans appear to have no other adaptation to the cold.

Animals that have adapted to cold climates have a continual flow of warm blood to their extremities and lack the intense vasoconstriction reflex found in humans. They also lack the propensity towards frostbite. If humans were appropriately cold-adapted, perhaps cold injuries would not be a major problem. Unfortunately, because we undergo marked peripheral vasoconstriction with cold exposure, we are not able to maintain peripheral tissue temperatures and, therefore, suffer cold injuries.

The type of cold injury depends upon the degree and nature of the cold to which the body is exposed, and the duration of exposure. For practical purposes, cold injuries may be divided simply into "freezing" and "nonfreezing" types. The former is the well-known frostbite (either superficial or deep). The nonfreezing types are chilblain, trench foot, and immersion foot.

## NONFREEZING COLD INJURIES

### Chilblain (Pernio)

Chilblain (pernio) is the mildest form of cold injury and may be divided into acute and chronic forms. This injury occurs with repeated exposure of bare skin to cold, wet, and windy weather ranging from 15.5 to 0°C (60 to 32°F). Chilblain is more commonly seen in England than in the United States.[5]

In the acute case, there is usually moderate to severe pruritis with red, dry, and roughened skin. Erythema, cyanosis, and

| Features of Chilblain | |
|---|---|
| Setting | Cold, wet, windy weather |
| | Temperatures from 32 to 60°F |
| Predisposing factors | Raynaud's phenomenon |
| | Sulindac administration |
| Onset | Seasonal |
| Symptoms | Pruritis and burning sensations |
| Signs | Erythema, cyanosis, edematous patches of skin |
| | Tender, bluish nodules on the face and dorsum of hands and feet after rewarming |
| Treatment | Protective clothing |
| | Topical lotions |
| | Avoidance of cold weather |
| Prophylaxis | Avoidance of exposure |

edematous patches are seen 12 to 24 hours after exposure to the cold. Primarily seen on the face and the dorsal surfaces of the hands and feet, it is frequent in young women. The lesions are usually bilateral and symmetrical, although they may be single or multiple. Patients frequently describe a burning sensation, particularly noticeable upon rewarming the areas. After rewarming, tender bluish nodules develop that last 10 to 14 days. This condition is frequently seasonal starting with the onset of cold weather and clearing up when warm weather returns.

Chronic pernio appears to occur more frequently in the middle ages of life and may evolve through a continued exposure to the cold in patients with acute chilblain. Symptomatic complaints are the same as in acute pernio with pruritis and burning sensations. Numerous clinical variants of chronic pernio have been described. Lesions may be annular, papular, or, rarely, hemorrhagic bullae and pustules. Scarring and postinflammatory pigmentation changes are common. Healing occurs during the summer months.

Histologically, chilblain is characterized by edema of the papillary dermis and a mild vasculitis of both the superficial and deep dermal vessels. Histological changes strongly favor vascular damage as the primary etiologic factor in the formation of the perniotic lesions.[6] It is associated with increased vascular tone, which results in prolonged vasospasm even after initial warming is begun.

Patients with Raynaud's phenomenon and those who take sulindac appear to be predisposed to chilblain.[7] A differential diagnosis for pernio or chilblain may include Raynaud's disease, lupus erythematosis, cellulitis, frostbite, herpes, traumatic injury, chronic myelocytic leukemia, vasculitis, and vascular thrombosis.[8,9]

To treat chilblain, the patient should be instructed to wear protective clothing and to apply a soothing topical lotion to the affected areas. For severe cases, avoidance of cold weather areas may be needed. Acute chilblain is self-limiting, and the lesions do not recur unless reexposure to cold occurs. Severe cases may demonstrate vesicles, bullae, petechiae, hemorrhage, and ulcers (although this presentation is rare).

## Trench or Immersion Foot

The term *immersion foot* was coined during World War I as a description of those patients who were shipwrecked and isolated in a lifeboat for a prolonged period of time. The patients would have their feet in a dependent position in the bilge water. The water temperatures were usually between 0 and 10°C (32 and 50°F), and the exposure often lasted many days. *Trench foot* was applied to a similar situation during World War I when the infantry would be pinned down in trenches filled with cold mud and water.

Although once thought to be different entities, trench foot and immersion foot are indistinguishable. They occur after prolonged exposure to wet and cold. The temperature usually ranges from just above freezing to about 50°F.[10] The duration of exposure to the wet and cold usually exceeds 10 to 12 hours. If the extremity is kept in an immobile and dependent position, the depth and extent of injury will be exacerbated.

There are three phases to this type of injury.

- First, the tissue becomes vasospastic and appears cold, swollen, white, or cyanotic. Pulses and sensation in the extremity are decreased. This initial phase results in tissue hypoxia leading to increased capillary permeability and edema.
- Warming the extremity initiates the second phase, a hyperemic response where the extremity appears hot, dry, and reddened with

| Features of Immersion (Trench) Foot | |
|---|---|
| Setting | Cold, often just above freezing, water |
| Onset | Usually greater than 10 to 12 hours |
| Description | 3 phases |
| | Cyanotic (acute phase) |
| | Hyperemic (4 to 10 days after rewarming) |
| | Recovery (slow healing after injury) |
| Symptoms | Loss of dexterity |
| | Aching or burning pains |
| | Reddened skin |
| | Numbness |
| | "Block of wood" feeling |
| Signs | Reddened skin |
| | Whitish coloration |
| | Cyanosis |
| | Decreased pulses |
| Treatment | Identical to frostbite |
| Prophylaxis | Avoidance of prolonged exposure to wet and cold |

*Note:* This describes only the first or cyanotic phase of immersion foot. See the text for further information and prognosis associated with the hyperemic and recovery phases.

bounding pulses and extreme pain. Bullae are also common. This phase may last from 4 to 10 days. Severe or repeated exposures can result in gangrene and extensive tissue loss. In many cases, after the patient has been rewarmed, it is difficult to distinguish the effects of trench foot from frostbite.

- The third and last phase is one of recovery, and it is characterized by decreasing edema and the return of normal pulses in a patient who has no complications. In severe cases, the result is an injury noted for extensive edema, pain, and slow recovery. Associated with the recovery phase may be skin depigmentation, hyperhidrosis, cold sensitivity, and pain on weight bearing. This phase may last for years after the initial insult. Late problems may include intermittent local ulcerations, painful cutaneous fissuring, and chronic infections.

Though not often seen in the civilian population, trench foot is an occupational hazard for those in the military, especially when troops are under fire during maneuvers in inclement weather.[11,12] In 1944, Patton commented to his commanders that trench foot represented a greater hazard to his soldiers than the German Army.

## FROSTBITE

## Pathophysiology

Frostbite occurs when tissue freezes. Since tissue is not composed of water alone, it will not freeze until it has been cooled to about $-3$ to $-4°C$. For the tissue temperature to drop this low requires the ambient temperature to be about $-6°C$ or less. Needless to say, the tissue temperature is influenced by the external cold stress as well as internal heat production. An exposure to extremely cold temperatures, such as Arctic winters, or exposure to liquified gases may cause rapid tissue freezing.

Experimental studies have implied that the mechanism of tissue injury in frostbite may either be ice crystal formation in the extracellular fluid compartment or microvascular aggregates and emboli formation with subsequent vascular stasis. There are proponents of both theories in the literature. Proper understanding of frostbite pathophysiology may well advance the treatment of this condition, presently limited to little more than adjunctive therapy.

| *Features of Frostbite* | |
|---|---|
| Setting | Temperature less than $-4°C$ (28°F) |
| Onset | Usually 7 to 10 hours of exposure but may be quite shorter with sufficiently cold ambient temperatures |
| Symptoms | Cold sensation<br>Numbness<br>"Block of wood" feeling |
| Signs | Whitish color<br>Frozen consistency with resilience<br>"Block of wood" consistency |
| Treatment | Rapid rewarming in warm water |
| Prophylaxis | Proper clothing and protection, avoidance of exposure |

## Ice Crystal Formation

As the tissue freezes, ice crystals form in the extracellular fluid compartment. As fluids are drawn from the intracellular space in an attempt to maintain osmotic equilibrium, the colloid osmotic pressure in the extracellular region decreases. The cell membrane is disrupted as the relative dehydration progresses. The extracellular crystallization also causes pressure on the surrounding tissues including the vascular structures and the cell membranes. These mechanisms can lead to cell death and rupture if they are severe enough or of long enough duration.

## Microvascular Changes

Associated with frostbite is red-cell sludging and microthrombus formation resulting in the diminution of the distal blood flow. These microvascular aggregates form within 1 to 2 hours after the tissues are thawed. Prominent in animal studies of even minimal frostbite is the endothelial damage noted. This initial insult is followed by increased vascular permeability, edema formation, and decreased circulation.[13]

It is felt that this injury to the microvasculature system probably plays a decisive role in the development of tissue destruction in frostbite. Weatherly-White and associates demonstrated the magnitude of this vasculature insult when they showed that normal skin transplanted to frostbitten tissue beds will slough, whereas frostbitten skin transplanted to a normal tissue bed will have a significant chance of survival.[14] Also, the decreased circulation can be detected by RISA studies and by serial angiographs of the affected extremity (Fig. 3.1.).[15] Local tissue hypoxia and death occur as a result of the decrease in circulation.

The causes of the resulting microvascular aggregates, intravascular sludging, and tissue damage are not well understood but may include the increased viscosity of fluids at low temperature, capillary membrane damage, an increase in the activities of clotting factors, and local vasospasm with hypoxia. Recent work has also implicated arachidonic acid, released from the damaged epithelial cells, as a direct cause of tissue damage.[16,17]

The major pathophysiologic problem after the vessel damage seems to be hypoxemia and microvascular compromise. Any factor that decreases oxygen transport will exacerbate the injury and lead to further damage. The surrounding cells then convert to anaerobic metabolism, producing lactic acid. This

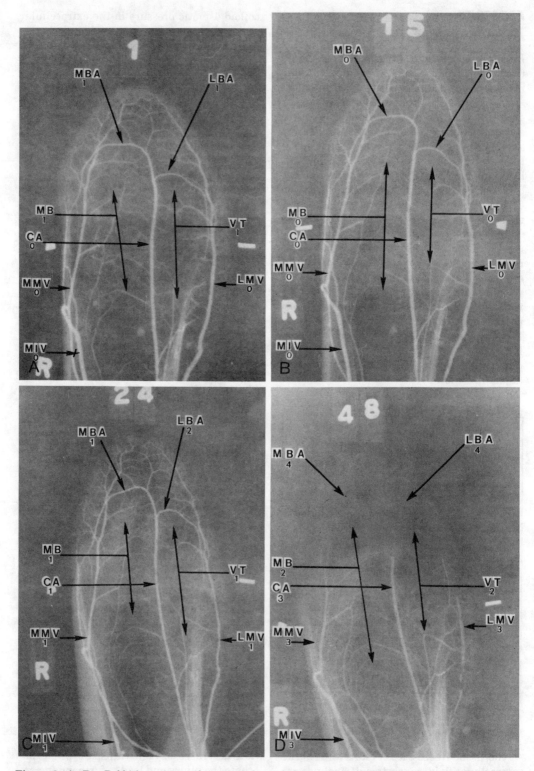

**Figure 3.1A–D.** Rabbit's ear interval angiography with demonstration of decrease in vascularity. (From Lazarus HM, Hutto BS. Electrical burns and frostbite: patterns of vascular injury. J Trauma 1982;22:581–585.)

leads to impaired enzyme function and further disruption and death of cells in an already compromised cellular milieu. It is important to remember that this process expands outward as the injury progresses. The peripheral region of injury is in a state of reversible damage, not death; therefore, proper care is important to limit the final tissue loss. Partial rewarming allows the circumferential tissue to temporarily revitalize, but refreezing the tissue will result in increased tissue loss. This may be caused by local blood trapping with more local fluid crystallization and further tissue destruction. This seems to be the basis of "freeze-thaw-freeze" injuries.

Tissues vary in their susceptibility to cold injuries. Those most sensitive include the nerves, blood vessels, and striated muscle. Skin, fascia, and connective tissue are relatively resistant to injury by cold, while bone and tendon are highly resistant. An exception appears to be juvenile bony epiphyses, which appear to be more sensitive to cold than other bony surfaces.

One problem in researching frostbite is that there are no completely satisfactory animal models to study.[12] Unfortunately, volunteers are few and far between, and most ethics committees rightfully frown on experiments that may lead to substantial tissue loss, even in educated and informed volunteer subjects. Current animal models include the rabbit (ears and hind feet), hairless mice (ears), and pig (back and abdominal skin). Another obstacle in the analysis of frostbite is the difference between the slow clinical onset in human subjects and the more rapid onset of frostbite by refrigeration techniques in the model.

## Risk Factors (Table 3.1)

### AMBIENT TEMPERATURE AND CLIMATIC FACTORS

Needless to say, the predominant risk factor in frostbite is exposure to cold. Cold exposure is directly related to the air temperature and the duration of the exposure. It also is related to the relative humidity and the local wind conditions. As thermal losses increase with decreased temperature, increased winds, increased humidity, and increased duration of exposure, there is a higher chance of cold injury.

**Table 3.1.**
**Risk Factors for Frostbite[a]**

| Good | Bad |
|---|---|
| White or Alaskan | Black |
| Northerner | Southerner |
| Healthy | Prior vascular or cardiac disease |
| No prior injury | Prior cold injury |
| Normovolemic | Hypovolemic, shock |
| Good clothing | Inappropriate clothing |
| Sea level | Altitude or hypoxia |
| Exercising | Sedentary or comatose |
| | Alcohol or drug use |
| | Mental instability |
| | Accidents |

[a]Christenson C, Stewart CE. Frostbite. Am Fam Phys 1984;30:111–122.

Perhaps the most dramatic recorded cases of frostbite occurred in the World War II B-17 and B-24 bombers as the waist port gunners had to open their doors to fire their weapons. They were exposed to very cold air rushing by at over 200 miles per hour. During the winter of 1943, frostbite caused more casualties in these bomber crews than all other sources combined, including enemy fire. In the civilian population, 90% of frostbite occurs at temperatures below $-6.6°C$ (20°F) after 7 to 10 hours of exposure. (Table 5.2.)

Increased heat loss is also seen when tissue is in contact with volatile liquids, such as kerosene or gasoline. Wet clothing or direct metal contact to skin dramatically decreases the time needed for frostbite to occur (Fig. 3.2). The wetness enhances the skin's conductive and evaporative heat losses. Exposure to very cold chemicals, such as liquid oxygen or liquid nitrogen, produces "instant" frostbite. This quick-freezing phenomenon may also be seen when the skin is in direct contact with ice or "dry ice."[19] The "instant" frostbite of liquid gases has the potential to produce not only cutaneous but deep and severe tissue injury.[20]

The direct contact of living tissue with cold objects will result in a quicker and more sig-

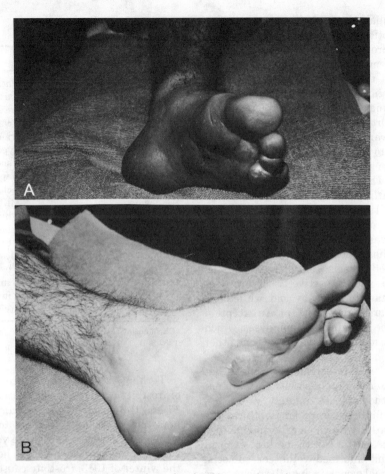

**Figure 3.2.** Cold transmission through sole of boot with steel shank (frostbite of foot).

nificant cold injury than mere exposure to cold surroundings. This may be particularly notable in patients who have been injured or are comatose and sustain cold injuries. Those body parts in contact with the snowbank or ground will show a deeper cold injury. Heat conduction by direct contact is increased across a wet surface.

The amount of tissue exposed plays a role in the overall recovery from the cold injury. The larger the surface area exposed, the greater the total heat loss.

## NUTRITIONAL STATUS

Because of the borderline metabolic status of the cells, severe malnutrition predisposes a person to cold injury. The cells have little reserve against injury, and the cold injury is deeper and more severe than in a person with normal metabolic reserves.

## RACE AND HEREDITY

Military studies have demonstrated that blacks are from 2.8 to 6 times more susceptible to a cold injury.[21] In the Korean War, blacks suffered 52% of the total cases of frostbite but numbered only 9 to 10% of the exposed population. In addition, their injuries appear to be both deeper and more severe than those of other races.[22,23]

Caucasian southerners are more than 3.7 times more susceptible to cold injuries than those from the northernmost states. It is not known whether this is related to birth, training, or acclimation.[24]

## PREVIOUS COLD INJURY

A previous cold injury increases the risk of a subsequent cold injury to the injured area. The prior cold injury leaves residual microvascular changes that can increase the morbidity of any additional cold injuries. Minor superficial cold injuries, when fully resolved, probably do not cause an increased risk.

## CONSTRICTING CLOTHES, SHOCK, AND BLOOD LOSS

Constricting clothes, shock, and hypovolemia may markedly decrease the peripheral blood flow and result in a decreased heat transfer and oxygen supply to the affected tissues. Heat flow into the extremity is also altered by a cramped position or direct pressure. As the peripheral blood flow decreases, there is less warming by the "metabolic furnace." These factors increase the chances of developing frostbite in the affected tissues and may increase the severity of the subsequent injury.

Trauma sustained in freezing and subfreezing conditions poses a special problem in management. The patient who is immobilized, with hypovolemia due to shock, and with possible vascular compromise due to fractures, is at high risk for frostbite and generalized hypothermia. Large amounts of heat can be rapidly lost through contact with the ground or snow. It is imperative to insulate the patient from the ground to minimize these losses.

## DRUGS AND MEDICATIONS

Any drug or medication causing a decreased peripheral circulation, impaired mental capacity, or altered thermal reflex arcs may increase the risk of cold injuries. The autoregulation of peripheral circulation is critical in the maintenance of body temperature, and an impaired response may decrease the blood flow to the extremities. This increases the risk of frostbite. Vasoconstrictive drugs, such as nicotine, can cause hypoxia and rapid heat loss in the extremities, increasing the extent of the frostbite and shortening the freezing times. The vasodilating effect of drugs, such as alcohol, causes increased blood flow to the cold extremities. The increased cooling of the blood increases the risk of hypothermia and obtundation. Cerebral functions are impaired as the body temperature drops, and it becomes difficult to solve more complex problems, such as how to get to someplace warmer. A paradoxical undressing is often found in patients with severe hypothermia. (See Chapter 4 for a more complete description of this phenomenon.)

In addition, drugs such as alcohol, narcotics, and barbiturates decrease baseline physical activity and central heat production with a resultant increased risk of cold injury. If mental function is further impaired due to pharmacologic or psychiatric reasons, improper clothing and shelter again may be chosen. This increases the risk of exposure.

## ALTITUDE AND HYPOXIA

If all other factors are equal, a frostbite injury at high altitude is more profound and deeper than at sea level. The decreased ambient oxygen tension found at high altitudes causes hypoxia, which increases the severity of the injury. Evidence from World War II, the Korean War, and mountain climbing expeditions support this finding.

## ACTIVITY

Activity and the subsequent increased heat production provides a protective effect for patients. Certainly, if the patient has been exercising in sufficiently cold weather, with insufficient insulation, frostbite may ensue. Generally, however, a dependent position with inactivity has been noted to have a marked increase in the rapidity with which frostbite occurs.

At least one author has proposed that anxiety and fear also predispose to cold injuries.[25] Sampson notes that behavioral immobility, disorganization, and carelessness were commonly associated with anxiety in combat. He further notes that anxiety and fear provoke sweating and vasomotor constriction in the extremities. These responses can certainly predispose the affected individual to cold injury. Perhaps similar situations may predispose lost or stranded civilians in cold environments to an increased incidence of cold injuries.

## Clinical Course

As frostbite begins, the patient may be unaware that it is occurring. As tissue temperatures drop to less than 10°C (50°F), afferent sensory impulses no longer warn of the impending danger.

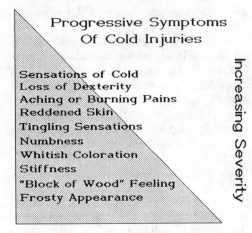

**Figure 3.3.** Symptoms of cold injury.

The initial symptoms are variable, but most patients describe a gradual subsidence of painful cold sensations followed by tingling and then numbness (Fig. 3.3). Frequently, this numbness is likened to "a block of wood" or "a club."

The tissues may first appear blanched and then progress through a doughy stage to "rock hard" indicating complete freezing. Frequently, a frosty rime will appear on the tissues after freezing.

After the extremity has been thawed, a throbbing pain is common and lasts for 2 to 4 days. It may last as long as several weeks in severe cases. Shortly after thawing, edema formation begins. With more severe injuries, blisters form within 24 to 48 hours.

In several days, edema and blisters begin to resolve. A dark black, dry eschar will form over the course of 2 to 3 weeks. Four or more weeks after the injury, the eschar will begin to gradually slough, and a demarcation will form between the viable and the nonviable tissues. Over a period of days, weeks, or months, demarcation between healthy and dead tissue becomes more pronounced, and the viable tissues separate from the mummified until spontaneous amputation occurs (Fig. 3.4).

Some patients describe a long-lasting tingling sensation. This may be mild, or it may be particularly unpleasant and similar to an electric current sensation. The feeling is generally intensified at night. Other patients may describe a burning sensation that slowly subsides over a 3 to 4 week period. This burning sensation may be intensified with the dependent position, activity, or wearing boots. It does not occur in patients who have no tissue loss.

All frostbite victims will lose sensation to touch, pain, and temperature just proximal to the line of demarcation. In extreme cases, the loss of sensation may extend as much as 4 centimeters proximal to the demarcation. This sensory deficit may persist indefinitely.

## Physical Findings
### DEGREES OF FROSTBITE

In the past, the extent of the frostbite injury was described by degrees as in thermal burns.[26] The authors who described frostbite in this manner were impressed by similarities between thermal burns and cold injuries.

### First Degree Frostbite

First degree frostbite is characterized by hyperemia and edema. After rewarming, the tissue becomes mottled, cyanotic, and painful with intense pruritis or burning sensations. There may be desquamation of superficial tissue 5 to 10 days after the injury (Fig. 3.5.)

### Second Degree Frostbite

In a second degree injury, there is hyperemia and vesicle formation. After rewarming, the skin becomes deep red and feels hot and dry to the touch. Within 2 to 3 hours after rewarming, the injured area begins to swell. Blebs, usually containing a clear fluid, form after 6 to 12 hours (Fig. 3.6.)

### Third Degree Frostbite

Third degree frostbite is associated with necrosis of the skin and cutaneous tissues. Again, bullae form, but these frequently appear violaceous or hemorrhagic. Within 6 days after rewarming, the entire region becomes edematous. This "degree" is frequently associated with early anesthesia followed by severe deep aching or throbbing in 1 to 2 weeks.

### Fourth Degree Frostbite

A fourth degree injury is characterized by complete necrosis and loss of tissue. In this

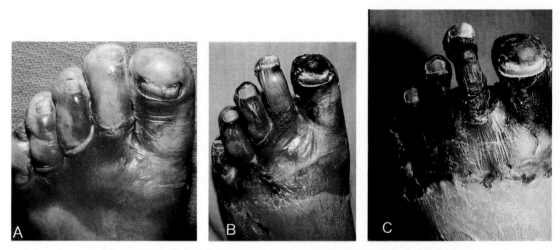

Figure 3.4 A–C. Serial changes in deep frostbite over 30 days' time (foot).

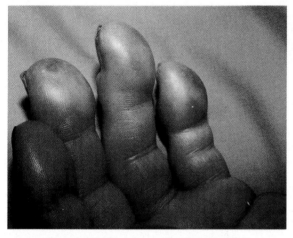

Figure 3.5. First degree frostbite (hand).

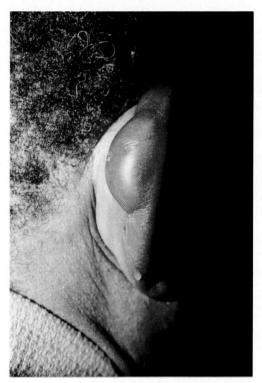

Figure 3.6. Second degree frostbite (ear).

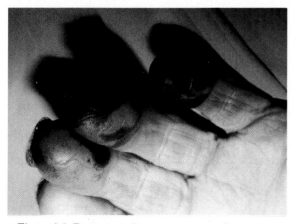

Figure 3.8. Postrewarming appearance and apparent severity of injury. (See also Table 3.2).

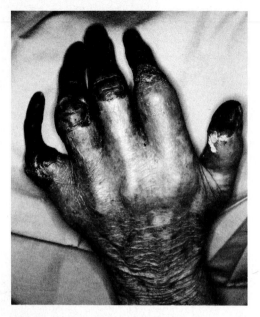

**Figure 3.7.** Fourth degree frostbite (untreated claw hand).

stage, the tissue, including the bone, is destroyed. After rewarming, the part becomes deep red, cyanotic, or mottled. There is anesthesia in the involved area, and after 6 to 12 hours, the proximal area begins to swell. The injured area does not become edematous. Dry gangrene and mummification rapidly develop (Fig. 3.7.)

## DEPTH OF FROSTBITE

The idea of "degrees" of frostbite is being replaced in emergency departments by simple differentiation into superficial and deep cold injury.[27] This is an attempt to more rapidly describe the depth and extent of the injury. In the hospital, after rewarming, it is often difficult to differentiate frostbite from trench foot or to determine the level of tissue destruction. Even after days of observation the early classification by degrees was often incorrect and misleading in prognostic value. Clinical differentiation between superficial and deep frostbite allows a more rapid description of the injury. The common old expression "frozen in January, amputate in July" illustrates the difficulty of determining the depth of the injury on the basis of clinical signs and symptoms alone.

### Superficial Frostbite

Superficial frostbite describes a sudden blanching of the skin which is followed by a white, waxy, frozen appearance. Beneath the superficial injury the tissues are resilient. This injury is often also called frostnip. It represents a reversible and superficial injury.

### Deep Frostbite

Deep frostbite occurs when the tissues are icy hard, without deep tissue resilience. The area resembles a piece of frozen meat. There is no sensation, and the patient frequently describes an extremity as "feeling like a block of wood." If the patient presents after the extremity has been thawed, these signs will not be present, and it will be difficult to classify the injury. Historical data from the patient may help in the classification process.

## PROGNOSTIC FACTORS

Damage is commonly overestimated in the early stages of frostbite, even by relatively experienced clinicians. An important part of management is to allow time for the resolution of the injuries before giving firm prognostic predictions.

### Blebs

Within 24 hours after thawing, blisters or blebs of various sizes usually develop. A relatively favorable sign is the development of blebs, filled with pinkish fluid, that extend to the ends of the affected digits. Blebs that are small, filled with purple or hemorrhagic fluid, and extend only partway to the ends of the digits are a poor prognostic sign.

In the most severe cases, the extremity is completely anesthetic, cold, bloodless, and without blisters or edema. Mummification will often begin within a few days.

## PRIOR TO REWARMING
### Mechanical Damage

Frozen tissues must be treated in a gentle fashion. Massage, rubbing with snow or ice, or ambulation are to be avoided. Patients with frostbite of the lower extremities should be considered litter patients, if at all possible.

## Freeze-Thaw-Freeze Injuries

Under no circumstances should the part be allowed to refreeze. The cycle of freeze-thaw-refreeze leads to a marked increase of tissue destruction. Indeed, this was the very point that Baron Larey had noted in his famous clinical observations quoted previously.

It should be noted that keeping the frozen part frozen without increasing the amount of frozen tissue is not an easy task. The extremity should be insulated from further cold exposure, while not so insulated that internal body heat provides a slow rewarming. Transport in heated ambulances or "snow cats" is frequently associated with slow rewarming over long transports. If the transport vehicle subsequently breaks down or becomes mired, the patient is at risk of the freeze-thaw-refreeze phenomenon. Judging the best time in a winter storm to evacuate a patient with severe cold injuries may require both judgment and experience.

## Adjunctive Diagnostic Procedures

The unpredictable necrosis and the time taken for demarcation present a dilemma to the physician. The desire to preserve as much extremity length as possible is offset by the duration of therapy required before definitive resolution of the problem. Of the physicians who have proposed classification schemes to attempt prediction, few have succeeded in any important way. Knize devised a complex scheme using many parameters to predict the extent of necrosis, but this scheme is not widely accepted.[28]

This search for quicker diagnostic classification techniques has yielded one fruitful technique—nuclear flow scanning.

### ANGIOGRAPHY

Arteriography has been used to assess tissue viability by demonstrating perfusion of the vessels in the distal part of the involved extremity. Routine angiography is relatively crude and inadequately demonstrates the smaller vessels or the microvasculature needed for continued cell life. Angiography catheters can also serve to instill vasodilating medications into the selected arterial perfusion tree.[29] This affords a "medical sympathec-

**Table 3.2.**

| Postwarming Appearance[a] (0 to 8 hours) | Probable Extent of Injury |
| --- | --- |
| Redness | Minimal |
| Tingling | Minimal |
| Local edema | Minimal |
| Sensation loss | Moderate |
| Delayed capillary filling | Moderate |
| Extremity edema | Moderate |
| Distal bullae formation | Moderate |
| Poor flushing after rewarming | Moderate |
| Severe extremity edema | Severe |
| Lack of pain or sensation | Severe |
| Lack of distal edema | Severe |
| No bullae formation | Severe |
| No capillary refilling | Severe |

[a]See also Figure 3.8.

tomy" without significant systemic effects if the total doses used are small. Serial microangiography has been used to show the changes in perfusion in the rabbit's ear, but no studies have been done with this technique in humans[30] (Fig. 3.8 and Table 3.2.)

### NUCLEAR SCANNING

Since vascular injury with subsequent interruption of blood flow is the major sequela in frostbite that appears to cause tissue death, flow studies of the region affected by the frostbite may be a useful indicator of tissue viability. Methods that have been tried include xenon[133] injected subcutaneously, bone scanning with technetium methylene diphosphonate ([99m]TcMDP), and [99m]Tc pertechnetate imaging.[31,32] Bone scanning with technetium is not a good prognostic indicator of the extent of tissue loss until at least 5 days and possibly 3 weeks have elapsed.[33] In many cases, it is the soft tissue injury that determines the extent of resection, not the bony injury that is estimated by the bone scan.

By combining the techniques of radionuclide scans and angiography, a good, early method of eliciting the depth and level of the frostbite injury has been [99m]Tc pertechnetate angiographic imaging within 24 to 48 hours after the injury is the current method of choice.[34] In multiple cases, there has been a good correlation between the flow scinti-graphic findings and the extent of deep tissue that ultimately required surgical resection. The nonviable tissue appears as a perfusion defect on the radionuclide angiogram and the subsequent static images. Persistent perfusion defects on follow-up scans 7 to 10 days after the injury are a good sign of nonviable tissue and of a need for surgical therapy. This technique has proved more accurate than Doppler flow studies or routine angiography.

### X-RAY

Plain film radiography is known to be relatively insensitive in assessing the degree of tissue damage in frostbite. Early indicators of tissue damage on x-ray are essentially non-existent.[35] Late indicators are further discussed in the section on sequelae of frostbite and are not useful in diagnosis or prognosis of the disease.

## Treatment

The treatment of a severe cold injury should begin in the field with proper management, and continue with evaluation of the situation that caused the cold injury and then rapid rewarming of the lesions in specific and the patient in general. After rewarming, there is a predictably long course of rehabilitation and demarcation of the lesions.

### FIELD CONSIDERATIONS

Rewarming should not be performed in the field if there is any danger that the extremity may be refrozen. An extremity that has already thawed should **NOT** be rapidly rewarmed. Field transportation should be by litter unless only upper extremities are involved.

Injured extremities are at very high risk for cold injury, particularly if they are splinted. Be certain to check the neurovascular status of a splinted extremity and the tightness of the splint frequently. Ensure that the ex-

tremity, if not already frostbitten, is well protected.

### AVOIDANCE OF AMBULATION

It is considered to be less damaging to walk on frozen feet to shelter than it is to stay out in the cold or to walk on feet that have been thawed and then allowed to refreeze.[36] Remember that in temperate climates, where temperatures often fluctuate daily, thawing is likely to occur spontaneously. When transporting the patient with unthawed frostbite, the patient compartment or cabin should be kept cool and the extremity kept away from the heater.

A cold-injured part should never be rubbed with snow or massaged. This can lead to irreversible mechanical trauma.

### TREATMENT OF HYPOTHERMIA

With very rare exceptions, patients who have sustained frostbite should be considered to have had such significant exposure to cold that they are at risk from generalized hypothermia. A rectal or other core temperature should be obtained on any patient who has sustained frostbite or immersion foot. Oral temperatures are usually not adequate, because some well meaning soul has frequently pressed a cup of hot drink into the victim's hands prior to recording the temperature. If the core temperature is less than 35°C (95°F), hypothermia needs to be treated before the frostbite or immersion foot.

The patient should have a thorough physical assessment with special attention to the presence of other conditions. Since many urban cases of frostbite are attributable in part to trauma or the effects of alcohol or drug use, the presence of these should be ascertained, if possible. Other conditions that should be considered include dehydration or hypovolemia, anoxia, carbon monoxide poisoning from faulty heaters or cars, and metabolic acidosis. The appropriate blood and urine determinations should be a part of the evaluation of any patient who presents with less than a completely normal neurologic examination. Under these less than optimal conditions, frostbite may easily affect more than one body part, so the emergency physician should examine other likely areas as well as the obvious injuries. (See cold injury treatment orders below.)

## REWARMING
### Warm Water

The ideal method of rewarming the freezing injury has not yet been found. Rapid rewarming by external means appears to provide better results than slow thawing but does not always give protection from tissue losses, particularly in deep or long duration freezing injuries. (See rewarming protocol below.)

The Alaskan frontier and winter military campaigns have been good testing grounds for various methods of treatment of cold injuries. In 1956, studies began to test the use of rapid rewarming of the injured area with water between 32 to 43°C (90 to 108°F) for 20 to 40 minutes.[37,38] This temperature range has seemed to provide the least amount of residual tissue damage and death.

The current preferred initial treatment for deep frostbite is rapid rewarming in a water bath at temperatures of 32 to 42°C (90 to 108°F). The temperature of the water is monitored closely. Additional hot water should be added to the bath only after the extremity has been temporarily removed. The hot water should be mixed with the cooler water and the temperature checked before replacing the extremity in the water bath.

Rewarming should be continued until a hyperemic flush extends completely to the ends of the extremities. This often takes 30 to 40 minutes. If the part has been quite deeply frozen, the flush may not extend completely to the ends of the digits. To encourage vasodilation, warm blankets and warm drinks should be offered to the patient if medically appropriate.

Rewarming is quite painful, and the patient often requires narcotic analgesia during the initial thawing phase. Intravenous narcotics are suggested for both speed of action and surety of effect. (See suggested rewarming protocol on p. 83.)

The part should not be massaged during rewarming. Do not use rapid rewarming if the part has been previously thawed.

### Nonrecommended Forms of Rewarming

Many other forms of treatment for frostbite have been tried including the following: thawing the tissue in water mixed with melting ice, rabbit or other animal fats, cods' heads, hot oil; rewarming the area with radiant heat; and massaging the affected part. The results of these methods were disastrous. They increased the incidence of gangrene, high-degree amputation, infection, and death from sepsis.

Spontaneous rewarming permits variable results that appear to be determined by the depth of injury, duration of the freezing injury, and the patient's activity during the rescue and thawing phases. Results of gradual rewarming at room temperature seem satisfactory for treatment of superficial frostbite.

Excessive heat should be avoided in the rewarming phase. Numerous anecdotal and published accounts have shown that excessive heat can lead to poor recovery. Sources of dry radiant heat at temperatures greater than 150°F (66°C) (such as found with wood fires, hair dryers, or radiant heaters) should be avoided.[39] Because the dry heat temperature is too difficult to control and the frozen part is too insensitive, the heat may cause further damage to the frozen part. Neither auto heaters nor engine exhaust should be used to rewarm a frostbitten area for the same reasons.

Unfortunately, most frostbite is not seen by physicians while still frozen. Indeed, wartime statistics revealed that less than 2% of the cold injuries were seen by a medical officer prior to rewarming.[26] In civilian practice, many of the patients with frostbite have tried one or another home remedy prior to seeking medical care. These do-it-yourself treatments can result in serious complications. Other patients will not seek care following a cold injury until bullae formation, marked cyanosis, or even gangrene of the ex-

*Routine Frostbite Orders*[a]

| | |
|---|---|
| *Diet:* | High-calorie, high-protein diet |
| | Push fluid |
| *Vital Signs:* | Every 2 hours for 24 hours then every 4 hours for 24 hours |
| | Include pulse and capillary fill of involved extremities using Doppler as indicated |
| *Isolation:* | "Reverse" with caps, gowns, and masks for 1 week |
| *No Smoking:* | Causes peripheral vasoconstriction that hampers healing |
| *Activities:* | 1. Bathroom and shower privileges |
| | 2. In hall to and from tub only |
| | 3. Whirlpool immediately following shower |
| | 4. For lower extremity injuries: |
| |    a. Use wheelchair or litter |
| |    b. Protect feet with stockinette |
| |    c. Shower sitting up only (*NO STANDING*) |
| | 5. For upper extremity injuries |
| |    a. Use plastic bags over mitts for bowel care, oral hygiene, and shaving |
| |    b. Whirlpool after shower |
| |    c. May require help in shower |
| *Wound Care:* | 1. Whirlpool b.i.d. at 95°F with Betadine followed by clear rinse and air dry |
| | 2. For lower extremity injuries: |
| |    a. Feet to air under sheet cradle |
| |    b. Cotton between digits |
| |    c. Cover feet with stockinette |
| |    d. Elevate foot of bed |
| |    e. Berger's exercises 20 minutes q.i.d. with two sessions just prior to whirlpool |
| | 3. For upper extremity injuries |
| |    a. Elevate hands on pillows |
| |    b. Wear stockinette mitts continuously |
| |    c. Constant digital exercises while awake |
| |    d. Cover mitts with plastic bags as in 5a above |
| *Consult:* | Physical therapy for whirlpool and for exercise program |
| *Lab:* | 1. Complete blood count, urinalysis, electrolytes, and blood glucose |
| | 2. Culture any purulent drainage |
| *X-ray:* | Chest x-ray |
| | X-ray of all affected extremities if any suspected trauma |
| *Medications:* | Ibuprofen or other NSAID |
| | Tetanus immunization as indicated |
| | Darvocet N-100 q. 4h. p.r.n. pain |
| | Valium 5 mg PO q. 6h. p.r.n. anxiety for 3 days |
| | Restoril 32 mg h.s. p.r.n. sleep |

[a]Stewart CE. Cold injuries. In Rakel RR, ed. Conn's current therapy. Philadelphia: WB Saunders Co., 1987:963.

tremities has occurred. It should be noted that those in Alaska have had good experience with a telephone treatment protocol for home therapy of frostbite, which is used when weather does not permit transportation to a medical facility. This telephone protocol follows the steps outlined for hospital treatment of cold injuries in this chapter.

After the patient has been rewarmed, it is frequently impossible to adequately stage the illness for hours to days. The patient's history may aid in classification, but prior inappropriate therapy may make any classification scheme unusable. These patients must be managed as appropriate for the presenting stage of their disease.

```
                    Rewarming Protocol
Before Thawing:   1. Protect the part
                  2. Do not massage or rub area
                  3. Take core temperature with hypothermia thermometer
Thawing:          1. Rewarm extremities in 100 to 108°F water
                  2. The only safe method of rewarming is a water bath with thermometer
                     control
                  3. Whirlpool is the best form of water bath
                  4. Debride all blisters and blebs
                  5. Administer morphine or meperidine for pain
                  6. Do not debride any tissue

   All patients with cold injuries of lower extremities should be treated as litter patients.

Postthaw:         1. See routine orders
                  2. Do not allow area to refreeze
                  3. Protect area from mechanical damage
```

## Postthaw Care

In addition to rewarming the frozen extremity, hospital-based treatment includes prevention of infection, promotion of healing, and preservation of function. Since much of the underlying damage of frostbite is related to the vasospasm and intravascular microemboli, substantial efforts have been directed towards the remedy of these problems.

### WOUND CARE
#### General

After thawing, the digits should be separated with cotton pledgets and the limbs elevated to minimize swelling. Most authorities agree that treatment of the cold-injured extremity should be open, although there is disagreement about this precept.[40] Occlusive dressings and wet dressings should be assiduously avoided. The injured tissue should be protected, clean, and dry. Success with dressing "bags" of flamazine in burn patients has prompted one group to use these antibiotic cream-filled bags for treatment of hand lesions with good success. Other groups are currently treating frostbite with aloe vera cream (Dermaid) and have also reported good successes. These techniques deserve a controlled study to establish their efficacy.

Reverse isolation should be practiced until the blebs rupture naturally and dry. When the injury is severe, the extremities should be protected by sheet cradles to avoid trauma and pressure. Feet should be elevated and may be covered with soft wrappings. This is not necessary for injuries to the upper extremities that may be laid upon sterile sheets on the bed over the chest and trunk. Hands may be protected with plastic bags for routine care, such as shaving, and during toilet functions.

### Antibiotics

In general, neither topical or systemic antibiotic solutions are required. Gentle debridement of superficial tissue can be adequately done by the twice daily use of a whirlpool using a Betadine solution at 30°C (90°F) temperature. This is followed by a clear rinse and air drying. Some clinicians disagree with this approach and start all nonallergic patients on penicillin until the edema resolves.[17] There are no controlled studies that validate this practice.

### Ambulation

If the lower extremities are involved, no ambulation should be permitted. Crutches or a wheelchair may be used for the first 1 to 2 weeks. If eschar limits a full range of motion or circulation, escharotomy may be performed.

### Surgical Debridement

Generally, blebs are left intact until they spontaneously rupture. Already ruptured blebs should be gently debrided. Whirlpool baths are used twice daily for 20 to 30 minutes at a time with water temperatures between 32 and 35°C (90 and 95°F). The whirlpool cleans the debris and superficial bacteria from the extremity. The gentle debridement of the whirlpool is the only surgical debridement until the demarcation is complete.

All authorities stress the absolute need to watch and wait before other surgical debridement is initiated. If given enough time (1 to 6 months), the dead tissues will demarcate and mummify—clearly delineating between dead and viable tissue. If one intervenes too early, this delineation will not be apparent and excessive tissue may be surgically excised. Splitting or bivalving of the eschar may be needed to promote joint movement and prevent stiffness.

If the extremity has remained frozen for a prolonged period of time or if significant trauma has been associated with the freezing injury, a compartment syndrome may be noted. This condition is usually found in the lower extremities, although it may be occasionally seen in the upper extremities. The diagnosis may be determined by measuring the compartment pressures; in serious cases, continuous compartmental pressure monitoring may be indicated. Fasciotomy may be required for resolution of this problem. Delay in performance of fasciotomy in the face of high compartment pressures may lead to the loss of the limb.

### Smoking

Nicotine should be avoided due to its vasoconstriction effects. Because it is vasodilating, alcohol should be avoided in the early phase of rewarming. Vasodilation of cold and frozen extremities may send a rush of cold blood to the heart. Combine this with a general hypothermia and the likelihood of fatal arrhythmias increases. Alcohol in moderation may be beneficial after rewarming is accomplished.

## ADJUNCTIVE THERAPY

### Sympathectomy

Surgical and medical regional sympathectomy have long been proposed for treating frostbite.

Surgical sympathectomy has been recommended in cold injuries severe enough to produce necrosis. Performed from 36 to 72 hours after thawing, it is thought to hasten the resorption of edema and reduce the spontaneous pain and hypersensitivity; it does not appear to increase the amount of tissue salvaged.[41,42] If a lumbar surgical sympathectomy is done, male patients must be counseled that a possible complication is permanent impotence. Sympathectomy does appear to confer some protection against subsequent cold injury.[43] It seems unlikely that the marginal improvement obtained would outweigh the risks of an additional operative procedure with its attendant complications.

Medical sympathectomies can be achieved using regional intraarterial guanethidine or reserpine.[44,45] Some studies have found that these agents cause a more rapid demarcation between viable and nonviable tissue. Onset of action of intraarterial reserpine is 3 to 24 hours after the injection with an effective duration of 14 to 21 days.[46,47] Studies using both intraarterial reserpine and tolazine do show some decreased tissue loss in the patient who has had slow rewarming, as is so often found in clinical practice. Unfortunately, neither agent is readily available in the United States.

Ganglionic-blocking agents, such as dibenzylene, can also be used to produce a systemic medical sympathectomy. They decrease vasospasm and increase the blood flow to the injured area. If systemic drugs, such as dibenzylene, are administered, the patient needs to be well hydrated to prevent orthostatic hypotension. The effects of medical sympathectomy are reversible.

### Dextran

Experimental animal model studies have shown that low molecular weight dextran, administered as soon as possible after a frostbite injury, helps to decrease red blood cell aggregation and microemboli formation.[48] These experimental results conflict with clinical studies that have failed to confirm any clear benefit in humans.[49]

## Anticoagulant and Thrombolytic Agents

Heparin and coumadin have also been tried in the early treatment with good results in animal studies but have failed to increase tissue survival in human subjects. Again, the human studies were not done in patients with controlled rewarming and may be subject to error.

Streptokinase and tissue plasminogen activator have been proposed as adjunctive agents in the treatment of frostbite, but have no clinical studies yet (unpublished communications with Genentech, Inc.) The idea of lysis of the microvascular emboli is appealing and may offer significant relief from the local hypoxic effects. Animal and human clinical studies are needed before this concept is validated. Both of these agents have significant side effects.

## Thromboxane Inhibitors

Recent studies have shown that a breakdown product of arachidonic acid, thromboxane, and the prostaglandins may increase dermal ischemia.[16] The presence of these products in the fluid obtained from the frostbite blebs of an experimental rabbit-ear model and the quicker healing after removal lead to this conclusion. In one study, aloe vera was used as a topical thromboxane inhibitor, and systemic aspirin was given to inhibit prostaglandin production. This study suggests some local perfusion benefit, but the study did not show increase in tissue survival. The quality of the healed tissue may be improved.

Since ibuprofen (and other NSAIDs) and topical aloe vera are relatively free of noxious side effects and are easily tolerated by most patients, even modest benefits in healing would justify a routine use in cases of frostbite. Further investigation using these and other similar agents is needed.

## Hyperbaric Oxygen

Hyperbaric oxygen has been used by some centers as an adjunctive therapy for frostbite. The reasoning is that if any part of the ultimate gangrene is due to a reversible vascular factor, measures that are designed to relieve local tissue anoxia will be helpful during the resolution of the vascular damage. It

is further postulated that the administration of hyperbaric oxygen will increase the oxygen content of the plasma up to 20 times, enhancing the oxygenation of the marginal tissues. Anecdotal reports have been equivocal.[50,51] Animal studies have been contradictory, and there are no controlled studies in humans.[52,53]

## Sequelae

The sequelae and amount of residual damage from frostbite are related to the extent of injury sustained during the acute episode (Table 3.3). It is important to remember that tissue damage is in proportion to the depth of the frostbite. After suffering from superficial frostbite, a person may have long-term problems, such as small muscle atrophy, fatty tissue loss, and cold sensitivity. Tissue damage follows vascular occlusion, which leads to tissue anoxia and hypoxemia. The muscle damage may partially resolve after blood flow returns to normal.

Late symptoms occur in as many as 80% of frostbite victims and may last as long as 4 years.[54] These symptoms include sensation of cold feet, excessive sweating (hyperhidrosis), and pain or joint discomfort.[55] The symptoms increase with cold weather. Color or nail-bed changes and vasomotor instability may also develop after frostbite of the distal extremities. An exaggerated vasomotor response to cold may increase the chances of another cold injury.

Urban frostbite victims may have significant psychosocial pathology that can interfere with rehabilitation efforts. These diseases range from alcoholism to drug dependence to suicidal ideation. The popular image of the cold injury amputee as the intrepid explorer, cross-country trekker, or climber caught in a blizzard is certainly not the case in urban environs.[56]

**Table 3.3.**
**Sequelae of Severe Cold Injury**

1. Small muscle atrophy
2. Scarring with possible stricture formation
3. Cold sensitivity
4. Phantom pain
5. Growth plate abnormalities
6. Arthritic changes
7. Tissue loss

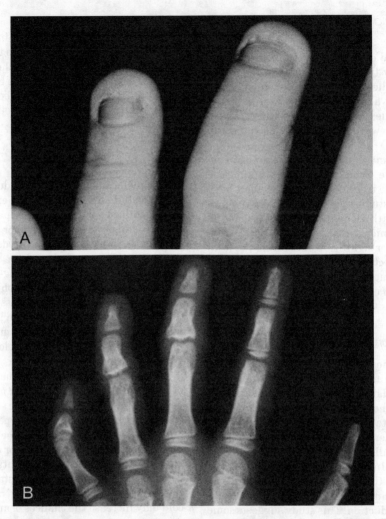

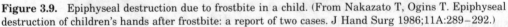

**Figure 3.9.** Epiphyseal destruction due to frostbite in a child. (From Nakazato T, Ogins T. Epiphyseal destruction of children's hands after frostbite: a report of two cases. J Hand Surg 1986;11A:289–292.)

If the injury involves the blood supply to the bones, distal bone death and subsequent amputation may ensue. Once an extremity has been amputated, phantom pain may be experienced. This is the sensation of pain or discomfort in the missing body part.

If the bone is frozen, joint space and growth plate changes may occur.[57] The basic pathophysiology appears to be the anoxia and hypoxemia suffered during the initial insult. About 50% of the patients with frostbite of the distal extremities will develop osteoarthritis months to years after the injury.[58] The radiographic findings show osteoarthritic changes similar to erosive osteoarthritis. The diagnosis is made by a history of preceding

frostbite and the asymmetric distribution of findings.

Frostbite in children may lead to epiphyseal growth abnormalities resulting in length discrepancies and deformity.[59] Epiphyseal changes in children due to frostbite are not immediately visible and do not seem to be widespread.[60] A significant x-ray finding is that the distal phalanges are the most affected, with the proximal phalanges affected only after the distal involvement.[61] Thumb damage appears to be rare, perhaps due to the clasping of the thumb in the palm of the hand found in cold weather.[62] (Figure 3.9 shows an x-ray of a frostbitten child's hands.) The exact mechanism for the epiphyseal destruction is, of course, unknown but presumed to be due to a combination of the direct freezing and the prolonged ischemia.[63]

Frostbite to the ears has rarely produced a condition known as a "petrified auricle." In this condition, the pinna becomes rock hard and develops ectopic sites of ossification. This condition also has been found in surfers who have had long-term exposure to very cold (16°C or less) water for extended periods of time.[64]

## Prevention

The prevention of frostbite requires good physical conditioning, good clothing, adequate rest, and the prevention of illness and trauma. Above all, it requires vigilance on the part of the potential victim and companions. In times of severe cold weather, activities should be planned carefully to minimize exposure times.

## OUTDOOR SPORTS

Close attention should be paid to weather and route when planning any outdoor sports. Although feeling "encumbered," the cross-country skier, hiker, or snowmobiler should pack survival equipment suitable for the worst weather encountered in the area and know how to use it. The mountain climber or hiker must also be prepared for the vagaries of the mountains and plan early withdrawal or have appropriate equipment to spend the night on the mountain in inclement cold weather. Friends, neighbors, or family should know the route taken, access points to the route, and likely shelters along the route. Once the route is decided, outdoor enthusiasts should not deviate from it without clear markings of the proposed changes.

Needless to say, winter outback sports are not appropriate for solo ventures. Even downhill skiers should use a buddy system while skiing.

Many cross-country skiers compete with exposed face, skintight clothing, and inadequate gloves and boots. Because of their grip on the poles, skiers may neglect their hands until frostbitten. Wetness from falling or perspiration should be attended to promptly with extra clothes or a change of clothes. Thin skier's racing uniforms and jogger's clothing may predispose to frostbite of the genitalia

in males and the breasts in females. This condition can be decreased by having racers and joggers don warming suits immediately after races or runs.

## PROTECTIVE CLOTHING

Protective clothing is extremely important in the prevention of both hypothermia and frostbite. Fortunately, current ski and outdoors fashions include clothes with excellent insulation and protection properties. If there is any question, dress for the weather, not for fashion. Protection is more important than looks in extreme weather.

Wear several layers of loose, warm clothing, rather than one bulky fitted layer. Polypropylene or Lycra undergarments allow moisture to escape from the layers next to the skin. Boots should be laced loosely and all tight-fitting clothes should be avoided. Boot liners must be kept dry at all times. Socks should be kept dry and wrinkle free. Extra dry socks in the survival pack may save wet feet from serious cold injury. Mittens are better in extreme weather than gloves for prevention of hand injuries. Exposure to liquids with low freezing points and direct flesh to metal contact should be avoided.

Children's winter outdoor clothing is, for the most part, not as well designed or as insulating as adult gear. This is not usually a problem for the urban child with a home to retreat to when the weather becomes too uncomfortable. With the advent of the family excursion to the great outdoors, this lack of proper gear becomes a more acute problem. The infant in the backpack carrier on the cross-country skier's back is not protected from cold and is not exerting at the same level as the parent. This seated, sedentary child becomes a setup for generalized hypothermia and for peripheral cold injuries, particularly of the lower extremities. The 6- or 7-year-old cross-country or downhill skier will lose heat more quickly because of the increased surface-to-mass ratio of childhood. This same child may have gaiters that do not adequately protect the legs, boots that are not well insulated, and gloves that are too tight or light. The unwary parent may ignore the child's subsequent complaints to the child's detriment.

Apply protective cream or petroleum jelly

to protect the child's tender skin. Ensure that extra garments are carried that can be draped about a child's carrier. "Space" blankets may be pinned to the carrier to block winds. Carry extra clothing for the young skier. With the increased frequency of falls at young ages, clothing may rapidly become wet, losing substantial insulation ability.

### WIND-CHILL

The wind-chill factor plays an important part in the development of conditions that lead to frostbite. The cooling effects of cold temperatures are markedly exacerbated by the presence of winds and are discussed in detail in Chapter 3 on hypothermia. It should be noted that exposed flesh will freeze in approximately 30 seconds with a 30 mile wind at 30 below zero Fahrenheit. This set of conditions is frequently encountered by persons approaching rescue helicopters in the mountains and less frequently by skiers and snowmobilers.

### DRUGS AND MEDICATIONS

Of course, it is much easier to discuss telling a patient to decrease consumption of alcohol or drugs than it is to have them actually do it. In one series of over 100 cases of frostbite, alcohol was implicated as a cause in over one third of the cases.[33] Likewise, the tobacco industry spends millions of dollars carefully undoing any medical advice to stop smoking. These two measures are certainly important preventative points for the physician counseling on avoidance of frostbite. Particularly important is the avoidance of smoking and subsequent vasoconstriction in the patient who has an associated diabetes or peripheral vascular disease.

Seizure and diabetic patients should be counseled on proper medication practices so that they are not caught unawares by complications of their illness while in cold weather. The subsequent unconscious period in contact with the cold ground may be sufficient to cause severe frostbite.

### CONCOMITANT ILLNESSES

Patients with peripheral vascular disease, Raynaud's phenomenon, and other concomitant illnesses should be counseled about their propensity for more rapid development of cold injuries. Patients with prior cold injuries are at particular risk for repeat cold injuries, and the injuries will be more severe than similar patients without such a history.

### SUMMARY

Frostbite is the freezing of a body part. It can be classified into superficial and deep frostbite depending on the depth of tissue destruction. The underlying mechanism of the injury is hypoxemia due to osmotic changes and/or microthrombus formation. Local metabolic changes also play a role in the extent of the injury. Certain predisposing factors are known to increase the severity of the insult. (See Table 3.1.)

Thawing is the most critical time in a frostbite injury. It should be postponed until there is no chance of refreezing. During thawing, the tissue must be protected from mechanical trauma. To thaw the injured part, it should be immersed in water, warmed to 108°F for 30 to 45 minutes. Rewarming will be painful, and analgesia should be offered to the patient. Vasoconstrictors, such as nicotine, must be avoided to maximize tissue survival.

After warming, the tissues must be managed very gently and care must be taken to postpone surgical intervention until demarcation of the injury has occurred. Demarcation may take as long as 6 months. Daily whirlpool with a povidone-iodine solution is one method used to debride eschar and nonviable tissue. Reverse isolation will protect the patient from secondary infection. Unless an infection develops, blebs should be left intact.

Although of questionable benefit, sympathectomy, aloe vera, heparin, dextran, and asprin have all been used in the care of frostbite. Sequelae depend upon the depth and extent of the injury. (See Table 3.3.)

Since the days of Napoleon, medicine has made impressive advances in the care of frostbite injuries. Mortality is rare and less tissue is lost as a result of manipulation, infection, secondary thermal burns, and early amputation than was lost only a few decades ago.

# References

1. Bishop HM, Collin J, Wood RF, Morris PJ. Frostbite in Oxfordshire: the impact of a severe winter on an unprepared civilian population. Injury 1984;15:379–380.

2. Richards T. Medical lessons from the Falklands. Br Med J 1983;286:790.

3. Larray DJ, Surgical memories of the campaigns of Russia, Germany and France. Philadelphia: Carey and Lea, 1832. (Translated by Hall.)

4. Dana AS, Rex IN, Samitz MH. The hunting reaction. Arch Dermatol 1969;99:441–450.

5. Percy EC, ed. Trauma rounds. CMA J 1972;106:261–263.

6. Jacob JR, Weisman MH, Rosenblatt SI, Bookstein JJ. Chronic pernio: a historical perspective of cold-induced vascular disease. Arch Int Med 1986;146:1589–1592.

7. Reinertsen JL. Unusual pernio-like reation to sulindac (Letter). Arch Derm 1981;117:1215

8. Herman EW, Kezis JS, Silvers DN. A distinctive variant of pernio: clinical and histopathologic study of 9 cases. Arch Derm 1981;117:26–28.

9. Kelly JW, Dowling JP. Pernio: a possible association with chronic myelomoncytic leukemia. Arch Derm 1985;121:1048–1052.

10. Barber FA. Cold injury in the military. Medical Bulletin of the US Army, Europe 1980; 37:22–27.

11. Vaughn PB. Local cold injury—menace to military operations: a review. Military Medicine 1980;145(5):305–311.

12. Dembert ML, Medical problems from cold exposure. Fam Phys 1982;25:99–106.

13. Bourne MH, Piepkorn MW, Clayton F, Leonard LG. Analysis of microvascular changes in frostbite injury. J Surg Res 1986;40:26–35.

14. Weatherly-White RC, Sjostrom B, Paton BC. Experimental studies in cold injury. II. The pathogenesis of frostbite. J Surg Res 1964;4:17–22.

15. Lazarus HM, Hutto BS. Electrical burns and frostbite: patterns of vascular injury. J Trauma 1982;22:581–585.

16. Raine TJ, London MD, Golucld L, et al. Antiprostaglandins and antithroboxames for treatment of frostbite. Surg Forum 1980;31:557.

17. McCauley RL, Hing DN, Robson MD, Heggers JP. Frostbite injuries: a rational approach based on the pathophysiology. J Trauma 1983;23:143.

18. Gadarowski JJ Jr, Esce JD. Acute systemic changes in blood cells, proteins, coagulation, fibrinolysis, and platelet aggregation after frostbite injury in the rabbit. Cytobiology 1984;21:359–370.

19. Peterson LR, Peterson LC, Peterson AK. French vanilla frostbite (Letter). N Engl J Med 1982;307;1028.

20. Hicks LM, Hunt JL, Baxter CR. Liquid propane cold injury: a clinicopathologic and experimental study. J Trauma 1979;19:701–703.

21. Sumner DS, Criblez TL, Doolittle WH. Host factors in human frostbite. Milit Med 1974;139:454–461.

22. Miller D, Bjornson DR. An investigation of cold injured soldiers in Alaska. Milit Med. 1962; 127:247–252.

23. Whayne TF. Cold injury in World War II: a study in the epidemiology of trauma. Washington, DC: US Government Printing Office, 1950.

24. Whayne TF, DeBakey ME. Cold injury, ground type. Washington, DC: US Government Printing Office, 1958.

25. Sampson JB. Anxiety as a factor in the incidence of combat cold injury: a review. Milit Med 1984;149:89–91.

26. Technical Bulletin 81. Cold injury. Department of the Army, 1976;1–13.

27. Washburn B. Frostbite. N Engl J Med 1962; 262:974–982.

28. Knize DM, Weatherley-White RC, Paton BC, Owens JC. Prognostic factors in the management of frostbite. J Trauma 1969;9:749–759.

29. Gralino BJ, Porter JM, Rosch J. Angiography in the diagnosis and therapy of frostbite. Radiology 1976;119:301–305.

30. Erikson V, Ponten B. The possible value of arteriography supplemented by a vasodilator agent in the early assessment of tissue viability in frostbite. Injury 1974;6:150–153.

31. Sumner DS, Boswick JA, Criblez TL, Doolittle WH. Prediction of tissue loss in human frostbite with xenon[133]. Surgery 1971;69:899–903.

32. Lisbona R, Rosenthal L. Assessment of bone viability by scinti-scanning in frostbite injuries. J Trauma 1976;16:989–992.

33. Miller BJ, Chasmar LR. Frostbite in Saskatoon: a review of 10 winters. Can J Surg 1980;23:423–426.

34. Salimi Z, Vas W, Tang-Barton P, et al. Assessment of tissue viability by 99mTc Pertechnetate scintigraphy. Am J Radiol 1984;142:415–419.

35. Tishler JM. The soft tissue and bone changes in frostbite injuries. Radiology 1972;102:511–513.

36. Mills WJ, Jr. Frostbite and hypothermia—current concepts. Alaska Med 1973;15:26.

37. Mills WJ, Jr. Out in the cold. Emerg Med 1979;March:211–229.

38. Mills WJ, Jr., Whaley R. Frostbite: experience with rapid re-warming and ultrasonic therapy. Alaska Med 1960;2:1.

39. Burkhalter EL, Burkhalter JA. A cold burn: a

third degree thermal injury complicating frostbite. Cutis 1984;34:82–83.

40. Page RE, Robertson GA. Management of the frostbitten hand. The Hand 1983;15(2):185–191.

41. Golding MR, Mendoza MF, Hennigar GR, et al. On settling the controversy on the benefit of sympathectomy for frostbite. Surgery 1964;56:221.

42. Golding MR, Martinez A, DeJong P, et al. The role of sympathectomy in frostbite, with a review of 68 cases. Surgery 1965;57:774.

43. Bouwman DL, Morrison S, Lucas CE, Ledgerwood AM. Early sympathetic blockade for frostbite-is it of value? J Trauma 1980;20:744–749.

44. Porter JM, Wesche DH, Rosch J, Baur GM. Intra-arterial sympathetic blockade in the treatment of clinical frostbite. Am J Surg 1976;132:625–630.

45. Kaplan R, Thomas P, Tepper H, Strauch B. Treatment of frostbite with guanethidine [Letter]. Lancet 1981;October:940–941.

46. Snider RL, Porter JM. Treatment of experimental frostbite with intra-arterial sympathectic blocking drugs. Surgery 1975;77:557.

47. Snider RL, Merhoff GC. Intra-arterial sympathetic blockade in the treatment of frostbite. Surg Forum 1974;25:237.

48. Mundth E, Long DM, Brown RB. Treatment of experimental frostbite with low molecular weight Dextran. J Trauma 1964;4:246.

49. Penn I, Schwartz SI. Evaluation of low molecular weight dextran in the treatment of frostbite. J Trauma 1964;4:784.

50. Smith G. Therapeutic applications of oxygen at two atmospheres pressure. Dis Chest 1964;45:15.

51. Cooke JN. Hyperbaric oxygen treatment in the Royal Air Force [Letter]. Proc Roy Soc Med 1971;64:881–882.

52. Okuboye JA, Ferguson CC. The use of hyperbaric oxygen in the treatment of experimental frostbite. Can J Surg 1968;11:78–84.

53. Gage AA, Ishikawa H, Winter PM. Experimental frostbite: the effect of hyperbaric oxygenation on tissue survival. Cryobiology 1970;7(1):1–8.

54. Blair JR, Schatzki R, Orr KD. Sequellae to cold injury in one hundred patients, follow up study four years after occurrence of cold injury. JAMA 1957;163:1203–1208.

55. Kumar VN. Intractable foot pain following frostbite: case report. Arch Phys Med Rhabil 1982;63:284–285.

56. Hunter J, Middleton FR. Cold injury amputees—a psychosocial problem? Prosthet Orthot Int 1984;8:143–146.

57. McKendry RJR, Frostbite arthritis. CMA J 1981;25:1128–1130.

58. Carrera GF, Kozin F, McCarty DJ. Arthritis after frostbite injury in children. Arthritis Rheum 1979;22:1082–1087.

59. Brown FE, Spiegel PK, Boyle WE. Digital deformity: an effect of frostbite in children. Pediatrics 1983;71(6):955–959.

60. Murray JJ. Pediatric aspects of nordic skiing. Ped Clin N Am 1982;29(6):1423–1429.

61. Nakazato T, Ogino T. Epiphyseal destruction of children's hands after frostbite: a report of two cases. J Hand Surg 1986;11A:289–292.

62. Bigelow DR, Boniface S, Ritchie GW. The effects of frostbite in childhood. J Bone Joint Surg [Br] 1963;45:122–131.

63. Kemp SS, Dalinka MK, Schumacher HR. Acroosteolysis: etiologic and radiologic considerations. JAMA 1986;255:2058–2061.

64. DiBartolomeo JR. The petrified auricle: comments on ossification, calcification, and exostoces of the external ear. Laryngoscope 1985;95:566–576.

# CHAPTER 4

# Generalized Hypothermia

## INTRODUCTION

Although hypothermia is usually associated with colder climates, it is not uncommon even in southern states.[1] It can happen indoors, among outdoor sports enthusiasts, or even to marathon runners on a summer day. Chronic hypothermia is becoming more common as a result of increasing heating costs among the elderly who often live on a fixed income. Hypothermia is also often unrecognized, can be caused by many situations and diseases other than environmental exposure, may complicate management of other problems, and is potentially reversible.

Hypothermia and the effects of winter have caused at least two modern commanders to lose military campaigns in Russia and have adversely affected numerous other battles from those of Alexander the Great to confrontations in Italy and Korea. Indeed, the Nazis used the excuse of battle-related hypothermic deaths as justification for experiments on concentration camp prisoners to find out better methods of management of hypothermia.[2] Hypothermia has claimed lives on every major peak in all continents and on both poles. Numerous trek leaders, marathon runners, cross-country skiers, and whitewater river runners have had firsthand experience with the effects of hypothermia.

## DEFINITIONS

Hypothermia is defined as a core body temperature of less than 35°C (95°F). Accidental

Acute—Usually reserved for submersion in near-freezing water
Subacute—Reserved for episodes involving exposure of 24 to 48 hours in cold ambient air temperatures
Chronic—Hypothermia found with extended periods of subnormal environmental temperatures or the effects of metabolic or pharmacologic changes over extended periods of time

hypothermia may be further defined by the apparent etiology of the hypothermia on the basis of duration of cooling.

## Clinical Categories of Hypothermia

The initial response to acute cold exposure is that of an intense sympathetic nervous system stimulation. It is characterized by intense shivering, generalized muscular tension, marked peripheral vasoconstricion, elevation of the blood pressure, and markedly increased respiratory rate and cardiac output. With this sympathetic outpouring, the total and myocardial oxygen consumption are markedly increased. This stress response will produce a short rise in core temperature. If the cold exposure continues, the patient's defenses will eventually be overwhelmed and hypothermia will result. The following divisions are based upon general physiologic responses to the hypothermic stress.

## MILD (32 to 35°C) [89.6 to 95°F]

This depth of hypothermia is characterized by an intense feeling of cold and subsequent shivering. Respiratory rates are increased. In cases of mild hypothermia, the body can usually mount an effective response to the cold insult by shivering, increasing vasoconstriction, and increasing the basal metabolic rate.

## MODERATE (26 to 32°C) [78.8 to 89.6°F]

With moderate hypothermia, there is a loss of the shivering reflex and a progressive decrease in the basal metabolic rate. Vasoconstriction is usually seen in the patient with moderate hypothermia.

## SEVERE (Below 26°C) [78.8°F]

In severe hypothermia, the capacity for defending the body against further heat loss is absent.

## Measurement of Temperature

A number of devices may be used to record the temperature, including liquid in glass thermometers, electronic thermocouples or thermistors, color changes in chemicals, and thermograms.

## LIQUID-IN-GLASS THERMOMETERS

The most commonly used liquid for medical thermometers is mercury, with an alcohol-water-coloring mixture following closely. The liquid is contained within a glass envelope that has a tight constriction so that the highest temperature attained may be read later.

By virtue of the glass envelope, they are fragile and broken frequently (usually just prior to being needed). The liquid in the thermometer must be shaken to move it below the constricting neck of the glass vessel. If this is not properly done, the thermometer will be broken or inaccurate. The glass thermometer must be inserted into an orifice, such as the rectum or the mouth, for accurate readings. Placing the thermometer in the rectum may mean exposing the patient repeatedly to a hostile environment. Since it measures the highest temperature in the vicinity, it cannot be used easily to follow a rapidly changing temperature. The common clinical thermometer only registers down to 35.5°C (96°F), which severely limits its utility in the care of the hypothermic patient.

Still, the glass thermometer is the least expensive temperature-measuring device available. Special low-reading clinical thermometers are easily procured and should be available in all emergency departments, ambulance services, and rescue groups. Trek leaders should have one among the first-aid equipment.

## ELECTRONIC THERMOMETERS

The most useful instrument for temperature measurement is the electronic thermometer. The temperature range of electronic thermometers is far greater than the best liquid-in-glass thermometer. They are more easily read and are far more accurate. Unfortunately, they require electric power, often in the form of batteries. Murphy, a noted authority on critical component failure, often expounds on the propensity of power supply failure.[3] This device may be used remotely, either with telemetry, or allowing a stretcher-side reading during an evacuation. The probes may be made in a number of shapes and sizes, allowing easier insertion into bodily orifices. The electronic thermometer can be used to accurately measure the skin temperature.

## COLOR CHANGES IN CHEMICALS

Certain chemicals will change color with a sharply defined temperature gradient and have been used to measure skin temperature. Unfortunately, the only systems available do not measure below the normal clinical temperature range.

## THERMOGRAPHY

Thermography records the radiant heat from a surface either by a camera with infrared film or with an electronic camera equipped with appropriate infrared optics. This method cannot measure well the absolute temperature of a body but can easily map "hot spots" over the surface. This has been used to record the areas of high heat losses but is generally only used as a research tool.

## CORE TEMPERATURE

Esophageal probes may provide the most accurate of the "core" measurements. The close proximity of the esophagus to the great vessels means that the esophageal temperature accurately reflects the temperature of the heart.[4] Measurement of the esophageal temperature requires an electronic thermometer probe placed below the level of the carina. Emergency personnel have little experience in the placement of these probes; hence they are often not used in the field.

The rectal temperature is the most often measured temperature in the field treatment of hypothermia. It is also the most frequent measurement in the emergency department. It is useful for an initial assessment of the subacute or chronic hypothermic patient but may not bear a good relationship to core temperature in the acutely hypothermic patient. Feces warms at a different rate than tissue, and the decreased pelvic circulation may mean that the rectal temperature lags substantially behind the true core temperature. As noted earlier, the patient must be exposed each time a glass thermometer is used rectally.

Tympanic measurements are also frequently touted as being the closest to the core cerebral temperature. Placement of these tympanic probes requires an otoscope and some clinical training. If improperly placed, they may perforate the tympanic membrane or give inaccurate results.

Recent technologic improvements have allowed development of an electric tympanic thermograph. This device allows rapid (15 seconds) determination of tympanic temperature without direct contact. The effect of cerumen or blood in the otic canal is touted as insignificant. The devices are battery powered and quite portable. Further field evaluation is indicated for this device.

The oral temperature is often criticized but is quite useful in the field. The true core temperature should not be lower than the mouth temperature so that the oral reading is a useful screening measurement. Provided that the patient has not recently consumed hot food or drink, an oral temperature of 37°C (98.6°F) should be considered normothermic.

## CLINICAL SUSPICION

Hypothermia should be considered in all patients who have been exposed to cold, and have a less than normal level of consciousness. It should also be suspected in any patient who has a temperature reading less than 35.5°C (96°F). (A reminder: Some thermometers will only measure to that temperature.) Shivering is an important clue but may be suppressed in the face of depletion of glucose stores or physical exertion. Hypothermia is frequently found in the patient who has sustained trauma in a cold environment and in the patient who has suffered a localized cold injury.

The astute physician can often appreciate clinical hypothermia on physical examination alone. When the patient's abdomen, axilla, or trunk, under the covering clothing, is cooler than the physician's exposed hand, the patient is hypothermic until proven otherwise. This finding may not be so useful in the completely unclothed patient, however. The emergency provider in a field or rescue situation may rapidly differentiate unconsciousness due to hypothermia from other causes with this finding.

An axillary temperature reading of greater than 35.5°C (96°F) will likewise preclude hypothermia. The rescue team leader can use this as a screening tool in care of multiple casualties. This skin temperature simply is a more accurate version of skin palpation described above.

Forgey recommends the "walk a straight line" technique for field diagnosis of hypothermia.[5] If the victim proves unable to walk a straight line for a distance of 10 meters, then ataxia from hypothermia is a likely problem. Unfortunately, ataxia is also noted in altitude illnesses and may be found associated with exhaustion, hypoglycemia, and dehydration (as postural hypotension), so this test is not pathognomonic. It does indicate that a member of the party has potential problems and needs immediate therapy. Generally, each member of a group should be monitored, but particular scrutiny should be made of the most fatigued, least conditioned, or most poorly equipped team member.

Hypothermia in the field may be a significant problem and early recognition is important. The initial signs may not be appreciated by leaders who are nearly as cold as subjects. As hypothermia increases, judgment fails, and the hypothermic patient may imperil others in the party as well as self.

## DEFENSES AGAINST THE COLD

Humans have evolved in the savannah and plains and are superbly designed to shed heat. Unfortunately, we are not well designed enough to maintain that heat against the fall of night or winter weather. Our endogenous defenses are limited, and until we were able to design and carry our microclimates with us, we were unable to venture easily into cold weather. We rely upon behavioral thermoregulation for these ventures.

An attempt to lower the body's temperature is met with mobilization of the body's defenses against cold, which produces a complex interaction between mechanisms against heat losses and simultaneous increase of heat production. These defenses are both passive and active and include the clothing worn by the victim. The body can be modeled in three layers to visualize the endogenous thermoregulatory mechanisms. At the innermost layer, the core, the temperature is defended stoutly against all temperature changes. This core consists of the central nervous system, heart, lungs, and abdominal organs. The outermost layer, the skin, subcutaneous tissue, and thermoreceptor sites may be the most important portion of the heat control mechanisms. Here, the temperature varies widely with blood flow, external (ambient) air temperature and flow, humidity, or water flow or evaporation. The outer shell may drop to nearly ambient surface temperature as blood flow plummets in an attempt to conserve the core temperature. The middle shell, the muscular layer, provides a marked heat production in times of need, albeit at enormous energy expenditure. To these shells must be added the insulative effects of the clothing worn by the victim. These, then, are the assets in the war against the fall of winter weather.

### Basal Heat Production

Heat is produced by the metabolism of food through normal enzymatic and metabolic processes of life. At the basal metabolic rate, heat is produced at about 50 kcal/m$^2$ of body surface area per hour or about 70 to 100 kcal/hr for the average person. This core heat is a relatively fixed asset in cold weather, changing within only small limits.

Thermal suppression and activation of the sympathetic nervous system by a cold-induced secretion of norepinephrine in humans will cause an initial increase in basal metabolic rate. Part of this rate increase is due to a general increase in muscle tone and increases the metabolic rate to about twice the normal amount.[6]

Unfortunately, basal metabolism is also suppressed by hypothermia. At 28°C (82.4°F), basal metabolic rate falls to 50% of the normal levels. This results in lower oxygen consumption and decreased use of glucose. Below 24°C (72.2°F), both autonomic and endocrinologic mechanisms for heat conservation are lost.

### Insulation Layer

Muscle and subcutaneous fat are excellent insulators, when not perfused, with a conductivity = 18 kcal/hr/°C gradient (similar to cork). More obese males and females have thicker mantles of this insulating layer. With the normal amount of insulation about the core at maximum vasoconstriction, only about 20 to 40 kcal/hr are transported to the surface by heat conduction from the core to the skin. The rest of the heat produced by metabolism is transported by movement of warm blood from the core to the skin and subcutaneous tissues.

### Vasomotor Tone

As the temperature falls, surface and subcutaneous vessels immediately constrict, effectively decreasing the circulation to the skin and increasing the insulation of the body. This mechanism is our fastest and earliest defense against cold. The vasoconstrictor mechanism is so effective that upon skin exposure to cold and subsequent vasoconstriction, the core temperature RISES about 0.5°C. Under these conditions of surface cooling, blood flow to the skin and subcutaneous tissues is reduced tenfold.

Vasomotor tone is lost at about 26 to 28°C (78.8 to 82.4°F), as the nerves are no longer able to fire and the muscles no longer able to contract easily.[7] There is some evidence that part of the lost vasomotor tone may be due to a cold-induced insufficiency of epinephrine and related analogs. This loss of vasomotor tone means that the human body is now effectively poikilothermic and unable to protect itself from the environment.

## Shivering

Shivering is the body's main involuntary defense from the cold. This uncontrolled rhythmic contraction and relaxation of the skeletal muscles is initiated by the hypothalamus or by skin temperature receptors.[8] The shivers are produced by the action of muscle antagonists at a rate of about 6 to 12 cycles per second. This pattern of muscle activity increases metabolic heat production to about 500 kcal/hr while minimizing the wide excursions of limbs that increase radiation and convection heat losses.[9] Shivering is initiated at about a 37°C (98.6°F) core temperature and plays both a fine-tuning and emergency role in maintenance of core temperature.

Shivering is abolished by any of four conditions: the core temperature rising above 37°C (98.6°F); the core temperature falling below about 30°C (86°F); the victim becoming hypoglycemic; or the victim taking a medication that abolishes the shivering response. When the core temperature rises, shivering is no longer needed and is shut down by the hypothalamus. When the core temperature falls to about 30°C (86°F), the shivering reflex is abolished. Likewise, when there is no further fuel in the form of glucose or glucose substrate, the hypothalmus abolishes shivering. Multiple medications, including barbiturates, beta-blocking agents, phenothiazines, and possibly alcohol, will suppress the shivering response, partially or completely.

Shivering is an inefficient form of energy production. It causes an increased blood flow to the muscles and shunts warm blood from the core. It also causes some skin vasodilation. This increases heat losses by about 25%. Shivering may double or treble oxygen consumption and carbon dioxide production.

## Exercise

The ability to voluntarily exercise is the most efficient defense against the cold that the body possesses. Exercise is not only more efficient than shivering, it can accomplish useful tasks. As noted in the chapter on heat injuries, strenuous exercise can produce as much as 1000 kcal/hr additional heat. Indeed, skiing cross-country uphill at maximal speed produces as much as 1100 kcal/hr. This extraordinary exercise capacity is possible for only world class athletes and then only for brief durations. Even the slowest running speeds can result in energy expenditures equivalent to eight or nine times the resting metabolic rates, but only well-conditioned athletes can tolerate expenditures of 700 to 800 kcal/hr for a long duration. It is obvious that one of the best preparations for an emergency in the cold is good physical conditioning.

Exercise brings with it the complications of increased sweating, peripheral vasodilation, and expenditure of energy reserves. Sweating wets clothes and temporarily wrecks the insulation value of many fabrics and insulation materials. Increased sweating also causes increased evaporative heat losses. Peripheral dilation increases radiation from the skin's surface areas and ruins the insulative values of the subcutaneous tissue. If exercise is continued, despite decreasing reserves of food and water, circulation in the muscles may be maintained at the expense of core temperature. When energy reserves are depleted, exercise and shivering produce no further heat.

## Clothing

At the heart of the behavioral thermoregulation that allows humans to venture into the cold is the accessory insulating layer we know as clothes. When adequately protected, humans can tolerate temperatures as low as −58°C (−72.4°F), but they can withstand only about a 4 or 5°C core temperature variation without impairment of working capacity. Adequate clothing maintains our "microclimate" surrounding the body. The following discussion of clothing should be considered only an introduction, and further information is available from multiple sources.

Air is a superb insulator, and the basis of

most clothing worn is to trap a layer of air about the body. The standard reference—a clo—is the amount of insulation provided by dress that will maintain comfort at room temperatures of 21°C (70°F) with a relative humidity of less than 50% and a wind of only 20 feet per minute. This corresponds roughly to standard business attire. By way of contrast, a runner moving at 6 to 7 mph will need insulation of only about 1 clo at temperatures as low as −34.3°C (−30°F). The winter jogger or cross-country skier can easily testify to the lack of clothing needed with these strenuous activities.

When the hiker or camper is not going to maintain an extensive level of exercise for a prolonged period of time, more insulation will likely be needed. To maintain the greatest flexibility of dress, layering has been used for centuries. This allows the removal or opening of a garment to vent excess heat during times of greater exercise.

Four layers are considered optimum for most camping or hiking activities. These four layers are the undergarments, clothing layer, insulation layer, and an outer shell. The undergarment layer maintains comfort next to the skin. The clothing layer absorbs moisture and provides some insulation, while the insulation layer provides the bulk of the insulation. Shells are used to protect against wind, rain, and snow. For active use, insulation should be effective, even when wet. In this respect, the synthetics are clearly superior to the natural fibers or products. Down, for example, is virtually useless when wet. A sole exception is the well-known insulation retained by wool, even when wet.

Clothing for children should be examined as critically as that for adults. With the higher surface-area-to-mass ratios, and relative inactivity, infants in backpack carriers are at increased risks of hypothermia compared to the parent carrying them. Older children should have extra dry clothing to change into after the inevitable fall or romp in the snow.

## Acclimation

Adaptation to the cold is poor or nonexistent in humans. Humans have a relatively constant resting heat production, which cannot be changed except by exercise or shivering. Humans also have little nonshivering ther-

mogenesis, perhaps due to the scanty deposits of brown fat. Anecdotal evidence suggests that we may reduce the discomfort of the cold by adaptation, but there is little physiologic adaptation to colder climates. Most adaptation cited is behavioral, with better shelter, clothing, and habits to keep warmer.

There is some adverse adaptation, however. With repeated exposure or slow onset of cooling, shivering responses may be reduced or even abolished at a set temperature. This may be one of the causative factors in chronic hypothermia of the elderly.

## MECHANISMS OF HEAT LOSS

### Conduction

Conduction is the direct transfer of heat from the human frame to the surrounding environment (or from the environment). Conduction is most important in immersion hypothermia, because water conducts heat nearly 30 times more rapidly than air, and water has a specific heat capacity of 1000 times that of dry air. This means, practically, that cold water will remove vast amounts of heat from the body quite rapidly. Conductivity is of great importance in the patient who is lying directly on the ground or pavement during the wintertime.

Exercise and shivering are not as effective in cold water as they are in cold air because they tend to increase the blood flow to the muscle groups. This increased blood flow, unfortunately, brings warmer core blood to the surface where it is rapidly cooled, which leads to increased conductive (and convective) heat losses from the uninsulated extremities.

### Radiation

Radiation is the transfer of heat by electromagnetic waves. The most familiar example of radiation is the warm sun's rays on an otherwise cold winter day. All objects radiate heat, and if there is a temperature differential, heat is transferred from higher temperature objects to lower temperature objects. At an ambient temperature of about 20°C (68°F), as much as 70% of basal heat production is lost by radiation. More heat is lost in the spread eagle position than in fetal position.

Blood flow to the head comprises about 20% of the body's total cardiac output and cannot be restricted significantly by vasocon-strictive responses. This means that heat loss from the uncovered head can account for as much as 50% of the body's total heat production at 4°C (39.2°F).

## Evaporation

Sweating is of lesser importance in the non-exercising patient in the cold. Some sweating is obligatory (insensible water losses), but normal sweating is inhibited by cold. In a cold environment, evaporation from insensible perspiration accounts for only 20 to 25% of the basal heat production. It becomes a major factor in those who are exercising heavily such as snow shovelers, cross-country skiers, and long distance runners. Evaporation is also of profound importance in patients who have become wet by other means and are now drying off. Each liter of water will cause the loss of approximately 580 kcal of heat from the body.

## Convection

Convection is the block movement of air or water from around the body. Still air or water next to the body is warmed. Movement strips this warmed layer away, necessitating the rewarming of a new layer of water or air. Convection thus carries away heat far more quickly than simple evaporation or conduction.

This wind or water chill depends upon the temperature and the velocity of the air or water, respectively. Dr. Paul Siple, in 1945, compared the time that it took water to freeze at varying temperatures and wind velocities. Those wind velocities and temperatures with similar freezing times were "equivalent."

## Transpiration

Cold air must be warmed to core temperature and completely humidified as it enters the lungs, in order to prevent drying of the mucous membranes. The evaporative heat losses caused by humidifying and warming the air during breathing are labeled transpiration. These heat losses amount to about 25 to 30 kcal/hr to warm air from 20°C (68°F) to body temperature. For −40°C (−40°F) air, the losses are about 60 kcal/hr. For a warm climate, this amounts to a minimal amount of heat loss for humans. Animals, such as dogs, frequently employ transpiration as a significant means to decrease a heat load. In winter, this insensible heat loss, even in properly insulated individuals, may be quite significant and is not easily modified.

## CAUSES OF HYPOTHERMIA

Factors leading to the development of hypothermia can be divided into three general causes:

Decreased heat production
Impaired thermoregulation
Increased heat loss

*Decreased heat production* commonly results from endocrine disorders, such as hypoglycemia, myxedema, or Addison's disease. Depletion of nutritional reserves by starvation, anorexia nervosa, or malabsorption syndromes may also contribute to decreased heat production.

*Impaired regulation* of the body's temperature results from the aging process, cerebrovascular accidents, skull trauma, neoplasms, and drug use. Obviously, an intoxicated patient incapable of seeking proper shelter will become hypothermic. Alcohol may also contribute to hypothermia by diminishing peripheral vasoconstrictive reflexes to cold. The causative role of drugs and alcohol in a large percentage of urban hypothermics is well known to most urban emergency departments. The use of phenothiazines, barbiturates, and tricyclic antidepressants also increases the risk of becoming hypothermic. These drugs impair the centrally mediated vasoconstriction response and may abolish the shivering reflex.

*Increased heat loss* can be easily attributed to environmental factors. What is not as well appreciated are the iatrogenic causes of heat loss: cool operating rooms, emergency departments, and intensive care units; lavage (both external and internal) with unwarmed or even iced solutions; or transfusion and fluid replenishment with cool solutions. Additional causes of increased heat loss can include skin diseases and burns.

Obviously, the cooler the ambient temperature, the easier an unprotected person becomes hypothermic. The two effects of wind and increased conduction of heat by water can be cumulative with marked heat loss in unprotected, wet individuals.

Organ failure, sepsis, shock, and myocardial infarctions may have multifactorial causes for the hypothermia that is commonly associated with them.

## PREDISPOSING FACTORS FOR HYPOTHERMIA

Although the cause of hypothermia can frequently be traced to purely environmental effects, predisposing factors contribute to the rapidity of the fall in temperature, the final temperature reached, and, most importantly, the possibility of recovery from the insult.

### Age

Certain groups are particularly vulnerable to hypothermia, including the elderly and children.

#### INFANTS

Hypothermia has been well studied in the newborn infant to include the potential of generalized hemorrhagic complications, implications for sepsis, and therapy. The total lack of ability to avoid the cold, high surface-area-to-mass ratio, minimal muscle mass, and wet surface of the newborn are sufficient causes for quite severe hypothermia. Pediatricians, obstetricians, and emergency providers are thoroughly briefed about the implications of hypothermia in the newborn and take immediate action to correct the problem. While not usually a significant problem in developed countries with the prompt recognition and easy therapy, this is not the case in undeveloped nations.[10] Both radiant heat and heated rectal and gastric lavage have been used to treat these miniature patients. Mortality is much lower with rapid rewarming than with slow external rewarming in the hypothermic newborn.

It is entirely conceivable that an unsupervised or emergent birth may present with mild or moderate hypothermia in the newborn. Wrapping the child in appropriate insulation, placing the child at the mother's breast if possible, and then further insulating both of them is the appropriate field therapy.

If transport is significantly delayed for any reason, 100 cc/kg of 10% glucose solution administered orally or via an umbilical catheter is indicated.

#### CHILDREN

In skiers, a disproportionate number of cases of hypothermia are found in children.[11,12] This disproportionate representation may be due to inappropriate insulation of children's clothing, to the increased body-to-surface-area ratio of children in comparison to adults, and to a tendency of the child to ignore the symptoms of hypothermia in games or play.

#### THE ELDERLY

There is a considerable difference in the mortality of the young, healthy athlete trapped outdoors in adverse weather conditions and the elderly patient. The difference is particularly dramatic in the case of those older than 75 years for whom the risk of death from hypothermia is about five times higher.[13] Differences in the ability to detect cutaneous temperature changes, varying degrees of autonomic dysfunction, decreased muscle mass and thus ability to shiver, and increased use of vasoactive medications all are implicated in the higher incidence of hypothermic geriatric patients.[14] Certainly, the inability to mount an appropriate cardiovascular response to the cold, coupled with medications designed to cause vasodilation—or to produce vasodilation as a major side effect—will hamper the elderly in maintaining their core temperature at even modestly cool ambient temperatures. When one couples the decreased responses with a decreased budget for food and fuel, inadequate or inappropriate clothing, and the potential use of alcohol, phenothiazines, or other mental-status-altering medications, one sets the stage for chronic hypothermia.

Secondary causes of hypothermia are likewise more common in the aged. Sepsis and hypoglycemia are important secondary causes of hypothermia and are discussed separately. Eighty percent of myxedematous patients are hypothermic, and the presence of hypothermia is clearly correlated to an increased mortality.

Unfortunately, although the elderly are a

high-risk group for morbidity with hypothermia and for development of hypothermia, little education is aimed at this risk group. The elderly should be considered vulnerable. Both the elderly and their caretakers should be informed of the dangers of hypothermia, the predisposing conditions, and the early clinical signs of hypothermia.

## Infection

Infection is frequently noted as a predisposing factor for patients with nonexposure hypothermia.[15-17] Indeed, numerous authors recommend empiric antibiotics in elderly hypothermic patients on this basis. A review of the cases of hypothermic patients who are not victims of obvious exposure does reveal a high percentage of occult infections. It is difficult for the physician to identify those patients with infection at the time of admission to the emergency department. Mortality in the septic patients will be much higher than in noninfected patients.

It should also be noted that cold adversely affects the defenses against infection. Pneumonia is recognized as a frequent complication as will be noted later. Ciliary motion in the pulmonary tree is decreased, lymphocyte motility is slowed, and resistance to endotoxins is lowered. All of these will predispose a hypothermic patient to infection.

Hypothermia may also obscure an infection. Past medical historical data are typically lacking in these comatose or obtunded patients. Chest x-rays may not reflect a pneumonia due to the dehydration following a cold diuresis. Warmth and erythema are lacking in the cold skin surfaces.

## Hypoglycemia

The occurrence of hypothermia together with hypoglycemia has been noted for more than 40 years. The cause of the hypoglycemia may be inappropriate doses of insulin, effects of alcohol, or exhaustion of available glucose stores by exercise or malnutrition.[12] Hypoglycemia can produce hypothermia by at least two distinct mechanisms: inhibition of shivering and involuntary increase in sweating. In light of these responses, all hypothermic patients should be treated with intravenous glucose immediately after a blood specimen has been obtained, unless serum glucose values are immediately available. Customary doses of glucose for age and body weight are appropriate. Central inhibition of shivering occurs when the plasma glucose falls below about 45 mg/dl.[18,19] The decreased shivering is apparently mediated by the hypothalamus.[20] Intravenous glucose will rapidly reverse this decrease in shivering.

Tachycardia and sweating frequently accompany the outpouring of catecholamines associated with hypoglycemia. This involuntary sweating, even when temperatures are low, can trigger hypothermia by evaporative heat losses. Needless to say, if the hypoglycemia is so profound as to produce unconsciousness, then hypothermia can be easily evoked by purely environmental means.

Paradoxically, in some hypothermic patients, serum glucose is elevated. It is thought that decreased pancreatic insulin release, decreased tissue consumption of glucose, decreased effects of insulin at lower temperatures, and possibly decreased liver function all contribute to the hyperglycemia noted in these patients. Diabetic ketoacidosis has been implicated in some of these hypothermic patients, but in view of the decreased action of insulin at temperatures below 30°C (86°F), it is clearly inappropriate to treat these patients until they have been warmed.[21]

## Trauma

A traumatized patient in a cold environment is at a higher risk of becoming hypothermic because of the decreased cardiovascular function associated with shock. If rescue time is prolonged, then severe hypothermia develops more rapidly than in untraumatized patients. This accelerated rate of onset of hypothermia has grave applications for rescue and emergency providers in the field.

There appears to be no little substantial difference in management of either trauma or hypothermia in these cases, but rewarming technique needs careful consideration. Heparinization for cardiopulmonary bypass or hemodialysis is probably not appropriate in the face of multiple trauma. Abdominal trauma precludes the use of peritoneal dialysis. Open lavage of the mediastinum may well be the technique of choice in these patients.

### Drug and Alcohol Use

The association between alcoholic intoxication and hypothermia is well known to urban emergency practitioners. The hypothermic homeless and drunken tramp found on the street after a sudden cold snap is a familiar site to paramedics and physicians alike. Indeed, in studies of hypothermia in Sweden, two thirds of fatalities are intoxicated.[22] The mean serum concentration of alcohol in this group was 160 mg/dl.

As noted earlier, much of our ability to tolerate cold weather is due to learned responses, not innate reflexic actions. It is certain that if the patient is so drunk as to be unable to make the judgment to remove himself from the cold environment, the "anesthetic" effects of alcohol will cause hypothermia. This is probably the major reason for the increased incidence of alcoholics in series investigating hypothermia. Whether the alcohol can cause a lesser abolition of the victim's responses resulting in an indifference to colder climates is open to some question. Alcohol, hypnotics, and barbiturates given in sufficient doses also will all abolish the shivering response, with subsequent increased rates of cooling noted.

Alcohol also supposedly causes an inappropriate peripheral vasodilation in the face of cold ambient temperatures, causing a more rapid cooling of the victim. Of the peripheral vasodilation theory of alcohol's actions in hypothermia, there are questions. Investigators have shown that ethanol has no major influence on the overall skin circulation, despite the multiple unsubstantiated theories to the contrary.[23] In fact, survival in alcoholics seems to be somewhat higher at the same low core temperature than in nonintoxicated persons, almost as if alcohol actually did act as an "antifreeze." Of course, more alcoholics put themselves into a position to become severely hypothermic, with subsequent higher rates of hypothermia noted among alcoholics.

Wernicke's encephalopathy is specifically notable as a cause of hypothermia among chronic alcoholics. Although coma and hypothermia are not common complications of Wernicke's encephalopathy, they are remarkable in their implications for ease of treatment. Use of thiamine in all hypothermic alcoholics or suspected alcoholics is appropriate therapy. Omission of thiamine will cause increased mortality in an otherwise treatable condition.[24]

It can be expected that other intoxicating drugs such as heroin and barbiturates would remove the patient's impetus to find a warm environment or take other self-protective measures. Indeed, operative anesthesia with all anesthetic agents is associated with perioperative hypothermia if the patient is not properly protected, whether or not paralytic agents are used.

### Exercise

Although exercise is one of the most efficient ways to produce endogenous heat, it is at times a distinct predisposition for hypothermia. The high levels of heat production in the trained athlete may cause the same athlete to shed clothing. The increased sweating and transpiration are also rapidly conducting the heat away. If the wind increases, or the athlete stops exercising, hypothermia rapidly results. This is not infrequent in marathon runners and cross-country skiers.[25,26] In heavily exercising patients, even with adequate clothing, the combination of wind and wetness from sweat may reduce the insulation of the clothing to nearly zero.

### Immersion Hypothermia

Many of the most pleasurable wilderness and outdoor activities involve the hazards of exposure to cold and sometimes even icy water. This can include sailing and boating and its variants, white-water rafting and boating, caving, ice skating, sport diving, and even hunting or fishing. Nor is play the only reason for submersion in cold water. Work environments for divers and sailors, in particular, may involve immersion in icy waters. Professional divers are subject to immersion hypothermia due to increased losses not only through the skin, but through the respiratory system. Most instances of immersion hypothermia are probably of brief duration, unreported, and are treated by companions or local medical authorities without either hospitalization or ill effects.

When a human is plunged into icy water from a fall, the shock from the immediate and intense cooling elicits several reflexes. The first reflex is an involuntary gasp as one enters the water. The tachypnea that follows the gasp is more severe than that of the patient suddenly exposed to dry cold air. There is a simultaneous profound outpouring of catecholamines with a rapid rise in heart rate and increase in blood pressure. The blood pressure is also increased because of the cold-induced peripheral vasoconstriction. In other patients, the plunge may cause a vagally mediated bradycardia, particularly if the face is immersed by the fall into cold water.

Unfortunately, all of these reflexes have potentially fatal results not caused by generalized hypothermia. If the victim is underwater when the initial gasp occurs, there is a high likelihood of aspiration. The elaboration of catecholamines combined with the tachycardia and increased blood pressure may overwhelm those who have marginal circulatory reserves, leading to myocardial infarctions or cerebrovascular accidents. The same factors may induce fatal tachydysrhythmias or ventricular fibrillation. These arrhythmias have even occurred in younger patients.[27] The vagal bradycardia may cause a syncopal episode, which can cause drowning. The sudden entry of cold water into the ear may cause a caloric labrynthitis with subsequent disorientation and vertigo. Cold-induced tachypnea may cause respiratory alkalosis and tetany with resulting decreased ability to swim. Finally, the profound tachypnea may rarely cause hyperventilation syncope, with fatal results in the water.

Few victims die of the immediate complications of accidental immersion in cold water. As the victim stays in the water, grave heat losses are occurring from conduction and convection. How well the victim fares after the first few minutes depends upon the balance of heat production with heat losses. Heat losses in still water are up to 25 times more than in still air, simply because of the differences in thermal capacity and conductivity of air and water. The heat loss is partially balanced by insulation, either from fat or from clothing and by metabolism.

Shivering alone is not sufficient heat production to balance the losses. When volunteer subjects were immersed in 10°C (50°F) water, Hayward found that skin temperatures dropped within 5 to 10 minutes to nearly that of the water.[28] Shivering-induced metabolic heat production rose to about twice basal rates. After 15 to 20 minutes, core temperatures fell

and shivering and metabolic rates rose to a maximum of four to five times basal levels as the core cooled to 33 to 35°C (93 to 95°F). Despite these increases, core temperatures continued to fall.

If the patient starts to exercise or swim, then increased convection losses cause quicker heat losses than in the still patient. Movement of the arms and legs sweeps away the layers of warmed water from the body, causing rapid heat losses. More efficient head down swimming is often very uncomfortable or impossible in cold water, leading to slow progress towards shore. Indeed, survival times for the inactive patient are about 50% longer than survival times of swimmers. Swimming becomes more difficult in the cold water as the muscles stiffen and the arms and legs become numb from the effects of hypothermia. Clothing presents an encumbrance if left in place and more rapid heat losses if removed. A widely taught technique, drown-proofing, will cause even more heat losses without significant movement towards shore as the arms are widely held from the body and then swept down.

Rescuing and resuscitating the victim of a cold water submersion is a complex problem. The victim is protected, to a degree, by the hypothermia from the hypoxic insult. Rewarming before maintenance of the airway and breathing will remove any hypothermic protection from hypoxia. Slow rewarming is advocated by some authorities to ensure that the protective effects of hypothermia are not eliminated before the patient has adequate protection of the respiratory system. It is in precisely this patient that rapid institution of cardiopulmonary bypass should be considered with the resultant ability to both rewarm and reoxygenate the patient expeditiously.

Further management of near-drowning, to include the protective effects of cold and of the submersion or mammalian dive reflex, is covered in Chapter 11. If the victim is near a tertiary center with availability of cardiopulmonary bypass, diversion of the hypothermic submersion patient to this center for rewarming and therapy should be a protocol.

## CLINICAL MANIFESTATIONS

When the patient is exposed to a cold environment, the initial reflex response of the body is to preserve heat in the core. The peripheral small blood vessels will constrict. At the same time, there is a release of circulating catecholamines. This sympathetic response will cause an increase in the heart and respiratory rate, the blood pressure, and, of course, the basal metabolic rate.

If the patient stays in the cold, the shivering reflexes are activated. Shivering, an involuntary reflex, will markedly increase the heat production of the body and is the major defense against cold. If heat losses continue to exceed the production of heat from shivering, the patient's core temperature will continue to fall. Shivering will continue until the core temperature approaches 30°C (85°F), until glucose or insulin reserves have been depleted, or until the patient warms to about 37°C (98.6°F). If the patient is no longer able to shiver and is still exposed to the cold environment, the core body temperature will fall rapidly.

Hypothermia's characteristic clinical manifestations correspond roughly with the drop in core temperature. Unfortunately, there is not a one-to-one relationship between core temperature and clinical signs. There is a general decline in the physiologic responses after the initial catecholamine response has waned. The respirations begin to decline slowly, and the pulse rate and blood pressure now decrease.

As the core temperature drops, so does consciousness and the ability to take further protective actions. Before coma intervenes, the victim is frequently unable to coordinate any swimming or other activities such as clinging to a raft. If the victim is not wearing a personal flotation device, at this point submersion and drowning occur. If an appropriate flotation device is worn, then unconsciousness and death will be caused by hypothermia. On land, the victim's requirements for self-protection may not be quite as acute as in immersion hypothermia, but self-protective actions are equally blunted. Numb fingers, slowed muscular responses, and poor judgment may make fire starting or shelter building nearly impossible.

## CARDIOVASCULAR EFFECTS

Progressive cardiovascular decompensation with both conduction defects and ventricular irritability poses the greatest danger in hypothermia. Below 30°C (86°F), the patient becomes increasingly susceptible to ventricular ectopy and ventricular fibrillation. Spontaneous ventricular fibrillation is common below 28°C (82.4°F). At higher temperatures, rough handling, or insertion of central monitoring lines, may precipitate ventricular fibrillation. The ventricular fibrillation of hypothermia is usually refractory to drugs and countershock below core body temperatures of about 28 to 30°C (82.4 to 86°F).[29,30]

In the severe hypothermic, myocardial contractility and rate decrease continually. Bradycardia classically appears in severely and moderately hypothermic patients. At a core temperature of about 30°C (86°F), the pulse falls to about 50 to 60 beats per minute. Below 28°C (82.4°F), it can fall as low as 20 to 30. The heart's stroke volume also decreases as the core temperature falls. Taken together, the decrease in stroke volume and the slowed pulse rate result in a decreased cardiac output and hypotension. If the hypothermia occurs quickly, the tissue oxygen consumption falls proportionately. If the cardiac output lags behind the tissue's metabolic needs, lactic acidosis results. Shivering and exertion may increase the lactic acidosis. This acidosis increases the potential for ventricular dysrhythmias.

Electrocardiographic changes include prolonged PR intervals, various types and degrees of block, widened QT intervals, prolonged QRS complexes, and sometimes inversion or elongation of the T waves. As the temperature continues to fall, the rhythm becomes progressively slower and culminates in asystole in the undisturbed patient.[31] An Osborne wave ("J" wave) on the downstroke of the QRS is present in many, but not all, patients. The J wave is thought to be related to the severity of the hypothermia by some.[31]

Atrial fibrillation is typically found below 30°C (86°F). This arrhythmia usually returns spontaneously to a normal sinus rhythm when the patient is rewarmed. A fine baseline artifact, due to muscle tremors and shivering, may dominate the electrocardiogram in hypothermic patients with lesser depression of the core temperature.

Peripheral pulses and blood pressure are often impalpable in the severe hypothermic and the pulse may be missed completely when the heart rate is only 15 or 20 beats per minutes in a severely hypotensive patient. Peripheral vasoconstriction is marked until about 28 to 29°C (82.4 to 84.2°F), when vasoconstriction reflexes are lost. With the decreased cutaneous circulation associated with peripheral vasoconstriction, the skin is cold and firm. Warm skin in a cold patient should make the physician search for sepsis, use of a vasodilatory drug, or erythroderma.

## RESPIRATORY EFFECTS

Early in the course of acute cold, respiratory rates are increased, with a subsequent respiratory alkalosis. Severe hypothermia is associated with profound depression of the medullary respiratory centers. Pulmonary function is maintained until the core temperature reaches about 32°C (89.6°F). The tachypnea associated with shivering gives way to slowed respirations at about 32°C (89.6°F). The slowed respirations decrease; carbon dioxide retention and respiratory acidosis then result. If the oxygen consumption is slowed sufficiently by hypothermia, respiratory needs may be met by the slowed respirations. The results may, therefore, be either a respiratory alkalosis or a respiratory acidosis. As the core temperature falls, spontaneous respirations will cease at about 24°C (75.2°F).

Pneumonia is a frequent and potentially lethal complication of hypothermia. Hypoventilation and subsequent atelectasis is also noted as the depth and frequency of respirations are found. Depressed ciliary reflexes, with subsequent accumulation of secretions, may be one contributing factor. An absent cough reflex, combined with depressed mental status, may increase the incidence of aspiration and also lead to pneumonia.

Pulmonary edema is also noted in hypothermic patients, but the cause remains unknown. A possible etiology is inappropriate iatrogenic fluid administration. Direct pulmonary injury due to cardiopulmonary bypass used for rewarming may be another cause.

Interpretation of arterial blood gases in this setting is controversial. Some authorities feel that the results of blood gases should be corrected for the decreased temperature.[32,33] Unfortunately, other authors feel that to properly interpret these blood gases, the normal arterial blood gases should also be corrected for the decreased core temperature.[34-38] If oxygenated blood is chilled, the oxygen content and the hemoglobin saturation do not change with the temperature, but the hemoglobin is more tightly bound to the oxygen ("left" shift of the oxyhemoglobin dissociation curve), and the carbon dioxide is more easily dissolved in the serum. These changes happen whenever any patient's blood is chilled. It is probably easier if the blood gas sample is rewarmed to 37°C (98.6°F), and the interpretation is made without correction for temperature. The ventilation status can be adequately monitored, and the clinician is more comfortable with the determination of the acid-base status.

## CENTRAL NERVOUS SYSTEM EFFECTS

The cerebral blood flow will decrease about 6 to 7% for each drop of 1°C in core body temperature. The patterns of the clinical manifestations due to decreasing body temperature are similar from patient to patient, but each person appears to have a different temperature threshold.

Initial signs of hypothermia are frequently missed by the victim. The patient becomes slightly confused, fatigues easily, and starts to shiver. As the patient's teeth chatter and the core temperature continues to fall, the coordination deteriorates. Increasing disorientation, loss of short-term memory, and inability to think rationally follow. These patients may want to "just stop and rest" when it is clearly inappropriate to do so. Initial signs of hypothermia, fatigue, and slight confusion may often go unnoted by victims.

A phenomenon known as "paradoxical undressing" may occur as the patient starts to lose the vasoconstricting reflexes and vasodilation ensues at about 29 to 30°C (84.2 to 86°F). The confused and disoriented patient notes that the skin temperature starts to increase as the warmer core blood suffuses into the skin. The patient presumably feels the warmth and starts to undress, believing that the ambient temperature is rising. This paradoxical undressing may cause suspicions of a sexual assault.

As the core temperature continues to drop, so does the level of consciousness. Severely hypothermic patients may be so neurologically depressed as to appear dead. As the core temperature falls below 26 to 27°C (78.8 to 80.6°F), the patient becomes comatose and areflexic. The pupils become dilated and unresponsive. As the core temperature falls below 20°C (68°F), the electroencephalogram becomes flat.

The central nervous system depression, coupled with the falling requirements for oxygen, protect the hypothermic patient from ischemia or anoxic injury. Indeed, early cardiac surgeons (prior to cardiopulmonary bypass techniques) would deliberately induce profound hypothermia in order to operate on the heart for periods up to 20 minutes. Particularly in young patients with rapid immersion cooling, the prognosis is good even after prolonged periods of anoxia, without cardiopulmonary resuscitation (CPR). Patients have been resuscitated after 4 hours of cardiopulmonary arrest without CPR with core body temperatures of 19 to 24°C (66.2 to 75.2°F) with good recovery. These fine outcomes prove the adage that the physician should continue resuscitation efforts on the severe hypothermic until the patient is "warm and dead."

Marked muscle tonus occurs in the lower temperature ranges. These patients appear as if they are in rigor mortis. The patients are cold, cyanotic, pale, stiff to touch, and often feel frozen. Coarse facies and a husky voice may suggest myxedema. Nuchal rigidity, coupled with impaired consciousness, may require a lumbar puncture to rule out meningitis.

## METABOLIC EFFECTS

Metabolic acidosis develops secondary to decreased tissue perfusion and production of lactic acid from shivering. As the core temperature drops, the respiratory alkalosis due to tachypnea gives way to respiratory acidosis from respiratory depression and increased $CO_2$ solubility in the blood. Arterial blood gases should be corrected for temperature effects.

Electrolyte imbalances occur but do not demonstrate a consistent pattern. Potassium and sodium may be either markedly elevated, depressed, or normal.

Serum glucose levels are in part dependent upon the temperature and other underlying conditions. Insulin becomes enzymatically ineffective below 30°C (86°F), and the patient will theoretically be hyperglycemic.

In patients with marked or prolonged shivering, the body stores of glucose may be depleted with subsequent hypoglycemia. Alcoholics will frequently be hypoglycemic. The individual patient may be hypo-, hyper-, or euglycemic at any temperature. If insulin is given to the patient before rewarming, it will be ineffective and may accumulate with disastrous results later. The effects of hypoglycemia mandate that all unconscious hypothermic patients should receive intravenous glucose.

## EFFECTS ON FLUIDS AND RENAL STATUS

The hypothermic patient will have a decrease in the glomerular reabsorption with a subsequent increase in urine flow. This "cold diuresis" may cause significant dehydration. As warming occurs, the patient has a sharp onset of oliguria, probably mediated by ADH (antidiuretic hormone) but may remain hypovolemic.

Fluid shifts from the intravascular spaces to the interstitial spaces may contribute markedly to the dehydration and hypovolemia. The hypothermic patient may shift as much as 20% of intravascular fluid into the interstitial spaces. This relative dehydration may require a significant fluid replacement during resuscitation. Below 26°C (78.8°F), the skin appears puffy, and the patient may appear myxedematous. This edema will resolve as the patient is warmed.

The fluid shifts and diuresis cause a hemoconcentration and increased plasma viscosity. The extreme effects of this phenomenon may lead to intravascular thrombosis and subsequent embolization. As a patient is rewarmed, release of thromboplastins into the circulation may cause a disseminated intravascular coagulation.

## GASTROINTESTINAL

Intestinal motility decreases below 34°C (93.2°F). Frequently, ileus is found in these severely hypothermic patients. Bowel sounds are decreased, and the abdominal musculature is rigid, making examination of the abdomen difficult.

Since the detoxification and conjugation activities of the liver are also slowed, drugs may remain in the circulatory system for significantly longer periods. For example, the half-life of morphine is about 4 minutes in a normothermic patient, whereas it increases to 98 minutes in a patient with a temperature of 25°C (77°F).

About half of hypothermic patients develop hyperamylasemia. Some of these patients may have pancreatic injuries or go on to have pancreatitis.[39]

## TREATMENT
### Hazards of Field Rewarming

There is little question that the most dangerous time for the hypothermic patient is during rewarming. Deaths often occur during rewarming. The key to a successful resuscitation is in carefully controlled prehospital care, followed by control of the patient's environment as the physician rewarms the patient. The best survival rates have been achieved by rewarming in an intensive care situation with close monitoring and careful attention to oxygenation, ventilation, serum electrolytes and glucose, and fluid replenishment.

Rapid, uncontrolled, surface rewarming may allow vasodilation of the peripheral vessels. The resulting flow of cold, acidotic, potassium-laden blood to the core may cause a cardiovascular collapse ("rewarming shock") in the already fragile patient. The obligatory hypothermic diuresis and subsequent hypovolemia may increase this potential.

The cold heart has a decreased fibrillatory threshold, and any rapid motion or jolt may precipitate ventricular fibrillation. Patients with core temperatures of less than 32°C (89.6°F) are in imminent danger of spontaneous and often fatal ventricular dysrhythmias.[40] Insertion of central monitoring lines, hypocapnia, hypercapnea, unnecessary stimulation of the patient, and CPR can all precipitate ventricular fibrillation.

### Prehospital Care

The most important aspect of prehospital care is to realize that routine use of advanced cardiac life support guidelines is clearly inapproprate for the hypothermic patient. Until the patient reaches the controlled environment of the emergency department, careful handling and rapid transport are paramount considerations. Blind defibrillation or CPR of the hypothermic patient with bradycardia and hypotension may cause the patient to develop intractable ventricular fibrillation.

Rescue teams likely to encounter cases of severe hypothermia should be equipped with low reading thermometers, portable oxygen heaters, and cardiac monitoring devices. Insulation for the patient is crucial and some of the commercially available insulation devices and rescue packs are less bulky and more efficient than the traditional blankets. Heating pads are useful to ensure that intravenous lines do not freeze.

### PREHOSPITAL REWARMING CONSIDERATIONS

In dealing with hypothermia in the field, one must specify the situation. Field emergency care is the "art of the possible" and hypothermia is no exception to this philosophy. Measures clearly inappropriate for a patient who is going to be in a hospital setting within 20 minutes are perhaps appropriate for patients on a 5-day cross-country ski trek. Many authorities do not advocate rewarming until within the confines of the emergency department, feeling that the physiologic effects of the hypothermia place the patient in a "metabolic icebox" with little deterioration during transport. This attitude suffices for the patient who is only a few hours away from the hospital but is not necessarily appropriate for the patient who is many hours, or even days, evacuation from hospital medical care.

The essential and immediate action in treating hypothermia in the field is to prevent any further heat loss by providing shelter, dry clothing and adequate insulation. The patient should be sheltered, have wet clothing removed, and be covered with blankets or other insulating devices. If heated, humidified oxygen is available, it should be used to minimize heat losses. An intravenous line of warmed 5% glucose in normal saline should be started. These simple measures will prevent further heat loss as well as combat the commonly found dehydration and hypoxia. Spontaneous rewarming should be allowed to take place within the confines of the shelter as described later. For most cases of moderate hypothermia due to exposure, spontaneous rewarming is a safe and effective technique. It has been recommended by many authors for routine use.[41–44]

Other techniques have been shown in a large prospective field study to increase afterdrop and the possibility of ventricular fibrillation.[45] Most techniques of rewarming patients are simply not suitable for treatment of the patient in the field, on a mountainside, or far from monitoring devices.

## FLUID AND METABOLIC SUPPORT

In addition to the warmed intravenous line, the patient should receive intravenous glucose (50 cc of 50% glucose), naloxone (Narcan 2 mg IV), and thiamine (100 mg IV).[46] As noted earlier, Wernicke's encephalopathy can cause hypothermia and is probably more common than realized.

Small, insulated thermos containers with chemical heating packs can prevent fresh intravenous fluids from freezing. If possible, intravenous fluids should be heated prior to transport in the field container to ensure the highest possible starting temperature. Intravenous lines should be insulated in the field and should be checked frequently to ensure that they do not freeze. In minimally hypothermic and trauma victims, a stocking cap can both hold an intravenous bag and simultaneously insulate the patient's head. The severely hypothermic patient is not producing enough heat to prevent freezing of the intravenous solutions in subzero weather for this method.

## RESUSCITATION

The indications for cardiopulmonary resuscitation in the severely hypothermic patient are controversial, and little hard data exist to support most contentions.[47] The following discussion is, therefore, a product of anecdotal personal cases and distillation of the literature. If further *field* data are forthcoming, recommendations given may be validated or refuted, but readers should be wary of blindly applying hospital-based data collections and reports to field situations with prolonged transport/rescue times.

Profound bradycardia and markedly slowed respirations are common in the severe hypothermic. When the pulse and respirations are inapparent, the inexperienced, enthusiastic rescuer may start CPR, causing the irritable cold myocardium to fibrillate. A careful check for the presence of respirations and pulse is always indicated, but this may be difficult on a windswept, snow-covered slope during the field rescue. There is simply no question of cardiac activity if monitoring equipment is available, however. If the patient's core temperature is below 28°C (82.4°F), chest compressions and invasive procedures should probably be withheld until the patient can be monitored.[48,49] This is felt to be particularly true in field emergency medicine, where transport times may be hours or days, instead of the minutes associated with the urban environment. This position is controversial and at least one authority strongly disagrees, feeling that the hypothermic patient should always receive CPR.[50]

For normothermic cardiac arrests that occur in urban emergency services, survivals are rare after 30 minutes of CPR and essentially nonexistent after 1 hour of CPR. In a rescue with a *minimally* hypothermic patient, it makes little sense to initiate CPR when the transport time to the nearest roadhead is over 3 hours. This is particularly true when there is no monitoring or other advanced life support equipment available.

This may not be true in the *severely* hypothermic patient, however. Various authors have recorded survivals after resuscitations as long as 4 hours in severely hypothermic patients.[51,52] It should be stressed that these "arrests" were completely unmonitored, and there is a significant possibility that the patient had a nonpalpable but intact circulation. It is particularly important to withhold CPR when the severely hypothermic patient shows any signs of movement, because motor activity is presumptive evidence of some cardiopulmonary activity.[53,54]

EMS providers are regularly reminded that the only criterion for death in hypothermia is that the patient is "warm and dead," but this is not always the case. If the victim is frozen solid so that it is not possible to move the body, or if the nasal passages and mouth are blocked with ice, it is reasonable to assume death has occurred. Likewise, if the core temperature is equal to the ambient temperature below 10°C (50°F), it is unlikely that a resuscitation will be successful.

If CPR is necessary, hypothermic patients may require a slowed rate of respirations and cardiac compressions, even with fibrillation or asystole.[55] Reduced rates of ventilation avoid respiratory alkalosis and subsequent increased ventricular irritability. The stiff cold heart fills more slowly than a warmer one. About half the usual rate of respirations and compressions will be adequate in severely hypothermic patients.

Intubation should be performed by the first competent provider available. Not only does intubation provide the usual protection of the airway from aspiration, but it allows heated, humidified mist to be used in the treatment of the hypothermia. Intubation has been described by many authors as inducing ventricular fibrillation. There have been anecdotal cases of patients developing fibrillation at the time of intubation, including one treated by this author, but large series of well-documented and monitored patients show no consistent trends.[56–58]

## REWARMING METHODS

Rewarming of the human frame is a physical process subject to simple laws of physics. If the specific heat of tissue is assumed to be 0.83, it takes 60 kilocalories to rewarm a 70 kilogram human 1°C. This energy must either be added or produced by internal processes. Without the added heat, there will be no change in temperature. Unfortunately, this simplistic viewpoint does not take into account the effect of warming of the various "shells" previously described. Warmed muscles start to produce heat, warmed hearts start to beat, and warmed blood vessels dilate, skin insulation decreases as heat is added, each with positive and negative effects on the rate of rewarming.

As with the overall experience in hypothermia, rewarming therapy suffers from a regrettable lack of well-founded studies. Due to obvious ethical constraints, the degree of hypothermia induced in human subjects in an experiment of this type must be relatively mild. Few of the studies involve exhausted or hypoglycemic subjects. Most studies involve immersion hypothermia using physically fit volunteers. It is unlikely that the hypothermic responses of the exhausted, sedentary, alcoholic patient are going to mimic the 20-year-old college student volunteer.

Other studies neglect the effects of internal heating and insulation and concentrate only on the perceived effect of the therapy touted. These studies note the surface area of the lung, skin, and intestinal tract and relate the rate of heating to the surface area

of the area of interest. It should be clear that the rate of heating of the body is related to the amount of energy added, not the surface area where it is added (within broad limits, of course; one could burn a small area with high heat flow). The actual heat added by a process can be measured relatively easily. What cannot be measured easily is the body heat lost and gained during the rewarming process by other means.

Warming methods can be described by general nature:

1. **Peripheral passive measures**
   Blankets, etc.
2. **Peripheral active measures**
   "Buddy" rewarming
   Heating pads and "plumbed garments"
   Hot packs
   Warm baths
3. **Simple core rewarming measures**
   Lavage of stomach or urinary bladder
   Heated intravenous fluids
   Warmed, humidified oxygen
   Peritoneal lavage with warmed dialysate
4. **Invasive core rewarming techniques**
   Hemodialysis with heat exchanger
   Cardiopulmonary bypass
   Thoracotomy with lavage of mediastinum

The rewarming method chosen for the severe hypothermic patient should depend upon the skills of the physician and the equipment readily available. Transportation of the severe hypothermic to a properly equipped trauma center makes more sense than attempting to rewarm a critically ill patient with less than adequate equipment. Obviously, this judgment must be based upon reasonable transport times, well-equipped transport vehicles, and properly trained attendants. Transporting the same critical patient with a "pool" nurse in a hearse-like ambulance in inclement weather for long distances is a formula for disaster.

### Field Rewarming Techniques

Countering mild hypothermia in a field situation, before formal treatment is necessary, may be difficult when the bivouac is on the side of a mountain face. Nevertheless, it is far easier to treat the mildly hypothermic patient early than to transport a litter patient. In the field situation, for example, only dry clothing, blankets, warm beverages, hot fires, and close application of other, hopefully warmer, human bodies may be available. Only in specialized rescue units are either more efficient or more invasive heating techniques found.

Buddy rewarming is often advocated for treatment of mild field hypothermia. Body-to-body contact has been studied by Harnett and colleagues, who discourage its use when treating the profoundly hypothermic patient.[59] They cite a greater afterdrop with the moderate surface heating provided by the buddy. Chest-to-chest contact was noted to shorten the rewarming time and provide subjective improvement in cases of mild hypothermia. It has only modest enhancement over simple, passive rewarming as described later. The use of heating pads to back or chest fared only minimally better in their study.

Rewarming by radiant heat (campfires) may cause extensive damage to frostbitten skin and should be used with great caution. Hotpacks, as noted later, are associated with skin burns and are ineffective for heat transfer. They may be used well for heating intravenous lines, however.

## Passive or Spontaneous Rewarming

The use of dry clothing and blankets is suitable only for the patient with mild hypothermia (temperature greater than 32°C [89.6°F]). This method is slow, the patients rewarm at their own metabolic rate, and they must be hemodynamically stable and able to generate heat by shivering or by voluntary exercise. This method should be considered only as a basic field expedient for mild hypothermia.

All studies of experimental subjects cooled to mild hypothermia levels would be well advised to use passive rewarming as a baseline therapy. A therapy that touts rapid rewarming should provide a significant and reproducible improvement over simply insulating the "patient" and allowing basal metabolism to provide the heat.

The normal metabolic rate provides about 70 kcal/hr. The heat production is decreased as the patient's temperature and consequent basal metabolism are lowered, however. Resting heat production at a core temperature of 28°C (82.4°F) has been estimated at only 30 kcal/hr.[60] This decreased resting metabolic rate may be augmented by shivering, but most patients with profound hypothermia do not shiver.

## Active Surface Rewarming

This method, which includes warm baths, plumbed garments, and hot packs is widely used but has many severe disadvantages. Conduction of the heat to the skin warms the periphery first allowing vasodilation with subsequent return of cold, potassium-laden, acidotic blood to the central core and afterdrop.

Transfer of heat from the skin to the core varies with the blood flow to the skin and with the insulation of the subcutaneous fat. It is this insulation that allows obese men and normal women to tolerate cold immersion better than lean men.[61] Blood flow to the skin is under both local and central nervous control. These variables of insulation and blood flow make calculation of the heat gain more formidable than the simple calculations of core rewarming. Measurements of the water temperature before and after rewarming may be made and then corrections added for the normal cooling of the same body of water without the addition of the human. This is analogous to finding out how long it takes for an ice cube to melt in a pan of water in a cool room. More elaborate mathematical models have been developed if the water is heated during the test.[60]

The heat transfer from skin temperature to core temperature may be approximated by Newton's law as:

$$H = A * K_s * (T_s - T_c)$$

where A is the skin area in contact, $K_s$ is a composite constant derived from the thermal conductivity of blood, skin, and fat, coupled with the volume and flow of the subcutaneous blood. The rate of heat transfer is represented by H, while the skin temperature and core temperature are $T_s$ and $T_c$, respectively. $K_s$ has been estimated to be between 6 and 26 calories/100 cm²/min/°C.[60] Higher figures for $K_s$ are found when the blood vessels are maximally dilated, lower when the blood vessels are maximally constricted.

Active surface rewarming is not particularly recommended for critically ill patients. It may be suitable for rewarming of young, active patients with acute or semiacute hypothermia. If active surface rewarming MUST be used, then the patient should be warmed about the thorax and abdomen only, leaving the extremities exposed and vasoconstricted until the core has been rewarmed. The use of vasodilators will increase the rate of rewarming but may do so at the expense of increasing colder blood flow from the extremities.

## AFTERDROP

As one warms the cold extremities of the severely hypothermic patient, the intense vasoconstriction is relieved, allowing cold, acidotic, potassium-laden blood to flow toward the core.[59] This is the probable basis of rewarming "afterdrop" and is a major disadvantage of every method of rewarming that attempts to rewarm from the skin toward the core. Shivering will likely tend to promote afterdrop by the increased blood flow to the muscles. The genesis of afterdrop through vasodilation and liberation of pooled cold extremity blood has been generally accepted but has been challenged and should be considered controversial at this point.[62,63]

Whatever the reason, afterdrop of up to 4°C is noted with all external forms of rewarming. Afterdrop is defined as the greatest reduction in rectal temperature seen during rewarming. A comparison of studies shows that afterdrop is greatest when the extremities are heated in a water bath, less with heating pads or trunk-only immersion, and least when core rewarming techniques are used. Therapeutic regimens that include only surface heating exhibit the largest mean afterdrops.

## WATER BATHS

The use of warm water baths for treatment of hypothermia is advocated by many.[64] A hypothermic patient with a core temperature of 28°C (82.4°F) immersed except for his extremities in a well-stirred water bath of 45°C (113l°F) would be expected to have heat transfer of between 600 and 2400 kcal per hour from the water. If the surface area exposed to the water is estimated at 1 meter square:

$$H = 1M^2 * (6) * (45 - 28)$$

$$= 10.2 \text{ kcal/min (612 kcal/hr)}$$

$$H = 1M^2 * (26) * (45 - 28)$$

$$= 44.2 \text{ kcal/min (2652 kcal/hr)}$$

The higher figure would be found under conditions of maximum vasodilation. The water bath, not surprisingly, is considerably more efficient than most methods of core warming.

Management of the critically ill patient in a water bath of any sort is fraught with hazards. Not only is monitoring for ECG, pulmonary artery, or central venous pressure difficult, but simply taking vital signs on a patient suspended in water is hard. When the patient has ventricular fibrillation, countershock becomes hazardous to both staff and patient. Water bath rewarming is probably impractical for field use in any form due to the mass and weight of the tub, water heating apparatus, water, and fuel required to heat the water.

Water temperature must be kept within reasonable limits or the patient will sustain burns. Use of water temperature of greater than 45°C (113°F) may be associated with skin scalding burns.[65]

## HOT PACKS AND HEATING PADS

Surface rewarming with plumbed garments, hot packs, or heating pads (both electrical and chemical) are used in smaller hospitals or in the field to warm hypothermic patients. These may all be lumped under the designation of topical heating devices.

Chemical heating pads, heated towels, and plumbed heating pads have all been applied to smaller areas to rewarm patients.[66] The smaller units are far less efficient than rewarming in a tub of hot water and they warm surface areas only. In the hypothermic patient, cool skin is poorly perfused, and local heat applied to a relatively small area of skin does little to either reverse this perfusion deficit or rewarm the core. Lesser surface area in contact, decreased visibility of the patient, and skin burns are all noted with these methods of rewarming.[67] Skin burns are particularly common when the heating pad is hotter than 45°C (113°F). Singular care must be used in applying these topical heating devices to immobile, anesthetized, or unconscious patients.

Fluidized bead beds with heated airflow may provide external rewarming without the dangers and complications of water immersion. Anecdotal reports are good, but no controlled studies exist.[68]

Hypothermia sarongs and other large plumbed garments warm a larger surface area.[69] The self-contained heating sources used in some units may make them servicable for rescue work, but fuel requirements may be excessive for these same purposes. Safety records are unproven, and there are little data supporting use in actual patients. There is no contraindication to using these units in awake and alert victims of mild hypothermia.

## RADIANT HEATING

Radiant heat from a campfire or the sun may have been the earliest artificial rewarming technique used by man. Radiant heat has been recently used to rewarm hypothermic newborn infants and to prevent heat losses perinatally and intraoperatively.[70-72] It has not been well studied in adults for treatment of hypothermia, although it has been used anecdotally since prehistorical times.

Since radiant heat is poorly controlled, extreme care must be taken to avoid tissue damage, particularly when frostbite is present. This method of rewarming is generally not recommended for hospital use, except for the mildly hypothermic newborn.

## Simple Core Rewarming Techniques

Core rewarming decreases the possibility of afterdrop by warming the viscera before the periphery. The myocardium and pulmonary circulation are warmed in advance of the rest of the body in order to meet the increasing circulatory and respiratory demands as the body temperature rises. Core rewarming can be performed safely in hospitals of any size. More than one method can and should be used simultaneously in these critically ill patients. The best methods are those that the physician is familiar with and the hospital has the equipment and personnel to institute safely.

In smaller hospitals, simple core rewarming techniques are still available. Although not as quick or technically elegant as later mentioned techniques, they are, nonetheless, effective. If weather, personnel, or transportation precludes transport to a larger hospital of more invasive capability, it is important to start rewarming in the most practical and timely fashion available.

## PERITONEAL DIALYSIS

Peritoneal dialysis is routinely used in the treatment of renal failure and toxic overdosages of drugs that diffuse easily into the peritoneum. It is also used in the United States as a technique to diagnose the presence of a ruptured vessel or viscus following blunt abdominal trauma. The technique consists of inserting a flexible catheter into the peritoneal cavity and instilling a suitable liquid into the peritoneum. After a short period, the fluid is drained from the peritoneum and fresh fluid instilled. Warmed peritoneal dialysis is widely advocated for treatment of accidental hypothermia.[73-75]

Warmed peritoneal dialysis is easily administered, with few complications, and is the method of choice for the small hospital. The fluid should be a potassium-free neutral dialysis fluid and should be heated to about 42 to 44°C (111.2°F). Rates of about 5 to 6 liters per hour are achievable. For more rapid exchange, two catheters may be placed—one used as input and one used as output.

> The actual heat gain from peritoneal dialysis is easily calculated by subtracting a known outflow temperature from the known inflow temperature and multiplying the result by the amount of fluid used. Thus for a rate of 6 liters per hour with dialysate at 40°C (104°F) inflow temperature and 28°C (82.4°F) outflow temperature, the total heat added would be $(40 - 28) \times 6 = 72$ kcal per hour.

The procedure conducts the heat through the mesenteric, portal, and caval veins to the heart and lungs. This means that the liver, heart, great vessels, kidneys, and lungs are warmed preferentially by peritoneal dialysis. The procedure has some theoretical benefits in the patient who has had a concomitant overdose of certain drugs and in the patient with renal failure. Peritoneal dialysis may be used in addition to other rewarming techniques and does not interfere with any monitoring techniques.

The contraindications of rewarming with peritoneal dialysis are the same as those of the procedure in general. Recent abdominal surgery or abdominal trauma are major contraindications. Dialysis with an inappropriate solution may cause electrolyte imbalances and electrolytes should be monitored frequently. Infection and bleeding are infrequent but reported. One must take the greatest aseptic precautions in order to avoid peritoneal contamination. Perforation of a viscus is very rare, unless a patient has had prior peritonitis or surgical procedures. Peritoneal dialysis is not suitable for field rewarming.

## LAVAGE OF OTHER ORIFICES

Warmed lavage of the stomach or bladder supplies heat to the core in a less invasive manner than peritoneal lavage. The usual technique is to introduce fluid and then withdraw it in a manner similar to lavage for toxic overdoses. A modified Sengstaken tube has also been used with Ringer's lactate at 41°C (105.8°F) lavage solution.[76] Lavage of the stomach can lead to electrolyte imbalances and fluid overload. Regurgitation of fluid may result in aspiration of gastric contents. CPR would be expected to increase the chances of aspiration.

Colonic lavage is impractical in all critically ill patients, since feces and fluid may egress from the colon and present a hazard to monitoring or defibrillation. Traumatic injury is possible, particularly with deep insertion of the rectal tube in the cold, stiff patient. This method cannot logically be recommended, particularly when other, better techniques are available.

## RADIO WAVE REGIONAL HYPERTHERMIA

Experimentally, radio wave regional hyperthermia (diathermy) has produced more rapid results than aggressive peritoneal lavage for rewarming hypothermic dogs.[77] It is touted as safe, simple, and rapid. There have been no clinical studies in the English literature on this method.

## Complex Core Rewarming Techniques

### CARDIOPULMONARY BYPASS

Cardiopulmonary bypass with extracorporeal rewarming may be the method of choice for the severely hypothermic patient, although this is controversial.[78,79] The first use of this technique in accidental hypothermia was in 1967.[80] External rewarming of the blood and body before removal from bypass following cardiac surgery has been used since the 1950s, however.

Not only does cardiopulmonary bypass warm the heart, it oxygenates the blood and provides adequate perfusion pressure even when the patient is in ventricular fibrillation. The warmed blood returning to the heart directly warms the myocardium, decreasing irritability and potentiating antiarrhythmic medications. Oxygenation and circulatory pressures are restored immediately, despite cardiac dysrhythmias and myocardial depression. Patients with severe myocardial depression due to hypothermia may be resuscitated and warmed despite the absence of normal blood circulation. Fluid and electrolyte corrections may be easily made during the bypass procedure. If flow rates of 3 to 4 liters per minute are maintained, and incoming blood is warmed just 2°C, 600 kcal/hr of added heat may easily be given to the patient.

Extracorporeal circulation is most simply done with femoral vein catheter insertion. The blood is warmed, oxgenated, and then returned through a femoral artery catheter. Systemic heparinization is required and may preclude its use in patients with other trauma. Patients with head injuries or cerebrovascular accidents are at particular danger from the heparinization.

Disadvantages of extracorporeal circulation include the necessity for a specialized team and sophisticated equipment. This specialized equipment precludes its use in most emergency departments and rural hospitals. If a rescue or ambulance crew has the choice between taking a severely hypothermic patient to a hospital without bypass capability or to a farther hospital with bypass capability, they should clearly choose the hospital with the capability to place the patient on cardiopulmonary bypass.

The risks of extracorporeal circulation are related to the problems of the machine and the plumbing needed to institute bypass. Hemolysis, air leaks, vessel destruction, embolization, and distal limb ischemia have all been reported following use of this equipment in cardiac surgery. It can be expected that with increased use of cardiopulmonary bypass these problems will be noted in treatment of the hypothermic patient.

### HEMODIALYSIS

Hemodialysis with an in-line heat exchanger provides a superior means of rewarming a patient. If available, it provides rapid central rewarming and control of both fluid and electrolyte status. The general benefits, heat exchange, and dangers are similar to those found with cardiopulmonary bypass. Hemodialysis machines and competent operators are more readily available than cardiopulmonary bypass machines.

## OPEN THORACOTOMY

Open thoracotomy with mediastinal lavage with warmed saline not only rapidly rewarms the heart, it allows cardiac massage with subsequent increased flow rates.[81,82] The technique is useful but has largely been supplanted by hemodialysis and cardiopulmonary bypass in larger hospitals in the United States. Thoracotomy is more frequently used in Europe than in the United States for rewarming.

The procedure requires surgical skills, backup facilities and staff, and intubation of the patient prior to performing the procedure. Warm, sterile water is poured into the pleural cavity, warming the heart, pulmonary circulation, and systemic circulation, simultaneously. A less invasive but similar technique is to insert one or two chest tubes and use these for thoracic irrigation.[83] With 42°C (107.6°F) saline added to the 28°C patient at a rate of 1 liter every other minute, one could reasonably expect to add 400 kcal per hour, at least for the first hour or so.

Open thoracotomy may be a useful "last resort" for the hypothermic patient who has intractable asystole or ventricular fibrillation or for the patient who is not rewarming rapidly with either hemodialysis or cardiopulmonary bypass. Open thoracotomy would be totally unsuitable for field rewarming in any setting.

Any open technique carries with it a risk of infection. Emergent thoracotomy for other reasons has low infection rates and would be expected to have similar rates when performed for hypothermia.[84] Since the usual negative pressure of the thorax is destroyed, positive pressure ventilation is mandatory and requires endotracheal intubation.

### Adjuvant Techniques

Warmed intravenous fluids and warmed, humidified oxygen should be administered to all patients with hypothermia. Although the actual heat gain by either of these methods is minimal, they tend to decrease the amount of heat loss.

## HEATED INTRAVENOUS FLUIDS

If intravenous fluids are heated beyond 112°F (45°C), at the site of delivery, cell damage will occur when the fluid is infused. The limiting effect of water overload precludes significant volume exchanges in this method, and the overall result is but a small contribution to the increase in the patient's temperature when compared with other methods.

> If a 70-kg human at 28°C core temperature receives 1 liter of water at 45°C, the total added heat is 17°C × 1 kg = 17 kcal. Thus each liter of water will warm the human approximately (17 kcal × .83)/70 kg = 0.20°C change.

All hypothermic patients receiving intravenous fluids should have those fluids warmed to prevent further heat losses. The fluids may be warmed by thermal bath, microwave, hot packs, or an examiner's body to 37°C (98.6°F).[85-87] Precalibration of a microwave oven is needed to prevent overheating of the fluids. Red blood cells and blood should not be heated in a microwave oven because of the hemolysis that results.[88]

## HEATED, HUMIDIFIED OXYGEN

Heated inhalation therapy is often proposed as a noninvasive core rewarming technique or to minimize heat losses.[89-91] Heat is thought to be supplied directly to the core and the advantage of warming the core first is cited. The vast surface of the lung is considered a large heat exchanger and the technique adds supplemental oxygen.

Heat exchange surface area and added heat are two different quantities and should not be used interchangeably. The true rate of patient rewarming with heated mist is unclear, and the amount of heat added by this technique is not easy to calculate.[92] There are few experimental or clinical studies that contrast rewarming rates of insulated patients or experimental subjects with and without use of heated mist, although many studies impart an advantage without such logical comparisons. Also there are few studies that address the comparison between this technique and other techniques in relatively matched patients. In one study, in dogs, peritoneal dialysis showed significantly more rapid rewarming than did warm, humidified inhalation for the treatment of experimental severe immersion hypothermia.[93]

The temperature of the mist must be less than 45°C (113°F) or tissue damage will result. Fully saturated mist with a high ventilatory rate is necessary for maximum heat transfer. This is logical, as the specific heat of dry air is about 0.001, so dry air will transfer very little heat to the tracheobronchial tree. Since dry air and oxygen have similar specific heats, there is little difference in heat transfer capability between the two gases. The water vapor in the inhaled gas carries much more heat than the gas itself. Much of the heat content is due to the roughly 540 kcal/L latent heat of vaporization of the water vapor, which is given up only when the vapor condenses within the body. Shanks and Marsh estimated that with a ventilatory rate of 10 L/min that the total heat input from heated mist is about 10 kcal/hr from 100% saturated 45°C (113°F) mist.[94] Meyers and coworkers felt that the heat transfer rate was somewhat higher, about 30 kcal/hr, in their calculations with similar flows and temperatures of heated mist.[60]

If this rate of heat exchange were the only effect of heated, humidified mist, it would scarcely be worth the trouble. Fortunately, one additional effect of warming the inspired gases is that the effluent gases do not carry heat away. As noted earlier, transpiration may be responsible for as much as 13 kcal/hr heat losses. Heated, humidified mist will also prevent this heat loss mechanism, resulting in perhaps as much as 43 kcal/hr heat gain, using the highest available heat exchange calculations. (One fourth of the heat gain is from endogenous heat sources, however.)

Again, with a 70-kg person, and 43 kcal/hr heat gain, the person would rewarm at (43 kcal × 0.83)/70 kg = 0.50°C/hr from heated mist. This corresponds well to published rates touted for heated mist rewarming and assumes that the transpiration heat losses are eliminated by this method.

It should be noted that as the patient's temperature rises, this and all such methods of heat exchange become inherently less efficient. If the calculations are repeated with the patient's core body temperature at 32°C (89.6°F), the heat delivery rate is 16% slower, because transfer of heat works best when the two objects are most widely separated in temperature.

The advantages of this method are the relative simplicity and availability of the equipment, rapidity of application, and the low cost. A minor disadvantage to this technique is the obviously slow rate of rewarming.

The major disadvantage of heated mist is that the addition of water vapor directly to the lungs should be contraindicated in the patient with pulmonary edema. Severe hypothermia is often associated with pulmonary edema. Condensation of water vapor in the lung can increase this pulmonary edema. Given the ability to suction the patient via an endotracheal tube, the reduction of heat losses by transpiration, and the ability to administer high-flow oxygen, this disadvantage becomes more theoretical than practical.

Although the equipment to provide heated, humidified mist is easily available in hospitals, few ambulance services have it ready or available, and fewer rescue services even have the capability. Small, portable units have been developed but are not universally used or available.

The major contraindication for the use of humidified mist would be massive facial trauma. In this case, humidified mist could be applied via a surgical airway. It is assumed that in the treatment of this particular patient, the airway management would take precedence over the rewarming technique.

Heated, humidified mist should be used for all severely hypothermic patients as an adjuvant technique. Current clinical trials easily indicate that it adds a small amount of heat and prevents respiratory heat losses. Since it does not interfere with any other heating technique and has no substantive contraindications, it should be used for every patient, if available. It should not, however, be used as the sole rewarming technique. If the patient's endogenous heat production capability is depressed, heated mist will be less effective.

## OTHER ADJUVANTS

The cautious use of vasodilators, such as nitroglycerin or nitroprusside, may decrease peripheral vasoconstriction and increase heat transfer. These have been used in recent episodes of hypothermia, but there are no controlled studies attesting to their use or efficacy.[95]

## Medications

Medications are generally less effective when the subject is severely hypothermic. This decreased effect includes many of the medications used in the treatment of life-threatening cardiac dysrhythmias and hyperglycemia.

Intravenous glucose solutions may restore shivering and increased metabolic warming in hypoglycemic patients, particularly at core temperatures greater than 32°C (89.6°F).[96] Patients who are thiamine depleted may develop Wenicke's encephalopathy. Since alcoholics constitute a large part of urban hypothermia, routine administration of thiamine is probably appropriate for hypothermia.

### ANTIBIOTICS

The question of "prophylactic" (better termed empiric) antibiotics in the hypothermic patient is unresolved. Certainly, the physician should carefully examine all patients for the presence of infections. Particularly, the non–exposure-related hypothermic patient should be evaluated for at least 72 hours for sepsis. Blood cultures, sputum and urine cultures, and chest x-rays are minimal. Throughout hospitalization, soft tissue infections in dependent areas should be watched for. Although the proper use of antibiotics in these patients is not yet resolved, the high percentage of sepsis and the increased mortality in these septic patients indicates that antibiotics are probably indicated in this select subset of hypothermic patients. Antibiotic therapy should be directed against the Gram-negative causes of urosepsis, and the Gram-positive cocci and mouth anaerobes found in aspiration. If all cultures are negative at 72 hours and no clinical evidence of infection has been found, antibiotics should be discontinued.

### INSULIN

Insulin is a polypeptide that is not active below 30°C (86°F). Hypothermia further inhibits pancreatic insulin release as well as peripheral glucose utilization.[97] Insulin therapy is frequently not needed in the hypothermic. As the patient is warmed, spontaneous correction of hyperglycemia is noted. The patient with profound hypothermia and hyperglycemia should be warmed to at least 30°C before insulin is given. As in all critically ill patients, insulin should be given by the in-travenous route and never by subcutaneous injection in the hypothermic patient.

### ANTIARRHYTHMICS

A large number of antiarrhythmic agents have been tried in the hypothermic patient with little substantive results. These agents have included lidocaine, procainamide, quinidine, magnesium sulfate, and bretylium.

Bretylium tosylate is the only antiarrhythmic that has been found to be anecdotally effective in the severely hypothermic patient.[98] Animal studies are promising when bretylium is used either for prophylaxis or for treatment of hypothermia-facilitated ventricular fibrillation. Unfortunately, all evidence is in animal studies, and good human studies are unavailable.[99,100] Lidocaine has not been clinically effective for either treatment or prophylaxis of ventricular fibrillation in severe hypothermia. Procainamide reportedly increases the incidence of ventricular fibrillation in hypothermia victims. Both magnesium sulfate and quinidine have been used with some success in the treatment of ventricular fibrillation in this setting.

If ventricular fibrillation develops during treatment of hypothermia, bretylium tosylate is the current agent of choice. Use of bretylium as a prophylactic agent for ventricular fibrillation in the hypothermic setting is a venture into unknown territory, and appropriate animal and clinical studies are needed before recommendations can be made. Toxicity, optimal dose, and ideal rate of infusion of bretylium in the severely hypothermic patient are unresearched and unknown. Unfortunately, even this agent is typically ineffective until the patient has been warmed to at least 28°C (82.4°F) and preferably 30°C (86°F)

## PROGNOSIS

In most cases of hypothermia treated in civilization, survival is thought to be better correlated with the presence of an underlying disease than with a core body temperature attained by the patient. Certainly, this is arguable. Profoundly hypothermic patients have an unfortunate prognosis, whatever the underlying health status. Likewise, minimal hypothermia carries a favorable prognosis, despite the presence of underlying diseases.

It is in the severely hypothermic patient with core temperatures above 25°C (77°F) that underlying health problems will contribute the most to mortality.

In hypothermic infants, studies are conflicting and usually published from the lesser developed countries, where advanced life support tools and techniques may not be available.[101,102] Slow, passive, external rewarming has been advocated, but quick rewarming appeared to be more satisfactory in these children with improvement from 70% mortality to 33% mortality.

## ADMISSION CRITERIA

All patients with a core temperature of less than 33°C (91.4°F) should be admitted for observation. If the patient has additional pathology, the need for admission should be considered at higher temperatures. Prior to discharge, physicians should understand and document the CAUSE of the hypothermia. If a street alcoholic is returned to the street without adequate food or shelter, that patient has had no benefit from the hospital therapy. If an elderly patient on phenothiazines, cardiac medications, and barbiturates who is also hypothyroid is returned to a minimal care facility without adequate diagnostic workup and therapeutic intervention, the patient has experienced only an expensive hospital stay. A marathon runner or cross-country skier with a similar temperature may be able to safely proceed to his home after adequate rewarming and observation. Appropriate disposition should, therefore, include ensuring heat, clothing, light, and proper administration of medications.

## PREVENTION

A major objective in this book is to prevent environmental illnesses. The timeworn precepts that are often bandied about are found frequently in reference to hypothermia: "Wear your boots and your scarf." "Be prepared." Mother Nature is unforgiving to those who ignore her rules. "Dress warm, stay dry, eat well, and avoid intoxicants." There is, of course, great truth to the hackneyed aphorisms, but application is different from knowledge. A weak climber, a slip on the mountain, an overturned raft in the rapids, or a sudden summer snowstorm can pin the party on the mountain or an island, exposed to wind, wet, and cold.

The following principles may help the outdoorsman or woman in avoiding the ravages of the cold:

---

In addition to the recommended peelable layers of clothing designed to sustain more than adequate warmth, every trekker should carry a wind- and waterproof outer layer of rubberized nylon or one of the newer water-shedding fabrics. A hooded jacket is not enough. A poncho or poncho and rain pants is ideal and should be carried in the pack at all times when not actually needed.

Remember that wool and the artificial insulating fabrics provide insulation even when wet. Cotton and down lose insulation ability when dampened. Skiers, particularly, should remember that wet jeans provide little protection from the cold.

Ensure that extra food is carried. Remember that the fire goes out when the fuel is exhausted. Carry sugars, such as candy, carbohydrates, and proteins. Emergency foods should be compact and require no preparation. Hikers who miss breakfast or have restricted their food intake are at increased risk for hypothermia.[103]

Carry emergency bivouac equipment. A poncho, tube tent, or tarp is ideal. Extra dry socks, hat, and mittens should be carried at all times. Hike or ski with a partner.

Stop early. Set turnback times and hew to them. An emergency bivouac made while all are exhausted and after dark has fallen ensures that the snow cave will collapse, the tent will be blown away by the wind, the gear will fall down the mountain, and the fire will be impossible to start. (Remember that Murphy was an optimist.) Alternative shelter is best found or made while reserves are intact and daylight is still present. As Pugh's studies have shown, an emergency shelter offers a better chance for survival by preventing exhaustion and restorating clothing insulation than pressing on to a specific destination.[26,104,105] Plan for survival shelters before the need is desperate. Remember that as hypothermia intervenes, judgment will fail. "Pressing on" is frequently a fatal judgment error.

Elderly patients should be visited on a daily basis by someone able to recognize a change in affect or habits. Elderly patients who are posturally hypotensive have been noted to be more susceptible to hypothermia.[106]

## References

1. Altus P, Hickman JW, Pina I, Barry PP. Hypothermia in the sunny south. South Med J 1980;73:1491–1492.
2. Alexander L. The treatment of shock from prolonged exposure to cold, especially in water. Combined Intelligence Objective Subcommittee, Item No 24, File No. 26–73, London 1945. 1945.
3. Murphy I. If it possibly can go wrong, it will (unpublished).
4. Hayward JS, Eckerson JD, Kemna D. Thermal and cardiovascular changes during three methods of resuscitation from mild hypothermia. Resuscitation 1984;11:21–33.
5. Forgey WW. Hypothermia: death by exposure. Merrillville, IN: ICS Books: 1985;52.
6. Gerry RC. Control of the temperature of the body. Med Sci Law 1969;9:242–246.
7. Chernow B, Lake CR, Zaritsky A, et al. Sympathetic nervous system "switch off" with severe hypothermia. Crit Care Med 1983;11:677–680.
8. Lim TPK. Central and peripheral control mechanisms of shivering and its effect on respiration. J Appl Physiol 1960;15:567–74.
9. Muza SR, Young AJ, Sawaka MN, et al. Power spectral analysis of the surface electromylogram during shivering. Aviat Space Environ Med 1986;57:1150–1153.
10. Racine J, Jarjoui E. Severe hypothermia in infants. Helv Acta Pediatr 1982;37:317–322.
11. Sherry E. Richards D. Hypothermia among resort skiers: 19 cases from the Snowy Mountains. Med J Aust 1986;144:457–461.
12. Murray JJ. Pediatric aspects of Nordic skiing. Ped Clin North Am 1982;29:1423–1429.
13. Anonymous. Action needed to prevent deaths from hypothermia in the elderly [Editorial]. JAMA 1980;243:407–408.
14. Kurtz KJ. Hypothermia in the elderly: the cold facts. Geriatrics 1982;37:85–93.
15. Lewin S, Brettman LR, Holzman RS. Infections in hypothermic patients. Arch Intern Med 1981;141:920–925.
16. Morris DL, Chambers HF, Morris MG, Sande MA. Hemodynamic characteristics of patients with hypothermia due to occult infection and other causes. Ann Intern Med 1985;102:153–157.
17. Doherty NE, Fung P, Lefkowitz M, Ellrodt AG. Hypothermia and sepsis [Letter]. Ann Intern Med 1985;103:308.
18. Gale EAM, Bennett T, Hilary-Green J, MacDonald IA. Hypoglycemia, hypothermia and shivering in man. Clin Sci 1981;61:463–469.
19. Hanson PJ, Loughridge LW, Mulhall BP, Packham DK. Hypothemia in hypoglycemia. Br Med J 1984;288:1212–1213.
20. Fitzgerald FT. Hypoglycemia and accidental hypothermia in an alcoholic population. West J Med 1980:133:105–107.
21. Gale AM, Tattersall RB. Hypothermia: a complication of diabetic ketoacidosis. Br Med J 1978;2:1387–1389.
22. Albiin N, Eriksson A. Fatal accidental hypothermia and alcohol. Alcohol Alcoholism 1984;19:13–22.
23. Vanggaard L. Alcohol (ethanol) and cold. Nordic Council Arctic Medicine Research Reports 1982;21:82–92.
24. Kearsly JJ, Musso AF. Hypothermia and coma in the Wernicke-Korsakoff syndrome. Med J Aust 1980;2:504–506.
25. Smolander J, Louhevaara V, Ahonen M. Clothing, hypothermia, and long distance skiing. Lancet 1986;July 26:226–227.
26. Pugh LGCE. Clothing insulation and accidental hypothermia in youth. Nature 1966;209:1281–1285.
27. Balfour AJC. No drowning mark upon him. Aviat Space Environ Med 1983;54:1021–1022.
28. Hayward JS. Immersion hypothermia. In: Wilkerson JA, Bangs CC, Hayward JS. eds. Hypothermia, frostbite, and other cold injuries. Seattle: Mountaineers: 1986:66–83.
29. Da Vee TS, Reinbert EJ. Extreme hypothermia and ventricular fibrillation. Ann Emerg Med 1982;9:100.
30. Welton DE, Mattox KL, Miller RR, et al. Treatment of profound hypothermia. JAMA 1978;240:2291.
31. Rankin AC, Rae AP. Cardiac arrhythmias during rewarming of patients with accidental hypothermia. Br Med J 1984;289:874–877.
32. Reuler JB. Hypothermia: pathophysiology, clinical settings, and management. Ann Intern Med 1978;89:519–527.
33. Zell SC, Kurtz KJ. Severe exposure hypothermia: a resuscitation protocol. Ann Emerg Med 1985;14:339–345.
34. Stapczynski, JS. Resuscitation from severe hypothermia [Letter]. Ann Emerg Med 1985;14:1126–1127.
35. Hansen JE, Sue DY. Should blood gas measurements be corrected for the patient's temperature? N Eng J Med 1980;303:341.
36. White FN. Reassessing acid-base balance in hypothermia—a comparative point of view. West J Med 1983;138:255–257.
37. Wong KC. Physiology and pharmacology of hypothermia. West J Med 1983;138:227–232.
38. White JD. Hypothermia therapy [Letter]. Ann Emerg Med 1985;14:1036.
39. Mackan D, Griffiths PD, Emslie-Smith D. Serum enzymes in relation to electrocardi-

ographic changes in accidental hypothermia. Lancet 1968;2:1266.

40. White JD. Hypothermia: the Bellevue experience. Ann Emerg Med 1982;11:417–424.

41. MacLean D, Emslie-Smith D. Accidental hypothermia. Oxford:Blackwell, 1977.

42. Anonymous. Rewarming for accidental hypothermia [Editorial]. Lancet 1978;1:251–252.

43. Stewart CE, ed. Safe and effective management in severe accidental hypothermia. Emerg Med Rep 1986;7:17–24.

44. Winter First Aid Manual, 4th ed. Denver: National Ski Patrol System, Inc., 1984.

45. Harnett RM, O'Brien EM, Sias FR, et al. Initial treatment of profound accidental hypothermia. Aviat Space Environ Med 1980;51:680–687.

46. Kurtz KJ. Hypothermia in the elderly: the cold facts. Geriatrics 1982;37:85–93.

47. Manigas PA, DeGuzman LR, Hollenbach SJ, et al. Regional blood flow during hypothermic arrest. Ann Emerg Med 1986;15:390–396.

48. Zell SC, Kurtz KJ. Severe exposure hypothemia: a resuscitation protocol. Ann Emerg Med 1985;14:339–345.

49. Stewart CE. Cold injuries. In Rakel R., ed. Conn's Current Therapy. Philadelphia: WB Saunders Co., 1987.

50. Steinman AM. CPR and hypothermia. Response 1982; Fall:3–6.

51. Althaus U, Aeberhard P, Schupbach R, et al. Management of profound accidental hypothermia with cardiorespiratory arrest. Ann Surg 1982;195:492–495.

52. Lloyd EL. Resuscitation. In Hypothermia and Cold Stress. Rockville, MD: Aspen Systems Corp., 1986:240.

53. Gunby P. Cold facts concerning hypothermia (news). JAMA 1980;243:1403–1404, 1409.

54. Rudikoff MT, Meaughan WL, Effrom N, et al. Mechanisms of blood flow during cardiopulmonary circulation. Circulation 1980;61:345–352.

55. Martyn JW. Diagnosing and treating hypothermia. Am Med Assoc J 1981;125:1089–1096.

56. Ledingham I, et al. Teatment of accidental hypothermia: a prospective study. Br Med J 1980;280:1102.

57. Miller JW, Danzl DF, Thomas DM. Urban accidental hypothermia: 135 cases. Ann Emerg Med 1980;9:456.

58. Danzl DF, Pozos RS, et al. Multicenter hypothermia survey. Ann Emerg Med 1987;16:1042.

59. Harnett RM, O'Brien EM, Sias FR, Pruitt JR. Initial treatment of profound accidental hypothermia. Aviat Space Environ Med 1980;51:680–687.

60. Myers RAM, Britten JS, Cowley RA. Hypothermia: quantitative aspects of therapy. JACEP 1979;8:523–527.

61. Carlson LD, Hsei ACL, Fullington F, et al. Immersion in cold water and body tissue insulation. Aviation Med 1958;29:145–152.

62. Savard GK, Cooper KE, Veale WL, Malkinson TJ. Peripheral bood flow during rewarming from mild hypothermia in humans. J Appl Physiol 1985;58:4–13.

63. Lloyd EL. Hypothermia: the cause of death after rescue. Alaska Med 1984;26:74–76.

64. Zachary L, Kucan JO, Robson MC, Frank DH. Accidental hypothermia treated by rapid rewarming by immersion. Ann Plast Surg 1982;9:238–241.

65. Feldman KW, Schaller RT, Feldman JA, et al. Tap water scald burns in children. Pediatrics 1978;62:1–7.

66. Sturm JT, Logan MA. Microwave aids in external rewarming of hypothermia patients [Letter]. Ann Emerg Med 1985;14:277.

67. Feldman KW, Morray JP, Schaller RT. Thermal injury caused by hot pack application in hypothermic children. Am J Emerg Med 1985;3:38–41.

68. Miles JM, Thompson GR. Treatment of severe accidental hypothermia using the Clinitron bed. Anaesthesia 1987;42:415–418.

69. Arnold JW, Eichenberger CM. The hydraulic sarong: emergency treatment device for accidental hypothermia. JACEP 1975;4:438–439.

70. Kaplan M, Eidelman AI. Improved prognosis in severely hypothermic newborn infants treated by rapid rewarming. J Pediatr 1984;105:470–474.

71. Motil KJ, Blackburn MG, Peasure JR. The effects of four different radiant warmer temperature set-points used for rewarming neonates. J Pediatr 1974;85:546.

72. Levinson H, Linsao L, Swyer PR. A comparison of infrared and convective heating for newborn infants. Lancet 1966;2:1346.

73. Johnson LA. Accidental hypothermia: peritoneal dialysis. JACEP 1977;6:556–561.

74. O'Connor JP. Use of peritoneal dialysis in severely hypothermic patients [Letter]. Ann Emerg Med 1986;15:162–163.

75. Davis FM, Judson JA. Warm peritoneal dialysis in the management of accidental hypothermia: Report of five cases. New Zealand Med J 1981;94:207–209.

76. Ledingham IM. Clinical management of hypothermic patients. In: Pozos RS, Wittmers LE, eds. The nature and treatment of hypothermia. Croom Helm/London: University of Minnesota Press, 1983:165–181.

77. White JD, Butterfield AB, Greer KA, et al. Controlled comparison of radio wave regional

hyperthermia and peritoneal lavage rewarming after immersion hypothermia. J Trauma 1985;25:989–993.

78. Moss JF, Haklin M, Southwick HW, Roseman DL. A model for the treatment of accidental severe hypothermia. Trauma 1986;26:68–73.

79. Maresca L, Vasco JS. Treatment of hypothermia by extracorporeal circulation and internal rewarming. J Trauma 1987;27:89–90.

80. Davies DM, Miller, IA. Accidental hypothermia treated by extracorporeal blood warming. Lancet 1967;1036–1037.

81. Coughlin F. A heart-warming procedure (Letter). N Engl J Med 1973;288:326.

82. Linton AL, Ledingham IM. Severe hypothermia with barbiturate intoxication. Lancet 1966;1:24.

83. Paton BC. Accidental hypothermia. Pharmacol Ther 1983;22:331–377.

84. Mattox KL, Jordan GL. The emergency center as a site for major surgery. JACEP 1974;3:372.

85. Ausman RK, Kerkhof K, Holmes CJ, et al. Frozen storage and microwave thawing of parenteral nutrition solutions in plastic containers. Drug Intell Clin Pharm 1981;15:440–443.

86. Leaman PL, Martyak GG. Microwave warming of resuscitation fluids. Ann Emerg Med 1985;14:876–879.

87. Gong V. Microwave warming of IV fluids in management of hypothermia [Letter]. Ann Emerg Med 1984;13:645.

88. Werwath DL, Schwab CW, Scholten JR, Robinett W. Warming nondextrose crystalloid in a microwave oven [Letter]. Ann Emerg Med 1986;15:228–229.

89. Hayward JS, Steinman AM. Accidental hypothermia: an experimental study of inhalation rewarming. Aviat Space Environ Med 1975;46:1236–1240.

90. Linko K, Honkavaara P, Nieminen MT. Heated humidification in major abdominal surgery. Eur J Anesthesiol 1984;I:285–291.

91. Lloyd EL. Accidental hypothermia treated by central rewarming through the airway. Br J Anaesth 1973;45:41–47.

92. Slovis CM, Bachvarov HL. Heated inhalation treatment of hypothermia. Am J Emerg Med 1984;2:533–534.

93. White JD, Butterfield AB, Almquist TD, et al. Controlled comparison of humidified inhalation and peritoneal lavage in rewarming of immersion hypothermia. Am J Emerg Med 1984;2:210–214.

94. Shanks CA, Marsh HM. Simple core rewarming in accidental hypothermia. Br J Anaesth 1973;45:522–525.

95. McCann J. Mt. Hood disaster shows bypass valuable in severe hypothermia. Emerg Dept News 1986;July:1,8.

96. Maclean D. Emergency management of accidental hypothermia: a review. J R Soc Med 1986;79:528–531

97. Thredfall CJ, Yates DW, Barton RN, et al. Metabolic aspects of hypothermia in the elderly. Clin Sci 1980;59:9–27.

98. Danzl DF, et al. Chemical ventricular defibrillation in severe accidental hypothermia. Ann Emerg Med 1983;11:698.

99. Buckley JJ, Bosch OK, Bacaner MB. Prevention of ventricular fibrillation during hypothermia with bretylium tosylate. Anesth Analg 1971;50:587–593.

100. Murphy K, et al. Use of bretylium tosylate as prophylaxis and treatment in hypothermic ventricular fibrillation in the canine model. Ann Emerg Med 1986;15:1160.

101. Tafari N, Gentz J. Aspects of rewarming newborn infants with severe accidental hypothermia. Acta Pediatr Scand 1974;63:595.

102. Racine J, Jarjoui E. Severe hypothermia in infants. Helv Pediatr Acta 1982;37:317–322.

103. Andrew PJ, Parker RS. Treating accidental hypothermia [Letter]. Br Med J 1978;9 Dec:78.

104. Pugh LGCE. Accidental hypothermia in walkers, climbers, and campers: report to the Medical Commission on Accident Prevention. Br Med J 1966;1:123–129.

105. Pugh LGCE. Cold stress and muscular exercise, with special reference to accidental hypothermia. Br Med J 1967;2:333–337.

106. Kallman H. Protecting your elderly patient from winter's cold. Geriatrics 1986;40:69–81.

# CHAPTER 5

# Management of Radiation Injuries

## INTRODUCTION

Perhaps nothing in modern technology incites greater fear than the thought of a radiation accident.[1] Whether the fear is from the effects of monster bombs, a silent death, or changes in generations unborn is quite immaterial. In reaction to this fear, the news media have sensationalized any damage, injury, or fatality from a nuclear "spill" or accident. Fictional portrayals, such as "Dr. Strangelove," "On the Beach," and "The China Syndrome," help create this unmitigated horror about radiation accidents. (Strictly speaking, an accident refers to release of radioactive substances or radiation, while an incident is an event with the potential for radioactive contamination. If things get out of hand, an incident may become an accident.)

To get some idea of the rarity of serious radiation injuries, and the media exaggeration of the consequences, a look at some statistics is in order. During the 32-year period from 1943 to 1975, there were 10,086 accidents in the nuclear-related industries reported to the Atomic Energy Commission. Of these 10,086 accidents, 0.4% (41) were due to radiation exposure. There were three fatalities. From 1945 to 1986, there were fewer than 1000 persons worldwide involved in serious radiation accidents (in about 11,000 incidents), and, of these, about 500 people received medically significant doses of ionizing radiation, resulting in 50 fatalities.[2]

There have also been a few major power reactor spills or accidents with fatalities; at Los Alamos in 1945 and 1946 and at the National Reactor Testing Station in Idaho in 1961. In England, in 1957, a fire occurred in the graphite-moderated reactor in Windsdale. This reactor fire was contained within the reactor and had only a minimal release of radiation to the outside environment. In the United States, the damage to the Three Mile Island reactor systems in 1979 is still being decontaminated. Again, there was minimal release of radioactive material to the outside and absolutely no injuries due to the accident.[3] Nuclear power has had a superlative safety record, worldwide, when compared with chemical spills, fires in plants, coal mining, or any construction industry.

Of course, this all changed on April 26, 1986, in the northern Ukraine town of Chernobyl when at least 30 people died in history's worst nuclear accident.[4,5] Due to Soviet restrictions on reporting, perhaps the toll this accident took will never be known. The ill effects of this accident will be with us for years to come as more than 100,000 people were exposed to high levels of radioactive fallout. The accident should serve as a warning to all that the power of the atom can damage far from the source, when appropriate precautions are not met. The sensationalists had a field day with this unmitigated disaster, yet other "natural" disasters have had more fatalities or injuries (e.g., Pompeii, the Johnstown flood, the San Francisco earthquake, the 1988 Armenian earthquake, or even the chemical spill in Bhopal).

Many of the problems associated with nuclear power have been exacerbated and exploited by critics, who are using the accident at Chernobyl as an excuse to call for shutdown of all nuclear power plants. They fail to acknowledge that over the long run, every industrial nation, including the United States, will need the electric power supplied by the nuclear power plants. They also fail to acknowledge that coal, oil, and all other power sources have their associated dangers. These critics should also take note that the feared devastating genetic effects of nuclear war or nuclear power have not materialized in more than 40 years after Hiroshima and Nagasaki.

This is not intended to unrealistically minimize the potential hazards of a nuclear power plant accident. The possibility of a radioactive spill or nuclear power plant accident is real and all nearby medical facilities should be ready to manage such an accident. Hospitals and other medical care facilities near nuclear power plants are designated to handle the potential problems from such an accident and have prepared approved radiation accident protocols.[6]

Other sources of radiation are far more prevalent than bombs or reactors.[7] The use of radioactive materials and radiation-producing equipment has infiltrated American industry at all levels. The most common radiation source is the familiar diagnostic x-ray unit in hospitals and physician's and dentist's offices. Radiation sources are also used in thickness gauges, moisture gauges, and sterilization of medical supplies, food, and materials. Radioactive tracers and sources are used in pipelines and nondestructive testing of aircraft and machined parts. Radioactive tags are common in research in all fields of chemistry. In short, sources of radiation exposure for the emergency provider may be far greater than usually realized. Radioactive sources are NOT confined to weapons and reactor materials.

The transportation of radioactive isotopes presents the greatest risk of exposure for the emergency provider. These radioactive sources range from industrial and medical isotopes to spent fuel from reactors and, of course, nuclear weapons material. The substances should be clearly marked and appropriately packaged.

The problems associated with nuclear warfare—including the large-scale release of very active isotopes, disruption of organized medical care and government, and the threat of "nuclear winter" or annihilation of life as we know it—will not be discussed in this book. Abundant well documented and referenced texts describe these scenarios already.

Fortunately, the greatest risks for accidents do not occur with the nuclear weapons material and related items. Military security and military nuclear accident/incident control (NAIC) teams are stationed throughout the United States. Two designated military Radiologic Advisory Medical teams are further available 24 hours a day to aid the NAIC teams should they need additional medical help or consultation. The NAIC teams closely monitor the movement of nuclear weapons and weapons material because of the obvious terrorist threat with these items. They also respond rapidly to any accident involving aircraft or ships that carry nuclear weapons.

Although it is unlikely that any untoward events should happen, emergency departments that serve major transportation hubs must be ready to handle such transportation accident casualties. A civilian emergency department is more likely to have a problem with industrial or medical radioactive sources than from a military source or transportation accident. Such accidents may involve other trauma to the victim besides the effects or radiation. The most common medical scenario is a spill occurring within the hospital's own nuclear medicine department or as a result of transportation of materials within the vicinity of the hospital.[1]

## IMMEDIATE RESPONSES

The emergency management of radiation casualties depends upon the type of exposure and the amount of exposure. A person may be irradiated with x-rays or gamma rays, incorporate radioactive material into his body, or be contaminated with radioactive material.

The first question that the emergency provider needs to answer is:

Is the exposure continuing?

If the answer is yes, then the rate of exposure is ascertained, and an appropriate tolerable exposure time for rescue workers calculated, BEFORE entry into the area of exposure. If the source is a $Co^{60}$ radiation therapy or sterilization machine, shielding the source stops further exposure for all. If the source is an x-ray machine, removal of power stops radiation production.

The emergency worker's first priority should be to his/her own safety. If the radiation source is continuing, and the emergency worker becomes seriously exposed, he or she has just become a patient, not a rescuer.

After the exposure has ceased, or a tolerable time of exposure has been established, the next question that needs to be answered is:

Was the exposure irradiation or contamination (incorporation)?

The contaminated person continues to pose a danger to the medical staff because the contamination can be washed off, brushed off, or rubbed off onto the medical staff. Irradiated patients are not a danger to the staff.

It is essential for someone to measure the type and amount of the incident or contaminating radioactivity. If the source cannot be shielded or removed, then the allowable radiation exposure times must be calculated. The need to determine safe exposure times has influenced hospitals to designate a radiologist or radiotherapist as the chief physician when dealing with accidents from radioactive sources.

Facilities that include a radiation therapy unit are likely to have a medical health (radiation) physicist on staff, while all facilities with a Nuclear Regulatory Commission license must have a designated Radiation Control Officer. Either of these two people are also likely to be able to provide concrete advice about the management of radiation sources.

When the accident is purely from irradiation, the designation of a radiologist or nuclear medicine physician as the physician in charge may be appropriate. Unfortunately, and practically, these physicians may have had little experience beyond training with the management of radioactive materials or calculations of absorbed radiation doses. Few radiologists understand the constraints and vagaries of the field environment. When blast, trauma, or burns are included, a radiologist is most manifestly an inappropriate physician to coordinate all activities. The emergency physician or general surgeon who is coordinating the management of the traumatized, contaminated patient would be well advised to solicit the help of those physicians experienced with the management of radiation sources, however.

## Radiation Physics

In order to concisely discuss the management of the radiation emergency, a short review of the physics of radioactivity and radioactive materials is needed.

Radiation can be produced or occur naturally. Natural radiation occurs as the nucleus of a spontaneously occurring unstable isotope decays. Artificially produced radiation may occur as an artificially produced unstable radioisotope decays, or as a stream of electrons, protons, or neutrons hits a target and causes a naturally occurring element to decay or to emit excitation radiation.

Radiation is generally classified into two varieties: particulate and electromagnetic. Particulate radiation has mass; electromagnetic radiation has no mass but is, rather, an energy "wave" like light but in a different part of the spectrum. Particles may also have electrical charge and may travel at different speeds.

### ELECTROMAGNETIC RADIATION

Electromagnetic radiation has no mass or charge and can be thought of as an extension of light in its physical properties. Conceptually, electromagnetic radiation is at the high end of the energy spectrum that includes light, microwaves, infrared rays, ultraviolet rays, and x-rays or gamma rays. Electromagnetic radiation can be focused, deflected, blocked, and refracted by various materials. Electromagnetic radiation decreases in intensity according to the inverse square law—e.g., as the distance increases by 2, the intensity falls off by 4. (See Table 10.1. and Fig. 5.1.)

Electromagnetic radiation is emitted when electrons in the atom are shifted in their orbits, by either a nuclear decay (gamma rays) or by added external energy (x-rays). If this electromagnetic energy is greater than 100 electron volts, it is arbitrarily termed an x-ray. The only difference between gamma rays and x-rays is the source. (See Fig. 5.1.)

An electron volt is the kinetic energy of an electron accelerated through a potential difference of 1 volt.

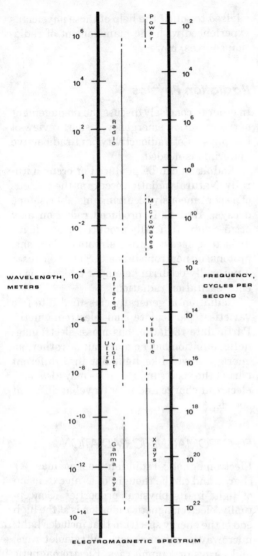

**Figure 5.1.** Electromagnetic spectrum.

## PARTICULATE RADIATION

Each radioisotope has a characteristic pattern of alpha, beta, neutron, and gamma emission. The energy of the alpha and beta particles can be measured and the spectrum of the gamma emissions analyzed. When these are measured, a radiation physicist can identify the isotope or isotopes causing the radiation. Lamentably, this identification may take substantial time. Fortunately, most radiation accidents involve well-known sources and the radiation physicist is more concerned with calculating the effects of the various emission spectra rather than trying to identify an un-

known mixture of isotopes from the emission spectra. (See Fig. 5.2.)

### Alpha Particles

Alpha particles consist of a helium nucleus with two protons and two neutrons that have been ejected from a decaying nucleus. The sum of the masses of the ejected alpha particle and the remaining product nuclei equals the mass of the parent nuclei.

Because the mass of the alpha particle is so great, it is easily stopped by other matter. It can cause significant cellular damage because of this same mass, however. This means that alpha particles cannot penetrate the skin but, if ingested or incorporated, present a very serious hazard.

### Beta Particles

Beta particles are equivalent to an electron emitted or ejected at high speed from the nucleus. The charge on this particle may be either negative (an electron) or positive with the negative charge much more common. The charge and energy of the ejected beta particle varies with the particular isotopic reaction.

Again, the mass of this particle means that it is easily slowed by thin shielding. With their greater speed and lesser mass, the beta particle can penetrate more deeply than the alpha particle. The beta particle, therefore, represents both an external and an internal hazard. The internal hazard is far greater than the external hazard, however.

### Protons

Protons are the stripped nuclei of hydrogen atoms with a single positive charge. Although particle beam accelerators use protons, and protons are prevalent in the Van Allen radiation belts, proton radiation is not a significant problem for emergency providers.

### Neutrons

The neutron is a particle of the nucleus that has no charge. Neutrons are emitted by reactors, neutron beams, and some radioactive isotopes. The neutron is usually found only with fission reactions. The rate at which a fission reaction proceeds is regulated by con-

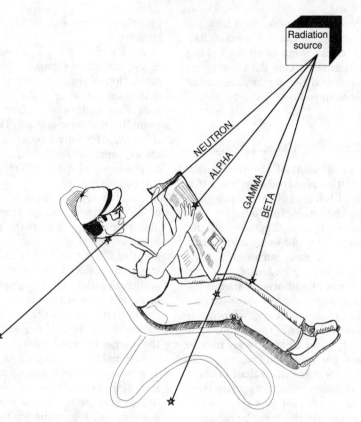

**Figure 5.2.** Penetration of particle radiation.

trolling the number of neutrons available to interact. The atomic bomb is an uncontrolled nuclear fission reaction.

Neutrons impinging upon another nucleus can be captured, making that nucleus into an unstable and, therefore, radioactive element, or they can destroy the nucleus. Fast-moving neutrons react primarily with hydrogen atoms, destroying them and causing an emission of protons that then causes secondary cellular damage. This cellular damage is the basic principle of the "neutron" bomb. (Actually a neutron bomb is a fission bomb that generates large numbers of neutrons). Slow-moving or thermal neutrons are captured by the collision with the atom's nucleus, resulting in a new radioisotope. The new element can decay and cause damage from the secondary radioactivity.

This slow neutron capture produces many of the medical isotopes, such as radioiodine or radiotechnetium. Unfortunately, if a sufficiently powerful slow neutron "flux" strikes the human body, many of the elements, such as gold fillings, sodium, chlorine, and phosphorus, will become radioactive. This residual induced radioactivity is proportional to the number of neutrons that hit the material and can be used to measure the dose of neutrons received. It is rarely significant enough to cause a danger to medical providers.

## MEASUREMENT OF RADIATION

The amount of instantaneous radiation may be measured at the moment it strikes an object or a cumulative dose can be determined. Two different systems are used to measure these two types of units.

### Flux Measurements

The classic radiation flux meter is the Geiger counter or the scintillation counter. These devices measure the number of flashes or ionized sparks caused by the impinging radiation per unit of time. They describe how much radiation would be absorbed if the flux stays at the same level for the prescribed time period. (One point that radiation physicists like to emphasize is that there is no such thing as a "Geiger counter." (One does not count Geigers!) Properly, these devices are called survey meters equipped with Geiger-Mueller [GM] probes.)

## Absorbed Radiation Measurements

The usual measurement of absorbed radiation is the radiation absorbed dose (rad). It is the deposition of 100 ergs of energy per gram of material by the impinging radiation. Another term often used is the roentgen (R), which is the deposition of 87 ergs of radiation per gram of air. For most purposes, the rad and the roentgen are equivalent.

Different types of radiation damage tissues in different ways, and the absorbed dose of radiation in rads does not always correlate with the apparent effects of the radiation on the tissues. This effect on the tissues may be correlated with the radiation that impinges on tissue by the roentgen equivalent in mammals (REM). The tissue effects of specific types of radiation are expressed as a relative biologic effectiveness (RBE) times the measurement of absorbed radiation, the rad. For example, the RBE for neutrons is about 2 since 150 rads of neutron radiation is thought to be equivalent to 300 rads of gamma rays in effects on the tissue. Both would be expressed as a 300 REM dose. For most exposures, the millirem (mrem) is used. RBEs vary from 1 for most x-rays, gamma rays, and beta emitters to about 20 for alpha particles.[3]

The usual measuring device for radiation absorbed doses is the dosimeter. The dosimeter provides a measurement of the total amount of radiation received by the **dosimeter** during the time measured. (It won't measure the radiation received if it wasn't worn by the person.)

The dosimeter may consist of a small film badge that increases in "fog" with absorbed radiation. The density of the fog can be measured and correlated to known radiation doses for similar film held in a controlled environment. Inside the case are three shields that allow different radiation energy levels to be measured when the film is processed. Carbon[14] and tritium ($H^3$) release insufficient energy to be detected by the film badge, while phosphorus[32] and iodine[131] ($I^{131}$) are easily detectable.

Film badges provide a permanent record of the radiation exposure. Indeed, close examination of the film may provide evidence of contamination or of direction of the exposure. Film badges suffer from fogging due to humidity and temperature. They are usually collected after only a month's wear (or a single exposure for an incident). The film must be processed at a laboratory before the dose can be determined.

Another type of dosimeter uses the decay of an electrical charge from radiation-induced ionization. This is the principle of the familiar pencil dosimeter. A movable filament is fixed to a hollow tube. An electrostatic charge is placed on the chamber wall and on the filament, causing the filament to be repelled toward the center of the tube. As the radiation causes the charge to decay, the filament falls toward the wall. The travel of the filament toward the wall is measured and is proportional to the amount of radiation. The reading from a pencil dosimeter is immediately available so it can be used to minimize exposure or when a worker will be exposed to very high radiation fluxes. The pencil dosimeter is sensitive to impact and will give false readings if dropped. For this reason, film badges are often used in conjunction with the pencil dosimeter.

A third type of dosimeter that is replacing both the pencil dosimeter and the radiation badge dosimeter is the thermoluminescent dosimeter (TLD). This latest and most sophisticated entry into the field of dosimetry is a small chip made of lithium fluoride crystals. The principle behind the TLD is that the lithium fluoride crystal gives off light in an amount proportional to the amount of radiation impinging upon it. When excited by radiation, some of the electrons are raised to a higher energy level and remain at that level until they are heated. The TLDs are inserted into badge holders containing filters to help determine the type and energy of the ionizing radiation to which the badge was exposed.

When the TLD chip is heated, the electrons return to the base state and release energy as light. A TLD reader heats and reads the subsequent light release in one operation. The electrons are then returned to their base state and the TLD chip is ready again. The reader is portable and field measurements can be readily made. TLDs are sensitive, measuring as low as 10 mREM. They have a long shelf life and may be worn for as long as 3 months. The major drawback to the TLD system is that once read, the information is lost, and there is no permanent record of the person's exposure.

## Biologic Dosimetry

The effects of radiation upon animals and humans have been well described as the result of our experiences following the bombing of Hiroshima and Nagasaki, in the infrequent radiation accident, and especially the experience at Chernobyl. These biologic effects form a crude "biodosimeter." (See Table 5.1.)

An early and important clinical indicator of radiation damage is the lymphocyte count. As the absorbed radiation dose increases, the magnitude and rapidity of the lymphocytopenia increases. If the patient has fewer than 500 lymphocytes per cc at 48 hours, the prognosis is poor. If the lymphocyte count is above 1200 per cc, the chances of survival are excellent. Lesser counts at 48 hours suggest more serious exposures.

Skin erythema, akin to a sunburn, also can act as a biodosimeter. The amount of erythema may be unreliable because it varies substantially with the type of radiation. Erythema that develops within minutes to hours after exposure to gamma rays does suggest serious exposure and possible systemic injury.

Gastrointestinal symptoms, such as nausea and vomiting, can also serve for biodosimetry. The severity of symptoms varies tremendously from person to person and is, therefore, not particularly useful. The timing of the symptoms is more useful. Early fever, diarrhea, decreasing level of consciousness, and/or hypotension are associated with extreme doses. Absence of gastrointestinal symptoms connotates a minimal exposure.

## TYPES OF EXPOSURE AND RESULTANT EFFECTS

### Irradiation

Irradiation occurs with either x-rays, neutrons, or gamma radiation and in lesser amounts with the relatively nonpenetrating beta particles. (See Figure 5.2.) Penetrating radiation can produce damage only in the portion of the body exposed. Most injuries and fatalities from radiation have been of this nature. Usually, the patient has been working and will know that he or she has been exposed to an x-ray source, a radiation sterilizing device, or a radiation source. The estimate of damage and need for treatment is likely to be a more difficult problem than the initial diagnosis or the nature of the injury.

**Table 5.1.**
**Recommended Exposure Limits**

| Exposure | Yearly Dose |
|---|---|
| Occupational exposure whole body including gonads lens of eye, and red bone marrow | 5000 mREM |
| All other organs including thyroid | 15,000 mREM |
| Hands | 75,000 mREM (25,000 per quarter) |
| Forearms | 30,000 mREM (10,000 per quarter) |
| General public | 500 mREM |
| Occasional radiation worker | |
| Fertile women | |
| Minors | |
| Emergency workers (one time) (whole body) | 25,000 mREM |
| Lifesaving actions (one time) | 100,000 mREM |

| Nominal Radiation Exposures | |
|---|---|
| Living near normally functioning reactor | < 1 mREM/yr |
| Watching color television | 1 mREM/yr |
| New York to San Francisco flight | 5 mREM |
| Chest x-ray | 50 mREM |
| Natural background radiation (Denver) | 150 mREM |
| Intravenous pyelogram | 500 mREM |
| Acute lymphocytopenia | 25 REM |
| Nausea and vomiting | 100 REM |
| $LD_{50}$ (untreated human) | 450 REM |
| $LD_{100}$ (100% death in humans) | 1000 REM |
| Acute CNS/ cardiovascular death | 5000 REM |

Please note that it is generally agreed that radiation exposure should be kept as low as reasonably achievable.

There are occasional exceptions where the diagnosis is not obvious, however. Symptoms typical of flu, nausea, vomiting, skin burns or ulcerations, or bone marrow depression have been noted when a history of radiation exposure was not known or suspected immediately. This may be a very difficult differential diagnosis, when the radiation exposure was days or weeks previously and the patient is completely unsuspecting of the event.

It should be emphasized that an irradiated person has the equivalent of a burn. Just as a person with a thermal burn does not give off heat, an irradiated patient does not give off radioactivity. Cells have been damaged or killed, but the person is not radioactive. They do not glow in the dark. The sole exception to this rule is exposure to exceptionally high levels of neutron radiation. The neutron radiation can induce secondary radioactivity in such places as fillings and prosthetics. Exposure to this level of neutron radiation is exceedingly rare. *The irradiated person generally presents no danger to the medical staff.*

## PROTECTION

Protection of the medical personnel involved in a continuing irradiation accident revolves around three factors: duration, distance, and defenses.

The **duration** of the exposure can be carefully monitored to ensure that any scene responder does not receive a dangerous irradiation. In this manner, the first responder may carry a piece of equipment into a hallway and then retreat. The next responder may carry the equipment farther into the building and retreat and so on. Any single responder will not receive a dangerous level of radiation, but if one responder were to perform the whole task, the yearly or lifetime limits may be exceeded.

The remainder of the personnel can interpose **distance** so that the inverse square law will afford protection. As noted earlier, the inverse square law means that doubling the distance decreases the radiation to one fourth of the original intensity.

**Defenses**, such as lead shielding, can be used by those who must enter an area to perform a technical task. These defenses may allow a surgeon to perform an amputation or a technician to lower a high-intensity source into a shielding well.

| *Clinical Radiation Injury Classifications* | |
|---|---|
| Mild exposure | Fewer than 125 rads |
| Intermediate exposure | About 400 rads (probably nonlethal) |
| High level exposure | About 400–600 rads (may be lethal) |
| Very high level exposure | About 600–1500 rads (probably lethal) |
| Extreme exposure | Greater than 1500 rads |

It should be emphasized that the approximate dose values may vary as much as 50% in individual patients.

## Mild Exposure

The mild exposure case (fewer than 125 rads whole body exposure) will generally require only reassurance that there are no serious effects anticipated. White and red blood cell counts will be lowered in most people with over 25 rads exposure. Nausea will be a problem for about 5 to 10% of those exposed to over 50 rads and the percentage of those nauseated will increase with increasing exposure. The nausea and vomiting will usually last no longer than 48 hours. Ten percent of the population will have a transient hair loss with exposure of 100 to 200 rads.

The patient should be advised that this dose may slightly increase the relative risk of developing cancer or leukemia. There is no known early preventative measure that will eliminate the slight increase in risk of the late effects (cancer and leukemia) for any significant exposure to radiation.

Males should be advised to employ a form of contraception for about 6 months following exposure to avoid potential congenital malformations if conception were to occur during this period. After this period, precautions should not be needed.

## Intermediate Exposure (Treatment Likely)

Exposure in the 100 to 400 REM range will cause symptoms of nausea, vomiting, and often diarrhea. The bone marrow is suppressed, often completely with later neutropenia, lymphopenia, and decrease in platelets. Hemorrhage from the thrombocytopenia may occur but more often infection supervenes.

Those cases in the intermediate dose range will require medical observation and possibly active treatment. Without appropriate medical therapy, 5 to 50% of those exposed to 200 to 400 rads will die within 60 days. The time of greatest risk will be during the bone marrow depression phase 3 to 4 weeks after exposure. The problem, quite simply, is one of keeping the exposed patient alive for the 5 to 6 weeks until the bone marrow begins to recover.

Therapeutic requirements for these patients fall into three categories:

1. **Control of infection**—protection from exogenous and nosocomial infections during the first 5 weeks. The use of strict isolation or "clean" room environments, use of appropriate antimicrobial drugs, and possible use of immunoglobulins are all indicated.
2. **Control of bleeding**—use of blood, platelets, and blood products as needed to control bleeding diatheses. Of course, the patient should be protected from trauma.
3. **Supportive Therapy**—psychological support, rest, and counseling about the genetic and personal effects of the dose received. For the health physicist, radiologist, or radiation therapy technician that has just received a total lifetime exposure, and must seek new work, this counseling cannot be emphasized enough.

Just as the complex burn is best managed by a burn team, the complex course of a severely irradiated patient is best managed by a "radiation injury team." The long-term care of these patients, quite properly, is outside the province of the emergency provider.

## High Level Exposure (Maximal Lifesaving Effort Required)

An exposure in the 600 to 1000 REM range will primarily produce hematologic and gastrointestinal effects. The early course of the patient will be marked with severe and persistent nausea, diarrhea, and vomiting. Occasionally, GI bleeding will be noted. As the nausea abates, the profound hematologic effects become manifest. The marrow is completely suppressed, often with early neutropenia, lymphopenia, and thrombocytopenia.

The above-mentioned therapeutic requirements and concerns regarding infection and bleeding in the intermediately exposed pa-

tient are now mandatory for these high level exposures. Use of "clean" rooms or filtered laminar airflow rooms is mandatory.

Heroic efforts to save the patient's life in suspected lethal or near lethal exposures (500 to 1000 rads) might include the use of marrow transplantation during the first 10 days postexposure. This is about 2 weeks before the period of maximal bone marrow suppression expected. Cross circulation of a patient with another has also been proposed.

Fortunately, there is a period of about 1 week to arrange for special consultations and advice on the needed hospital services. Dur-

---

*Sources of Help for Radiation Injuries*
Department of Energy
Regional Coordinating Offices for Radiologic Assistance
Brookhaven Area Operations Office   516-282-2200
Responsible for Connecticut, Delaware, Maine, Maryland, Massachusetts, New Hampshire, New York, New Jersey, Pennsylvania, Rhode Island, Vermont, Puerto Rico, and the Virgin Islands.

Oak Ridge Operations Office   615-576-1005
Responsible for Arkansas, Kentucky, Louisiana, Missisippi, Missouri, Tennessee, Virginia, and West Virginia.

Savannah River Operations Office   803-726-3333
Responsible for Alabama, Georgia, Florida, North Carolina, South Carolina, and the Canal Zone

Albuquerque Operations Office   505-844-4667
Responsible for Arizona, Kansas, New Mexico, Oklahoma, and Texas

Chicago Operations Office   312-972-4800 and 312-972-5731
Responsible for Illinois, Indiana, Iowa, Michigan, Minnesota, Nebraska, North and South Dakota, Ohio, and Wisconsin

Idaho Operations Office   208-526-1515
Responsible for Colorado, Idaho, Montana, Utah, and Wyoming

San Francisco Operations Office   415-273-4237
Responsible for California, Hawaii, and Nevada

Richland Operations Office   509-373-3800
Responsible for Alaska, Oregon, and Washington

ing this time, the patient may be transferred to a "radiation injury team" facility staffed to provide the needed expertise, hematologic, oncologic, and laboratory services.

### Very High Level Exposure (Probable Lethality)

A constellation of immediate symptoms including mental confusion, nausea, vomiting, diarrhea, and shock will be seen with exposures greater than 1000 rads. Nausea and vomiting may be seen within minutes. The neutrophil count rises rapidly and then falls equally rapidly to fewer than 100 within 24 hours. Lymphocyte counts approach zero within 24 hours.

These large doses of radiation may produce acute CNS and cardiovascular deterioration. Previously, it was thought that CNS effects accounted for most rapid deaths, but recent experience has shown that cardiovascular deterioration may also be rapid following these supralethal doses. The rapid neurologic and cardiovascular deterioration is the basis for the effectiveness of the so-called "neutron bomb." A neutron bomb is a low-yield antipersonnel thermonuclear device specifically designed to produce maximal amounts of high-energy neutrons with low blast and fallout damage.[9]

These surely terminal patients will require symptomatic therapy during what will probably be a short course (at most 2 to 10 days). Treatment will be supportive and palliative and includes sedation, antiemesis, and fluid replacement. The maximal survivable radiation doses may be significantly higher with current therapy, and if there is even a remote chance of success, vigorous therapy should be given.

## LOCAL EXPOSURES

Possibly, the most frequent type of irradiation accident seen in the emergency department is the local exposure of a hand in a high level radiation field. These accidents often occur with gamma source x-ray cameras or sterilizing devices. A technician deliberately defeats the safety precautions (usually to service the machine), accidently exposes himself, and presents for therapy.

The amount and depth of damage are proportional to the level of exposure. Fortu-

nately, only infrequently will a technician receive a total body irradiation in this manner. Since the gastrointestinal tract and the bone marrow are not irradiated, the patient does not develop the symptoms of whole body irradiation. Soft tissue exposed to radiation has far greater resistance than more rapidly reproducing tissues.

With a dose of fewer than 500 REM, the patient may have local erythema. There may be a slightly increased level of localized neoplasms as a late complication, but early complications are few.

With doses of about 2500 REM, the patient may develop localized depilation, followed by a temporary but slowly healing ulcer. Skin atrophy, telangiectasia, and localized vitiligo may be late complications. At doses of greater than 5000 REM to a localized area, ulcers are permanent, and a marked increase in neoplasms is noted. Doses greater than 50,000 REM cause great destruction in the path of the beam, with severe necrosis resulting.[10] Management of these lesions is frustrating because deep vascular damage often precludes successful grafting. (See Table 5.2.)

Early treatment of these localized lesions should proceed as if the patient has incurred a skin burn. The patient should be dressed with a common burn ointment, such as silver sulfdiazine. Referral to a surgeon knowledgeable in the management of these difficult and

**Table 5.2.**
**Skin Effects of Localized Exposure to Radiation**

| Dose | Early Effects | Late Effects |
|---|---|---|
| < 500 REM | ? Erythema | None (may be slight increase in neoplasms) |
| > 500 REM | Erythema Depilation | Usually, minimal increase in neoplasms |
| 2500 REM | Ulcerations Depilation | Local atrophy, telangiectasia Altered pigmentations |
| 5000 REM | Ulcerations | Chronic ulcerations Substantial carcinogenesis |
| > 50,000 REM | | |

frustrating patients may be accomplished at leisure.

## CONTAMINATION

If the patient is radioactive, this may be due to contamination or induced activity from a neutron source. Induced radiation from neutron exposure does not produce any hazard to medical workers and serves mostly to aid in an estimation of the size of the dose to the patient.

Perhaps the most important point for medical personnel to realize is that radioactive contamination is similar to a chemical burn. Until the radioactive or chemical contaminant is removed, it will continue to burn. If it is spread to a medical worker, it will burn the medical worker also. If it is a weak source of radiation, it will burn at a slower rate, just like weak solutions of chemicals will burn at a slower rate than strong solutions.

To continue the comparison with the better known chemical burn, radioactive contamination may be external, may be ingested, or may be incorporated in a wound. The radiation and contamination exposure may be complicated with other injuries such as blast injury or burns. When treating a chemical contamination, there is often no way of knowing when the chemical has finally been diluted or washed out. This is not true in radiation emergencies. In the treatment of radiation contamination, we have the ability to measure the residual contamination with appropriate instruments.

## Protection

For contaminated cases, ambulance and rescue personnel should don the appropriate protective gear for the scene. Filtration-type masks or self-contained breathing apparatus are minimal appropriate gear in most scene responses for radioactive contamination. Continuing exposure to high level radiation should be managed as outlined above with limits to duration, increased distance, and defenses as indicated. A radiation biologist will usually determine these needs.

Protection of the environment of the ambulance may be quite a problem. It is unlikely that word of an accident will be received in such time and such detail that all nonessential equipment can be removed from the ambulance and the interior covered with plastic or paper. Ambulances and ambulance personnel should be considered as contaminated. Scene responders should not be released until both they and their vehicles are decontaminated and cleared by the radiation biophysicist.

If the hazard area involves multiple casualties, the decontamination of the vehicle and crew will be at the joint discretion of the radiation biophysicist and the mass casualty scene commander (usually a physician). A minor level of contamination may be tolerated in order to transport further patients, particularly those who also may be contaminated.

The medical staff should handle the patient with (at the least) masks, scrubs, gowns, and gloves to avoid exposure to themselves. Medical staff must be decontaminated after care of the patient, just as if a chemical agent were involved.

Medical attendants are permitted 5 R for routine treatment and decontamination of patients. For emergency treatment, up to 25 R are permissible. This level of exposure will constitute a lifetime's exposure for a radiation physicist and will preclude work in that or a related field. For lifesaving treatment, up to 100 R are permitted in 1 year's time. Pregnancy should preclude participation in any voluntary radiation exposure.

### NOTIFICATION

Although these patients or their coworkers may notify the hospital of all details, it is imperative that the hospital have as much advance notice as possible. The scene response crew must gather as much information as possible to ensure proper and prompt notification of both hospital and state authorities. The responsibility for notification of state and federal authorities should be outlined for all hazardous materials response teams, hospitals, and nuclear laboratories.

An important point to note for all medical personnel is that if the agent is known, such as in a power plant, radioisotope treatment facility, or nuclear laboratory, the personnel working with the isotope often know more about the exposure than most emergency providers. Guidance given by these nuclear workers (even as patients) may well limit the spread of contaminants, decrease absorption

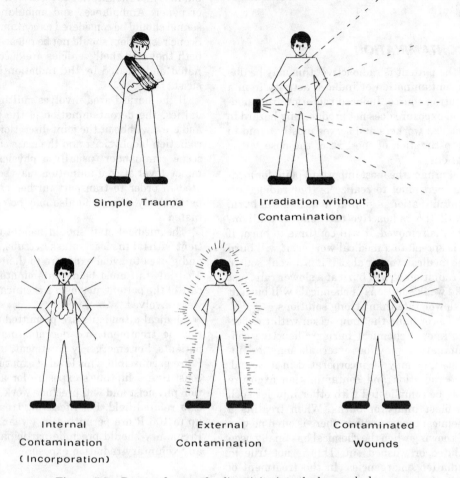

Simple Trauma

Irradiation without
Contamination

Internal
Contamination
(Incorporation)

External
Contamination

Contaminated
Wounds

**Figure 5.3.** Routes of entry of radioactivity into the human body.

of radioisotopes, or limit exposure to all concerned. This source of information and guidance must not be neglected.

### Internal Contamination (Incorporation)

Internal contamination can occur by either ingestion or inhalation of radioactive compounds. (See Figs. 5.3 and 5.4.) Incorporation may also result from particles driven into the body by a blast effect. Although the incorporation of radioactive agents may be lethal to the patient, incorporated agents pose little risk to emergency providers. The sole exceptions to this would be, of course, handling of bodily wastes and disposal of the fragments from wounds.

The seriousness of internal contamination is determined by:

1. The route of the contamination
2. The half-life of the isotope
3. The chemical nature of the isotope
4. The location of the isotope within the body
5. The level of exposure to the isotope
6. The specific therapy indicated for each radioactive isotope

The level of exposure must be assayed by the radiation physicist. This can be done by gastric washings, urinalysis, nasal smears, and, if available, whole body counters. The location of the isotope can be determined in the patient's body by a gamma camera assay, if, of course, the isotope emits gamma rays.

There are multiple agents that prevent the

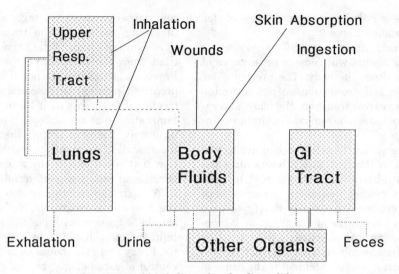

**Figure 5.4.** Metabolic paths of radionuclides.

uptake or hasten the excretion of a radio-isotope. The first few hours after the incorporation of a radionuclide may be crucial for effective treatment. A radiation physicist or physician experienced in nuclear medicine should be consulted in all cases of suspected incorporation of radioisotopes.

Ipecac, charcoal, and magnesium citrate or sorbital will all enhance excretion or interrupt gastrointestinal absorption. Metals, such as copper, iron, or plutonium, are generally better absorbed in an acid environment such as the stomach. Neutralizing stomach acids with antacids may cause the formation of hydroxides or reduce the solubility of these metals.[11-13] Sorbital, sodium alginate, or aluminum salts should be used for strontium ingestions.

Bronchoalveolar lavage may be used for inhaled contaminants but has significant side effects and complications. It is customarily reserved for those who have far exceeded the maximal allowable body burden of the isotope.

Isotope competition can reduce the absorption of an isotope by providing an excess of a similar but nonradioactive form of the element. A familiar example would be the use of iodine salts to prevent the uptake of $I^{131}$ by the thyroid. If given within 2 hours of exposure to $I^{131}$, 100 mg of stable iodine will reduce the uptake in the thyroid by about 90%.[14] The agent used in this technique is often called a blocking agent.

A related technique is isotopic dilution, in which large quantities of a stable isotope are added in order to decrease the statistical possibility of incorporation of a specific atom of the radioactive form. The usual example is the use of ordinary water when faced with a radioactive dihydrogen (tritium) oxide incorporation. Sometimes, the dilution is done with a completely different element that shares chemical properties with the radioactive isotope. An example of this technique, called displacement therapy, is the use of calcium to block radioactive strontium uptake or iodine to block radioactive technetium uptake.[15] Contact your department of nuclear

| *Chelation Therapy for Incorporation of Isotopes*[19] | |
|---|---|
| *Isotope* | *Chelating Agent* |
| Iron | Deferoxamine |
| Cesium | Prussian blue |
| Copper, gold, lead, mercury, and cobalt | Penicillamine |
| Rubidium | Chlorthalidone |
| Polonium | Dimercaprol (British Anti-Lewisite BAL) |
| Cadmium, chromium, lead, and zinc | Calcium—EDTA |
| Transuranic rare earths* | Zinc DPTA |

*Americium, californium, cerium, curium, lanthanum, plutonium, promethium, scandium, and yttrium.

medicine or radiologist for specific agents for specific radioisotopes.

For some isotopes, specific heavy metal chelating agents will remove all isotopes of that type from the body. The prototype for this action is the medical use of deferoxamine to remove excess iron from the body, and radioactive iron can be removed in similar manner.

If these various blocking or chelating agents are used in the first 1 to 3 hours after the ingestion, absorption can be reduced. In order to supply prompt treatment, the emergency department must have a well-defined plan based on knowledge of the plant or lab operations, the radionuclides used, and the medications required. This may not be possible when a "street" accident is the cause of the exposure.

After treatment, the patient should have repeat assay of the isotopes, including both gamma camera and whole body counter assays to document the decontamination. The radiation physicist can then calculate the total absorbed radiation dose in order to determine whether a clinical radiation syndrome is likely.

## Decontamination

The decontamination effort is started at the scene. If the patient's condition permits, the ambulance personnel should remove the patient's clothing and wash contaminated areas with soap and water. This action alone will remove the bulk of surface contamination and will quickly decrease the exposure to medical staff. The effluent and clothing should be stored in plastic bags in order to ensure that the contamination does not spread.

Medical providers should ensure that de-

contamination does not take priority over lifesaving measures. The traumatized patient is more likely to die from the trauma than from the radioactive contamination. Providers, at all levels, should complete appropriate primary and secondary surveys, treating life threats as if there was no contamination. The sole exception to this might be invasive bodily procedures that could cause incorporation or mouth-to-mouth resuscitation that could expose the rescuer to incorporation of radioactive materials.

A separate decontamination area within the hospital is essential. Walls and floors should be covered with plastic sheeting, and light switches should be protected with plastic. Entry and exit should be only under the control of a radiologist or radiation biophysicist who can check for radioactive contamination. If an installed decontamination shower with holding tank is not available, portable showers with large plastic holding tanks should be considered. All refuse water from the shower should be considered contaminated until cleared by a radiation biophysicist.

A single person, preferably a radiation physicist, should assume responsibility for ensuring that all personnel have and wear a dosimeter and ensure that the dosimeter readings are recorded. The same person should ensure than all nonessential personnel are excluded from the area and that only verified uncontaminated supplies and personnel go from the "dirty" area to the clean area.

The patient's clothes and bedding should be removed and then put in plastic bags if this has not previously been done. All jewelry and metal items should also be removed and placed in plastic bags. These plastic bags should be labeled "Radioactive material—DO NOT DISCARD."

Areas of contamination should be measured and recorded on an anatomic chart. A Lund and Browder burn chart is excellent for this recording. (See Chapter 2.) A second reading at the end of decontamination will verify the adequacy of the effort.

The use of specific agents for skin decontamination is determined by the properties of the contaminant, and this information should be readily available to the health physicist. If there is no specific chemical or diluent that will remove, stabilize, or aid in

---

*Protection from Continuing Radiation*
*Duration*
Keep the duration of exposure to the lowest possible limits.
*Distance*
Doubling the distance between you and the radioactive source decreases exposure to one fourth the original exposure.
*Defenses*
Shielding can markedly attenuate the radiation.

dissolving the agent, then the use of detergent solution is indicated. Vigorous scrubbing should be avoided because it tends to break down the skin barrier. Copious amounts of water or other diluent are appropriate. Tepid water should be used rather than hot water because hot water will open pores and allow internal contamination.

Decontamination solutions that have been used successfully include soap and water, green soap and water, phosphate-based detergents such as Tide or Cheer, chelating agents such as EDTA and DPTA, and potassium permanganate followed by sodium bisulfite and titanium oxide.[16]

Surgical debridement and decontamination is best done by a surgeon who has been trained in the treatment of radioactive wounds. Additional surgery staff may be needed if a patient has been contaminated with a very high level source or if multiple patients have been injured. In extreme cases, the surgeon may operate behind a lead shield while removing fragments.

Decontamination should start, if medical status permits, with cleansing and scrubbing the areas of highest contamination first. Gentle washing is mandatory, as scrubbing and denuding skin will allow entry of particles. Give special attention to skin folds, creases, hair, and body orifices. Remeasure after each washing and showering and record the results.

Measurements of the amount of contamination that has been removed, and, most importantly, the amount yet remaining must be obtained. The radiation biophysicist will need nasal and oral swabbings to estimate the amount of ingested contamination. Also 24-hour urine and 72-hour fecal collections will prove helpful. All sputum, vomit, debrided tissue, particles and fragments, shaved hair, and exudates must be collected and saved separately. Extra samples of blood should be drawn for the use of the radiation biophysicist in estimation of exposure. Whole body radiation counts and radioiodide counts may be indicated.

When all patients have been decontaminated, the medical staff will need to be decontaminated themselves. All clothing, masks, booties, and linens should be bagged and labeled. Showers should be taken and fresh scrubs donned. A radiation biophysicist should monitor the medical staff and record any sites of radiation, ensuring that all is removed.

Finally, the suite, ambulances, litters, gurneys, etc., used need to be decontaminated, under strict control by radiation physicists. All disposable materials will be discarded, used or unused, as contaminated. Severely contaminated equipment may need to be replaced. Any articles that are contaminated will be either decontaminated, stored for a length of time until the isotope decays, or disposed of as radioactive waste in accordance with Federal Regulation.

## LABORATORY DATA

Laboratory data may provide clues to the extent of exposure, the nature of the radioactive agent, and the prognosis of the exposed person. Minimal laboratory tests should include:

Complete blood count with platelets every 6 hours
Urinalysis (save all urine from the time of the accident)
Fecal analysis for affected radionuclide (save all feces from the time of the accident)
Nasal swabs before blowing nose, washing face, or showering
Patient's dosimeter, if any

Laboratory specimens should be handled as if radioactive, until proven otherwise. Personal effects, such as jewelry and clothing, may be decontaminated and returned to the patient after approval of the radiation control officer. Never let the patient touch laboratory specimens or other objects until the patient has been decontaminated and verified free of residual contamination.

## PROPHYLAXIS

One of the most biologically important fission products released by reactor accidents is $I^{131}$. Public health authorities have recommended two methods to prevent the uptake of this isotope, including evacuation of the downwind area and administration of stable iodine. Evacuation from the path of the fallout will decrease any uptake of radioactive iodine but may be impractical, unfeasible, or too time consuming. Administration of iodine can be preplanned and the civilian population can self-administer the dose upon public health recommendations.[17]

---

*Problem Areas*

Wounds—If a wound is involved, prepare and cover the wound with a self-adhering disposable surgical drape. Cleanse the surrounding areas until decontaminated. Remove the wound covering and irrigate the wound with sterile water. Catch the irrigating fluid and store it in a large marked plastic container. Each step of the decontamination procedure should be monitored and the extent and location of contamination recorded.

If a wound is grossly contaminated, both wet debridement as described above, and sharp surgical debridement, may be indicated. Again, at each step of the decontamination process, the extent and location of contamination should be measured and recorded.

If contamination persists, further surgical debridement may be indicated. Do not mutilate to decontaminate, without *very* good reason. Check with the radiation biophysicist about the nature and extent of the injury if the contamination was not removed and use appropriate judgment.

Ears, Mouth, and Eyes—Irrigate the area with saline or water and save the irrigation for analysis. Be sure to get swabs of these areas before irrigation and save them in plastic bags for the use of the radiation biophysicist.

Hair—Hair may retain some isotopes and should be cut in such cases. Do not shave the scalp if possible as the skin injury may increase absorption and later incorporation into the body.

Inhalation—About half of the contaminated material that has been inhaled is returned to the pharynx by ciliary action in the trachea. This portion is often swallowed. Save all sputum for analysis. Lung lavage may be indicated; check with the radiation biophysicist.

---

According to Federal Drug Administration recommendations, this prophylactic treatment should be given only when the estimated radiation exposure to the thyroid will be greater than 10 to 30 REM.[18] There is some controversy both about public application of this therapy and about the threshold of radiation for administration of iodine. Blocking therapy with stable iodine was used in the wake of the Chernobyl accident with good effect.

## SUMMARY

As we have noted, most small hospitals will never be faced with the possibility of a serious radiation incident. Our increasing use of radioisotopes and transportation of them puts all emergency departments in jeopardy, however.

The usual "radiation emergency protocol" should be updated by a manager or physician director on a yearly basis. Personnel may receive training on management of a radiation accident upon initial orientation in some hospital and emergency services. Unfortunately, what is not used is lost, and training on radiation emergencies is no exception. All emergency providers should receive initial and annual training in the management of radioactive accident victims.

## References

1. Milroy WC. Management of irradiation and contaminated casualty victims. Emerg Med Clin North Amer 1984;2:667–686.
2. Federal Emergency Management Agency. Course for radiological monitors. Washington, DC: U.S. Government Printing Office, 1979.
3. Fabrikant JI. The effects of the accident at Three Mile Island on the mental health and behavioral responses of the general population and nuclear workers (special report). Health Physics 1983;45:579–586.
4. Associated Press. The Pueblo Chiefain, Associated Press, August 3, 1986.
5. Geiger HJ. The accident at Chernobyl and the medical response. JAMA 1986;256:609–612.
6. Bores RJ. The scope of nuclear regulatory commission requirements for arrangements for medical services for contaminated injured individuals. Bull NY Acad Med 1983;59:956–961.
7. Stasiak RS, Stewart CE, Redwine RH. Symptoms and treatment of radiation exposure. Emerg Med Serv 1986;15:21–26.
8. Casarett AP. Radiation biology. Englewood Cliffs, NJ: Prentice-Hall, Inc., 1968.
9. Taylor TB. Third generation nuclear weapons. Sci Amer 1987;256:30–39.
10. NCRP Report No. 39. Basic radiation protection criteria. Bethesda: National Council on Radiation Protection and Measurements, 1971.
11. Baxter DW, Sullivan MF. Gastrointestinal absorption and retention of plutonium chelates. Health Phys 1972;22:785.
12. Tompsett SL. Factors influencing the absorp-

tion of iron and copper from the alimentary tract. Biochem J 1940;34:961.

13. Jacobs AG, Rhodes DK, Peters H, et al. Gastric acidity and iron absorption. Br J Haemat 1966;12:728.

14. Ramden D, Passant, FH, Peabody CO, Speight RG. Radioiodine uptakes in the thyroid studies of the blocking and subsequent recovery of the gland following the administration of stable iodine. Health Phys 1967;13:633.

15. Lincoln TA. Importance of initial management of persons internally contaminated with radionucleides. Am Ind Hygiene Assoc J 1976; 37:16–21.

16. Saenger EL. Radiation accidents. Ann Emerg Med 1986;15:1061–1066.

17. Fowinkle EW, Sell SH, Wolle RH. Predistribution of potassium iodide—the Tennessee experience. Pub Health Rep 1983;96:123–126.

18. Saenger EL. Radiation accidents. Ann Emerg Med 1986;15:1061–1066.

19. NCRP Report No. 65. Management of persons accidentally contaminated with radionucleides. April 15, 1980. Washington, DC: National Council on Radiation Protection and Measurements, 1980.

# CHAPTER 6

# Management of Altitude-Related Emergencies

## INTRODUCTION

As long as people have climbed mountains or gone to high places for reasons of trade or war, they have recorded tales of the difficulties that are encountered at altitude. Examples of altitude-related illnesses have been described by Romans and Carthaginians in the Alps, by the Chinese in the Himalayas, and by the Spanish in the Peruvian Andes. In 1913, T. M. Ravenhill noted the effects of the rapid ascent to high altitude by new miners in the Chilean Andes. He noted the differences between a high-altitude pulmonary edema and a lesser sickness, and he puzzled as to how strong healthy men could be stricken in hours by these diseases.[1] This question has not yet been adequately answered.

During the last two decades, a tremendous increase in recreation in mountainous areas has caused a corresponding increase in the prevalence of altitude-related illnesses. Prior to the 1960s, only a few hearty adventurers would brave the trek to the base camp at Mt. Everest. This trek involved 3 weeks of arduous approach that acclimated all in the party. Today, over 5000 travelers each year in the Himalayas alone reach altitudes that are potentially dangerous. Some 3600 people visit the top of Pike's Peak (14,213 feet—4332 m) each day. Millions more will trek to stateside mountain resorts for skiing, hiking, and, of course, climbing. The major difference now is that the trekker may fly to the resort, spend only a few days skiing or hiking, and then return to sea level. These same folks return to their homes where physicians who are inexperienced in environmental medical problems do not consider the altitude exposure in their diagnostic patterns.

Altitude-related illnesses are not discrete separate entities but, rather, a spectrum of illness caused by inappropriate compensation to continuing relative hypoxia. The diseases may be lethal, usually occur when man ascends above 8000 feet (2400 m), and are best treated with descent to lower altitude.

The usual illnesses that accompany travel into high altitudes include the following:

1. *Acute mountain sickness (AMS)*. This is a common disease that affects up to 25% of travelers that ascend rapidly to any altitude greater than 8500 feet (2590 m). Headache, nausea, vomiting, dyspnea, fatigue, work intolerance, and sleep disturbances are common. AMS is usually a self-limited disease that requires only supportive therapy or descent to lower altitude.

2. *High-altitude pulmonary edema (HAPE)*. This unusual but always serious disease is rarely seen above 8500 feet (2590 m). The common early symptoms include headache, rales, dyspnea, fatigue, and a nonproductive cough.

3. *High-altitude cerebral edema (HACE)*. This rare, life-threatening disease is manifested by headache, fatigue, ataxia, confusion, and hallucinations. This disease will rapidly progress to coma and subsequent death if not treated.

4. *High-altitude retinal hemorrhage (HARH)*.

This is a relatively common and usually innocuous finding of travelers at the upper limits of very high altitude and beyond. It does not usually require therapy.

## DEFINITIONS

**High altitude**. High altitude is usually defined as an altitude greater than 8000 feet (about 2400 m) to about 14,000 feet (4300 m). About 12% of the world's population (40 million people) live at or above this altitude.[2] Because a large number of individuals visit locations within this altitude range, *most cases* of altitude-related illnesses occur at these elevations. The most serious forms of altitude-related illnesses have a lower incidence at the lower altitudes in this range.

**Very high altitude**. Very high altitude is the range of altitude from 14,000 feet (4300 m) to 18,000 feet (5500 m). Although most cities frequented by tourists are located lower than this range of altitude, a significant number of base camps and towns exist at these altitudes. Indeed, the highest known continuously inhabited town on earth is located at 16,732 feet (5100 m) (Wenchuan on the Chianghe-Tibet road).

In this range of altitudes, any known altitude illness can occur. Rapid ascent to these heights without prior acclimation is dangerous.

**Extreme altitude**. Extreme altitude is the range of altitude from 18,000 feet (5500 m) to 29,000 feet (8800 m). There is a substantial risk of altitude-related illnesses at these higher altitudes. Ascent to these heights without substantial preparation is exceedingly dangerous. Fortunately, most climbers at this altitude have been properly acclimated. Those climbers who are susceptible to altitude illnesses have usually turned back or have been evacuated.

Above 18,000 feet (5500 m) one does not become acclimated to the altitude. Rather, there is a gradual increase in physical and mental deterioration.

## COMPOSITION OF THE ATMOSPHERE

### Standard Atmosphere

In terms of pressure, one standard atmosphere is equal to 760 mm Hg at sea level. This atmospheric pressure decreases linearly with increasing altitude at all terrestrial elevations (Fig 6.1).

The actual atmospheric pressure varies somewhat with the weather, the seasons, and the latitude, although these changes seldom are greater than 10 mm Hg. The atmospheric pressure is somewhat higher at the equator and lower at the poles due to the shape and rotation of the earth and the presence of a dense cold air mass above the equatorial earth.

Except for water vapor content, the composition of the atmosphere is constant throughout this range of altitudes and over the entire surface of the earth. When completely dry, the atmosphere is composed of 20.94% oxygen, 79.02% nitrogen, 0.04% carbon dioxide, and trace amounts of inert gases. The only substantial variable is the water vapor content, which is dependent upon a number of factors.

For medical purposes, the water vapor contribution may be presumed to be the vapor pressure of water at tracheal temperatures (47 mm Hg at 37°C). This assumption is safe, because the air is completely saturated with water vapor by tracheal moisture by the time it passes into the alveoli. The vapor pressure of water is primarily dependent upon temperature and will be higher with higher temperatures or fever. (At 39°C, water vapor pressure is 50 mm Hg.)

### Partial Pressures

The pressure exerted by each component of a mixture of gases is termed the gas tension or the partial pressure of that gas. The total pressure of a gas mixture is the sum of the partial pressures of the individual gas components of that mixture. The partial pressure of each component can be given by the formula:

$$Pp = (\%gas) \times (\text{total pressure}) / 100 \qquad (1)$$

As noted previously, the air is fully saturated with water at the level of the alveolus. In the medical case, therefore, the above equation must be modified to account for the vapor pressure of water. The resultant equation is expressed by:

$$P = (\%gas) \times (\text{barometric pressure} - \text{vapor pressure})/100 \qquad (2)$$

# Barometric Pressure at Altitude

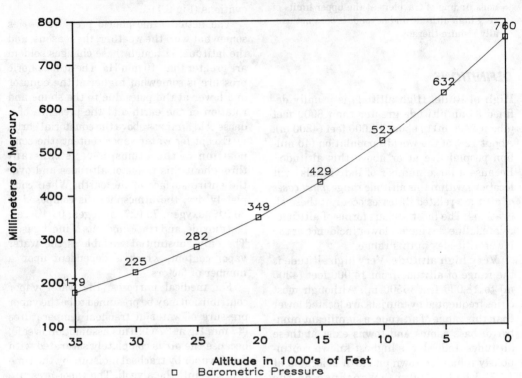

**Figure 6.1.** Altitude versus pressure graph shows the variation of barometric pressure with increasing altitude at the terrestrial altitudes.

Thus, the partial pressure of oxygen at the level of the alveolus is:

$$P = (0.21) \times (760 - 47)$$

$$= 149 \text{ mm Hg at sea level} \qquad (3)$$

Since the barometric pressure decreases as a function of altitude, the partial pressures of its constituents will decrease also. The oxygen partial pressure at 18,000 feet (5500 m) will be half that at sea level. An inevitable consequence of ascent to high altitude is the decrease in the amount of oxygen available to use (Fig 6.2).

## ADAPTATION TO LIFE AT HIGH ALTITUDE

Much of our early knowledge of altitude-related problems came from balloon, aircraft, and decompression chamber ascents. When the partial pressure of oxygen supplied to the human body is reduced abruptly, the compensation mechanisms are grossly inade-

quate. Indeed, the U.S. Air Force notes that the time of useful consciousness at 25,000 feet (7600 m) is only 3 to 5 minutes. This means that if a plane is flying next to Mt. Everest, and a window blows out, the occupants of the plane have only 3 to 5 minutes to do something about it before they lose the ability to start corrective actions. A gradual ascent to the same altitude does not carry the same connotations, or Messner and Habeler would never have been able to ascend to the summit without supplementary oxygen in 1978.[3] The hypoxic experiences learned in flight simply have little application to the trekker who reaches altitude in hours or days.

A gradual ascent, on the other hand, allows the body to adapt and acclimate in multiple ways to the decreased availability of oxygen. Man's survival and effective function at 18,000 feet (5500 m) and toleration of 28,000 feet (8535 m) without supplemental oxygen are examples of these acclimation responses. Such acclimation begins to be evident at altitudes greater than 6562 feet (2000 m).

# Tracheal Oxygen Tension at Altitude

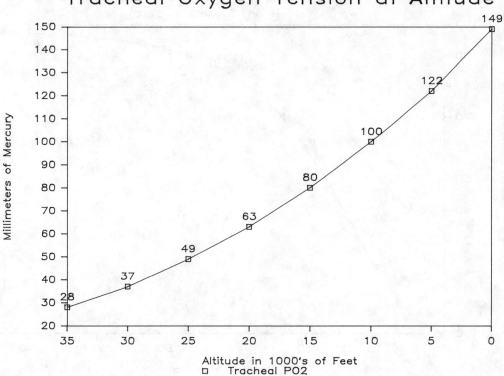

**Figure 6.2.** Barometric pressure versus available oxygen graph shows the decrease in available oxygen as the barometric pressure decreases.

## Effects of Altitude

The primary consequence of breathing air with a reduced partial pressure of oxygen is hypoxemia due to the decrease in available oxygen. The degree of tissue hypoxia tolerated is determined in part by feedback mechanisms that regulate respiratory and cardiovascular compensatory responses and, in part, by the characteristics of the hemoglobin dissociation curve. Because of the sigmoid shape of the oxygen-hemoglobin dissociation curve, a considerable increase in altitude is needed before the arterial oxygen saturation falls to below 90%. The precise elevation required to produce this fall varies among individuals and is influenced by concurrent or preexisting illnesses.

### FEEDBACK MECHANISMS

The carotid body chemoreceptors sense the decrease in arterial oxygen saturation and stimulate an increase in both depth and rate of breathing. In patients with a decreased sensitivity to hypoxemia, such as those with chronic obstructive pulmonary disease, breathing rates may not rise and the hypoxemia will be worsened.

### WORK OF BREATHING

As one climbs, the maximum useful and productive work that a human can do is reduced markedly. The reasons for this reduction relate directly to the hypoxia of altitude. The resting oxygen consumption of the various tissues in the body remains relatively constant at altitude. Unfortunately, there is a decreased amount of oxygen available per inhalation due to the decreased atmospheric pressure. This means that an increased rate of breathing is needed to meet tissue oxygen demands, even at rest. Oxygen consumption of the intrinsic muscles of respiration is therefore increased. Respiratory rates at the top of Mt. Everest were in the 60s to 70s, even at rest. The climbers who are breathing ambient air near the summit of Mt. Everest are

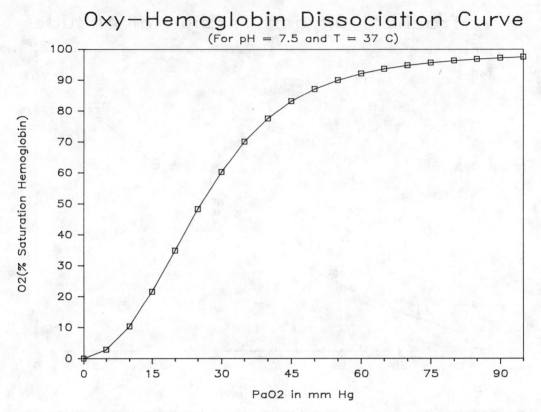

**Figure 6.3.** Hemoglobin dissociation curve. Note the shape of the oxygen-hemoglobin dissociation curve and the effects of increasing altitude on oxygen availability.

very close to the hypoxic limits of human survival.[4]

Maximum cardiac output remains constant for an individual at a given time, but a larger proportion of the cardiac output is now used "merely" to provide oxygen to the tissues. This leaves less cardiac output available for "useful work."

During exercise at low altitude, the arterial oxygen saturation does not change at all in healthy people. On the other hand, exercise at high altitude results in a distinct fall in arterial oxygen saturation, which is thought to be due to two factors:

1. The proximity to the steep part of the oxy-hemoglobin dissociation curve means that a small fall in the arterial oxygen tension will cause a large decrease in the oxygen saturation of the hemoglobin (Fig. 6.3).

2. As the respiratory exchange, and cardiac rate increases, the limits of maximum pulmonary diffusing capacity may be reached. In fact, it is possible to make a useful estimate of the dif-

fusing capacity of the lung at high altitude from the fall in oxygen saturation on exercise.[5]

Exercise at altitude contributes to the risk of acute mountain sickness, but no data are available to show just how much. It is well documented that those who exert themselves strenuously at altitude are more likely to become sick and are likely to have more severe symptoms.

## EFFECTS ON DIET

Not only is the shortness of breath a problem, but the sojourner to high altitudes will frequently be somewhat nauseated. Dietary preferences may change markedly, and there is often a craving for carbohydrates.[6,7] Fatty foods may be particularly unappealing.

## EFFECTS ON SLEEP

Another challenge to adequate oxygenation at high altitude is sleep. The normal respiratory drive will decline during sleep, with a subsequent slight reduction in the arterial oxygen saturation. At high altitude, this effect is greatly magnified. Periodic breathing (Cheyne-Stokes respirations) occurs with sleep and also may be seen at rest in awake subjects exposed to higher altitudes. The exact mechanism that produces periodic breathing has not yet been determined.

Along with this periodic breathing is a fairly profound arterial oxygen desaturation as the climber sleeps. During sleep with periodic breathing, the oxygen saturation of the hemoglobin may drop as low as 50%.[8] This periodic breathing and subsequent hypoxia may lead to severe sleep disturbances. The resultant exhaustion may cause judgment errors, poor concentration, and irritability.

Despite fatigue, many patients with altitude-related illnesses have difficulty sleeping. They wake frequently and have bizarre, unpleasant dreams. Sleeping at altitude seems to predispose climbers to the genesis of all of the illnesses of high altitude. People who spend their days above 8000 feet (5500 m) but sleep below this level are seldom ill, giving rise to the skier's adage of "ski high, sleep low."

Sedatives given to induce sleep will worsen the hypoxemia by decreasing the sensitivity of the oxygen chemoreceptors.[9] Reversal of the respiratory alkalosis with drugs, such as acetazolamide, appears to result in improved oxygenation and better sleep.[7]

## Respiratory Compensation and Effects

The first adaptive mechanism is an immediate increase in the respiratory rate and volume. This change begins at about 3200 feet (1000 m) and may not reach a constant value until several days at the target altitude. The net effect is to deliver more oxygen to the alveoli. This adaptation is obvious as a marked shortness of breath during exercise at altitude by a new arrival.

### RESPIRATORY ALKALOSIS

A natural consequence of the increased respiratory rate is a respiratory alkalosis. This coincides with the increasing hypoxemia during the first 24 to 48 hours after an ascent. The hyperventilation and subsequent respiratory alkalosis are profound at the extreme terrestrial elevations, with measured alveolar $PCO^2$ about 7 torr and calculated pH of 7.70 at the summit of Mt. Everest in one subject.[3,10] Reversal of alkalosis with drugs, such as acetazolamide, that induce the kidney to excrete bicarbonate result in improved oxygenation.

### CHRONIC ADAPTATION

Long visits at high altitude lead to a decrease in the ventilatory drive to breathe, particularly in response to hypoxemia.[11] Ventilation in native mountain dwellers is only one half that of acclimated lowlanders and the ventilatory response to exercise is lower.[12] When exercising, the highland natives will experience substantially less dyspnea than a lowlander.

A shift to the right on the oxyhemoglobin dissociation curve will occur shortly after ascent to high altitude. This is due to an increased level of 2,3-diphosphoglycerate (2,3-DPG) and a resultant decreased affinity for hemoglobin.[13,14] The immediate effect is thought to be improved oxygen unloading from hemoglobin at the tissue level. This may be offset by a decreased affinity of hemoglobin for oxygen due to pH (the Bohr effect), so the net effect is uncertain. Certainly, oxygen saturation is maintained within narrow ranges up to an altitude of 20,000 feet (6300 m).[15]

During chronic exposure to altitude, the pulmonary arterial pressures are elevated.[16] This will "force" open the capillaries in all portions of the lung and maximize perfusion to improve the capacity of the pulmonary circulation to absorb oxygen. While little effect on diffusion and pulmonary circulation is seen in lowland visitors to high altitude, a fully adapted native will show improved diffusion, increased pulmonary capillary bed size, and a relative redistribution of blood flow to the upper lobes of the lung.[17]

### Cardiovascular Compensation

As a person is subacutely exposed to decreasing barometric pressure and hypoxia, the cardiac rate and cardiac output increase.[18] The work of breathing increases markedly as noted above, causing more cardiac output to be diverted to life-sustaining processes. The maximum cardiac output, of course, is unchanged. This adaptation serves, in moderate hypoxemia, to oxygenate systemic organs. Needless to say, as the hypoxic insult is increased, target organs such as the brain become hypoxic despite the adaptive mechanisms.

The increased cardiac output at high altitude appears to be primarily a result of tachycardia rather than a change in the volume of blood ejected with each beat (stroke volume). As the cardiac rate increases with exercise, the net effect is to further decrease the stroke volume. This decreases the ability of the patient to accomplish useful work at high altitude.[19]

### Renal Compensation

After about 36 hours at altitude, an alkalotic diuresis usually spontaneously occurs as compensation for the respiratory alkalosis. The respiratory alkalosis found at high altitude is never completely compensated, even in high-altitude natives.[20,21]

With the loss of bicarbonate, an obligatory fluid loss occurs, predisposing the patient to dehydration and a decreased plasma volume.[22] In the 1981 American Medical Research Expedition to Mt. Everest (AMREE II), this fluid loss was studied. At 6300 m, the urine output is significantly greater than it is at 5400 m or at sea level. Osmolar clearance, creatinine clearance, and the urinary excretion of vasopressin were not changed. This increase in excretion despite increasing serum osmolarity may be due to a decrease in osmoreceptor sensitivity or a decrease in release or synthesis of vasopressin.[23]

In the same study, electrolytes and osmolality were also observed with changes in altitude. At an altitude of 5400 m, the serum concentration of chloride is above the upper limits of normal and the total $CO_2$ is below the lower limits of normal. At 6300 m, the serum concentrations of chloride were significantly greater than at lower altitudes. The total $CO_2$ concentration was significantly lower at 6300 m than at 5400 m. This sodium retention may in part be due to a blunted response to the renin-angiotensin-aldosterone system noted after 2 weeks or more at extreme altitudes.[24]

In other studies, test subjects at altitude with the most severe symptoms of acute mountain sickness appear to have the greatest decrease in aldosterone secretion.[25,26] The reason for this change in the renin-angiotensin-aldosterone system is not known. Japanese investigators have felt that the increase in osmolarity may be attributable to a fluid shift from extra- to intracellular spaces mediated in part by increased cortisone and aldosterone.[27]

In addition to the fluid shifts, the investigators of AMREE II noted the lack of subjective complaints of thirst that would be normal with a serum osmolarity of 302 mOsm/kg. These observations document a serious potential hazard of dehydration for mountaineers at extreme altitudes.

### Hematologic Compensation

As a chronic adaptive response, the total red cell mass will increase. A chronic hypoxia will stimulate production of the hormone erythropoietin by the kidneys, which stimulates an increase in the production of red blood cells by the bone marrow. The response will occur over the course of several weeks and is reflected in the higher hematocrit of the long duration high-altitude dweller.[14] Excessive elevation of the hematocrit (greater than 60%) may also be found with continued stimulation. This excess is associated with chronic mountain sickness. Over a longer period of time, increased capillary density, increased intracellular mitochrondria, and increased cytochrome oxidase enable the more efficient use of available oxygen stores.[28]

### Altitude Tolerance

The climbers who have reached the summit of Mt. Everest and other major peaks have been found to have certain physiologic attributes not predictable by sea level studies or performance at lesser altitudes. Some of these attributes include (1) high ventilatory response to hypoxia,[29] (2) effective cerebral function during severe hypoxia, (3) effective muscle function during severe hypoxia,[28] (4) high pulmonary diffusing capacity, (5) unusual ability to perform sustained physical work.[30] Again, these attributes have been noted in successful climbers at extreme altitudes and the physiologic basis is not yet understood.

It should be emphasized that fitness alone does not protect the individual from the problems encountered at high altitudes.[31] Indeed, by allowing a rapid ascent, a high level of fitness may predispose a subject to altitude-related illnesses. In this aspect, the older more sedentary trekker or skier who takes but a single holiday per year may be at an advantage over the younger and more fleet of foot.

## ACUTE MOUNTAIN SICKNESS

### Epidemiology

Acute mountain sickness is the most common manifestation of the altitude-related illnesses. Some symptoms are likely to appear in any lowlander that ascends to greater than 12,000 feet (3660 m). Severe symptoms rarely occur below 8000 feet (2440 m). As with the other altitude-related illnesses, the incidence of acute mountain sickness appears to be exacerbated by rapid ascent and vigorous exercise soon after arrival at altitude.

Some people become sick each time they visit a moderate altitude, no matter how slowly they travel. Others appear never to be affected until extreme elevations are reached. Infants and adolescents are more vulnerable. The reasons for the individual differences in sensitivity to altitude changes are not well understood.

| Features of Acute Mountain Sickness | |
|---|---|
| Setting | > 8000 feet (2440 m) |
| Predisposing factors | Rapid ascent |
| Onset | Within hours |
| Symptoms | Headache (most common) |
| | Nausea |
| | Vomiting |
| | Malaise |
| | Dyspnea |
| | Insomnia |
| Signs | Tachycardia |
| | Tachypnea |
| | Cheyne-Stokes respirations |
| | Sleep disturbances |
| Prophylaxis | Gradual ascent |
| | Acetazolamide |
| Treatment | Descent |
| | Low-flow oxygen |
| | Dexamethasone |

### Presentation

The most common initial symptom is headache, which may vary from a mild light-headedness to a severe, incapacitating pain. Lassitude, drowsiness, malaise, weakness and dyspnea on exertion are common. Anorexia is also common and, particularly in children, nausea and vomiting may occur. Observers may note facial pallor and cyanosis of lips and nailbeds. After arrival at altitude, a feeling of warmth and flushing of the face may be noted for the first 24 to 48 hours. Even slight physical effort may produce an annoying dyspnea, even in the physically fit. Weakness, tachycardia, and palpitations may also be associated with effort.

In addition to symptoms acquired with acute mountain sickness, sudden increases in altitude may also be accompanied by decreased performance in athletic endeavors. Such changes were observed in athletes at the 1964 Olympic games in Mexico City (elevation 6000 feet or 1830 m). The degree of athletic conditioning appears to have little or no influence upon the occurrence of symptoms with rapid changes in altitude.

Sleeping problems at altitude may be a major source of discomfort. Sleep, particularly for the first few nights, is difficult, with frequent periods of wakefulness and, at the higher altitudes, Cheyne-Stokes breathing. During the apneic phase of the periodic breathing, the episodes of hypoxia may be quite profound.

### Physiology

It has been suggested that the headache of acute mountain sickness is due to cerebral edema, but cerebral edema in other conditions is not surely associated with headache. A more plausible suggestion is that the headache of AMS is due to hypocapnea with concomitant spasm of the cerebral blood vessels or to hypoxia.

### Complications

#### SLEEP HYPOXIA

Occasionally, recent arrivals to high altitude are found to be very weak and drowsy. They may be found in a semicomatose state, hallucinating or behaving in an irrational pattern. The other members of the trek may note that the new arrival is deeply cyanotic. Improvement can be quickly achieved by awakening the person and encouraging deep breaths. Because of decreased respirations during sleep, a profound hypoxia may be noted. This is relieved by voluntary deep respirations when the individual is awake.

## HAPE AND HACE

It needs to be emphasized that acute mountain sickness is part of a spectrum of diseases of altitude and shares many of the attributes of the more serious high-altitude cerebral edema and pulmonary edema. Indeed, it is difficult to differentiate between minimal high altitude cerebral edema and AMS on a windswept slope in the snow. For these reasons, it should be clearly understood that evacuation of the patient with serious acute mountain sickness is preferable to allowing unnecessary progression of the patient's cerebral edema or pulmonary edema. It is often difficult to tell the trekker who has invested considerable time and money in a "once in a lifetime" trip that he or she is going "down the hill," but it is also a lot easier than telling the bereaved family that you did not think the illness was that serious.

## Treatment

Moderate or mild symptoms of AMS are best treated by rest, increased fluid intake, and symptomatic relief. Headache may be treated with aspirin, acetaminophen, mild narcotics such as codeine or propoxyphene, or combinations of any of these. A light diet should be followed, but anorexia and nausea may preclude any solid food intake. Alcohol and smoking should be strictly avoided.

Barbiturates or stronger narcotics should be avoided. Either class of drugs may depress respiratory efforts with subsequent catastrophic results. Barbiturates may make rest and sleep possible but may increase symptoms upon awakening. Oversedation may mask HACE. Diazepam may occasionally cause hypoxia, disorientation, and hallucinations. It has been suggested that if sleeping medications are to be used, the benzodiazepam class should be avoided; a medication such as Halcion is preferable because of the short duration of action.

Dexamethasone has been recently used for treatment of AMS with excellent effects and little incidence of side effects during the relatively short courses needed for this disease. Army troops brought to altitude on Denali (14,000 feet or 4270 m) and then treated with 4 mg of dexamethasone had good amelioration of symptoms. When the medication was discontinued, the symptoms returned. This medication has interesting promise and needs further study.

The use of antiemetics may be helpful. There is some evidence that prochlorperazine (Compazine) may be one of the few drugs of its category that does not dull the respiratory response to hypoxia. Calcium carbonate tablets have also been advocated for the treatment of AMS. There appears to be little additional gain by the use of Rolaids, but there also seems to be no harm done by this medication.

Some temporary relief of AMS may be achieved by forced voluntary hyperventilation. Ten to twelve deep breaths every 10 to 15 minutes will suffice. If the patient overdoes the "remedy," the symptoms of hyperventilation syndrome with dizziness and paresthesias about lips and distal extremities soon appear. For severe symptoms of AMS, descent and supplemental oxygen are recommended. Continuous administration of 1 to 2 liters per minute of oxygen during sleep may relieve symptoms and help the patient to obtain effective sleep.

## Prevention

### ACCLIMATION

The single most effective method of prevention of AMS is by appropriate acclimation to altitude. This may be done in one of three ways:

1. *Intermediate staging.* Prior to ascending to exercise at an altitude above 12,000 feet (3660 m), a program of gradually increasing exercise at an intermediate stop (6000 to 8000 feet or 1800 to 2400 m) for 3 to 4 days will provide sufficient acclimatization to prevent most problems at the higher altitude. For climbers to the 15,000 to 18,000 foot (4570 to 5500 m) range, a second acclimation stage at 12,000 to 13,000 feet (3660 to 4000 m) is helpful.

2. *Graded ascent.* In many areas of the Himalayas, a long approach march is made to reach the high elevations. During the classic approach to Mt. Everest, for example, both acclimation and physical conditioning take place. At altitudes above 14,000 feet (4200 m), ascents should be limited to 500 to 1000 feet (150 to 300 m) between sleeping elevations, and every third or fourth day should be a rest day.

3. *One stage ascent.* For the trekker with no time to waste, an ascent directly to 12,000 to 14,000 feet (3660 to 4200 m) without stopping is usually planned. The trekker should plan on spending at least 3 days at the altitude before engaging in strenuous activity. The risk of all altitude illnesses after such an ascent is high, and heavy exertion prior to acclimatization is foolhardy. It is usually more pleasant to spend the 3 to 4 days planned for acclimation at the lower altitudes.

## ACETAZOLAMIDE

Acetazolamide is a carbonic anhydrase inhibitor that increases the urinary excretion of bicarbonate, sodium, and potassium. The metabolic consequence of the forced bicarbonate diuresis is acidosis. This metabolic acidosis is felt to promote the sensitivity of the peripheral oxygen-sensitive chemoreceptors and stimulation of the medullary chemoreceptors. The beneficial effects of this increased sensitivity to hypoxia include increased ventilation at altitude, increased alveolar oxygen tension, and possibly improved sleep patterns.

Acetazolamide may be given in a dose of 125 to 250 mg once or twice a day beginning on the day prior to ascent. It should be continued until the patient is at the same or lower altitude for 5 days. Treated persons at high altitude have higher arterial oxygen tension, a lower arterial carbon dioxide tension, and a lower pH than control subjects.[32] Field studies of troops show that AMS at 14,200 feet (4330 m) can be ameliorated by a combination of staging at 5500 feet (1675 m) and administration of acetazolamide for the last 2 days of staging and the first 2 days of the new altitude. Hornbine also demonstrated an overall higher success rate in achieving the summit of Denali in those individuals using acetazolamide as compared to placebo.[33] This was apparently due to a combination of decreased symptoms of AMS

and improved ability to breathe. It does not appear to improve exercise performance at extreme altitudes.

Side effects of acetazolamide are common and may be incapacitating for a climber, although less troublesome for a trekker or skier. The most common side effects include paresthesias and hyposthesias about the lips and fingertips. The paresthesias in a climber who depends upon touch for climbing ability or for clutching an ice axe or ski pole may be exceedingly troublesome. This symptom complex is attributed to a transient peripheral neuropathy that may vary from a mild discomfort to a major annoyance. Other side effects, such as a flat taste to beer and cola drinks and myopia, may occur after a few days of medication.

## FUROSEMIDE

Furosemide has been recommended for the prevention and treatment of AMS and HAPE. The drug does not reduce the symptoms of AMS.[34] In normal persons, it has been noted that even small doses of furosemide may result in a substantial incidence of postural hypotension and near syncope at high altitudes.[35]

## EMERGENCY DESCENT

If the patient's symptoms worsen despite therapy, the patient should be returned to a lower altitude. The picture of a nauseated, vomiting, coughing, complaining climbing or hiking associate is nearly enough to motivate the homicidal. With the added stimulus of insomnia, Cheyne-Stokes breathing, and snoring respirations, one often can hope that one's tentmate simply doesn't take another breath.

Throughout this and subsequent discussions, it should be remembered that although emergency descent is often recommended, it is more easily proposed than performed. With a small party, evacuation of a litter casualty to a lower altitude may take the entire resources of the party. If the patient can travel under his or her own power, descent may be managed with 2 people for observation and aid. If a litter is required for a prolonged descent over rough terrain, no less than 12 will suffice for transportation and more will be appreciated by all. Hence, it is advisable to make the decision to descend early in the patient's course, before the individual is incapacitated. This will be a more acute decision if there is no supplemental oxygen available.

## HIGH-ALTITUDE PULMONARY EDEMA

### Epidemiology

High-altitude pulmonary edema occurs with rapid ascent without acclimation to altitudes greater than 8000 feet (2440 m). The overall incidence of clinically significant HAPE ranges from about 0.6% to 4% following a rapid ascent to 12,000 feet (3660 m) in those who are older than 20 years.[36] In those who are younger than 20, the incidence of HAPE during the same climb is sixfold higher than in adults (from 2.5% to as high as 38%).[37] The higher figures are derived from populations that live at high altitude and visit sea level periodically. Such high-altitude dwellers seem to be at increased risk of developing HAPE upon return to high altitude (Table 6.1).

HAPE usually begins 24 to 72 hours after ascent to an altitude of greater than 10,000 feet (3050 m). Fatal cases have been noted as low as 8000 feet (2440 m). Cases are rare on the day of arrival and very few cases are reported after more than 10 days at altitude.

Onset frequently is noted at night, but it is uncertain whether this is connected with the sleep disturbances of altitude or whether this is just when the tentmate first notes the cough that keeps both patient and companion awake.

### Predisposing Factors

HAPE most often occurs in young individuals who rapidly ascend to altitude, and then engage in strenuous exercise at altitude.

**Table 6.1.**
**Incidence of High-Altitude Pulmonary Edema**

| | |
|---|---|
| Colorado skiers | 0.1–0.01% |
| Everest trekkers | 1–2% |
| McKinley climbers | 3% |
| Indian soldiers | 0.6%–16% |
| High-altitude residents | 0.4% (adult) |
| | 1–6% (children) |

**Table 6.2.**
**Grading of High-Altitude Pulmonary Edema**

Grade I (mild)
  Mild cough
  Dyspnea on moderate exertion
  Heart rate: < 110
  Respiratory rate: < 20
  Chest x-ray shows minor infiltrates involving
    less than one fourth of one lung field
Grade II (moderate)
  Weakness
  Fatigue
  Headache
  Nonproductive cough
  Dyspnea on moderate exertion
  Rales in axilla (right most commonly)
  Heart rate: 110–120
  Respiratory rate: 20–30
  Chest x-ray shows infiltrates about involving
    half of one lung
Grade III (serious)
  Weakness
  Headache
  Nausea
  Dyspnea at rest
  Productive cough
  Rales and/or wheezes
  Slight cyanosis
  Heart rate: 120–140
  Respiratory rate: 31–40
  Chest x-ray shows infiltrates involving at least
    half of each lung field or all of one lung
    (rarely seen)
Grade IV (severe)
  Severe dyspnea at rest
  Frothy or bloody sputum
  Decreasing level of consciousness
  Death if untreated
  Heart rate: > 140
  Respirations: > 40
  Chest x-ray shows infiltrates involving more
    than half of each lung field

### AGE

The greatest percentage of HAPE victims are young, with adolescents and preadolescents comprising about one half of the cases. Children under 5 are considerably more susceptible, although the incidence in newborns appears to be lessened. There appears to be no great difference between sexes, although more males are climbers or skiers and, hence, exposed to the etiologic conditions more frequently.

## RAPIDITY OF ASCENT

The only known protective factor for HAPE is slow acclimation to ambient altitude. Indeed, in the early phases of the Sino-Indian border wars of 1962, Indian troops traveled by rail to altitude from sea level and suffered enormous casualties from HAPE.[38]

## EXERTION

Multiple studies have shown that exertion at altitude carries a marked predisposition to HAPE, although the actual increase in incidence is not known. Cross-country skiers, backpackers, and mountaineers who carry heavy loads and ascend rapidly are particularly at risk. Downhill skiers, who are not encumbered with packs and can rest while ascending, have lesser incidence of HAPE.

## GEOGRAPHICAL INCIDENCE

There may be some geographic variation in the incidence of HAPE, as there appears to be a somewhat greater incidence on Denali and in Peru than in other places. This apparent geographic variation may also be due to the difficulty in reaching other highlands and the subsequently slower ascent (RB Schoene, unpublished data).

## REASCENT TO HIGH ALTITUDE

The highest incidence of HAPE is among the acclimated highlanders who return home after a short trip or vacation at lower elevations. The low-altitude trip may be for only a few days, but the incidence of HAPE upon return to the highlands is high.[39]

## PRIOR HISTORY OF HAPE

There is good evidence that the condition has a relatively high recurrence rate. One study reported that 20% of HAPE victims had repeated episodes.[36] The mechanisms of this apparent predisposition have not yet been determined.

## PULMONARY ARTERY ATRESIA

A very high rate of development of HAPE has been reported among persons with unilateral pulmonary artery atresia.[40]

## Pathophysiology

The etiology of HAPE is uncertain. The low incidence, the remote locations where it most commonly occurs, and the lack of an animal model make it difficult to study.

High-altitude pulmonary edema has been described in the past as pneumonia or congestive heart failure but was recognized as a noncardiogenic pulmonary edema in the early 1960s. Catheterization studies show that HAPE is a noncardiogenic form of pulmonary edema associated with high pulmonary artery pressures and normal pulmonary capillary wedge pressures.[41] Recent data indicate that HAPE is a high-protein, high-permeability type of pulmonary edema, similar to that found in adult respiratory distress syndrome (ARDS).[42] The cause of the injury to the pulmonary vasculature in HAPE remains unknown. It is theorized that it is in part due to hypoxia and inordinately high pulmonary vascular pressures that may lead to vascular leakage.

Unlike patients with ARDS, HAPE victims improve rapidly with proper treatment and may return to climb under close supervision within 10 to 14 days of the original insult.

## Symptoms

The onset of symptoms of HAPE is somewhat slower than in AMS. Normally, the onset of symptoms occurs within 12 to 96 hours after arrival at altitude. The most common symptoms are a nonproductive cough, gradually increasing dyspnea, and fatigue. Dyspnea becomes marked, even with only modest exertion. The individual with pulmonary edema is usually more tired than other members of the climbing or skiing party. He or she may have a sense of "tightness in the chest" or a feeling of impending suffocation at night. Occasionally, a patient might note wheezing sounds with breaths and a burbling feeling in the chest. Headache, anorexia, nausea, and vomiting are frequently present, particularly in children.

An important indication of the severity of HAPE is the level of mental acuity. Confusion, delirium, and irrational behavior are signs of profound hypoxia. If the patient becomes unconscious, death will follow in 6 to

12 hours unless prompt descent or oxygen therapy are initiated.

## Signs

Signs are both cardiac and respiratory in nature. Tachycardia and tachypnea are always seen. The pulse rate is usually rapid (110 to 160/minute), even after several hours of rest. The respirations are usually greater than 20 per minute (typically 20 to 40). Cardiac signs of pulmonary hypertension may include a right

| Features of High-Altitude Pulmonary Edema | |
| --- | --- |
| Setting | > 8000 feet (2400 m) (rare) |
| | > 12,000 feet (3600 m) (common) |
| Predisposing factors | Youth |
| | Rapid ascent |
| | Vigorous exercise |
| | Reascent (highland dwellers) |
| | Sedatives for sleep ?? |
| Onset of symptoms | 1 to 3 days after arrival |
| | Often at night |
| Symptoms | |
| Early | Fatigue |
| | Cough |
| | Dyspnea |
| Later | Severe dyspnea |
| | Orthopnea |
| | Frothy sputum |
| Late | Confusion |
| | Coma |
| | Death |
| Signs | Tachypnea |
| | Tachycardia |
| | Rales (first in right axilla) |
| | Rhonchi and wheezes |
| | Cyanosis |
| Prophylaxis | Proper ascent procedures |
| | Limited early exercise |
| | Acetazolamide ???? |
| | Early descent with symptoms |
| | Climb high—sleep low |
| Treatment | Descent |
| | Oxygen |
| | Bed rest |
| | PEEP (severe cases) |

ventricular heave and an increased intensity of the pulmonic component of S2.

Rales are considered diagnostic of the condition and may best be heard in the early course about the right axilla (Hackett, unpublished communications). As the disease progresses, the rales become audible to the tentmates and may be heard several feet away. The cough is usually dry and intermittent at first but then becomes persistent and productive of a white, watery, or frothy material. Late in the course, the sputum becomes pink tinged or bloody.

The temperature may be slightly elevated but not markedly so. Cyanosis may be marked.

The severity of HAPE ranges from mild dyspnea at rest to severe respiratory embarrassment with production of frothy pink sputum. Rarely, coma or alteration of consciousness is seen as the first sign of HAPE, with little or no respiratory manifestations. Both signs and symptoms often become worse at night. Progression of the disease may be quite rapid and frequent examination of patients who present with minimal signs is important. Any worsening should mandate immediate oxygen therapy and descent.

Grading the severity of high-altitude pulmonary edema is advocated by many and may be useful. Patients with lesser severity (grade I) HAPE may have only mild symptoms, such as fatigue or exertional dyspnea. These patients typically recover after only a day or so at lower altitude and may proceed with the climb after a week or so. Patients with higher grades of pulmonary edema should be considered as major medical emergencies and require prompt treatment and evacuation to lower altitudes (Table 6.2).

## Laboratory and X-ray Findings

Radiologic findings include patchy infiltrates and alveolar infiltrates common to other adult respiratory distress syndromes (Fig 6.4). There are usually multiple small, irregular infiltrates with poorly defined margins in a patchy asymmetrical distribution. The infiltrates may be unilateral and appear first in the upper lobes, although in severe disease, infiltrates are often confluent and extensive. The pulmonary vascular pattern is often widened. Heart size appears normal and will not usually change with the clearing of infiltrates.

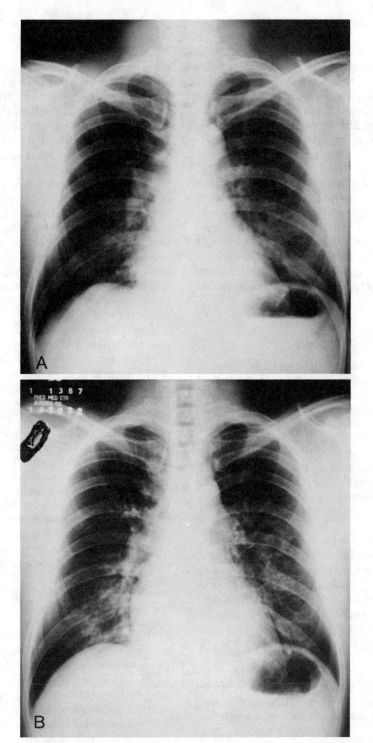

**Figure 6.4.**   Radiograph shows a high-altitude pulmonary edema with classic findings. The heart is of normal size, and there is a bilateral "butterfly" pattern pulmonary infiltrate.

With recovery, there is rapid clearing of the infiltrates.

Electrocardiographic findings are those of acute right heart strain with right ventricular overload. It is often difficult to differentiate the electrocardiographic findings of HAPE from those of a pulmonary embolus.

Pulmonary arterial catheters will show severe pulmonary hypertension, normal capillary wedge pressure, and normal left atrial pressure.

Only a few abnormal laboratory findings occur in patients with HAPE. The white blood cell count is frequently elevated with a leftward shift. Severe hypoxia is generally present with HAPE, and arterial blood gases will reflect this hypoxia. Administration of supplementary oxygen will improve the abnormalities but often does not completely correct them.

### Differential Diagnosis

When the history of high-altitude exposure in a young athlete is known and the typical findings of a noncardiogenic pulmonary edema are noted, the diagnosis of high-altitude pulmonary edema is relatively easy. When the symptoms develop on the mountainside, the whole party is usually aware of the potential for HAPE and acts accordingly. Indeed, the dry hacking cough that is often caused by the relative dehydration at altitude may trigger overzealous expedition leaders to order a descent.

The diagnostic problem occurs when the patient with cough, slight fever, and signs of pulmonary congestion presents to a practitioner AFTER returning from the ski trip or short climbing expedition. The pattern of right ventricular strain on the electrocardiogram and the clinical signs of pulmonary hypertension may also suggest a pulmonary embolism.

When the patient is a resident of high altitude who has a short stay at lower altitudes and then returns to the heights, the diagnosis may be missed if he is not returning to home.

### Treatment

Once high-altitude pulmonary edema is diagnosed, the best treatment is immediate descent. As in acute mountain sickness, a relatively small descent of 1000 meters can improve the patient's status immensely.

Oxygen administered on site is a *temporizing* measure and is not a substitute for and should not delay prompt descent. With full flow oxygen, the respiratory and heart rates drop, and the patient will feel better. Unfortunately, very few parties carry enough oxygen to treat a victim of HAPE with 6 to 10 liters of oxygen flow per minute for 12 to 48 hours. Even if the available oxygen supplies will not last that long, it may permit a completely debilitated patient enough recovery to allow him to ambulate to a lower altitude.

Positive pressure breathing is helpful in severe cases but is often unobtainable on the mountainside. Positive end-expiratory pressure (PEEP) by mask or endotracheal tube will improve gas exchange, although there is some controversy that PEEP will increase the incidence of HACE.

Drugs other than oxygen are not of much use in treating HAPE. Since the pathophysiology is that of a leaky membrane pulmonary edema that is similar to ARDS, it can be expected that morphine will have only limited effect, and this is borne out by clinical experience. The vasodilator effects of morphine may precipitate hypotension, although this is usually only postural. The central nervous system tranquilizing effects of morphine may be useful in calming the anxious dyspneic patient, but morphine and other opiates carry the risk of decreasing respiratory drive with catastrophic results.

A profound diuresis is often necessary in the treatment of pulmonary edema of cardiogenic origin, and a clinician may be tempted to employ furosemide for HAPE. Unfortunately, there is little rational basis for the use of furosemide in the noncardiogenic pulmonary edema of altitude. The etiology of HAPE appears to be from a leaky capillary membrane and is most certainly not from volume overload. Furosemide will have no effect on the membrane leak of HAPE and, therefore, will not substantially help in its treatment. Indeed, furosemide may precipitate either a profound orthostatic hypotension or a significant nonpostural hypotension as a result of the brisk diuresis. Orthostatic hypotension with use of furosemide may be so debilitating as to prevent the patient from walking, thus complicating the already formidable problem of evacuation.

Digitalis derivatives and rotating tourniquets are likewise ineffective since the left atrial pressure is normal. Steroids and sympathomimetics also have no proven efficacy. Antibiotics neither adversely affect nor help the course of HAPE.

On some recent Himalayan expeditions, there have been attempts to treat HAPE using small, portable hyperbaric chambers. Although the chambers appear relatively lightweight and portable, it is obvious that this therapy is suitable only for larger expedition groups or well-established treks, but these chambers may be useful in high ski areas in the United States, and bear further research.

The patient with HAPE should be considered to have a reversible physiologic disorder. All except those with the most advanced cases will recover with descent, rest, and oxygen unless iatrogenic complications ensue. Long-term, high-altitude residents who have returned to altitude after a visit to the lowlands represent a special case. These patients may be treated with rest and low-flow oxygen. They do not need to be evacuated to a lower elevation unless their illness is critical.

## Prevention

The single best way to prevent the problem is by acclimation to altitude as explained above.

Many outdoors persons are afflicted with strange (large) senses of ego that encourage them to press on despite all personal discomforts. Others see the plans of a trek disappearing in coughing spasms and vow to make the best of their hard-earned vacation money. The climber, cross-country skier, or hiker who reacts in this manner is likely to reach a state of collapse before his illness comes to the attention of his companions.

Early recognition is essential in dealing with high-altitude pulmonary edema because if it is diagnosed and treated early, the disease is more reversible. The trip physician should examine every member of the party every day at high altitude. This should include noting whether they are consistently falling behind or if they have a headache, shortness of breath, or unusual weakness. The physician should listen to the chest and check for resting pulse and heart rate. If the heart rate is above 110 in a fit climber at altitude, or the respiratory rate is above 20 or rales are present, the patient should be restricted to bed rest, observed closely, and evacuation considered. If mildly affected individuals are returned to lower altitudes promptly, the incidence of serious complications and death should be reduced to almost zero.

## HIGH-ALTITUDE CEREBRAL EDEMA

In 1959, Chiodi described a patient who had neurologic signs and symptoms with exposure to high altitude in the Andes.[43] The signs and symptoms disappeared promptly with descent. A cerebral angiogram and flow studies were normal. This syndrome has been found repeatedly since that time. Data from small numbers of patients have shown that increased cerebral spinal fluid pressure, retinal hemorrhages, and papilledema have been present. Cerebral edema was verified in one instance by craniotomy performed for a suspected subdural hematoma.[44]

Although the term "high-altitude cerebral edema" has been used for this complex of symptoms and signs, a better term might be "high-altitude encephalopathy." Cerebral edema may well be a consequence of the profound cerebral hypoxia and not the cause of the various clinical manifestations of this syndrome.

## Epidemiology

For an abrupt ascent to an altitude greater than 20,000 feet (6000 m), such as might occur in a decompression chamber or an unpressurized aircraft, there are good data that describe the physiologic effects of such an ascent. Within a few minutes the exposure results in a loss of higher mental functions, unsteady gait and posture, collapse, and finally coma. Return to sea level will relieve the symptoms in most individuals.

Climbers on Mt. Everest who did not use supplemental oxygen were evaluated with psychometric testing before and after the climb. All showed some neurologic deficits similar to those persons who ascend by unpressurized aircraft. HACE appears to have many of the same symptoms, with a longer and more severe course. Local circulatory factors, such as excessive vasoconstriction in portions of the brain, may be required for the full development of the syndrome termed HACE.

In rare instances, high-altitude pulmonary edema may appear as coma or unconsciousness without cough or shortness of breath and may simulate cerebral edema.

## Symptoms

Headache is the usual presenting symptom, although in some patients, it is curiously absent. The usual headache is a dull, severe, constant ache that requires narcotics for relief. The patient may complain of loss of memory, hallucinations, and confusion. Companions may note an inability to use proper judgment or psychotic behavior.

| Features of High-Altitude Cerebral Edema | |
|---|---|
| Setting | > 12,000 feet (3660 m) |
| Predisposing factors | Rapid ascent |
| Onset of symptoms | Hours to 2 to 3 days after ascent |
| Symptoms | Headache |
| | Ataxia |
| | Vertigo |
| | Confusion |
| | Hallucinations |
| | Lethargy |
| Signs | Lethargy |
| | Papilledema |
| | Coma |
| | Death |
| Treatment | Rapid evacuation to lower altitude |
| | High-flow oxygen |
| | Steroids (controversial) |

## Signs

The first sign noted on physical examination is usually ataxia. This may be followed by ataxia of gait, mental confusion, and somnolence. The climber may also "just want to stay in bed." Loss of memory, hallucinations, and lethargy may also be noted by the examiner. In the most severe cases, the patient can not be aroused and does not respond to verbal or even painful stimuli. Death will follow shortly if treatment is not emergently provided.

Funduscopic examination may reveal papilledema and retinal hemorrhages. On neurologic examination, the patient may have focal neurologic deficits and upgoing Babinski's reflexes. Ataxia is the single most consistent neurologic sign. The most common form of ataxia is truncal, where the patient is unable to maintain balance. In severe cases of ataxia, the patient cannot walk or stand without falling and may be unable to hold a cup or plate. Increasing heart rate, respiratory rate, and central cyanosis may signal concomitant HAPE.

## Treatment

The optimum treatment for HACE is not yet well established but appears to be similar to that of HAPE. Prompt descent, high-flow oxygen, and bed rest are the mainstays of therapy. As in HAPE, the best, mandatory, and most therapeutic treatment is descent while the disease is in an early phase.

Based upon long-standing recommendations of our neurosurgical colleagues, hyperosmolar solutions have been commonly employed. Unfortunately, there are no good controlled studies, and only anecdotal observations bolster these clinical studies. Mannitol and glycerol may reduce the cerebral blood flow and worsen HACE's effects. Acetazolamide and other diuretics may be useful but are unproven. Steroids may also be useful and will not reduce cerebral blood flow. Dexamethasone appears to be the current drug of choice for this disorder.

The heart and respiratory rate should be determined and the chest examined carefully in all cases to ensure that the rare case of HAPE with coma is not missed. A chest x-ray should be obtained as soon as practical.

## Complications

The neurologic deficits that are seen with this disorder will usually resolve slowly with the increase in oxygen pressure and supportive treatment. Recent studies do show that climbers of Mt. Everest who do not use oxygen will have residual hypoxic neurologic deficits, even if they did not have any symptoms of HACE. The longer that the high-altitude cerebral edema victim remains at high altitude, the greater the propensity for permanent nervous system damage or death.

## Prevention

Any confusion or ataxia combined with a severe headache in a member of a climbing or skiing party should raise the possibility of cerebral edema. These individuals should be assisted to descend, with oxygen if possible. Assistance is mandatory in view of the ataxia and the possibility of rapid progression with subsequent falls and injuries. The unconscious patient needs to be evacuated and hospitalized as soon as possible.

A simple test for early cerebral edema that may be performed even by lay trek leaders is the heel-to-toe gait test. The victim is observed as he walks a straight line with a heel-to-toe gait and is observed. If the victim loses balance and falls over, then he or she must descend. This test will help to detect the trekker who conceals symptoms in order to continue.

## HIGH-ALTITUDE RETINAL HEMORRHAGE

### Epidemiology

High-altitude retinal hemorrhages occur in half of all people who travel above 17,000 feet (5200 m).[45,46] Retinal hemorrhages are probably associated with an increase in retinal blood flow measured at high altitude.[47] They are uncommon below 15,000 feet (4570 m) but may be precipitated even at lower levels by strenuous activity.

| Features of High-Altitude Retinal Hemorrhage | |
|---|---|
| Setting | > 14,000 feet (4270 m) |
| Predisposing factors | Heavy exertion Valsalva's maneuvers |
| Symptoms (rare) | Blurring Floaters Scotoma (rarely) |
| Signs | Retinal hemorrhages on funduscopic examination |
| Prophylaxis | None known |
| Treatment | Descend for central scotoma or if examination indicates serious involvement |

## Symptoms

In most cases, the retinal hemorrhages of HARH cause no visual difficulty and are seldom symptomatic. Only when the macula is affected is the individual aware of a scotoma.

## Signs

To an examiner with an ophthalmoscope, the hemorrhages appear as small, flame-shaped markings or as large pools or blobs. Rarely, cotton-wool retinal edema markings are noted. The vessels show increases in tortuosity and in diameter. Hyperemia near the disk is also seen. Rarely, vitreous hemorrhages have been noted.[48]

## Etiology

The etiology of retinal hemorrhages is not known. Theories proposed include a defect in vasoregulation, increased venous pressure due to Valsalva's maneuvers with strenuous exercise, and decreased intraocular pressure associated with exercise.[49,50] Available evidence suggests that retinal hemorrhages are due to an increased capillary permeability. Capillary permeability is increased as confirmed by fluorescein leakage in the region about the optic disk in 8 of 20 subjects.[45]

## Treatment

No treatment or preventative medication is known. Acetazolamide does not appear to prevent HARH, but slow ascent or long stays at altitude do appear to reduce the daily incidence of retinal hemorrhages.[44,46] Macular hemorrhages and cotton-wool spots with scotomas probably should mandate descent. Retinal hemorrhages are not seen as contraindications to ascent, have not been shown to mark a hemorrhagic diathesis, and do not portend an abnormal vascular fragility.

The smaller lesions resolve without sequelae, but cotton-wool spots and macular hemorrhages often leave a permanent scotoma. Most lesions resolve within 6 weeks after descent to sea level.

## Prevention

There is no apparent ability to predict or prevent this disorder of altitude. Gradual ascent

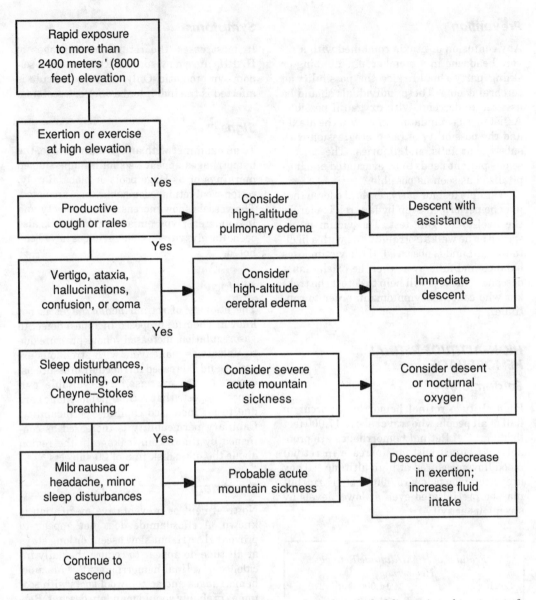

**Figure 6.5.** Flow chart for high-altitude illnesses shows a logical method of diagnosis and treatment of the serious high-altitude illnesses while in the field.

appears to reduce the rate at which HARH develops, but it is unclear as to whether it will reduce the incidence.[44]

### MISCELLANEOUS ALTITUDE-RELATED PROBLEMS

#### High-Altitude Flatus Expulsion

HAFE is the natural consequence of trapped intestinal gases following the dictates of the combined gas laws. The combined gas laws state that the volume of a gas is directly pro-

portional to the pressure and inversely proportional to the temperature of the gas. Since we are homeothermic and the temperature in our abdomen is relatively constant, this component can be neglected. The result is that as we ascend, our bowel gas is subject to less pressure and, hence, has greater volume. This can result in intraabdominal discomfort and the passage of large amounts of flatus. The syndrome has been associated with colonic rupture in at least one case.[51]

Fortunately the gastrointestinal (GI) tract has an egress to the outside world, so that the trapped gas may escape and not rupture the relatively fragile intestines.[52] Our tent-mates and comrades may not always agree. Simethicone may provide some relief. Descent is curative.

## Thromboembolic Disease

When the dehydration that is common at high altitude, the polycythemic response to hypoxia of altitude, and the inactivity noted during storms and when preparing for the climb are added together, the high-altitude sojourner has developed a high risk for thromboembolic disease.

The most frequently noted sites are the leg veins, but the deep veins of the upper extremities and the pelvis have been involved. As is true for lowlanders, pulmonary embolism is a risk for patients with deep vein thrombosis. Under field conditions, little can be done for the patient with a pulmonary embolus except to administer oxygen if available. For the patient who has been evacuated to a hospital, the standard therapies for pulmonary embolus should not be modified.

## Dysbarisms

Dysbarisms are disorders that are related to changes in atmospheric pressure. Although they are not related to the hypoxia of high altitude, they are discussed in this section for completeness. Most physicians will see these disorders in patients who have been flying recently, not climbing, skiing, or hiking. The disorders are loosely grouped into two classes: barotrauma and decompression sicknesses. (See Chapter 12.)

### BAROTRAUMA

Barotrauma in general involves what is known as the "trapped gas" phenomenon. Undissolved gas within body cavities that has no exit to the ambient pressure will follow the physical laws governing gases. During ascent, the gas in these areas will expand. If the opening to the outside world is occluded, the increased gas pressure will cause pain and occasionally damage. During descent, the enclosed gas will contract. This is not usually a problem unless a thin membrane, such as the tympanic membrane, collapses.

### BAROTITIS MEDIA

As noted above, as the patient ascends, the gas trapped behind the tympanic membrane will attempt to equalize with the ambient pressure. Usually, this gas can easily escape through the eustachian tube. As the patient descends, the eustachian tube, if partially blocked, will collapse, and the venting will not occur. The difference in pressure is felt with increasing pain and pressure on the tympanic membrane.

On physical examination, the tympanic membrane is retracted in mild cases. In severe cases, the tympanic membrane is ruptured and blood is noted in the canal. The pain may be quite intense until the tympanic membrane ruptures. Hearing may be disrupted.

Treatment is usually a long-acting nasal decongestant such as Afrin or cocaine. If practical, ascent to higher altitude and subsequent slow descent is often helpful. Swallowing, chewing gum, or yawning may open the eustachian tube and allow equilibration. Valsalva's maneuver (forced expiration against a closed mouth and nose) will also often help.

### BAROSINUSITIS

Poor drainage of the paranasal sinuses may lead to the trapped gas phenomenon within the sinuses. The frontal and maxillary sinuses are most frequently involved. Predisposing factors include an underlying chronic or acute sinusitis, edema of the nose from trauma or allergies, and a deformity of either septum or turbinates. This condition frequently occurs on descent and the patient will bitterly complain of pain about the affected sinuses. Blood may be present in the nose or mouth, and the sinuses will be markedly tender to palpation. X-ray studies will show the opacified sinus if fluid or blood is present.

Treatment consists of administration of both oral and nasal decongestants. The use of cocaine or another equally powerful vasoconstrictive nasal decongestant is the quickest way to relieve the pain.

### BARODENTALGIA

Those patients who have had a recent filling or capping of a tooth may have trapped air between the filling and the nerve root. As the atmospheric pressure is decreased, the increased pressure of the trapped air on the nerve root causes an exquisite pain. This pain is readily relieved with descent. Patients with barodentalgia should be advised to return to the dentist and have the filling or cap redone at leisure after the pain has been relieved by repressurization.

Rarely, the patient with an apical tooth abscess or severe caries may develop a similar pain. This dental pathology must be corrected as soon as practical.

| *Features of Altitude-related Peripheral Edema* | |
|---|---|
| Setting | > 8000 feet (2440 m) |
| Predisposing factors | Unknown |
| Onset of symptoms | 2 to 4 days after ascent |
| Symptoms/signs | Extremity swelling (common) Facial swelling |
| Prophylaxis | Acetazolamide ?? Furosemide ?? |
| Treatment | Cautious use of furosemide |

## GASTROINTESTINAL BAROTRAUMA

Ascent causes the intraluminal bowel gases to expand. The use of carbonated beverages or "beans" (legumes) prior to ascent will serve only to exacerbate the condition (see also HAFE). Belching and flatus are typical complaints. Since the GI tract is open at both ends, the condition is self-correcting to the consternation of those next to the patient and the embarrassment of those afflicted. The condition is an annoyance only at terrestrial elevations but may be serious at over 30,000 feet (9000 m) or in those who have had recent bowel surgery. If the patient has an ileus or has had a recent bowel anastomosis, the expansion of the trapped gas may cause a rupture of the affected portion of the intestinal tract.

Treatment is descent to the usual ambient elevation for the patient. Those with recent bowel surgery should not fly.

### Peripheral Edema

Systemic edema of high altitude is seen after 4 to 10 days at high altitude (Table 6.7). The overall incidence in one study of peripheral edema at 14,000 feet (4243 m) was 18%.[53] It appears in females more frequently than males but is not related to the menstrual cycle. The condition appears to be due to salt and water retention, which disappears spontaneously after returning to lower levels. The disorder is usually seen with both facial and peripheral swelling. It may make the patient quite uncomfortable but is not dangerous. It is often recurrent in the same patient each time he or she returns to high altitude.

Treatment may be delayed in most cases, and the edema will resolve after the trek is over. If the edema is marked, small doses of furosemide (40 mg daily) may be cautiously employed if there is no evidence of cardiac disease.

### Sickle Cell Crisis

Sickle cell disease is well known to be worsened by hypoxemia of any cause. Needless to say, the hypoxemia of high altitude can precipitate a sickle cell crises. Certainly at 15,000 feet (4570 m), the arterial oxygen tension is low enough to precipitate a massive sickle cell crisis, but crises have been observed at altitudes as low as 11,500 feet (3500 m).

### PREVENTION

Extensive investigations into the altitude-related illnesses have included attempts to predict susceptible individuals and to define the early indications of the more severe forms of altitude-related illnesses. These efforts have included written graded examinations, physical examinations, psychometric testing, self-assessment, leader review, and peer review of the performance of the subjects.[54]

In general, physical examination is rather unrewarding in prediction and in noting the EARLY effects of any of the altitude-related illnesses. Of course, it is an effective measure of more severe forms of any of the diseases. Heel-to-toe gait (as a test for ataxia) has been noted previously as a good objective test for the presence of HACE. It is easily performed by even lay leaders and is accurate as long as the subject is not on skis or crampons. Auscultation for the presence of rales is a similar test that is easily performed with a minimum of equipment and is relatively objective. Likewise, if a subject develops fatigue that is out of proportion to exercise and altitude or lassitude, these symptoms are easily observable. Subjects with any of these findings should be accompanied to a lower altitude. The literature is replete with references to tragedies of patients who were sent alone to lower altitudes but did not arrive.

Recent work by Fletcher and colleagues showed that peer review, interview, and self-assessment all seemed equally effective at rating the effects of high-altitude illness but are good only for identifying the more severely and least severely affected individuals.[54] Daily interviews and examinations by a qualified medical observer were felt to be the safest procedures by which to identify illness.

### Who Should Not Go High

A number of diseases that occur at low altitude will be predictably worsened by the hypoxia of high altitude. There are three groups of patients for whom this hypoxia is a major consideration.

1. Individuals with chronic pulmonary disease, congestive heart failure, or cyanotic congenital heart disease with chronic hypoxemia and low arterial oxygen saturation will have a marked risk associated with ascent. The presence of hypoxemia at the lower altitude appears to be a major risk factor for all of the above diseases. This is due to the lack of reserves available for the extra work of breathing and by the shape of the oxyhemoglobin dissociation curve.

The arterial oxygen desaturation caused by the relative hypoxemia of the disease places the patient at a downslope on the oxyhemoglobin dissociation curve. Once the blood is less than 90% saturated with oxygen, the curve is steeper and even small changes in the oxygen available will cause a marked change in the amount of oxygen that the blood can deliver to the tissues.

Even among permanent residents at high altitudes, mortality is higher in the mountains than in the nations as a whole. Deaths from emphysema occur at a lower age, after shorter durations of illness, and more commonly involve cor pulmonale than at lower altitudes, where pneumonia is a more common cause of death.[55]

2. Another group of patients who should not ascend are those patients with severe angina or heart failure. At the same time that the patient has decreased his available oxygen supply by ascending, the work of breathing is increased, and consequently the myocardial oxygen consumption has increased. This may have disastrous results for the patient with marginal coronary blood flow.

3. Patients with primary pulmonary hypertension may be at the highest risk. In addition to the arterial desaturation noted in the other risk groups, these patients have a primary disease process that is worsened by the normal vascular response to high altitude. In fact, one of the highest risk factors for HAPE is the presence of only one pulmonary artery.

In general, persons who are active at sea level, who have no uncontrolled illnesses, who are sensible enough to be careful, slow, and alert to the problems discussed should not be banned from the mountains. They may not be able to tolerate the expedition to the very high and extreme altitudes, however.

### SUMMARY

Four major variables appear to determine the susceptibility to altitude illnesses: rate of ascent, altitude reached, length of stay, and amount of vigorous exercise. The altitude sicknesses are a continuum of symptoms that are grouped into three major categories: AMS (headache, nausea, and dyspnea); HAPE (dyspnea, cough, and coma); and HACE (headache, ataxia, and coma). High-altitude retinal hemorrhages and peripheral edema are encountered at the higher altitudes but do not carry the serious connotations of the first three illnesses (Fig. 6.6).

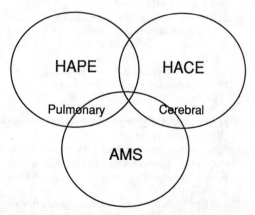

**Figure 6.6.** Venn diagram shows the relationships between the various serious high-altitude diseases.

Rate of ascent, if adjusted to the individual, is an excellent preventative measure. Acetazolamide may aid in acclimation to altitude and decrease symptoms.

Descent at an early stage of serious illness is the best therapy. Indeed, if descent is early, it may be the only therapy needed.

The final and most important point is that climbing or skiing at altitude is a sport of risks, and the individual responsibility and education of the climber or skier is the single most important preventative measure taken. This educational preventative is best taken at leisure prior to the climb, not learned in the schools of hard experience proctored by Mother Nature.

## References

1. Ravenhill TH. Some experiences of mountain sickness in the Andes. J Trop Med Hyg 1913;16:313–320.
2. Moore LG. Altitude-aggravated illness: examples from pregnancy and prenatal life. Ann Emerg Med 1987;16:965–973.
3. Habeler P. Everest: impossible victory. London: Arlington Books, 1979.
4. West JB, Hackett PH, Maret KH, et al. Pulmonary gas exchange on the summit of Mount Everest. J Appl Physiol 1983;55:678–687.
5. West JB, Lahiri S, Gill MB, et al. Arterial oxygen saturation during exercise at high altitude. J Appl Physiol 1962;17:617–621.
6. Smart J, Hunter D. Alpine travel: mountain sickness, the unwelcome companion. Med J Aust 1984;141:792–795.
7. Hansen JE, Hartley LH, Hogon, RP. Arterial oxygen increase by high carbohydrate diet at altitude. J Appl Physiol 1972;33:441–445.
8. Sutton JR, Houston CS, Mansell AL, et al. Effect of acetazolamide on hypoxemia during sleep at high altitude. N Engl J Med 1979;301:1329–1331.
9. Sutton JR. Sleep disturbances at high altitude. Phys Sports Med 1982;10:79–84.
10. West JB, Lahiri S, Maret KH, et al. Barometric pressures at extreme altitudes on Mt. Everest: physiological significance. J Appl Physiol 1983;54:1199–1194.
11. Sorenson SC, Sveringhouse JW. Irreversible respiratory insensitivity to acute hypoxia in man born at high altitude. J Appl Physiol 1968;25:217–222.
12. Lenfant C, Sullivan K. Adaptation to high altitude. N Engl J Med 1971;284:1298–1309.
13. Lenfant C, Torrance J, English E, et al: Effect of altitude on oxygen binding by hemoglobin and on organic phosphate levels. J Clin Invest 1968;47:2652–2660.
14. Lenfant C, Torrance JD, Reynafarje C. Shift of the oxygen-dissociation curve at altitude: mechanism and effect. J Appl Physiol 1971;30:625–631.
15. Winslow RM, Samaja M, West JB. Red cell function at extreme altitude on Mount Everest. J Appl Physiol 1984;56:109–116.
16. Banchero N, Sime F, Penaloza D, et al. Pulmonary pressure, cardiac output and arterial oxygen saturation during exercise at high altitude and at sea level. Circulation 1966;33:249–262.
17. Scoggin CH, Miller Y, Tate R. Getting high: the pathophysiology of high altitude. Topics Emerg Med 1980;2(3):53–61.
18. Vogel JA, Harris CW. Cardiopulmonary responses of resting man during early exposure to high altitude. J Appl Physiol 1967;22(6):1124–1128.
19. Alexander JK, Hartley L, Modelski M. et al. Reduction of stroke volume during exercise in man following ascent to 3,100 meters altitude. J Appl Physiol 1967;23:849–856.
20. Lahari S, Milledge JS. Acid-base in Sherpa altitude residents and lowlanders at 4880 meters. Respir Physiol 1967;2:323–224.
21. Winslow RM, Monge CC, Statham CG, et al. Variability of oxygen affinity of blood: human subjects native to high altitude. J Appl Physiol 1981;51:1411–1416.
22. Surks MI, Chinn KS, Matoush LO. Alterations in body composition in man after acute exposure to high altitude. J Appl Physiol 1966;21:1741–1746.
23. Blume FD, Boyer SJ, Braverman LE, et al. Impaired osmoregulation at high altitude: studies on Mount Everest. JAMA 1984;252:524–526.
24. Milledge JS, Catley DM, Blume FD, West JB. Renin, angiotensin-converting enzyme, and aldosterone in humans on Mount Everest. J Appl Physiol 1983;55:1109–1112.
25. Hogan RP III, Kotchen TA, Boyd AE III, Hartley LH. Effect of altitude on renin-aldosterone system and metabolism of water and electrolytes. J Appl Physiol 1973;35:385–390.
26. Maresh CM, Noble BJ, Robertson KL, Harvey JS Jr. Aldosterone, Cortison, and Electrolyte responses to hypobaric hypoxia in moderate-altitude natives. Aviat Space Environ Med 1985;56:1078–1084.
27. Okazakin S, Tamura Y, Hatano T, Matsui N. Hormonal disturbances of fluid-electrolyte metabolism under altitude exposure in man. Aviat Space Environ Med 1984;55:200–205.
28. Heath D, Williams DR: Man at high altitude. London, Churchill Livingstone, 1977:54–55.
29. Schoene RB. Control of ventilation in climbers

to extreme altitude. J Appl Physiol 1982;53:886–890.

30. Schoene RB, Lahiri S, Hackett PH, et al. Relationship of hypoxic ventilatory response to exercise performance on Mount Everest. J Appl Physiol 1984;56:1478–1483.

31. Anonymous. See Nuptse and die [Editorial]. Lancet 1976:1177–1179.

32. Evans WO, Robinson SM, Horstman DH, et al. Amelioration of the symptoms of acute mountain sickness by staging and acetazolamide. Aviat Space Environ Med 1976;47:512–516.

33. Hackett PH, Schoene RB, Winslow RM, et al. Acetazolamide and exercise in sojourners to 6,300 meters: a preliminary study. Med Sci Sports Exerc 1985;17:593–597.

34. Hultgren HN. High altitude medical problems. West J Med 1979;131:8–23.

35. Wilson R. Acute high altitude illness in mountaineers and problems of rescue. Ann Intern Med 1973;78:421–428.

36. Foulke GE. Altitude-related illness. Am J Emerg Med 1985;3(3):219–226.

37. Hultgren HN, Marticorena EA. High altitude pulmonary edema: epidemiologic observations in Peru. Chest 1978;74:372–376.

38. Medical problems of man at high terrestrial elevations. TB Med 288. Department of the Army. Washington, DC: Government Printing Office, 1972.

39. Maldonado D. High altitude pulmonary edema. Radiol Clin N Am 1978;16:537–549.

40. Hackett HN, Grover RF, Hartley LH. Abnormal circulatory responses to high altitude in subjects with a previous history of high altitude pulmonary edema. Circulation 1971;44:759–770.

41. Hultgren HN, Lopez CE, Lundberg E, et al. Physiologic studies of pulmonary edema at high altitude. Circulation 1964;29:393–428.

42. Schoene RB, Hackett PH, Henderson WR, et al. High-altitude pulmonary edema: characteristics of lung lavage fluid. JAMA 1986:256;63–70.

43. Chiodi H. Mal de montana a forma cerebral: posible mechanism etiopatogenico. An Fac Med Lima 1960:43:437.

44. Roy S, Singh I. Acute mountain sickness in Himalayan terrain: clinical and physiologic studies. In Hegnauer A, ed. Biomedical problems of high terrestrial elevations. Natic, MA: US Army Research Institute of Environmental Medicine, 1969.

45. McFadden DM, Houston CS, Sutton JR, et al. High-altitude retinopathy. JAMA 1981;245:581–586.

46. Rennie D, Morrissey J. Retinal changes in Himalayan climbers. Arch Ophthalmol 1975;93:395–400.

47. Frayser R, Houston CS, Bryan AC, et al. Retinal hemorrhage at high altitude. N Engl J Med 1970;282;1183–1184.

48. Singh I, Khanna PK, Srivastava MC, et al. Acute mountain sickness. N Engl J Med 1969;280:175.

49. Lempert P, Cooper KH, Culver JF, et al. The effect of exercise on intraocular pressure. Am J Ophthalmol 1967;63:1673–1676.

50. Shults WT, Swan KC. High altitude retinopathy in mountain climbers. Arch Ophthalmol 1975;93:404–408.

51. Davis EY. HAFE in Nepal. West J Med 1981;134:366.

52. Auerbach P, Miller E. High altitude flatus expulsion (Correspondence). West J Med 1981;134:173–174.

53. Hackett PH, Rennie D. Rales, peripheral edema, retinal hemorrhage and acute mountain sickness. Am J Med 1979;67:214–218.

54. Fletcher RF, Wright AD, Jones GT, Bradwell AR. The clinical assessment of acute mountain sickness. Q J Med 1985;54:91–100.

55. Moore LG, Rohr AL, Maisenbach JK, et al. Emphysema mortality is increased in Colorado residents at high altitude. Am Rev Respir Dis 1982;126:225–228.

# CHAPTER 7

# Bites and Stings

## Part 1
## Arthropods: Things That Sting, Jaws That Bite, and Other Creatures of the Night

### INTRODUCTION

Throughout history, insects, mites, and other arthropods have been one of the plagues of humans. Biblical punishment for the Pharaoh included a grevious swarm of flies (Exodus 8:24). Insects annoy us by their very presence with injurious bites and stings. Flies at home or at work, ants at the family outing, mosquitoes at the campsite are all examples of the annoyances these animals bring. The cyclist and the motorist with a bee in the car can both testify to the hazards of flying insects at speed.

These small arthropods are found everywhere—from the tropics to the tundra, in water, wood, plants, soil, decaying matter, and even in the bodies of other animals. Nearly a million different species of arthropods have been identified, more than all of the other animal species combined. They compete with all other organisms for food and in turn are a major food source for other animals and for each other.

In the process of feeding on other animals and defending themselves, many arthropods have developed the ability to deliver noxious substances or poisons through a variety of weapons and mechanisms. It is these arthropods and their "weapons systems" that we will concern ourselves with. Annually, more deaths occur due to envenomation from the arthropods than from any other venomous source. The venom or irritant may be delivered by sting, bite, skin secretions, hairs, or spray. (Arthropods bite with their front parts and sting with their rears.) The venom delivered by arthropods is complex in chemistry and pharmacology.

An additional source of trouble for humans lies in the mechanisms of feeding developed by some arthropods. Unfortunately, some of us provide the very best food for some of them. Equally unfortunately, in the process of acquiring their favorite dish, they may admit other unwelcome guests into us when they inject their salivary secretions. In this regard, the arthropods serve as major vectors for life-threatening diseases.

### ARACHNIDS

Arachnids comprise the largest noninsect class of arthropods and, perhaps, the most feared. They include 11 different orders with over 75,000 species identified worldwide. This class of arthropods includes spiders, ticks, mites, and scorpions. The arachnid class is ancient, first appearing over 350 million years ago.

### Spiders

There may be as many as 20,000 species of spiders in the world, and perhaps 18,000 of those spiders are venomous. Statistics are unavailable to determine just how many humans are bitten by spiders each year, yet death from a spider bite is rare in this country. Fortunately, only a few spiders have both the capability to penetrate human skin, the inclination to bite, and the venom potent enough to cause a reaction.

Unlike insects, spiders have only 2 distinct body parts, the cephalothorax (a combined head and thorax) and the abdomen. There are from six to eight eyes on the cephalothorax, depending upon the species. Spiders are thought to be relatively shortsighted and rely more upon touch for location of both enemies and prey. Spiders have a pair of jaw-like or fang-bearing appendages (chelicerae) in front of the mouth. These chelicerae contain the venom-delivery apparatus. They also have a pair of leg-like pedipalps between the chelicerae and the first walking legs.

Spiders have a venom that is, volume for volume, more potent than that of a rattlesnake. The venom is designed to paralyze the prey and then liquify the prey's tissues. The spider can then ingest the liquified tissues and hemolymph for nourishment. With this in mind, it is easy to predict the two types of reactions of spider venom: local tissue necrosis and neurotoxic reactions. Each species of spiders has venom that induces these reactions to a greater or lesser degree.

Their natural enemies are wasps, birds, internal parasites, natural disasters, and other spiders. In general, most spiders are shy and will run away when approached by humans. Despite their fearsome reputation, they are not usually aggressive. Indeed, some species have been kept as pets and will not bite unless held or squeezed.

## BLACK WIDOW (LATRODECTUS SPECIES)

Of all spiders, the black widow is probably the most feared in the United States. The black widow is found throughout the continental United States and is usually recognizable by the typical glossy black and orange coloring. The range is from Massachusetts to Florida, and west to Texas, California, Oklahoma, and Kansas. It is most common in the south but may be found in cooler climates and up to the 8000 foot level.

There are five species of "black widows," yet only three of them are black (*Latrodectus.*

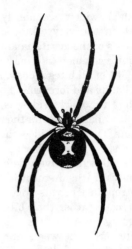

**Figure 7.1.** Black widow spider.

*mactans, L. variolus,* and *L. hesperus*). One other species is known as the red-legged spider (*L. bishopi*) and another is brown (*L. geometricus*). The widow spider has a species-specific red marking on the ventral surface of the abdomen (see Fig. 7.1). In only one species is this the classic orange-red hourglass shape. In most species, the equilateral triangles do not quite meet. Newly hatched widow spiderlings may be almost entirely red or orange, and the younger spiders may retain broad reddish markings on their abdomen for several moltings.

The female of the species is one of the largest of spiders with a body ranging up to ½ inch (1 to 1.5 cm) long with a leg span of up to 2 inches (4 to 5 cm). It is precisely this large size that allows the female black widow's fangs to be able to penetrate human skin. The female black widow may live as long as 3 years.

The male is only one third the size of the female (3 to 5 mm long). Contrary to myth, the male usually mates safely with the female. Because of his small size, the male's fangs are incapable of penetrating human skin, so most bites are from the female of the species. The female is capable of storing sperm and need not mate before producing each egg sac.

### Habitat

The black widow favors woodpiles, sheds, basements, and garages. In the days of privies, many unfortunates found the hard way that the black widow frequently built its shaggy web in the privy. Indeed, the frequency of bites of the genitalia and buttocks was once quite common and may have been as high as 50% of all bites. Today, most bites are on the hands and forearms.

The web of the black widow is an extensive, irregular, shaggy trap for the insects she normally eats. The black widow rarely leaves the web and stays close to her egg masses if present. She will aggressively defend the egg mass and bites if it is disturbed. Despite its aggressive reputation, this spider often attempts to escape rather than bite when she is not guarding eggs.

Most bites occur between April and October and usually in adult men.[1] Females hibernate during the winter, and bites are rare during that time. It is estimated that nearly half of all black widow bites could be prevented if articles of clothing and toilets were inspected before use.

## Venom

*Latrodectus* venom is considered to be one of the most potent venoms secreted by any animal.[2] It is manufactured by a pair of venom glands in the cephalothorax that contain an average of only about 0.2 mg of venom. The venom has a median lethal dosage ranging from 0.005 to 1 mg per kg. An 18-month-old black widow spider has enough venom to kill a 30-pound child.

The venom's toxic factor appears to be a neurotoxic protein with a molecular weight of about 5000 daltons that acts on the neurotransmitters.[3] In this neurotoxin's action, the majority of the signs and symptoms reflect the excitation and stimulation of the central nervous system and muscles due to presynaptic stimulation. The toxic factor causes a massive release of acetylcholine and norepinephrine at the synaptic junction. The continued release of neurotransmitters at the synaptic junction causes excitation of neural junctions and stimulation of muscle contraction. Eventually, the acetylcholine supply is exhausted and further synaptic transmission is blocked by depolarization of the membrane.

## Symptoms

The bite of the female black widow spider has been described in various terms ranging from no more than a pinprick to moderately painful. After 20 to 40 minutes, the bite site will often develop a small wheal and flare. Often the only finding may be local swelling and 2 small fang marks about 1 mm apart. Multiple bites effectively rule out spider envenomation since spiders rarely bite more than once.

After about 15 minutes to an hour, a crampy pain begins about the site of the bite and gradually spreads. The pain increases and comes in excruciating waves that often cause the patient to writhe on the bed. Normally, the thighs, shoulders, and back muscles are affected first, although all muscle groups may be involved. A classic finding is a severe board-like abdominal pain from muscle spasm of the abdominal wall. The pain often subsides after a few hours but recurs in mild form for 2 to 3 days. Weakness, tingling, and transient muscle spasms may persist for weeks to months as residual symptoms.

Often, fine muscle fasciculations can be seen if the room lights are dimmed and an indirect light is shown upon the face. Occasionally noted is facies latrodectismica: a flushed diaphoretic facies with a painful grimace and trismus.

Paralysis and respiratory arrest may occur, particularly in children. Nausea, vomiting, headache, weakness, increased salivation, and anxiety are common. The reflexes are often hyperactive and cerebrospinal fluid pressure has been noted as high. Priapism has been reported but is rare.

The most important finding is not the crampy abdominal pain but, rather, the marked hypertension that may progress to a hypertensive crisis. This hypertensive response is fortunately rare.[4] It is thought to be caused by an activation of the vasomotor centers of the bulbar and spinal medulla.[5]

Severe envenomation may produce shock, coma, or respiratory failure. These severe cases may also have electrocardiographic changes that are similar to those of a digitalis overdose. Deaths are usually due to cardiac or respiratory failure or a hypertensive crisis and are, fortunately, quite infrequent now that antivenin is available.

Those at high risk for severe morbidity from envenomation include patients who are:

1. Less than 16 or greater than 60 years of age

2. Have hypertension or hypertensive heart disease

3. Have signs or symptoms of severe envenomation with respiratory difficulty or uncontrollable muscle spasms

In high-risk individuals, the cardiovascular manifestations may lead to stroke, exacerbation of heart failure, and myocardial ischemia.

Because the bite may not be noted by the patient, the symptoms may be attributed to an intra-abdominal crisis, perforated peptic ulcer, pancreatitis, or tetanus. The abdominal pain from widow spider bites does not have associated rebound or deep tenderness. The bite of the black widow and the subsequent muscle spasms and trismus may also mimic poisonings from substances, such as cocaine, strychnine or lead.

## Treatment

Treatment of black widow spider bites consists of palliation of the pain, inactivation of the venom, and muscle relaxation for the muscle spasms. Muscle relaxants as described below often will relieve the pain, but if the pain is severe, narcotic analgesics may be needed. Hypertension may be controlled with muscle relaxants and pain medications, but antihypertensive agents may be needed in severe cases. All patients in high-risk categories should be hospitalized.

**Antivenin.** Antivenin is usually given only to children or to patients with preexisting cardiovascular disease. Antivenin may be given to adults between 16 and 65 if the patient has unusually severe symptoms, is pregnant, or has preexisting hypertensive or cardiac disease. For the majority of patients, the treatment is supportive. At least one study suggests that the administration of calcium and muscle relaxants may be as effective as antivenin, even in severe envenomations.[4]

The antivenin is a horse serum antivenom (Lyovac *Latrodectus mactans*, Merck, Sharp, and Dohme), and preadministration testing for sensitivity should be performed if possible. The usual dose is 1 vial of antivenin given intravenously. It will give relief of symptoms within 1 to 3 hours. Although one dose is usually adequate, a second dose may be needed in severe cases. The pediatric dose is the same as the adult dose. A frequent complication of this antivenin (and all horse serum-based antivenin) is serum sickness.[4]

**Calcium Gluconate.** Muscle relaxation is best achieved with calcium gluconate intravenously in doses of 10 cc of the 10% solution with relief of symptoms in about 50% of cases. Cardiac monitoring is essential with administration of this drug intravenously. If the patient is treated in the first 3 hours, there is better relief than if the patient's bite is greater than 3 hours old. Some authorities feel that the administration of calcium and subsequent relief of abdominal pain is diagnostic and will surely separate peritonitis from the effects of the black widow's venom.

**Diazepam.** Diazepam also appears to be effective in controlling the muscle spasms. The dose for adults is between 5 and 10 mg intravenously every 3 to 4 hours as needed. Children require proportionately smaller doses.[2]

**Sodium Dantrolene.** Sodium dantrolene has also been tried with good effect. Initial intravenous administration followed by oral dosage may be better than oral administration alone.[6]

**Methocarbamol.** Robaxin (methocarbamol) has been used, but results show less efficacy than calcium gluconate. Methocarbamol does not require cardiac monitoring for intravenous or intramuscular administration. The usual dose is 1000 mg (10 cc) intravenously followed by another 1000 mg in 250 cc of saline by drip infusion. The drug should be given in a widely patent IV at a rate no faster than 100 mg per minute.

**Local Care.** Local wound cleansing is done with any number of suitable solutions. Antibiotic therapy is not usually needed. The tetanus immunization status should be checked and corrected as needed.

## Prevention

Frequent cleaning to remove spiders and their webs from outbuildings, buildings, and outdoor living areas will decrease the chance of accidental contact with this spider. Routine hose washings of privies and woodpiles will also decrease the spider population. Insecticides may decrease the population of the food for the black widows but do not usually affect the spiders.

## Recluse Spider

Recluse or *Loxosceles* spiders are found in South, Central, and North America and in

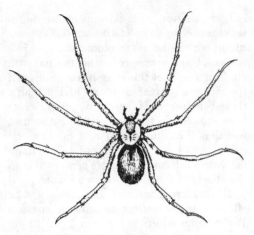

**Figure 7.2.** Recluse spider.

Europe. There are 13 species of this spider in the United States alone. "Brown recluse" refers only to the *Loxosceles reclusa*, which is the most prevalent in the United States.

Other names for this species have included the "violin or fiddleback" spider. The spider got these two names from a characteristic violin-like marking on its cephalothorax. The violin is not nearly as well defined as one would like it to be, and several of the species do not have this mark (see Fig. 7.2).

Recluse spiders are large, up to 1.2 cm long with a leg span of up to 5 cm. The bodies are fawn to dark brown and most North American species have a somewhat violin-shaped marking colored dark brown to yellow. The larger end of this marking is towards the head of the spider. The distal body is an elongated oval. The abdomen is grayish to dark brown with no obvious pattern.

## Habitat

The recluse spiders are generally found throughout the southern half of the United States. In the natural habitat, they hide under woodpiles and rocks. *Loxosceles* spiders tend to be found in close association with humans in the cooler climates. They appear to prefer a sheltered, darker habitat, such as closets and basements. Their reclusive nature makes them difficult to eradicate.

Localized populations of these spiders are reported in Arizona, Wyoming, California, Florida, New Jersey, North Carolina, Pennsylvania, and Washington, DC. These con-

centrations probably represent importation of the spider in baggage and household goods of our mobile population. In South America, the *Loxoscles laeta* species predominates and has caused many confirmed bites. It is found in up to 40% of urban houses in central Chile.[7,8]

Members of this species are nonaggressive and normally attempt to escape whenever they are threatened. Most bites occur when the patient traps the spider in clothing that is being donned, steps on the spider at night, or cleans an area where the spider resides. Multiple bites are not associated with this spider and are due to some other form of envenomation.

The diagnosis of necrotic lesions due to recluse spider bites is probably overestimated in the medical literature and certainly exaggerated by the lay press. In many areas, almost any necrotic lesion may be blamed on the recluse spiders by the lay population and uninformed medical staff. In Northern Colorado, for example, the brown recluse is not found, and yet during the summer months is frequently blamed for various skin lesions. In a review of about 600 "spider bites" between 1950 and 1980, 80% were caused by other arthropods, widow, *Phidippus*, or wolf spiders.[9] Further examination of the data indicated that only 10% were due to the recluse spiders. The remaining 10% were diseases unrelated to arthropod envenomation. Unless the arthropod is brought in with the patient, the physician should be exceedingly leery of attributing a necrotic lesion to the recluse spider. Certain identification of an arthropod envenomation requires the physical presence of the offending arthropod.

## Venom

*Loxosceles* venom is a complex mixture of at least eight separate venoms among which hyaluronidase, protease, esterase, and hemolysins have been identified.[3,10] The major action appears to be endothelial damage to the smaller blood vessels.[11] This leads to thrombosis with subsequent infarction and necrosis. Further tissue damage may be caused by lysis of the polymorphonuclear leukocytes liberating kinins and possibly histamine release by mast cells. The toxin produces a slowly healing necrotic lesion and an array of systemic effects.

**Local Effects.** The sequence of the recluse spider bite is thought to be characteristic and unique.[12] The bite is often relatively painless at first. After 2 to 8 hours, the area becomes indurated, erythematous, and painful. The start of tissue destruction is heralded by the development of a bleb over the bite site and erythema surrounding the site. For a while during the development of the necrotic lesion, the central portion is surrounded by halos of blanching and rings of erythema quite like a bull's eye target. The bleb becomes indurated 3 to 4 days later, forming a firm swelling that can measure as large as 1.5 cm in diameter.

The induration ruptures 7 to 8 days later and forms a crust that sloughs. When the crust sloughs, it leaves a necrotic ulcer that progressively enlarges and may be covered with a blackish or brownish eschar. The ulcer is often indolent with ragged edges and a necrotic base. The lesion may become quite extensive (as much as 15 cm greatest diameter) and involve underlying muscle and fascia.

No commercially available diagnostic test exists for the recluse spider's envenomation, although a serodiagnostic test has been experimentally developed.[13,14] Occasionally, a biopsy may be helpful and will demonstrate nonspecific endothelial damage, necrosis of the dermis, and possibly evidence of hemolysis.

**Systemic Reactions.** In mild envenomation, the patient may have chills, fever, and scarlatiniform rash. The rash may be quite like that of toxic shock syndrome. Young children and older adults may also have arthralgias, chills, nausea, and vomiting. The combination of high fever and scarlatiniform rash, together with a typical lesion, should be a strong clue to the diagnosis of systemic loxoscelism.

The systemic symptoms that may accompany severe envenomation include hemolysis, disseminated intravascular coagulopathies, renal failure, and death.[15] Hemolytic anemia has also followed the bite of recluse spiders.[16] Systemic reactions and intravascular hemolysis have been noted from 24 to 48 hours after the bite and before the development of the necrotic ulceration.[17] If there is no evidence of hemolytic symptoms after 24 to 48 hours, the prospects of survival are excellent. Fortunately, these severe cases are not common and fatalities are very rare.

## Treatment

Treatment depends upon the severity of the bite. The patient with a mild bite can be treated with an analgesic and an antihistamine to relieve pain and itching. Severe local reactions that are seen promptly may be decreased by the use of phentolamine wound infiltration (Regitine) of about 5 to 10 mg in 10 cc of saline.

Some authorities recommend steroids in doses of 4 mg of dexamethasone intravenously or intramuscularly every 6 hours during the inflammatory stage.[18] It probably has little systemic side effects and may decrease inflammation and tissue loss. Steroid therapy, as usual, has no conclusive evidence about its efficacy and remains controversial.

Early excision of the lesion is also recommended, but this is not universally accepted. Excision after 8 hours or so does not appear to be of much benefit. Eventually, the lesions heal, but sometimes with scarring that requires reconstructive surgery.

Dapsone has also been used to decrease the intensity and magnitude of the inflammatory reaction. This drug has been used anecdotally with excellent effect and prompt resolution of the ulcer. Use of dapsone is not without complications or danger, as dapsone can cause a hemolytic anemia.[19,20]

There is no antivenin for the venom of the recluse spider, yet. Systemic reactions should be treated as appropriate for the manifestation.

Local wound care of the ulcers can include soaks with Burrow's solution, hydrogen peroxide, triple aqueous dye, scarlet red, and antibiotic solutions. There is no good evidence that links decreased tissue losses with any specific local therapy, so the wound care that the physician is most comfortable with is the one that is most appropriate.

## MISCELLANEOUS SPIDERS

### Jumping Spiders

While the black widow and the recluse spiders get all the bad publicity, the most common biting spider in the United States is the crablike jumping spider, the *Phidippus* species.

Some species of this small, furry, aggressive spider are confused with the black widow, because they are black and have red or orange markings. Other species have white stripes with greenish fluorescent mouth parts, are hairy, and may be mistaken for baby tarantulas.

This spider will bite and hang on to the victim. The patient may bring in the spider still attached or squashed against the arm. Indeed, if the bite is not from a recluse spider, most spiders are brought to the emergency department attached to the victim or the victim describes pulling the spider off.

The bite of the *Phidippus* has a local reaction with swelling, pruritis, and irritation. The pain is dull and throbbing and may take days to subside.

Treatment is local wound care and minimal analgesia with aspirin or ibuprofen. Pruritis may be treated with antihistamines in usual doses. Localized cellulitis is uncommon.

## Tarantula

Another common spider bite is from the "tarantula." The name tarantula bears no zoologic significance and is used interchangeably for several species of large spiders. The common tarantula of the Southwest is a member of the genus *Avicularia* (bird spiders). Another species often called a tarantula is a wolf spider of genus *Lycosa* that has migrated from the south.

The desert tarantula of Arizona and New Mexico may reach a body size of 2¾ inches (70 mm) and have a leg span as large as 5 inches (100 mm). The male has longer legs and is more active than the female. Males are short-lived and do not molt after maturity, but the female may live as long as 20 years.

The tarantula from the American Southwest, although fearsomely large, does not produce a toxin with systemic effects. The mild venom produces a local inflammation and swelling that lasts for only a few hours. Indeed, these spiders are gentle and may be kept as pets. For these spider's bites, local wound care as outlined above will suffice.

The South American tarantula and the banana spiders do have an effective venom and are very aggressive. The red-legged, orange-kneed tarantula of South America is considered dangerous. These two spiders are not usually seen in the United States, except as stowaways. An antitoxin has been developed for the bite of the South American tarantula.

## SCORPIONS

Some authorities consider scorpions to be the most menacing of the desert animals. They are an ancient, but not particularly large, group of arachnids (some 1500 to 2000 species worldwide). It is apparent that scorpions are dangerous and not merely a "nuisance," but not all scorpions are deadly. More than 20 species of scorpions occur in Arizona alone, where detailed studies have been made of the American species.

## Identification

Identification of scorpions as a group is relatively easy. They appear like miniature lobsters with lobster-like pincers but have a long upcurved "tail" with a poisonous stinger. Like all arachnids, they have eight legs, with the first two being developed as pincers and the other six as walking legs.

## CENTRUROIDES

The deadly *Centruroides sculpturatus* (also called *C. exilicauda*) can be found mainly across the southern part of Arizona, New Mexico, in the bottom of the Grand Canyon, along the California side of the Colorado River, and at lower points across Colorado. As far as is now known, no other deadly species occur in the Southwest, although there are several in Mexico. The *Centruroides suffusus* (the Durango scorpion) is found in western Mexico and, until recently, was responsible for many yearly deaths. These scorpions and the majority of lethal scorpions throughout the world belong to the *Buthidae* family (see Fig. 7.3).

*Centruroides* is a small, narrow, brownish-yellow scorpion with thin pincers (chelicerae). It reaches a maximum size of 2 inches. The entire body, especially the joints of the legs, pincers, and tail are long and slender. This is in contrast with the stubby or chunky appearance of the many nondeadly species (see Fig. 7.4).

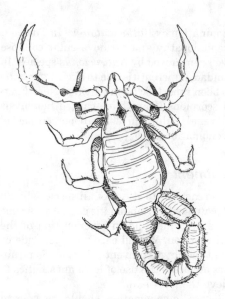

**Figure 7.3.** The giant hairy scorpion.

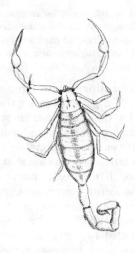

**Figure 7.4.** Centruroides scorpion.

## WHIP SCORPIONS

There is an even smaller subset of arachnids, the whip scorpions, that are similar in shape but possess no sting. These are not true scorpions, have no venom apparatus, and are quite rare.

### Habitat

Scorpions like warm and dry climates. They are nocturnal animals and, during the day, will hide under rocks, bark, and in the crevices of rocks and in debris. As many a camper will testify, they will explore boots and clothing left out overnight and may attempt to hide in sleeping bags, clothes and shoes during the day. Scorpions are generally shy and will sting only if disturbed. They hunt by night and may be observed with an ultraviolet light.

*Centruroides* species are commonly found under bark on old stumps, in lumber piles, or in firewood piled in dark corners. It is not unusual to find them in basements or linen closets.

### Venom

The scorpion stings with a venom apparatus located in the terminal portion of a six-segment abdomen called the telson. The telson terminates in a curved barbless sting and contains a pair of venom-producing glands and a poison reservoir. The sting is driven into the flesh of the victim by a quick motion of the tail. Muscles in the poison reservoir express the venom below the victim's dermis through two small ports in the distal end of the sting.

The pincers at the head end of the body hold the prey. The venom may be used to kill prey or for defense, but this is inconsistent among species. It appears as if the venom of those with large powerful chelicerae is weak, compared with those with smaller chelicerae. The nondeadly scorpions produce venom that has local effects only. The site of the sting swells and becomes red and painful immediately.

The smaller *Centruroides sculpturatus* produces little local reaction. The venom is a potent neurotoxin that may result in cranial nerve dysfunction and severe neuromuscular hyperactivity. This venom has been found to contain four separate neurotoxins that act on the activation process of sodium channels and increase spontaneous impulse firing. A fifth toxin causes a prolonged action potential. The combined results of this toxic mixture include:

Catecholamine release from adrenergic neurons

Increased neurotransmitter release
Catecholamine release from the adrenal gland
Catecholamine-induced cardiac hypoxia
Action at the juxtaglomerular apparatus, causing increased renin secretion

The untreated sting has been reported to be lethal to 25% of patients under the age of 5 but only 1% of the adults that are stung. This scorpion has been reported to have been the most lethal venomous animal in Arizona.[21] Prior to the late 1950s, this scorpion may have caused more than twice as many deaths as all other American venomous animals combined. There have been no reported deaths, however, since 1968.[22] This improvement has been attributed to improved control of the scorpion population, advances in medical care, and the development of antivenom.

After a typical *Centruroides* envenomation, there is immediate local pain with numbness or tingling in the area of the sting soon after. The involved part becomes sensitive to touch, pressure, or temperature. The majority of patients have a short duration of pain (less than 4 hours).[23] There may also be quite severe radiating pain from the site of the sting. The patient may complain of weakness in the involved extremity.

Symptoms of severe envenomation occur usually in children under 2 years old. After a severe envenomation, the following phenomenon generally appear in order: hyperexcitability, increased salivation, increased respirations, muscle twitching and contractions leading to convulsions, spastic paralysis, and respiratory failure. These may occur from a few minutes to several hours after the sting. These symptoms may be partly due to the massive outpouring of catecholamines elicited by the toxin. Autopsies of patients stung by a variety of scorpions show microscopic myocardial changes similar to those found in animals deliberately overdosed with catecholamines.[24]

Other dangerous species of scorpion throughout the world appear to have similarities in their venom and signs and symptoms following envenomation follow similar clinical patterns.[25] Some exceptions do occur, and there are species-specific differences. *Buthus quinquestriatus*, the toxic scorpion found in Israel, causes neurotoxicity and cardiotoxicity.[26] Myocarditis and pulmonary edema have been reported from India following envenomnation by *Buthus talamus*. In Tunesia, encephalopathy and cardiovascular collapse have been caused by *Androctonus* species. In Trinidad, pancreatitis due to *Tityus trinitatis* has been reported.[27] Unidentified Near Eastern scorpions (Iran) have caused hemolysis and renal failure in a small percentage of envenomations.[28]

## Treatment

Local reactions to stings of all species should be treated with symptomatic care. An ice cube to the area may aid in amelioration of the local reaction. Wound care with peroxide or an antibiotic will prevent infection. Some authors advocate the use of local anesthetics to relieve the local pain.

Severe envenomation should be treated with the scorpion-specific antivenin if possible. The *Centruoides* antivenin is available at the Poisonous Animals Research Laboratory of Arizona State University (Tempe, Arizona) as an "orphan" drug. Several hospitals in southern Arizona keep supplies of antivenin, and the patient should be taken to one of these hospitals if they are readily accessible.

The antivenin must be given intravenously with usual skin test precautions in a dose of 1 to 2 vials. Dramatic results are usually seen within 1 hour of the administration. Delayed reactions may be expected, but the incidence of such reactions appears to be less than with snake antivenin. The scorpion antivenin is made from a goat serum unlike the horse serum antivenin used for snake and black widow bites.

Theoretically, sympathetic blocking agents, such as propranolol, may be effective in controlling the tachycardia and cardiac irregularities. There have been no good controlled studies on humans with propranolol or other beta blockers for this indication, however.[29]

Although there have been reports of contraindications to narcotics in treatment of the *Centruroides sculpturatus* sting, there appears to be no substantial risk to the use of narcotics. It should be noted that earlier therapies for scorpion stings often included truly massive doses of barbiturates and narcotics, with the subsequent complications of barbiturate and narcotic overdose. Narcotics may be used prudently for the treatment of radiating limb pain. The patient should be warned that the pain and paresthesias may last for days after the sting.

Sedatives, such as phenobarbital or diazepam have been used in the past with varying degrees of success. For severe envenomation, the effects are transient with requirements for excessive doses. If the antivenin is subsequently given, the abrupt reversal of symptoms may also leave the physician with an iatrogenic sedative or narcotic overdose as the antivenin inactivates the venom. The usual dose of phenobarbital is about 5 to 10 mg per kg, intravenously. Larger phenobarbital doses may cause an iatrogenic respiratory depression. The dose of diazepam is 5 to 10 mg intravenously, although diazepam may cause less respiratory depression in larger equivalent doses than phenobarbital.

If no antivenin is used, careful bedside monitoring is essential for maintenance of cardiac and respiratory functions. Protection of the patient from self-injury from agitation or convulsions is also needed.

### Prevention

To avoid unpleasant surprises, boots, shoes, blankets, sleeping bags, and clothing should be shaken out before using. Shoes should be worn whenever walking at night. Leather gloves and long-sleeved shirts will decrease the number of stings while clearing rocks or debris.

Careful removal of debris around housing and camping areas will decrease the numbers of scorpions. Legs of cribs and children's beds may be placed in wide mouth glass jars. Children's cribs should be screened and parents should pull the sheets clear back before putting youngsters to bed. Insecticides help, but may cause certain species of scorpions to become hyperactive before death.

### TICKS

There are two types of ticks: soft (argasid) and hard (ixodid). The most frequently encountered tick in North America is the ixodid tick. It is more difficult to remove and is the commonest vector of tick-borne diseases in the United States (see Fig. 7.5).

Clearly, not everyone who is bitten by a tick becomes ill and not all persons who de-

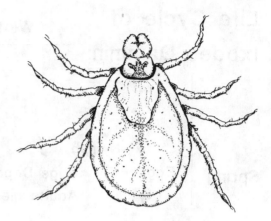

**Figure 7.5.** Ixodid tick.

velop a tick-borne disease can recall being bitten. We do know that handling ticks or crushing ticks can result in a disease transmission even in the absence of a tick bite. Tick saliva, tick feces, tick blood, and tick tissues all can contain rickettsia and other organisms if the tick happens to be infected.

### Development and Anatomy

Ticks are unusual in that they mature to adulthood through a six-legged larval stage and an eight-legged nymph stage (see Fig. 7.6). The larvae of *Ixoides dammini*, for example, will normally feed on mice, squirrels, rabbits, and other small mammals that may harbor a microorganism, such as tularemia. At the next stage, the nymphal form, the tick goes after another blood meal. This meal is usually one of the smaller animals but may be a larger animal, such as a dog or human.

In the adult stage, the tick normally feeds on a larger mammal, such as a deer or human. If the tick has ingested a microorganism at any phase in its development, that "bug" can be transmitted to the next host, where it can also be picked up by another tick or even another vector.

Ticks have sense organs that enable them to detect warm-blooded mammals as far as 25 feet away. They respond to shadows, touch, and odor and will drop onto or attach as the victim passes. Once on the victim, the tick seeks a comfortable spot, imbeds the mouth parts, and starts to suck blood. Females will remain attached for 5 to 13 days and then detach themselves. The most common season

# Life Cycle of Ixodes Dammini

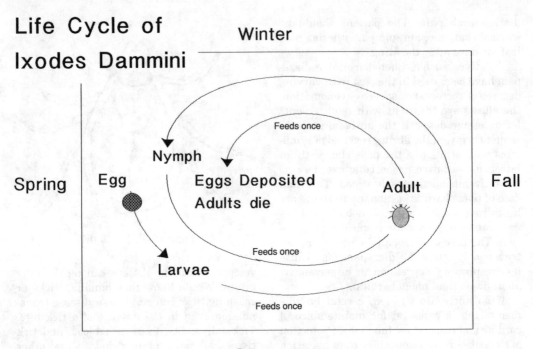

Figure 7.6. Life cycle of ixodes dammini.

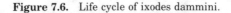

for tick infestation is between March and August, when the tick is sexually active.

The mouth parts consist of two retractile jaws, a pair of short appendages (palps), and a central probe with recurved teeth (the hypostome). These structures are attached to a plate called the capitulum. The tick attaches to the host with its mouth parts, which not only are imbedded in the skin but are also glued into place with a cement-like secretion. The tick can voluntarily detach from its host but, when forced off, may leave the capitulum and attached mouth parts imbedded in the skin.

## DISTRIBUTION AND HABITAT

Much of the United States and Mexico from sea level to tree line will be infested with ticks. High woodlands and meadows are common sites. The tick may be found on grasses, weeds, and low shrubs as well as trees.

## Local Reaction

A tick's bite is painless. The site of attachment may become reddened and indurated. Local petechial hemorrhages may be noted.

Days, weeks, or even months after a tick's bite, the area may develop a hard, localized granuloma. The lump may be as much as 3 cm in diameter and may last for months before it disappears.

## Systemic Reaction

### TICK PARALYSIS

Tick paralysis appears to affect young children or elderly people most often. Humans are not the only victims of this disorder, however; sheep, dogs, and cattle may also be stricken. The onset of the initial symptoms occurs 9 to 16 days after a pregnant female tick attaches itself.

The clinical presentation of tick paralysis is similar to Guillain-Barre syndrome, with an acute ascending weakness, areflexia, and often ataxia. The patient may complain initially of a weakness and tingling sensation in the legs. Paresthesias are somewhat less common. Once paralysis begins, the progression of the disease is rapid and the patient may be immobilized within 24 hours. The paralysis may have pronounced facial and tongue involvement. If untreated, the disease can progress to bulbar involvement with a fatal respiratory paralysis within hours to days.

The neurologic deficits are thought to be caused by a neurotoxin secreted in the salivary glands of pregnant ticks. This toxin appears to affect the peripheral nerves by causing a conduction block in the motor fibers with failure to release acetylcholine at the neuromuscular junction. There may also be a direct toxic effect on the CNS.

Diagnosis depends upon locating the tick, which may be hidden in scalp, axilla, or pubic hairs. Careful removal of the tick usually results in complete recovery within 24 to 48 hours. Mortality of this disease is about 11%, which is startling, considering that the treatment is simply removal of the tick.

Anyone who develops an acute weakness or ataxia during the spring and summer months may have this disease. Finding the tick may be difficult, particularly if the physician is not attuned to the possibility of tick paralysis or if the patient does not give a history of recent travels to tick-infested areas. The scalp and body should be searched for an attached tick. Ticks may be obscured by skin folds or hair-covered areas and may be mistaken for pigmented moles or other lesions.

## Vector for Diseases

### ROCKY MOUNTAIN SPOTTED FEVER

Rocky Mountain spotted fever is caused by *Rickettsia rickettsii*, an obligate intracellular parasite of several species of ticks, rodents, and possibly other mammals. The organism is transmitted to humans by the bite of the adult tick and, occasionally, by the nymph forms. Rarely, a crushed tick may transmit infection through open sores or wounds on the therapist's hands.

### Epidemiology

This disease is seen in three fourths of the United States and accounts for more illness than any other tick-borne disease. It is common in areas in the southeast including Virginia and North Carolina and not uncommon in Maryland. Oklahoma and Kansas are the two midwestern states with the highest rates (see Fig. 7.7). The tick vector for Rocky Mountain spotted fever varies from region to region. In the western United States, the wood tick (*Demacentor andersoni*) is the principle vector. In the eastern and southern parts of the United States, the dog tick (*Dermacentor*

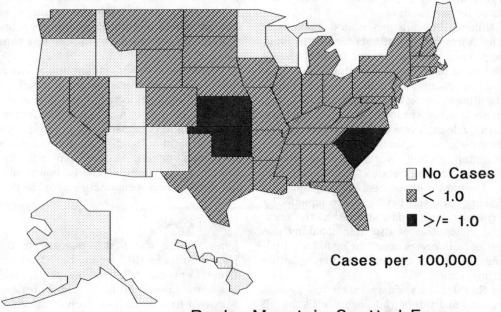

Cases per 100,000

## Rocky Mountain Spotted Fever

**Figure 7.7.** Rocky Mountain spotted fever distribution.

*variabilis*) is the major transmitter of the disease.

## Clinical Presentation

Rocky Mountain spotted fever produces a serious systemic infection. The average onset of the illness is from 5 to 7 days after exposure to the infected tick. If the disease is promptly treated, the mortality and morbidity are minimal. If there is a delay in treatment of 7 to 10 days, the mortality is related to a number of factors and may range from 3 to 7%.

The hallmark of Rocky Mountain spotted fever is a triad of fever, edema, and rash. In the early stages, the rash may not be present, may be overlooked, and may not be particularly obvious, particularly in Blacks and other darker skinned individuals. The rash starts on the wrists, palms, ankles, or soles of the feet and has a fine macular appearance. As the disease progresses, the rash deepens in color and then becomes maculopapular. It progresses into petechiae as the rickettsia multiply. As the endothelium of the vessels is progressively damaged, the patient may develop frank purpura and then vascular collapse.

The fever of Rocky Mountain spotted fever is usually high, reaching 103 to 104°F. (39.5 to 40°C), and is often accompanied by chills. The temperature will usually remain elevated for several days.

Edema is usually generalized and nonpitting. Virtually all patients have it to some degree as a result of damage to blood vessels and subsequent escape of serum. The edema is often so slight, particularly at the onset of the illness, as to be unrecognizable in patients that present to the emergency department. Edema, when present, is perhaps the most useful sign in the differentiation of Rocky Mountain spotted fever from other similar diseases, such as measles.

The most common neurologic symptom is lethargy. A severe headache, accompanied by myalgias, arthralgias, stiffness of the neck, and photophobia, is also often noted in these patients. In severe cases, the neurologic findings may mimic the findings of encephalitis or meningitis.

Renal failure, gastrointestinal hemorrhages, and interstitial pneumonitis are all seen in very severe cases but, fortunately, are relatively rare. Residual neurologic symptoms, ranging from nervousness to convulsions, have occurred in 21 of 37 patients who were followed from 1 to 8 years after their disease. The neurologic complications appeared to be related more to the duration of the fever than the clinical severity of the illness.

Unfortunately, there are few specific laboratory tests that provide a quick disease confirmation. Most serologic tests for *Rickettsia* do not become seropositive until the second or third week. There is an immunofluorescent antibody stain that can demonstrate the organism in a skin punch biopsy specimen but that is not widely available and often not positive until the fourth to seventh day of the disease.

Needless to say, the rash, headache, and fever triad is common to many illnesses, such as mononucleosis, meningitis, and measles. It can also be confused with a drug eruption. Without the history of a tick bite, the diagnosis could be quite difficult.

## Treatment

The treatment of choice is one of the tetracyclines, including doxycycline, for a known or suspected case of Rocky Mountain spotted fever. An alternative drug is chloramphenicol. In younger children, of course, tetracyclines are not appropriate because of the dental deposition and subsequent staining. The patient should be treated during the acute phase and for 3 to 5 days after the fever has subsided.

Prophylactic use of tetracycline or chloramphenicol is not recommended after tick removal or extrication.[30] The rickettsiostatic effect of either drug may modify the normal immunologic responses and precipitate a modified form of the disease after the drugs have been stopped. After removal of a tick, the family or patient should be informed of the signs of Rocky Mountain spotted fever.

## LYME DISEASE

Lyme disease was first recognized in the United States in 1975 around the city of Old Lyme, Connecticut.[31] It is now the leading tick-borne disease in the United States and is caused by a spirochete *Borrelia burgdorferi*. Lyme disease is transmitted primarily by ixodid ticks, but biting flies have also been implicated.[32] In the north and northeastern United States, it is transmitted to man by *Ixodes damminii* and by *Ixodes pacifus* on the west coast. Ninty percent of the cases have occurred in eight states: Connecticut, Massachusetts, New Jersey, New York, Rhode Island, Minnesota, Wisconsin, and California.[33] The majority of cases occur during the nymphal stage of the tick's life cycle, during the early and midsummer months.[34]

## Clinical Presentation

Lyme disease appears to be a three-stage disease based upon the clinical presentation. The first stage is that of cutaneous manifestations, stage two has either cardiac or neurologic manifestations, and stage three has arthralgias or neurologic manifestations.

**Stage I.** The earliest manifestation of Lyme disease is a pathognomonic skin lesion, erythema chronicum migrans.[35] The skin lesion begins as an erythematous macule or papule with gradual enlargement. When fully developed, the lesion has an erythematous border that surrounds a partially cleared central region. Skin lesions begin about 2 days to 2 weeks after the innoculation and usually last for 3 weeks. Unfortunately, only about 60 to 70% of victims exhibit the typical lesion. Variations on the theme are also common and may include target lesions and confluent lesions. The lesions may be confused with infected tick bites, summer exzemetoid rashes, or contact dermatitis from plants or pesticides. Early infection is often associated with malaise, flu-like symptoms, chills, fever, headache, myalgias, and arthralgias. Diagnosis is difficult during this stage of the disease and requires the examining physician to be constantly suspicious.

**Stage II.** The second stage of the disease is characterized by the development of acute neurologic or cardiac disease. The cardiac disease is seen in about 5 to 10% of infected patients and may include various heart blocks, myocardial dysfunction, and myocarditis. Neurologic dysfunctions seen include meningitis, encephalitis, or neuropathies. The acute neurologic findings are seen in about 15 to 20% of infected patients. The second stage is most often seen about 4 to 6 weeks after the initial infection.

**Stage III.** The third stage of Lyme disease was originally noted to be an oligoar-

thralgia, but recent work has also shown that late neurologic sequelae are also quite common in the untreated patient. The most common neurologic symptom is a long-term lassitude and fatigue. This fatigue is often associated with short-term memory lapses. Less frequently found are chronic peripheral neuropathies, chronic meningitis, or a multiple sclerosis-like syndrome.[36]

The most frequent late manifestation of Lyme disease is arthritis characterized by a sudden onset of monoarticular or polyarticular joint pain and swelling. The large joints are most commonly affected, and the knees are the most frequent target. The arthritis is brief in duration, resolving in about a week, and recurrent. Recurrence duration, severity, and intervals are quite variable both from case to case and recurrence to recurrence. About 60% of the infected patients who are untreated will subsequently develop arthritis; however, treatment decreases the incidence of arthritis. About 10% of the patients

---

*Diagnostic Criteria for Lyme Disease*

Definite Case
  Tick bite with engorgement
  Auxiliary clinical illness
  Erythema chronicum migrans diagnosed
    by a physician
  Positive serology
  Involvement of at least two of the three
    target organ systems
OR
  Isolation of *B. burgdorferi* from a clinical
    specimen
Probable Case
  Tick bite with engorgement
  Auxiliary clinical illness
  Erythema chronicum migrans diagnosed
    by a physician
  No serology
  Involvement of at least two of the three
    target organ systems
OR
  Tick bite with engorgement
  Auxiliary clinical illness
  Erythema chronicum migrans not present
  A positive serology
  Involvement of at least two of the three
    target organ systems
Possible case
  Any combination of the above criteria
    that cannot be ruled out as a negative
    case.

with acute arthritis will have long-term arthritic problems.

## Treatment

The treatment of Lyme disease remains controversial. Current recommendations for the treatment of early Lyme disease is doxycycline 100 mg twice per day or tetracycline 25 to 50 mg per kg per day in 4 divided doses for 10 days.[37] Alternatively, amoxacillin 500 mg 3 times per day plus probenecid 500 mg 3 times per day for 21 days may be used in the adult patient. Children may receive proportionately smaller doses. For patients allergic to tetracyclines or penicillins, erythromycin can be used in a dosage of 250 mg 4 times per day or 30 mg per kg per day for children. This appears to be less effective than the tetracyclines or penicillin and derivatives.[38] Treatment with amoxacillin or doxycycline early in the illness shortens the duration of the skin lesions and may attenuate or prevent subsequent sequelae.

Patients with relatively mild neurologic or cardiac disease may be treated with oral agents as discussed above. For late Lyme disease, intravenous penicillin is currently recommended in high doses (20 to 24 million units per day) intravenously for 10 days. As many as 50% of cases have been refractory to this agent. Ceftriaxone 2 to 4 grams, intravenously, daily for 2 weeks has been found effective in cases refractory to other agents.[39] Recalcitrant arthritis may resolve after retreatment with either the same or one of the alternative antibiotic regimens. Pacemaker insertion may be needed in severe cardiac disease.

All stages of Lyme disease may respond to one or more of the recommended antibiotic therapies. Unfortunately, few controlled trials exist that compare the various antibiotic therapies. The best therapy for late disease is still controversial, but both intravenous penicillin and intravenous ceftriaxone are promising.

## TULAREMIA

### Epidemiology

Tularemia has changed in presentation over the past few years. Humans are usually infected by handling, skinning, and cleaning infected wildlife. It used to be a disease of hunters, trappers, furriers, and farmers. With a decrease in rabbit hunting, the epidemiology of the disease has changed to a tick-borne disease. The causative organism, *Francisella tularensis* is a Gram-negative pleomorphic bacillus that can be carried easily by most hard ticks. It is also transmitted by deerfly bites.

### Clinical Presentation

Like the causative coccobacillus, the manifestations of the disease are pleomorphic with at least six different forms of the disease. The clinical forms of the disease are determined by the portal of entry of the coccobacillus.

Ulceroglandular
Glandular
Oropharangeal
Oculoglandular
Pneumonic
Septicemic (also called typhoidal)

Accompanying all of these forms of tularemia are the protean symptoms of headache, fevers, chills, myalgias, arthralgias, and malaise. Diarrhea, nausea, and vomiting often round out the flu-like syndrome's symptoms.

The most common forms are the ulceroglandular and the glandular forms. This accounts for 85% of the reported human cases in the United States. A localized lesion develops at the site of an insect bite, scratch, or cut with a contaminated knife. An ulcerating necrotic lesion develops about this local lesion. The lesions are found primarily on the extremities, and a suppurating lymphadenitis may follow. The glandular form has the lymphadenitis, without a primary lesion.

The oculoglandular form develops when the patient rubs an infected hand into the eyes. The primary lesion is located in the lower lid. This lesion may ulcerate and have regional lymph node involvement.

The most serious forms are the septic and the pneumonic. If not treated promptly, the course of these clinical forms may be short and lethal.

The typhoidal or septic form is thought to develop when the patient eats contaminated food or drinks contaminated water. The septic patient with tularemia has no special features to distinguish the sepsis from other causes of sepsis. They may have any of the manifold symptoms, such as diarrhea, abdominal pain, or fever. Ulcerative lesions about the mouth, pharynx, and intestines may also appear. These ulcerative lesions are often accompanied by swelling of the cervical lymph nodes.

The pneumonic form of tularemia is likewise nonspecific with congestion, shortness of breath, dyspnea upon exertion, fever, and cough that may or may not be productive. The pneumonic lesions frequently cavitate.

In this disease, as in so many, there is no good early diagnostic procedure. Lymph node aspirates can grow the typical bacillus and may be discovered in the routine culture of a fluctuant lymph node aspirate. Gram stains of the aspirate frequently will show the tularemia bacillus. A tularemia titer is helpful only after the patient has been sick for a week. A rising titer will confirm the diagnosis.

If the practitioner suspects tularemia, then ensure that the laboratory is notified of the suspicions. Tularemia can be inhaled off of the culture plates causing a laboratory worker to develop the pneumonic form of the disease from the cultures. Particularly if there is a history of a tick bite and fever, the laboratory workers need to be advised to exercise appropriate precautions.

The differential diagnosis should include cat scratch fever, bubonic plague, tuberculosis, psittacosis, *Legionella*, Q fever, histoplasmosis, mycoplasma, and blastomycosis, depending upon the manifestation of the disease.

## Treatment

The therapy for tularemia is streptomycin in doses of 30 to 40 mg per kg per day in 2 divided doses, usually given intravenously. The patient should be monitored carefully for ototoxicity. If a patient complains of tinnitus (either a ringing or roaring sound), the dose of streptomycin should be cut in half. An alternative to streptomycin is gentamicin given intravenously for 7 to 10 days. Again, the dosage and side effects must be monitored carefully.

## COLORADO TICK FEVER

### Epidemiology

Colorado tick fever is usually seen in the Rocky Mountain area and westward, including the mountainous areas in California. It is a viral disease with a double-stranded RNA virus and is transmitted by the common wood tick (*Dermacentor andersoni*).

### Clinical Presentation

Tick fever is a nonspecific flu-like disease. Common manifestations are fever, headache, photophobia, myalgias, diarrhea, and occasionally vomiting and abdominal pains. The fever ranges from 39 to 40°C (102 to 104°F) and is often described as "saddle backed." In 50% of the patients, the fever abates for 2 to 3 days, and then the symptoms recur and may even be more severe than the first attack. The disease lasts about 5 to 7 days and may have a period of 3 to 4 weeks where the patient is not completely well.

The diagnosis is often suggested by leukocytopenia (WBCs are frequently less than 2000). Platelets are likewise depressed in most cases. Unfortunately, many of the enteroviruses can produce similar clinical pictures and have the same hematologic findings. Direct fluorescent antibody tests can provide the final clue for this possibly difficult diagnosis. Needless to say, the differential diagnosis of this disease includes a plethora of viral diseases.

### Treatment

As with most viruses, there is no effective cure for Colorado tick fever. Treatment should be symptomatic and supportive.

## Q FEVER

A rare form of tick-borne disease is Q fever, caused by another rickettsia (*Coxiella burnetii*). It is found in the western and midwestern states and is usually associated with animal deliveries but can be carried by the wood tick (*D. andersoni*).

### Clinical Presentation

The typical symptoms include fever, chills, malaise, headache, myalgias, and occasionally arthralgias.

The diagnosis is made with agglutination and antibody testing. Unfortunately, there are no specific symptoms of Q fever and the disease resembles a plethora of other infectious diseases. The exposure to animals or tick bites is an important part of the history.

## Treatment

The treatment for Q fever is tetracyclines or chloramphenicol. Q fever, like Rocky Mountain spotted fever, should be treated until the patient is afebrile for about a week.

## Treatment of Tick Bites

Tick bites are painless and usually have little local reaction. Treatment is directed towards removal of the tick and prevention of tick infestation. Individuals who have had a tick removed should be counseled about the infectious complications associated with this arthropod.

### LOCAL

A variety of various plans, substances, strategems, and tools have been devised to aid in removing a tick. With millions of years of evolution in learning how to stay attached to moving animals, it is not surprising that the tick frequently remains attached despite our wishes. As long as the mouth parts are attached to the patient, the patient remains at risk for tick paralysis and tick fever.

There is no completely effective method for removal of ticks. One author evaluated five popular methods of removing ticks and felt that the tick would best be removed by grasping the tick close to the skin and exerting a steady even pressure.[40] Grasping the body of the tick with fingers, forceps or tongs, and then pulling it off may leave the mouth parts behind. Likewise, twisting or jerking the tick may cause the mouth parts to break off. When the tick is grasped, the squeeze may inject additional saliva and more microorganisms through the mouth parts. Crushing or puncturing the body of the tick may release additional infective agents with the tick's body fluids. One author freezes the tick with ethyl chloride and then removes it with forceps to decrease the risk of injection.[41]

Common folk remedies include application of heat or organic solvents to the tick's body. Application of a heated match, cigarette, or cautery to the tick body will occasionally cause the tick to back out of the skin but is more likely to cause burns to the victim. A very likely outcome is the death of the tick—prior to disengagement. Application of an organic solvent—such as chloroform, ether, gasoline, or fingernail polish—may also cause the tick to disengage itself but is more likely to result in the death of the tick. Needless to say, do not use a cautery or flame after application of such substances.

Finally, dead ticks (most often seen after one of the above methods has been tried and failed) should be removed by surgical excision of a small portion of the skin in order not to leave any mouth parts remaining.

While removing the tick, gloves should be worn because any minor abrasions may permit infection of the operator. Fingers should not be used to handle the tick or squeeze the tick, since tick feces and body fluids can also be contaminated. These precautions are particularly important for those who are "deticking" animals with multiple ticks.

### PREVENTION

Tick bites can be prevented by the use of effective tick repellents, such as butopyronoxyl, dimethyl phthalate, DEET, or benzyl benzoate. Exposed skin, shirt and trouser cuffs, collars, and the belt line should also be treated with the repellents.

People in high-risk areas should be cautioned to wear long-sleeved shirts buttoned at the neck and sleeves and trousers tucked into boots or high shoes. The skin should be inspected frequently and all ticks removed promptly. The examination should include a thorough search of the scalp, axillae, and perineal areas, particularly in children.

Pets should be promptly "deticked," to decrease the tick population near residences. Brush and grass should also be trimmed to decrease the tick populations. Locally infested areas can be sprayed with malathion to rid the premises of ticks.

## CENTIPEDES

The centipede is an elongated flat arthropod with a pair of legs for each of 15 or more body segments. The first segment has a pair of curved, hollow fangs with venom glands in the base. The last segment has a pair of long tail appendages. The tail appendages have no venom apparatus.

Species of centipedes of various sizes and

colors are found throughout the world. The largest of these species reach lengths of up to 30 cm. Fortunately, the majority of these colorful arachnids are small and harmless. Usually, they are found under boards, in cracks and crevices, and in other moist locations where they hide during the day and venture forth during the night to seek the smaller insects for food. The larger species occasionally eat small vertebrates.

The large poisonous desert centipede attains a length of 6 to 8 inches and has jaws of sufficient strength to pierce human skin and inflict a very painful bite. Glands at the base of this arachnid's jaw produce a poison that causes swelling and tenderness at the site of the bite. Most bites are on the hands and occur when a centipede is picked up.

The poison is primarily used to kill prey and not for defense and has not been studied in great detail. In experimental animals, the venom can cause local necrosis and respiratory paralysis, but in humans, symptoms appear to be limited to local pain, lymphangitis, lymphadenopathy, and, rarely, local necrosis. Secondary infection is common and local swelling and tenderness may persist for 10 to 14 days.

Because the bite of even a large centipede is usually a painful inconvenience rather than a serious injury, no specific treatment has been developed. The wounds should be cleansed and wound infection treated appropriately. The use of ammonia as a wash is reported to bring relief from the pain. Infiltration of the bitten area with lidocaine or other local anesthetic will certainly relieve the local pain. A local antiseptic applied to the bite site is also appropriate.

## MITES AND CHIGGERS

Mites are a small but important family within the class Arachnida. The family includes the grain mite, causing farmer's itch, the rat mite, the fowl mite, and the harvest mite (also called the chigger). Many of these mites use humans as a feeding source and reproductive habitat. Like some other arthropods, mites need a meal of blood in order to progress from one stage of development to another, so mammals (including humans) are integral to the life cycle of the mite.

The mites and chiggers produce a pruritic lesion that may be papular or vesicular. The lesion may have a small central ulcerated area surrounded by a typical flare reaction. Ankles, feet, belt line, collars, and intertrigonous areas are most frequently infested.

The general treatment is to eradicate the animal first by vigorous bathing with soap and water, then by application of 1% gamma-benzene hexachloride. Antihistamines may relieve the itching.

### Chiggers

The chigger burrows into a human's skin during its larval stage only. The nymph and the adult obtain food from insect eggs, vegetable matter, and other arthropods. They are found almost anywhere there is vegetation.

The chigger's bright red body is only about 0.4 mm in length and 0.25 mm in width. This tiny, nearly microscopic, mite of the *Trombicula* species may be devastating in the dermatitis that it causes (see Fig. 7.8).

The chigger larva crawls up vegetation, waits for a mammal to go by, then drops onto the mammal. It then searches for a soft spot and pierces the skin, releasing a saliva that digests epidermal cells. Chiggers do not burrow, instead they use the liquified epidermal cells as food, forming a tube behind the chigger as it feeds. After feeding for 3 or 4 days, the chigger falls off, leaving behind the tube full of secretions and irritants. The resultant inflammatory process may last for weeks.

During this sequence, there appears first

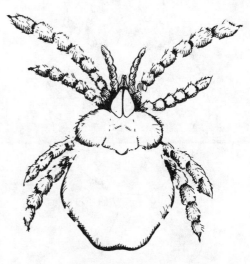

**Figure 7.8.** Chigger.

a bright red macule with the chigger at its center. Within 24 hours, the area becomes intensely pruritic and vesiculated. The lesions may resemble chickenpox and are usually found around the cuff and collar areas.

Treatment is symptomatic and directed toward minimizing the pruritis and preventing secondary infection. Various topical remedies, such as starch baths or calamine lotion, may decrease the reaction. Oral antihistamines may be useful if the patient has a large infestation. Children's fingernails should be trimmed closely to prevent excoriation and secondary infection.

The chigger mite is repelled by DEET and other insect repellents. Treatment of both clothing and skin is recommended.

## Scabies

A particularly troublesome mite and perhaps the most common infestation of the human body is the *Sarcoptes scabiei* or scabies mite. The scabies mite, an arachnid like the spider, appears to have about a 30-year cycle of eruptions but has been also called the "seven year itch" (see Fig. 7.9).

Most people associate scabies with poor hygiene, but they can also infest the well washed. Personal body contact or sharing a bed promotes transmission. Veterinarians and animal handlers may also contract scabies by handling animals with mange, which is also

caused by the scabies mite. Routine care of infested patients will put medical personnel at risk of infestation.

The nearly microscopic female burrows into the epidermis and deposits eggs over a period of 30 to 60 days. After hatching, the larvae mature to the adult stage within 2 weeks and continue the cycle.

Scabies burrows are threadlike with a small papule or vesicle at the far end. The adult female mite resides in this papule at the distal end of the burrow and may be scraped out with a scalpel or the edge of a needle. These skin scrapings show adult mites, larvae, and eggs, if treated with potassium hydroxide solution.

Unfortunately, the burrows are often obliterated by the excoriations from the pruritis. If no burrows are evident, then a dye may highlight the burrow. Apply any fountain pen ink to the skin, wipe away the ink with an alcohol swab, and look for small dark threadlike burrows. Occasionally, a skin biopsy may be needed for the diagnosis.

Lesions are most frequently seen in the web spaces of hands and feet, on the genitalia, and about the axillae and wrists. In adult females, the nipples are frequently involved. In small children, facial and head involvement is not uncommon, but this is rare in adults. Secondary infection due to excoriations is common.

Treatment is application of a 1% gamma-benzene hexachloride cream over the entire skin surface from the neck downward. The lotion should be left in place for 8 to 12 hours. Babies should be given a single application for only 6 to 8 hours. The agent enters the burrow and remains there for several days after the application. Two applications 24 hours apart should complete the treatment.

This will kill the adults but may not kill the eggs, so retreatment may be needed in about 1 week to complete the eradication of the pest, if symptoms persist. Even after effective treatment, a patient may continue to itch due to the secretions and feces remaining in the burrows.

Gamma-benzene hexachloride (lindane) may be neurotoxic if absorbed in sufficient quantities. Some authorities prefer crotamiton (Eurax), especially for infants and pregnant women, but that agent requires two applications.

The most common cause for recurrence is

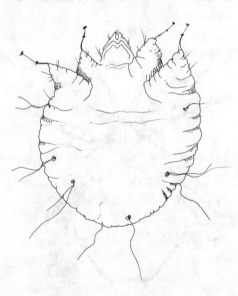

**Figure 7.9.** Scabies mite.

an untreated infested contact or sleeping partner. Close family members and intimate contacts should be treated, even if they are not symptomatic. Patients should be instructed to wash all bedding and recently worn clothing in hot water. Rarely, furniture and carpets may need to be cleansed, if recurrent infestations continue despite adequate treatment.

## INSECTS

Insects may deliver venom, act as vectors for disease, feed on human's blood, or merely be a nuisance.

Venom delivery of insects may be by stings or bites or by surface poisons. Few deaths or systemic illnesses are due to the direct effects of the microscopic amounts of venom delivered by most insects. The most common effect of venom delivery by insects is local irritation at the site of the sting or bite.

Blood-sucking insects feed in one of two ways: by slashing the surface with bladelike mouthparts or by a needlelike proboscis like the mosquito. It has been further noted that mosquitoes usually cause a local hemorrhage, while the bedbugs and cone-nose bugs commonly abrade a capillary and feed directly from the capillary.

## Hymenoptera

Everyone is familiar with ants, wasps, hornets, and bumblebees. There are few persons, indeed, that have not had at least one unpleasant experience with one or more of these insects.

The order Hymenoptera of the insects has four superfamilies: the *Apoidea* (bees), *Bombidae* (bumblebees), *Vespoidea* (wasps and hornets), and *Formicidae* (ants). In addition, there are two smaller families, the *Sphecidae* or thread-waisted wasps and *Mutillidae* or velvet ants, that are less well known.

### BEES

Of the superfamily *Apoidea*, the honeybee is of domestic concern to humans. The honeybee is not a native to the United states, having been imported from Europe. They are further separated into a gold "Italian" and a black and gray "Caucasian" race making up the

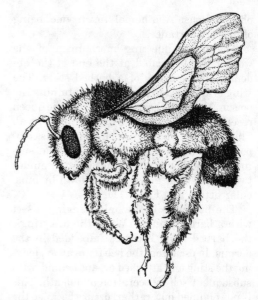

**Figure 7.10.** Honeybee (*Apoidea*).

majority of bees in the United States (see Fig. 7.10).

Bees kill more people each year in the United States than all other venomous animals combined (between 50 and 100 per year). Death from bee stings, however, is not generally from the envenomation but from an anaphylactic reaction. Since the bee leaves its stinger in place and other insects do not, bee stings can be readily identified. With this in mind, the yellow jacket has still been identified as the most common cause for allergic reactions.

Bees tend to sting when provoked and, like most stinging animals, usually do so in defense. The venom is not designed to kill but to discourage those who get too close from getting any closer.

Honeybee venom possesses several components, including histamine, dopamine, and norepinephrine. Hymenoptera venom also contains proteins and polypeptides, including mellitin, which is responsible for much of the local toxic effects. Mellitin alters cell wall permeability, resulting in the secondary release of vasoactive substances when the cell wall is destroyed. Bee venom also includes a mast cell degranulating peptide that has a potent effect on mast cells, again causing the release of histamine and other vasoactive substances. Another peptide, apamine, appears to be a minor neurotoxin. In bee venom, 58 enzymes have also been isolated with phospholipase A, a hemolytic enzyme, being of most importance.

The poison-injecting mechanism of the worker bee is located at the end of the abdomen and consists of a barbed sting. The sting is attached to a reservoir containing the poison. Male bees have no sting, and the queen reserves hers for possible use against a rival. The stinger is about $1/10$ inch long and is composed of a director and two lancets that surround a hollow stylus. The director guides two lancets that move up and down by muscular action (see Fig. 7.11).

The honeybee is the only stinging insect with a barbed stinger. When the bee stings, the barbed sting becomes imbedded in the dermis. In escaping, the bee tears away, leaving the sting and attached organs behind, with subsequent self-evisceration and death. This is not planned but, rather, occurs because the bee's thorax is less tough than the human's dermis. The bumblebee does not have this problem and, fortunately, does not often sting humans.

The muscles of the poison reservoir continue to spasm for as long as 20 minutes after the bee tears loose.[42] This means that the bee continues to sting even after leaving the scene of the crime.

Honeybees are social insects with a very highly developed colony structure consisting of thousands of sterile female worker bees, a few male drones, and a single queen. The workers care for the queen and young, gather food, and construct the nest. Hives may be found in trees, abandoned buildings, or crevices but, most frequently, are built on foundations constructed by men as part of an apiary (beekeeping).

The honeybee may be responsible for multiple stings, particularly when the hive is being defended. As the honeybee stings, it releases an alarm pheromone, a substance that alerts other bees, which then also sting and release more pheromone. The victim is marked with this odor and a chain reaction of more stings and more pheromone release then ensues.

Although systemic reactions are not likely unless there are more than 100 coincident stings, death becomes probable if there are more than 500 simultaneous stings. Death has occurred in small children or those who are stung myriad times but, generally, the bee's venom is a nuisance defense only. No one who has been stung will contest the effectiveness of this defense.

Symptoms of systemic toxicity include vomiting, diarrhea, faintness, and unconsciousness. These symptoms are often accompanied by edema (without urticaria), headache, fever, drowsiness or lethargy, involuntary muscle spasms, and occasionally convulsions.[43]

## Treatment

Treatment of stings of all of the bee and wasp species are essentially the same. The first thing that should be done for a bee sting victim is to scrape out the sting. This may be done with a knife blade or even with the fingernail. The sting should not be pulled out with fingers or forceps. By grasping the protruding poison reservoir with fingers or forceps, the reservoir is squeezed with injection of more poison.

Systemic reactions should be managed as discussed in the section on allergies and systemic reactions.

Antihistamines will decrease both the duration and the magnitude of the local reaction. Steroid creams may decrease the amount of swelling and may decrease the duration of the reaction. It should be noted that no topical agents have been found that are effective in treatment of test "stings" for other hymenoptera species, and there is no logical reason to believe that the bee is any different.[44]

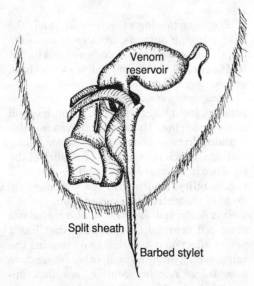

**Figure 7.11.** Picture of a stinger.

## BRAZILIAN (AFRICAN) HONEY BEES

Queens of Apies from Africa were taken to Brazil in 1956 with the objective of developing a race of bees better adapted to the Brazilian climate than the European bee. Both the desirable and undesirable features of the African bees were recognized at the time, and attempts were made to keep the queens and drones from escaping until a gentle cross-breeding could be effected. Unfortunately, the African bees swarmed and escaped in 1957.[45,46]

The outstanding features of swarms of Brazilian bees are their abundance and the viciousness with which they attack. Individual stings of Brazilian bees appear to produce effects comparable to stings from other strains of bees. The Brazilian bees appear to have a marked increase in their sensitivity to colony disturbances, their ability to communicate alarm within and between colonies, and their capacity to respond quickly with massive attack on intruders. There are reports of these bees attacking and killing animals and people.

## BUMBLEBEES (BOMBUS)

Bumblebees are 2 to 3 times the size of the honeybee but are not nearly so numerous or aggressive as the honeybee. The bumblebee is considered to be a relatively primitive social bee, whose colonies lack the order and highly evolved behavior of the honeybee. A bumblebee colony contains about 100 to 500 bees and consists of at least one queen, several males, and workers. Only the young and fertilized queens survive the winter to start a new nest each year, unlike the honeybee's survival throughout the winter. Nests are usually underground in areas that are undisturbed, such as fence rows. Bumblebees store pollen and honey just like honeybees.

## FIRE ANTS

This small reddish-brown to black ant lives in mounds with long radiating tunnels. Although it does not appear any more menacing than any of its less aggressive cousins, it does set itself apart by both virulence and behavior (see Fig. 7.12).

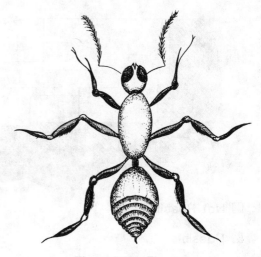

**Figure 7.12.** Fire ant.

## Distribution

Since the accidental and unwelcome arrival of the fire ant in the 1920s in Alabama, it has steadily widened its scope of infestation. At present, the fire ants have infested a small part of North Carolina, a larger part of South Carolina, most of Georgia, Alabama, Florida, Mississippi, and Louisiana. Some of Texas and Arkansas has been invaded, and the fire ant has the ability to move along the entire southern border of the United States (see Fig. 7.13).

To give some idea of the magnitude of this ant's domain, a survey in Mississippi, Georgia, and Alabama during 1971, reported over 12,000 stings. Of these, over 6,000 required treatment for secondary infection, 76 had anaphylactic reactions, 8 required skin grafting, and 5 required amputation of a limb. This survey was conducted 15 years ago, and the ant has continued to spread.

The reproductive capacity of these animals is truly phenomenal. In heavily infested areas, there may be as many as 100 nests per acre, each with 25,000 or more mature workers and several hundred winged males and females. The limiting factor to the ant's spread is climate. The ant apparently does not have the ability to survive much above the 10°F (−12.2°C) minimum isothermal line. The worry is, of course, that a genetic mutation will allow them to adapt to colder weather.

The nests are made in the ground and surrounded by a mound 18 inches to 3 feet in

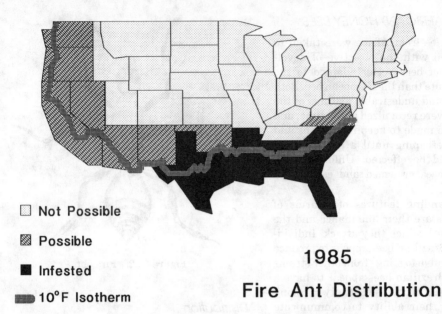

□ Not Possible

▨ Possible

■ Infested

▰ 10°F Isotherm

# 1985
# Fire Ant Distribution

**Figure 7.13.** Fire ant distribution (1985).

diameter but only an inch or 2 high. From the nest, five or six tunnels may radiate as long as 80 feet. These tunnels are only a quarter inch or so below the surface of the ground.

## Fire Ant Attacks

The usual time for fire ant envenomation is the warm summer months, when both the ant and victim are most active outdoors. The victim usually has shed some protective clothing or shoes. He or she steps on an ant colony and within half a minute, has hundreds of ants climbing on for the ride. Fire ants are unusual in two aspects. First, they do not run, they attack. Secondly, they not only bite, they sting. (Although other ants may be equipped with stingers, these ants have long enough stingers to pierce human skin.)

The attack of the fire ant occurs in two phases. First, the ant attaches itself to the skin with its sharp mandibles. This is typical behavior for all attacking ants and causes a small amount of pain. After the fire ant latches on, it thrusts the small (0.5 mm) stinger into the skin and injects a venom. It then pivots slightly and reinserts the stinger in another site. After a few minutes, there is a halo of stings around the site of attachment (see Fig. 7.14).

## Venom and Actions

Shortly after the venom has been injected, it causes a wheal and flare reaction, accompanied by intense burning pain and itching. The usual reaction lasts about an hour and the lesion ranges from only a 1 to 2 mm up to 10 cm or more, depending upon both the amount of venom injected and the severity of the reaction to the venom.

Over the next few hours, edema forms about the sting site. At about the same time, the area at the sting site itself becomes vesiculated with a clear small vesicle that slowly changes into a sterile pustule. In sensitive individuals, there may be marked edema formation and erythema about the sting. In most individuals, there is only a small amount of erythema about the area in the halo formation of stings about the bite site. The lesions are extremely pruritic for as long as a week after the injury.

## Treatment

Most people will do fine after the sting of a fire ant, although infants have been known to die after multiple stings. Treatment for the uncomplicated sting is minimal. Cold compresses or ice may decrease symptoms somewhat but are only palliative. Antibiotics, ste-

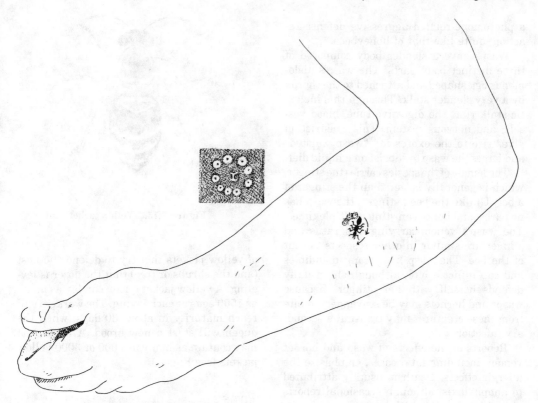

**Figure 7.14.** Halo of stings around site of attachment.

roids, and antihistamines have all been tried and found to be equally ineffective in both prevention of the pustule formation and relief of symptoms.

The real danger, as with bee stings, lies in the possibility of an allergic reaction. A sting reaction that extends for more than 10 cm or involves two or more joints is indicative of potential allergic reactions to the venom. Systemic allergic reactions have been fatal in a small number of patients. Systemic and locally exaggerated reactions should be treated as for any other allergic phenomenon.

Secondary infection of the pustules is the most common complication. The areas should be kept scrupulously clean and scratching discouraged. Children should have nails trimmed to the quick to decrease the excoriations from scratching.

Needless to say, the best treatment is prevention of the bites. This is not always easy as the mounds may be quite diffuse in sandy soils and difficult to avoid. Most residents are well aware of the dangers and visitors tend to suffer disproportionately.

## WASPS AND HORNETS

There are three species of social wasps that humans frequently encounter: the yellow jacket (*Vespula pennsylvania*), the bald-faced hornet (*Vespula maculata*), and the paper wasp (*Polistes*). These social wasps are considered dangerous because of their very aggressive defense and behavior, their large numbers, and their nesting habits.

All of the social wasps are papermakers. They chew up fragments of wood and leaves that they mix with saliva to construct the nests. Nests are built in eaves and corners of houses and cabins, in cavities of trees, underground, or out in the open attached to a branch of a tree. Nests have several layers of six-sided cells similar to the bees' cells but made of paper rather than wax. Like the bees, the queen will lay an egg in each cell, but the wasps usually place an insect into the cell for the larvae to feed upon. An open nest is often spherical or shaped like an inverted mushroom. There is usually only one entrance to the hive. Disturbance of the hive will provoke a pheromone-related aggressive defense reaction, quite like that of honeybees.

Wasps have a slender body composed of three distinct body parts. The wasp's abdomen is egg shaped and attached to the thorax by a very slender stalk. Through this inelastic stalk runs the digestive tube, blood vessels, and nervous system. This constriction gives rise to the expression "wasp waisted" and forces the wasp to subsist on a liquid diet.

The female of the species carries the stinger, which is generally larger than the stinger of a bee. Unlike the bee's stinger, the wasp has no barbs, and hence can sting multiple times. The wasp's venom-carrying apparatus and stinger are similar in other respects to that of the bee. The wasp has strong mandibles and can inflict a bite, although she usually defends herself with her stinger. Because wasps and hornets may be scavengers, a bite from these creatures may transmit a secondary infection.

Reports of the effects of wasp and hornet venom, including fatal cases, emphasize the allergic effects. Death is usually attributed to anaphylaxis, although occasional reports of toxicity due to multiple stings are found. Hemolysis and acute tubular necrosis have also been described. Greater than 100 stings may also cause rhabdomyolysis and subsequent renal failure.[47] It is thought that the muscle damage is due to a direct effect of one of the constituents of the venom.

Positive skin tests to multiple wasp and hornet venoms are common in patients with stinging insect allergies. Studies have shown that the venom from several species of hornets and yellow jackets had similar gel diffusion analysis. Yellow jacket venom appeared in these studies to provoke a greater reaction than any of the other wasp species.[48]

### Yellow Jackets

Yellow jackets are aggressive stinging pests that are attracted to food, sweet drinks, and bright colors. The yellow jacket is about a centimeter or so in length (0.6 inches) and has bright yellow and black stripes. They are persistent, aggressive, and bold and are frequent uninvited guests to outdoor social gatherings. The nests are often in tree hollows, gopher holes, shrubs, or buildings. Construction workers and bulldozer operators are often stung by very aggressive, nasty swarms

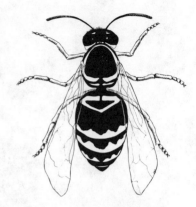

**Figure 7.15.** Yellow jacket.

of yellow jackets that try to defend the nest (and the shrubs or tree) that the dozer is leveling. A yellow jacket queen can lay as many as 1500 eggs at each laying. The workers will reach maturity in about 30 days, when the queen will start a new brood. A large nest may contain as many as 2000 or 3000 yellow jackets (see Fig. 7.15).

### Hornets

The distinctive football-shaped nest of the bald-faced hornet is often encountered high in the trees at the edge of eastern United States forests. Its smaller cousin, the European hornet, may nest on the sides of buildings, cabins, or barns or may be found in hollow trees. Normally, a relatively nonaggressive hunter, the hornet becomes irate if the nest is disturbed. Since there may be 2000 to 3000 hornets in a large nest, swarms of hornets may inflict many stings in short order (see Figs. 7.16 and 7.17).

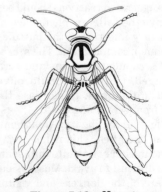

**Figure 7.16.** Hornet.

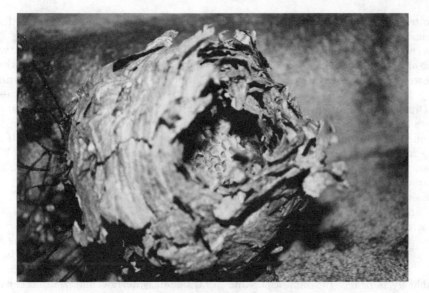

**Figure 7.17.** Wasp nest.

## Paper Wasps

*Polistes*, the paper wasp, is a long, slender, brownish-red wasp that frequents dwellings, such as cabins, outhouses, and attics. Polistes usually has a small colony of larvae that hibernate over the winter and emerge from the typical dwellings in summertime. The paper wasp is not as aggressive as the hornet or yellow jacket, and will usually sting only if provoked or if the nest is threatened. A paper wasp's nest may contain as many as 200 to 300 wasps (see Fig. 7.18).

## Diptera (Flies)

Flies and mosquitoes belong to the order of Diptera that is distinguished by having only one pair of wings. The second pair of wings has atrophied and become a pair of knobby in-flight stabilizers.

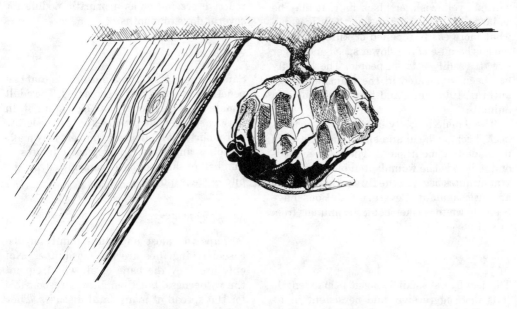

**Figure 7.18.** Paper wasp and nest (*Polistes*).

The bite of a fly is not a bite at all in the usual sense of chewing. The fly also does not have a venom or poison. The fly's proboscis stabs the skin and then she inserts saliva to break down tissues and make them easier to digest.

The Diptera will frequently feed on several hosts during the course of a few days. This frequent movement, coupled with swift and long-ranging flight, make them suspect or known vectors for disease transmission, both in animals and humans. It is this disease transmission that makes the diptera important to any discussion of environmental emergencies.

## STABLE FLY

The stable fly is nearly the same color and size as the common housefly. It can be distinguished only by its broader abdomen. This insect will feed on any warm-blooded animal but prefers the more docile animals, such as those found in a stable. If undisturbed, the fly may take as many as 3 to 4 minutes to complete a feeding. It has a bayonet-like proboscis that it thrusts into the skin to obtain food. The stable fly is suspect as a vector for disease but is otherwise only a nuisance.

## HORSEFLY

The horsefly is a large jet black fly with fine whitish, yellowish, or black hair. It may be as large as 2 to 2.5 cm in length. It is somewhat more easily repelled or killed than its cousins because of the slower speed and larger size. It readily attacks people. The horsefly has been implicated in the transmission of anthrax, tularemia, and trypanosomiasis in animals.

The female horsefly lands on the victim's neck, back, or head and slices the skin with its blade-like mouthparts. The fly then feeds on the blood. The wound often bleeds for several minutes because the fly's saliva contains an anticoagulant. Severe infestations have been known to weaken domestic animals from loss of blood.

## DEER FLY

The deer fly is a small fly about 1 cm in length. It is fast, aggressive, and persistent in its search for blood. Avoidance of this fly is difficult.

It has been implicated, together with the horsefly, in the transmission of anthrax, tularemia, and trypanosomiasis in animals.

There are over 80 different species in the United States. The male drinks plant juices, while the female seeks blood. The most common species, the Callidus deer fly (*Chrysops callidus*) has black on the thorax and V-shaped black marks on abdominal segments 2, 3, and 4.

## BLACK FLY

Biting adult black flies are the bane of many north country and mountain resorts, particularly early in the season. Some species can transmit waterfowl malaria that can account for nearly half of the deaths of natural waterfowl. North American black flies do not transmit human diseases, but in tropical areas some species may carry a roundworm disease that causes blindness.

This is one of the most difficult insects for humans to escape, primarily because of their enormous numbers. The female feeds exclusively on mammalian blood.

The saliva of the black fly may act as an anesthetic because the first thing that is noted may be a drop of blood at the site of the bite. Within an hour, intense pain, itching, and local swelling appear. The lesions last as a reactive eczema or as a pruritic nodule for several days to months.

## SAND FLY

Sand flies are tiny (1 to 3 mm) gnats that can penetrate most netting or screening. The adult female feeds exclusively on blood at night. In most cases, the bite produces only a moderate discomfort, but their sheer numbers may make camping an agony. In tropical climates, a number of diseases are transmitted by the bite of the sand fly.

## MOSQUITOES

Perhaps the most important family of disease-carrying flies are the mosquitoes. Not only are they the bane of all who frequent the wilderness, but their bite is responsible for the spread of many fatal diseases. They

**Table 7.1.**
**Major Mosquito-Borne Diseases**

| Disease | Vectors | Casual Organism |
|---|---|---|
| Malaria | *Anopheles* sp | Plasmodium |
| Dengue | *Aedes* sp | Arbovirus |
| Eastern equine encephalitis | *Culex* sp | Arbovirus |
| Filarisis | *Culex* sp | Wucheria bancrofti |
| St. Louis encephalitis | *Culex* sp | Arbovirus |
| Western equine encephalitis | *Culex* sp | Arbovirus |
| Yellow fever | *Aedes aegypti* | Arbovirus |

attack all warm- and some cold-blooded animals.

Unfortunately, little was known of the relationships of disease and insects prior to the invention of the microscope. The late 1800s brought the discoveries of the vectors of malaria, yellow fever, nagana (African sleeping sickness), and filariasis (see Table 7.1). Mosquitoes are two-winged flies (*Diptera*) that belong to the suborder *Nematocera* and the family *Culicidae*. Included in the mosquitoes are three subfamilies: *Anophelinae*, *Culicinae*, and *Toxorhynchitinae*. *Anopheline* mosquitoes include all the known vectors of human and simian malaria as well as the major vectors of filariasis. *Culicidae* mosquitoes include the vectors of yellow fever, rift valley fever, filariasis, St. Louis encephalitis, Murry Valley encephalitis, western equine encephalitis, and Japanese B encephalitis. Both sexes of *Toxorhynchinaous* mosquitoes are nectar feeding and hence not medically important (see Fig. 7.19).

The study of the life cycle of mosquitoes has been of great importance and has led to control of the diseases spread by them in some locations. The eggs are usually laid in water. They may be laid singly or floating together on rafts. Some species of mosquito will lay their eggs in dry areas that will be flooded at the first rain. When the eggs of these species are moistened, they will hatch. They may remain viable for years before moisture triggers hatching.

All mosquito larvae develop in water. Most feed on algae, but some species are predators, primarily on other larvae. Larvae, also known as wigglers, may be found anywhere there is standing water. This includes, but is not limited to, fresh and salt marshes, saline tide pools, empty containers, stumps, ponds, puddles, and plant boles. The wiggler has gills and breathes through a siphon at the end of the abdomen. The gills are not sufficient to sustain life. Larvae change to pupae in about 3 to 7. This varies with the species and the amount of available food.

Tumblers, as the pupae are sometimes called, are found in the same areas as the larvae. The pupae have a larger head than the larvae. A pair of siphons, also called trumpets, are found on the dorsal thorax of the pupae. These trumpets serve the same purpose as the siphons of the larvae. After about 3 days, the adult emerges from the pupae, again depending upon the species.

In the mosquito family, the female is the only bloodthirsty member. The male feeds strictly on nectar and fruit and plant juices. Females feed on both blood and nectar. The blood meal is needed for complete development of the eggs. In order to best obtain this blood meal, the female mosquito is attracted to the lactic acid that all warm blooded animals secrete through their skins (see Fig. 7.20).

The annoyance of mosquito bites is well known by all who go beyond the trailhead, and most urban dwellers. Many areas are

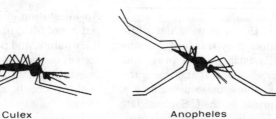

Culex                 Anopheles

**Figure 7.19.** Culex and Anopheles.

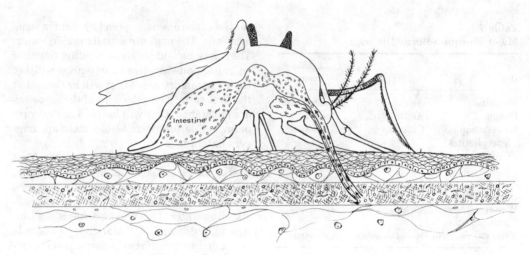

**Figure 7.20.** Potential inoculation of disease.

justly famous for their large swarms during the summer months, particularly about water recreation sites. Indeed, local residents may be known to fancifully brag that "it takes only x number of mosquitoes to carry off a small child." The reality of the mosquitoes may make it difficult for campers, backpackers, and others outdoors enthusiasts to fully enjoy themselves.

---

*Treatment of Mosquito Bites*

Topical antipruritics containing menthol or camphor

Topical steroids (not particularly effective)

Systemic antipruritics
 Diphenhydramine (5 mg per kg per day in 4 divided doses up to 300 mg per day)
 Chlorpheniramine (5 mg q.i.d. or 10 mg sustained release capsules b.i.d. for adults)
 Hydroxyzine (2 mg per kg per day in 4 divided doses)

Topical or systemic antibiotics for infection secondary to excoriations.

---

If annoyance of the bites were not sufficient, the mosquitoes may transmit encephalitis, malaria, filariasis, yellow fever, and dengue. With increased travel and immigration to the areas where these diseases are found, it is appropriate for the U.S. physician to have a basic familiarity with their prevention, recognition, and treatment. Since these diseases are well documented elsewhere, this cursory review serves only to whet the reader's appetite and to document current prophylaxis and treatment.

## *Siphonaptera*

### *FLEAS*

Flea bites are found in zigzag lines about the legs and waist. The lesions are hemorrhagic points surrounded by an erythematous patch and a flare reaction. Pruritis is intense after the flea's bite. The patterns are often obliterated by excoriations due to the pruritis. Secondary infection due to the self-induced damage is quite common.

Treatment consists of antihistamines to relieve itching. For very severe cases, topical steroids may be added to decrease inflammation. Secondary infections should be treated with both topical and systemic antibiotics.

### *LICE*

An infestation of lice carries with it connotations of filth, unwashed clothes, poor sanitary habits, and poverty. Unfortunately, lice are not respectors of race, sex, or social status. Infestations by the louse are rapid and thorough in schools, sports teams, and summer camps.

Lice come in three species: the head louse, the body louse, and the pubic louse. All of the species act similarly but have chosen different parts of the body to infest. Lice are so intensely inflammatory that the pruritis causes linear excoriations that should suggest the diagnosis.

## HEAD LICE

The white ova of head lice are often mistaken for dandruff and are the most prominent feature of an infestation. The egg or nit is 0.8 by 0.3 mm and is firmly attached to the hair with a cement-like substance. The nits hatch in 8 to 9 days, and the louse is mature at the end of 10 days. Eggs remain viable for as long as 30 days away from the human host, so infection of clothes is not unusual. Adult lice are difficult to find, except in severe infestations, but nits are easily found on the hair shafts. The favorite sites for deposition of nits appear to be around the ears and the occiput.

The adult male louse is about 1 to 1.5 mm long while the female is slightly larger at about 1.8 to 2 mm long. The louse has 6 claws that hook into the hair and provide enough motion so that the louse can pierce the skin, deposit saliva, and suck up lysed blood. Adult lice are usually grayish white with dark borders.

The adult female is fertile from maturity until senesence at age 30 days and lays four to six eggs every day. Her fertility varies with the abundance of food, and the host's temperature.

Head lice do not appear to transmit any diseases but secondary infection is not uncommon. Sensitization to the saliva and feces of lice is a frequent phenomenon, with subsequent scalp itching and excoriation of the scalp. Fever, cervical adenopathy, and malaise are common symptoms of the secondary infection. Rarely, streptococcal infections with nephritogenic strains can result in glomerulonephritis.

## PUBIC LICE

Pubic lice also cement their nits on the hair shafts. The nits are smaller than those of other lice and take about 15 days to develop into adulthood. Curiously, the adult pubic or "crab louse" is larger than the other types of lice. The crab louse deserves the name and looks quite like a small crab. The claws are heavy

and the louse stays in one spot for many days. The average life span of the pubic louse is about 35 days and the female lays about three eggs per day. The food for the louse is, of course, the host's blood.

Pubic lice are spread primarily by sexual intimacy, but infested clothing and bedding may also serve as sources of infection. Infants have been known to become infested during breastfeeding and may harbor the infestation about the head. In adults, the lower abdomen, thighs, and axillae may also be infested with this louse. Rarely, this louse takes up residence in the scalp in adults.

Pubic lice are not known to be the vectors for any disease. The presence of pubic lice should prompt a search for other venereally transmitted diseases, simply because of the association with sexual activity.

## BODY LICE

Body lice and their eggs are found in the seams of clothing, rather than about the hairy areas. Body lice tend to concentrate in feeding areas about the waist, shoulders, axillae, and neck. The body louse return to the skin four to six times per day and feed most commonly about the shoulders, belt line, and interscapular area.

Since the body louse is not found in skin, except for feeding, nits are not usually seen on the body. Usually, the nits and lice can be found about the inner seams of underclothing. In very heavy infestations, nits may be found on hair shafts.

Unlike the other forms of lice, the body louse has been found to be an important vector in the transmission of epidemic typhus, relapsing fever, and trench fever.[49]

The most common symptom of infestation with body lice is itching. The body louse leaves red maculopapular lesions in the feeding areas. Occasionally, these lesions may be urticarial, and they are always pruritic. Parallel linear scratch marks about the back are almost diagnostic of body lice infestation. Secondary infections are quite common and are due to the excoriations from the intense itching.

The body louse is transmitted by direct contact or by contact with infested clothing or bed linens. It is quite common in children's camps, among refugees, and on military campaigns due to the close contact and often crowded conditions.

## Treatment

Treatment for either head or pubic lice infestation consists of shampooing with gamma-benzene hexachloride shampoo, working it into a lather, and leaving it on the scalp for 4 minutes before washing it off. As always, gamma-benzene hexachloride must be used with caution in children and infants due to the possibility of systemic absorption and subsequent CNS toxicity. After shampooing, the hair should be combed with a fine-toothed comb to remove dead lice and nits. Alternatively, the hair can be shorn.

An alternative treatment is to apply gamma-benzene hexachloride cream or lotion for 8 to 12 hours before washing it off. The patient can use a second treatment in about 1 week. In young children and infants, care must be taken to limit the exposure and to ensure that no lotion is absorbed from mucous membranes.

For treatment of body lice infestation, the patient needs only a hot bath, care of secondary infections, and clean clothes. The louse is not normally found on the person but rather on the clothes. The clothing must be laundered in hot water, and the seams ironed to destroy residual nits. Be certain to include bed linens and all clothing that has been worn within 3 to 4 weeks in the disinfestation wash.

The treatment of lice infestation will not be complete until the source of the lice has been removed. Washing with hot water and soap will usually suffice for ridding clothes and bed linens of the infestation. Contaminated hats, coats, combs, and brushes should not be overlooked. Infested rugs and furniture should be washed with hot, soapy water, professionally steam cleaned, or dry cleaned.

## MISCELLANEOUS

### Kissing Bug

#### DESCRIPTION

The assassin bug, kissing bug, or western conenose bug (*Tiratoma protracta*) is a black or dark brown insect about 2.5 to 4 cm in length. It is a normal inhabitant of pacific western and southeastern states in brush and canyons. It enters houses, perhaps attracted by heat or light.

This bug is characterized by a long proboscis or beak that is used to pierce the skin of vertebrates and inject a saliva that lyses blood for food for the insect. When obtaining its meal, the kissing bug is often noted to stand beside rather than on the victim. The proboscis is extended to contact the skin and a hollow stylet is inserted. The meal is completed in 8 to 10 minutes, following which the proboscis is withdrawn. The bites are frequently multiple.

The bug is often found in bedrooms. Many bites are on the lips, suggesting the name "kissing bug." Since the bite is relatively painless, the victim is rarely aware of the attack.

The saliva acts as a foreign protein and can cause allergic reactions in humans, ranging from local pruritis and urticaria to nausea and chills. Rarely, it may cause anaphylaxis.

#### TREATMENT

Systemic reactions should be treated appropriately. Local reactions may be treated by relieving the pruritis with antihistamines or steroids. Secondary infections should be anticipated and treated appropriately.

Those individuals who become highly sensitized to the bite of the conenose should consider immunotherapy. There are enough recorded successful results with immunotherapy for this to be considered a fruitful enterprise to prevent anaphylaxis.

#### PREVENTION

Insecticide sprays such as lindane will eradicate the bug. Bed frames, springs, mattresses, baseboards, and carpets should be sprayed.

### Meloid Beetles (Blister Beetles)

Blister beetles are found frequently in the western United States. These beetles may exude large amounts of a blister agent (cantharidin) when disturbed. The vesicant penetrates the skin and causes bullae formation and irritation of the skin within a few hours of contact. Systemic reactions from skin absorption can include dysuria and hematuria.[50] The agent has been thought by some to be an aphrodisiac but, if ingested, will produce nausea, vomiting, diarrhea, and abdominal cramps, symptoms that tend not to be sensuous.

Treatment consists of protection of the bullae from infection. Large bullae may be drained and the open area covered with topical antibiotic ointments. If bullae occur on the feet, the patient should be considered to be a litter case and treated appropriately.

### Puss Caterpillars

Some species of caterpillars have a poison-delivery system within the hairs that cover their body. These hollow spines can contain poison that causes urticaria, allergic reactions, and systemic poisoning. The larval stage of the flannel moth, *Megalopyge opercularis*, is the best known and identified but is by no means the only such caterpillar. This puss caterpillar has a wooly surface and often is thought to resemble a small cat, hence the name. The wooly coat appeals to small children who become intrigued with it and thus handle it (see Fig. 7.21).

The dominant feature of the puss caterpillar's venom is an intense and rhythmic pain that immediately follows handling of the larva. The area becomes swollen and pruritic quickly and then develops a fine rash where the caterpillar's hairs made contact. Frequently, the rash will develop into whitish or red papules or small vesicles. The systemic symptoms include restlessness, fever, or muscle cramps. Shock has been reported rarely.

Treatment is immediate removal of the spines and control of the muscle cramps and pain. The spines can be removed with cellophane tape or other sticky tape. Calcium gluconate will relieve the muscle cramps and pain if given intravenously as 10 cc of the 10% solution for adults. Appropriate cardiac monitoring of the patient is essential during injection.

### Local Reactions

Unless complicated by infection, the trauma resulting from the action of the mouth parts of any blood-sucking insect is seldom severe enough to cause a serious disturbance in the host. The reaction to the bites of blood-sucking insects is an allergic reaction to the salivary fluid injected in the process of feeding.

### Allergic and Systemic Reactions

Systemic allergic reactions from insect stings are a common medical problem that affects about 0.4% of the population and results in between 50 and 100 deaths per year in the United States. About 33 to 40% of individuals suffering a systemic reaction have a personal history of atopic disease and there is a 2:1 male to female ratio. Allergy to insect venoms is mediated by specific IgE antibodies

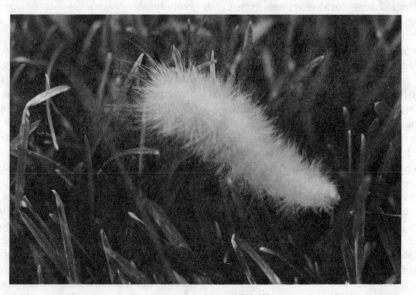

**Figure 7.21.** Puss caterpillar.

whereas immunity to insect stings is related to the presence of IgG antibodies.

## ANAPHYLAXIS

The most serious reaction after an insect envenomation is an immediate hypersensitivity reaction, also called acute anaphylaxis. The symptoms that occur are typical of anaphylaxis from any cause. Most reactions begin within 15 minutes after the sting, although there are anecdotal reports of reactions starting somewhat later. Generally, the sooner the reaction starts after the sting, the worse the reaction will be.

### Pathophysiology

The symptom complex of anaphylaxis is variable but may include generalized urticaria, flushing, angioedema, upper airway edema, bronchospasm, circulatory collapse, shock, and hypotension. Also seen can be gastrointestinal symptoms manifested by bowel spasms, diarrhea, and vomiting. The chief cause of death is upper airway obstruction involving the pharynx, larynx, and trachea, associated with copious secretions.[51] The next most common cause of death is a circulatory collapse with leaky vessels and hypovolemia—the anaphylactic shock syndrome.

Most patients have had no prior warning of their anaphylaxis. In several studies, only 18 to 25% of patients had a prior history of insect stings. Large, local reactions from insect stings have been noted in from 10 to 40% of patients who subsequently had a serious systemic allergic reactions. There seems to be little relationship between the time interval of this reaction and the subsequent life-threatening systemic reaction. Many patients note that the first remembered sting is the one that causes an anaphylaxis.

These reactions are also referred to as IgE-mediated hypersensitivity or atopic reactions. When two adjacent molecules of IgE are bridged by the right antigen, the release of histamine and similar substances, such as slow reactive substance of anaphylaxis (SRS-A) occurs and wreaks havoc on the organism. The pharmacologic action of histamine is to cause smooth muscle spasm, increased vascular permeability, and peripheral vasodilation.

The results of this histamine and SRS-A release at the level of the skin is urticaria or hives. If the vessel is more deeply seated, the result is angioedema. This release particularly affects the tongue, the lips, the scrotum, and all such areas with loose connective tissue.

Patients with a variety of allergies have been recently reported who have experienced refractory anaphylactic reactions while receiving beta blockers. The beta blockade has appeared to decrease the cardiovascular response to epinephrine with a relative bradycardia and hypotension. Physicians should be aware that beta blockers aggravate anaphylactic and anaphylactoid reactions, and alternative medications should be used in patients with histories of systemic insect sting reactions.[52]

### Treatment

Acute allergic reactions to insect stings are treated in the same manner as anaphylaxis from any other cause. The immediate drug of choice is epinephrine administered subcutaneously in doses from 0.2 to 0.5 cc in the 1:10,000 solution. Antihistamines, such as diphenhydramine 50 mg, may be given intravenously (preferred route) or intramuscularly. Bronchospasm, shock, or hypoxemia may mandate aminophyline, vasopressor sympathomimetics, or intubation with administration of 100% oxygen. In refractory cases, use of an epinepherine intravenous drip may be helpful.

**Airway.** Particularly careful attention should be paid to the upper airway since airway compromise has been identified as a common cause of death. If there is any doubt as to the airway status, the patient should be promptly intubated. The cardiac rhythm should also be monitored continuously.

**Prevention.** The best therapy for anaphylaxis is prevention of the insult. Those patients who have had a past history of systemic reactions following an insect sting should be considered at risk for subsequent reactions. These individuals should be cautious during all outdoor activities. Allergic patients should be wary of outdoor cooking and eating, since food and odors attract insects. These patients should wear shoes and long pants while walking during the summer. They should not use perfumes or hair sprays since these attract insects. The use of darker blues or browns in dress is preferable to the use of bright or pastel clothes. An identification bracelet or necklace will aid the emergency physician if the diagnosis is in doubt.

**Self-medication.** Specific medications for anaphylaxis should be issued to the known allergic patient and the family and friends taught to administer these medications. Kits containing these medications are readily available and should be prescribed to these patients at high risk. Whether nonmedical leaders of treks and expeditions should carry these kits is debatable and controversial. Wilderness-trained independent emergency medical technicians and paramedics should be trained to recognize the symptoms and be credentialed and equipped to take appropriate action.

**Immunotherapy.** Since immunotherapy is not an emergency procedure, discussion of this possible solution to the problem in a selected set of patients will be deferred to the allergist specialist who handles the therapy on a routine basis.

## References

1. Parrish HM. Deaths from bites and stings of venomous animals and insects in the United States. Arch Intern Med 1959;104:198–207.
2. Kobernick M. Black widow spider bite. Am Fam Phys 1984;29:241–245
3. Russell FE. Arthropod venoms. In Gluck L, Cone TE, Dodge RR, et al., eds: Current problems in pediatrics. Chicago: Yearbook Publishers, 1973.
4. Moss HS, Binder LS. A retrospective review of black widow spider envenomation. Ann Emerg Med 1987;16:188–191.
5. Hunt DW. The bites and stings of summer. Part 2. Spider bites. Emerg Med Serv Mag 1986;June:75–81.
6. Ryan PJ. Preliminary report: experience with the use of dantrolene sodium in the treatment of bites by the black widow spider *Lactrodectus hesperus*. J Toxicol Clin Toxicol 1984;21:487.
7. Schenone H, Rojas A, Reyes H, et al. Prevalence of *Loxosceles laeta* in houses in central Chile. Am J Trop Med Hyg 1970;19:564–567.
8. Schenone H, Prats F. Arachnidism by *Loxosceles laeta*. Arch Dermatol 1961;83:1193–1196.
9. Russell FE. A confusion of spiders [letter]. Emerg Med 1986;June 15:6–13.
10. Harves AD, Millikan LE. Current concepts of therapy and pathophysiology in arthropod bites and stings. Part I. Arthropods. Int Dermatol 1975;14:543–562.
11. Rees RS, Schack RB, Withers E, et al. Man-

agement of the brown recluse spider bite. Plast Reconstr Surg 1981;68:768–773.
12. Dillaha CJ, Jansen GT, Honeycutt WM, and Hayden CR. The gangrenous bite of the brown recluse spider in Arkansas. J Arkansas Med Soc 1960;60:91.
13. Burnett JW, Calton GJ, Morgan RJ. Brown recluse spider. Cutis 1985;36:197–198.
14. Barrett JT, Campbell BJ, Finke JH. Serodiagnostic test for *Loxosceles reclusa* bites. Clin Toxicol 1974;7:375–382.
15. Chu J, Rush CT, O'Connor DM. Hemolytic anemia following brown spider (*Loxosceles reclusa*) bite. Clin Toxicol 1978;12:531–534.
16. Eichner ER. Spider bite hemolytic anemia: positive Coombs' test, erythrophagocytosis and leukoerythroblastic smear. Am J Clin Pathol 1984;81:683–687.
17. Taylor EH, Denny WF. Hemolysis, renal failure, and death, presumed secondary to bite of brown recluse spider. South Med J 1966;59:1209–1211
18. Stochosky B. Necrotic arachnidism. West J Med 1979;131:143–148.
19. Rees RS, Altenbern DP, Lynch JB, King LE Jr. Brown recluse spider bites: a comparison of early surgical excision versus dapsone and delayed surgical excision. Ann Surg 1985;202:659–663.
20. Lang P Jr: Sulfones and sulfonamides in dermatology today. J Am Acad Dermatol 1972;1:479–492.
21. Stahnke HL. Arizona's lethal scorpion. Ariz Med 1972;29:490–493.
22. Rachesky IJ, Banner W Jr, Dansky J, Tong T. Treatments for *Centruroides exilicauda* envenomation. Am J Dis Child 1984;138:1136–1139.
23. Likes K, Banner W, Chavez M. *Centruroides exilicauda* envenomation in Arizona. West J Med 1984;141:634–637.
24. Gueron M, Yaron R. Cardiovascular manifestations of severe scorpion sting: clinicopathologic correlations. Chest 1970;57:156–162.
25. Glenn WG, Keegan HL, Whittemore FW Jr. Intergeneric relationships among various scorpion venoms and antivenins. Science 1962;135:434–435.
26. Amitai Y, Mines Y, Aker M, Goitein K. Scorpion sting in children. Clin Pediatr 1985;24:136–140.
27. Bartholomew C. Acute scorpion pancreatitis in Trinidad. Br Med J 1970;1:666–668.
28. Malhotra KK, Chadha JS, Mirdehghan M, and Tandon HD. Acute renal failure following scorpion sting. Am J Trop Med Hyg 1977;27:623–626.
29. Gueron M, Adolph RJ, Grupp IL, et al. Hemodynamic and myocardial consequences of scorpion venom. Am J Cardiol 1980;45:979–986.
30. Linnemann CC. Rapid recognition and specific

intervention in Rocky Mountain spotted fever. EM Reports 1987;8:105–112.

31. Steere AC, Malawista SE, Snydman DR, et al. Lyme arthritis: an epidemic of oligoarticular arthritis in children and adults in three Connecticut communities. Arthritis Rheum 1977;20:7–17.

32. Ryan CP. Selected arthropod-borne diseases: plague, Lyme disease, and babesiosis. Vet Clin North Am 1987;17:179–194.

33. Satalawich FT. Ticks in Missouri. Missouri Epidemiol 1989;11:3–4.

34. Steere AC, Pachner AR, Malawista WE. Cases of Lyme disease in the United States: locations correlated with distribution of *Ixodes dammini.* Ann Intern Med 1979;91:730–733.

35. Steere AC, Bartenhagen NH, Craft JE, et al. The early clinical manifestations of Lyme disease. Ann Intern Med 1983;99:76–82.

36. Halperin JJ, Colye PK, Little BV, et al. Lyme disease: a treatable cause of peripheral neuropathy. Neurology 1987;37:1700–1706.

37. Dattwyler RJ, Golightly M. Lyme disease. Emerg Decisions 1987;3:26–32.

38. Treatment of Lyme disease. Med Lett 1988;30:65–66.

39. Dattwyler RJ, Halperin JJ, Pass H, Luft BJ. Ceftriaxone as effective therapy in refractory Lyme disease. J Infect Dis 1987;155:1322–1325.

40. Needham GR. Evaluation of five popular methods for tick removal. Pediatrics 1985;75:997–1002.

41. Kumar RP. Tick trick [letter]. Consultant 1987;27:80.

42. Arena J. Poisonings. Springfield Il: Charles C Thomas, 1979.

43. Frazier, C. The hazards of hymenoptera. Am Fam Phys 1977;15;91–96.

44. McLeod LJ, von Witt RJ, Roberts MS. Consequences of wasp stings [letter]. Med J Aust 1986;144:220–221.

45. Kerr WE. The history of the introduction of African bees in Brazil. Apiculture West Aust 1967;2:53–55.

46. Kerr WE. The history of the introduction of African bees in Brazil. South African Bee J 1967;39:3–5.

47. Shilken KB, Chen BT, Khoo OT. Rhabdomyolysis caused by hornet venom. Br Med J 1972;1:156–157.

48. Reisman RE, Wicher K, Wypych J, Mueller M, et al. Comparison of the allergenicity and antigenicity of the yellow jacket and hornet venoms. J Allergy Clin Immunol 1980;58:200.

49. Parish LC, Witkowski, JA. Lice can happen to anyone. Consultant 1978;Sept:34–40.

50. Browne SG. Cantharidin poisoning due to a "blister beetle." Br Med J 1960:Oct 29;1290–1291.

51. Barnard JH. Studies of 400 hymenoptera sting deaths in the United States J Allergy Clin Imunol 1974;52:259–1264.

52. Awai LE, Mekori YA. Insect sting anaphylaxis and beta-adrenergic blockade: a relative contraindication. Ann Allergy 1984;53:48–49.

# Part 2
# Mammalian Bites

## INTRODUCTION

Animal bites, particularly those of dogs, cats, and humans are common problems. It is estimated that about 1 to 1 ½ million people are bitten by dogs each year in the United States.[1] In the locations where animal bites are a reportable condition, dogs account for 90%, cats about 5%, fellow humans and rodents for about 2 to 3% each, and all other animal species less than 1% of all bites.[2] It is estimated that animal and human bite wounds account for about 1 to 2% of all emergency department visits annually.

The vast number of animals that are capable of inflicting injury make it impossible to address every type of animal bite in a single chapter. This discussion has been limited to the more common of these injuries.

Although many bites appear to be minor at the time that they are inflicted, they frequently have devastating effects. The most common complication is infection, which may lead to systemic sepsis, joint injury, tendon injury, or even amputation of the limb. Many physicians do not appear to recognize this potential for disaster and do not obtain an adequate history or provide adequate treatment, particularly with human bites.

## BACTERIOLOGY

Whether it is from a dog, cat, fellow human, or other animal, when a tooth penetrates human skin, it carries with it high concentrations of bacteria. The mammalian mouth is a microbial incubator that supports over 200 species of bacteria.[3] Gingival material contains large numbers of anaerobic streptococci, spirochetes, and *Bacteroides* species in most mammals.[3] Other organisms commonly recovered from many mammals include

*Streptococcus viridens, Staphylococcus au-reus,* and *Pasteurella multocida.*

Infections that result from animal bites may have a wide variety of organisms responsible for the infections and mixed bacterial infections often predominate. Although any of the plethora of organisms that abound in the oral flora of the animal may cause the infection, some infections are species specific.

## ANATOMIC LOCATION

The anatomic location aids in determination of the risks involved in treatment of a mammalian bite. Generally, wounds that involve deep structures, such as bones, joints, tendons, vessels, nerves, or viscera, are at high risk of infection and other complications. Puncture wounds are generally considered high-risk wounds because they are so difficult to irrigate. Cat and human bites of the hand are at particular risk. Human bites in particular tend to be ignored until late, partly due to the influence of alcohol and partly due to social embarrassment.

In infants and small children, scalp and facial wounds are at risk of penetration through the thin membranous bones of the skull. In adults, these same areas are at low risk for infection because of the good vascular flow.

## SPECIFIC ANIMAL SPECIES
### Dog Bites

Dog bites are the most common of mammalian bites. One author estimates that there are more than 1000 patients per day who seek emergency care for dog bites and that there may be a much greater number who do not.[4] It is truly amazing that, despite this vast amount of clinical material on a daily basis, the only controlled studies have small numbers of patients and these studies are few in number.

Most authors feel that a disproportionate number of these bites are from German shepherds. Most dogs that bite are in a household rather than strays, and more than half of the victims are children.[5,6] It is estimated that dog bites account for about 80% of all animal bite injuries in the United States. In one study, about 5% of dog bites returned to the emergency department with a complication.[6]

Many dog bites are not simply a trivial contusion or laceration. Dog bites may be delivered with a force of 150 to 450 pounds per square inch, which is enough to create a crush injury, along with puncture and tear wounds.[7] Severe injury, including penetrating wounds of the skull, facial avulsions, and avulsions of lip or ear has been reported. Trauma with significant blood loss, rib fracture, airway compromise, pneumothorax, or even death may result from dog bites of the larger breeds. One percent of victims of dogbites will require hospitalization.[8]

About three fourths of all bites involve the extremities with about equal occurrence in upper and lower extremities. People use their extremities to ward off bites or to provoke them. The extremities are easier for the animal to grab than the trunk.

Most dog bites in children are relatively minor, occur on an extremity, and are promptly seen in an emergency department. This is not always the case, however. Severe facial lacerations occur almost exclusively in children under 10 years of age, and most bites are on the cheeks and lips.[5] The short stature of children places them at higher risk of facial bites than adults, simply by accessibility for the animal. In addition, children are more likely to place their faces in close proximity to the dog in an effort to inspect or "kiss" the dog.

The microbiology of dog bite wounds is complex. Many authors have reported that the results of initial cultures of noninfected dog bite wounds do not correlate with subsequent cultures of the infected wounds.[9-12] Bacteria that are frequently cultured from newly infected wound infections include the following[12,13]:

> *Pasteurella multocida* (wound infections within 24 hours)
> *Enterobacter*
> *Pseudomonas*
> *Staphylococcus aureus*
> *Bacillus subtilus*
> *Streptococci* species, particularly *S. viridens*

There appears to be an increased incidence of *Pasteurella* infection in patients under 4 years and over 55 years of age.[10]

All of these authors have noted that infected dog bite wounds frequently have multiple bacterial species involved. This varied multiple flora limits the clinical usefulness of the Gram's stain. Routine culturing of the wound, likewise, yields minimal information regarding the proper antibiotic to administer. Since culture and sensitivity results typically takes 48 to 72 hours to return, close clinical observation of the wound yields more information.

These same authors have concluded that antibiotic administration does not reduce the likelihood of subsequent infection in the management of recent dog bite wounds. The sole recommended exception to this policy would possibly be in hand bites.

The incidence of wound infections following a dog bite does appear to be markedly increased if the patient is older than 50, has a puncture wound, or has a hand wound, or if the wound is sutured.[14] As may be easily predicted, there is an increase in the incidence of wound infections if the patient waited longer than 24 hours to seek medical care or if there was inadequate wound care at the time of the first visit.

### Cat Bites and Scratches

Although not the most common bites, cat bites have a higher incidence of infection than dog bites.[15] Of cat scratch and bite injuries, 29% develop infectious complications. Cat bites and scratches are more common in women than in men and one fourth of the injuries occur while playing with the animal.[6]

In cats, the most common organisms recovered include *Pasteurella multocida*, *Streptococcus viridens*, and the other strains of *Streptococcus*, *Staphylococcus aureus*, and strains of *Bacteroides*. Cat scratches appear to be bacteriologically similar to cat bites, perhaps because of the manner in which cats groom themselves. In general, wounds due to cat scratches are equivalent to cat bites in severity.

There seems to be a high incidence (50 to 75%) of *Pasteurella multocida* in cat bites.[16] This small, nonmotile, Gram-negative coccobacillus grows both aerobically and anaerobically and does not form spores. *Pasteurella* causes a rapidly spreading cellulitis within 24 hours. It is sensitive to penicillin, cephalosporins, and tetracycline but generally is not sensitive to erythromycin.

The potential for involvement of the tendons and tendon sheaths with *Pasteurella* infections is high. The sharp-pointed feline teeth

seem to act as hypodermic injectors of *Pasteurella* into the tendon. Such puncture wounds are impossible to debride.

Cat scratch disease is caused by an unclassified bacterium, inoculated by the scratch of cat or other animal's claws. After a 3- to 10-day incubation, a tender papule develops at the site of the scratch. A regional lympadenopathy, fever, malaise, and a headache follow. There is usually a spontaneous resolution after a few weeks. It is unnecessary to treat this infection with antibiotics. An identical illness is noted after scratches of other animals and thorny plants.

### Human Bites

Human bites are similar to dogs and cats with two notable exceptions: location of the bite and presence of *Eikenella corrodens* in the wound.

*Eikenella corrodens* is a slow-growing Gram-negative rod that has been commonly isolated from human bite infections (10 to 30%).[17] This organism has an unusual antibiotic sensitivity pattern. It is resistant to oxacillin, methicillin, nafcillin, and clindamycin. It appears to be sensitive to ampicillin, penicillin, and the cephalosporins.

To date, transmission of acquired immune deficiency syndrome by a human bite has not occurred, but there is no reason that this will not happen. Other diseases, such as hepatitis B, have occasionally been transmitted by the bite of a human.

The other problem specific to the human bite is the "human" factor. The victim frequently lies about the mechanism of injury, which confuses matters. The victim may be embarrassed and delay in seeking therapy. The most common reason for delay in hand bites may be "recovery time" from a binge during which the fight took place.

One contribution to the confusion is known as the "clenched fist syndrome." When a person strikes an opponent's mouth, an irregular laceration occurs over the dorsum of the metacarpophalangeal joint (see Fig. 7.22). The joint is not covered by dorsal expansion hoods, and teeth may easily penetrate the joint space or tendon sheath. When the victim extends his fingers, movement of the tendon carries the saliva further into the joint and tendon sheath. The entrance wound into the meta-

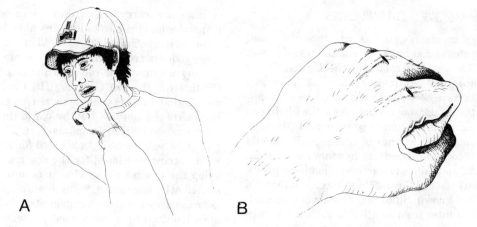

**Figure 7.22.** **A**, mechanism of bite injury; **B**, fight bite.

carpophalangeal joint is frequently over-looked. Even a small wound over the meta-carpals may conceal this multilayer violation of skin, subcutaneous tissues, joint capsule, and extensor tendons. Cartilaginous and bony injury have also been reported both from the effects of the original trauma and from the devastation of the infection.

These bites are most likely to occur during the summer months in men aged 20 to 35 and are on the dominant hand.[18] Unfortunately, the usual picture is that of a small draining wound over the third or fourth metacarpal in a patient who has delayed seeking medical care. Underlying the draining wound is often an infected joint space or tendon sheath that progresses to osteomyelitis or joint involvement.

Deep or full-thickness human bites of the hand have a high incidence of infectious complications, even when treated early. These infections are difficult to treat. Some services recommend that the patient be admitted and intravenous antibiotics started in **all** cases of suspected human bites to the hand that involve either the joint space or tendon.[19]

Older human bite wounds require exploration and drainage. This is best accomplished under anesthesia. Many will also need arthrotomy or drainage of the tendon sheath or both, if the joint space or tendon sheath has been violated. Some patients may require amputation. Intravenous antibiotics should be initiated as soon as possible.

Abrasions and contusions that do not penetrate the full thickness of the skin are unlikely to become infected. Wounds of the ex-

tremities other than the hand, or of the trunk have less propensity for infection.

## Other Animals

In addition to humans, dogs, and cats, other animals—both wild and domestic—may bite humans.

### PRIMATES

There is anecdotal evidence that bites by other primates and by pigs should be treated as a human bite. There are so few primate bites that even a cooperative study would be difficult to perform with any reasonable data.

### SKUNKS

The skunk is a frequent carrier of rabies and will bite when cornered. Wound care for the skunk bite should be as outlined for any other mammalian bite. There is an unfortunately high incidence of rabies in skunks, and these victims should recieve antirabies prophylaxis as discussed below.

Fortunately, most humans will avoid the skunk because of the foul-smelling spray that it employs in self-defense. Indeed, the spray can cause skin burning, nausea, vomiting, temporary blindness, and syncope. Care for the spray of musk includes rinsing of the eyes as if for a chemical burn. The musk can be neutralized with household bleach diluted 1:5, green soap, or tomato juice. The hair should be shampood with tomato juice and then thoroughly rinsed.

## SMALL, WILD CARNIVORES

Wild carnivores, such as bats, raccoons, foxes, coyotes and skunks, have accounted for most of the cases of rabies in the United States since 1960. Animals adopted as household pets have been found to be carriers of rabies. If the attack was not provoked, the likelihood of rabies is thought to be increased. Management of the wounds of these species should proceed as outlined for any other mammalian bite, and rabies prophylaxis should be given. The bacterial flora of these species in the wild is not known. Since there have been no studies of bites from small wild carnivores, reliable data on use of antibiotics are lacking.

## HERBIVORES

Cows, sheep, goats, horses, and other large herbivores frequently inflict blunt injuries by kicking or butting the victim. Goring injuries by the horned larger herbivores are often quite dirty.

An unknown and uncounted number of farm workers and equestrians also suffer bites from these animals. Generally, the bites are contusions with little skin damage. Management may be conservative—cleansing the area with antiseptic. It should be noted that most farmers and equestrians do not seek medical care for a simple bite, and the incidence is, therefore, unknown and most probably unknowable.

Camels have bitten humans to death.[20] The camel's bite is somewhat more dangerous than that of the other large herbivores since it has canine teeth that can rend flesh.[21] This animal has been known to sever a person's limb with a combination of biting and a whipping motion of the neck.

## RATS AND OTHER RODENTS

Despite the enormous numbers of rats, mice, and other rodents, they only account for 3 to 10% of all animal bites inflicted. Rat bites can transmit rat bite fever, plague, leptospirosis, murine typhus, and other diseases. The infection rate of rat bites has been routinely quoted at about 10%, but in one series, the resultant wound infections in a group of 50 bites was found to be only 2%.

Rats can carry rabies, but no cases of transmission of rabies to humans have been recorded in the United States.[22,23] The rat and other rodents are not thought to represent a risk of transmission of rabies to humans. The Centers for Disease Control (CDC) recommends that rabies prophylaxis not be given in cases of rodent bites, but the World Health Organization (WHO) recommends it.[24,25] Pet rodents who have been vaccinated for rabies with vaccine developed for the dog may develop the disease if the virus has not been sufficiently attenuated.[26] These animals appear to develop a more virulent strain of rabies. If bitten by a vaccinated pet who has had dog rabies vaccine, rabies prophylaxis is advised, despite the CDC recommendations. In rat bites sustained outside the United States, it would be prudent to follow the more conservative WHO recommendation and give rabies prophylaxis.

Rabbits have not been known to carry rabies, and rabbit bites should be treated as any other bite.

## OTHER WILD ANIMALS

The two major complications of domestic animal bites are local wound infection and rabies. Wild animal bites may include the attacks of carnivores intent on a meal on the hoof, animals in parks seeking an easy meal, animals disturbed by the trekker or camper, or animals defending their home or young.

## TREATMENT OF BITES

The patient needs to be carefully examined and all life-threatening problems attended to in the usual manner. The priorities of Airway, Breathing, and Circulation (ABCs) should be unchanged in the care of an animal bite. Life-threatening hemorrhage is controlled, and wounds that penetrate body cavities are cared for in customary fashion. The emotional care of the child who has just been attacked by an animal should be considered from the very start and the child properly comforted. Following these ABCs, the patient may be evaluated in a more leisurely manner.

## History

The following historical data are needed to properly evaluate and treat the dog bite:

| |
|---|
| *Historical data for dog bite evaluation* |
| Age of the patient |
| Species of animal biting |
|   (?? Domestic) |
| Time since the bite occurred |
| Health of the animal |
| Was the bite provoked or unprovoked |
|   (History of prior attacks) |
| Current location of the animal |
|   (?? Ownership vs stray vs wild) |
| Status of rabies prophylaxis for both animal |
|   and human |
|   (Animal—status of prophylaxis in |
|   domesticated animals) |
|   (Human—?? prophylaxis if patient is an |
|   animal handler) |
| Current and past medical problems of the |
|   patient |
|   History of immunocompromising disease |
|   or treatment |

## Physical Examination

Multiple bite sites are common, and the patient should be carefully examined to ensure that no lesions are missed. The wounds should be inspected for depth, and extent, and integrity of neurovascular and motor systems should be ascertained. Remember that, in a frightened child, it may be difficult to properly evaluate the neuromuscular and vascular systems. Verbal "sedation" of the child by parents and friends may help the examination.

### WOUND CARE

Perhaps the most important factor in the care of an animal bite is the proper care of the wound. Preparation should include mechanical cleansing to remove contaminated material, such as broken teeth and fragments of clothing.

Following this mechanical cleansing, the wound should be irrigated with a minimum of 250 cc of saline. Irrigation of the wound alone has been shown to decrease the rate of infection by a factor of five. Addition of antiseptics to the irrigation solution is contro-

versial, and there is no good proof that it increases the efficacy of irrigation alone.

Puncture wounds are very difficult to irrigate, and some clinicians recommend excising a small plug of tissue around the puncture wound or enlarging the puncture wound with scalpel or needle to facilitate the irrigation. These procedures have not been studied, information is anecdotal only, and the effectiveness is not known.

Where there is a high risk of rabies transmission, the wound should be irrigated with a 1% benzalkonium chloride solution. This solution has been shown to effectively kill the rabies virus.[27] The decisions regarding wound closure and use of antibiotics are made independently of decisions about rabies prophylaxis.

Debridement of the bite wound may remove embedded soil, clots, and organisms that are not removed by irrigation alone. Tissue that has potential vascular compromise may be removed at this time. A limited debridement is appropriate for wounds of the face, fingers, and areas where neurovascular or motor function can be impaired by extensive debridement. Sharp debridement in other areas will remove the crushed tissue and "tidy up" lacerations.

If the injury involves a body cavity, head, face, joint, or bone, x-ray films are appropriate. When swelling is present, from any cause, elevation of the area is essential. Particularly in hand and lower extremity wounds, immobilization may also be required.

Hyperbaric oxygenation has been advocated in human bite infections and the clenched fist injury from human teeth,[28] but this therapy remains controversial.

### INDICATIONS FOR HOSPITALIZATION

The decision regarding hospitalization is, in the vast majority of cases, either trivial or obvious. These guidelines will cover the cases that are either not obvious or controversial, as well.

### WOUND CLOSURE

Primary closure of animal bites is quite controversial. Fortunately, most wounds are minor and only 10% will require suturing or surgical care.[29] Wounds that may be sutured

---

*Indications for Hospitalization*

Massive blood loss or shock

Severe wounds that require surgical debridement or surgical airway management

Penetration of a body cavity, such as the chest, abdomen, or cranium

Major blunt injuries, such as goring

Signs of systemic sepsis

Injuries that involve bone or penetration of a joint space

Infected hand wounds

Hand wounds with human bites (controversial indication!)

Infected wounds or high-risk wounds in the presence of an immunocompromising disease, such as diabetes, liver disorders, chemotherapy for cancer, AIDS, or asplenia

---

relatively safely after they are appropriately cleansed include those to the face, trunk, or proximal extremities. Facial wounds may almost always be closed primarily, after appropriate cleansing, irrigation, and debridement. Wounds associated with risk factors are usually not sutured immediately. Certainly, in the case of human bites, the wound is best left open with a delayed primary closure at 48 to 72 hours after first care of the wound. In cases of cat bites or scratches to the hand, a similar policy should apply.

High-risk wounds, or wounds in high-risk patients, should not be sutured immediately. The wounds should be cleansed and debrided, then loosely packed with fine mesh gauze soaked in saline solution. If the wound remains uninfected for 48 to 72 hours, it can be reirrigated and closed on a return visit on the fourth postbite day. This delayed primary closure has produced excellent results in heavily contaminated wounds.[30]

"Loosely" suturing the wound, using surgical staples, or applying adhesive strips are functionally equivalent to suturing the wound. Wounds that are not amenable to closure by customary suturing techniques should not be closed by these techniques as an alternative.

If the wound becomes infected, then it should be opened if it was closed, sutures removed, and the wound irrigated with copious amounts of saline. The wound should then be debrided and packed open. Consideration should be given to admitting the patient to the hospital for treatment with intravenous antibiotics.

Extensive or multiple animal bite wounds are often better managed in an operating room under appropriate anesthesia. Particularly in children with facial wounds or extensive wounds, general anesthesia may be preferable.

## ANTIBIOTIC THERAPY

There has been no controlled, prospective, large-scale study of the role of antibiotics in the treatment of animal bites. The only studies have been small scale, confined to one institution, or retrospective. Accordingly, there is not a good data base upon which to build recommendations for antibiotic therapy in the management of animal bites. No single antibiotic agent is consistently active against all of the many potential bite wound pathogens. The recommendations below are based upon current information and are designed as a rational approach to management.

In abrasions, contusions, and other injuries that do not require sutures, antibiotics are probably not indicated. The major exception to this policy is the puncture wound, from either tooth or claw. Other low-risk wounds will also have little benefit from antibiotics.

In the rest of cases, although the term "prophylactic" antibiotics is used universally, this is not quite proper usage. Antibiotics are often given empirically, before a clinical infection is manifested, but truly prophylactic antibiotics would have to be given before the injury occurred. With this caveat, the customary usage is used in this chapter, i.e., prophylactic antibiotics are given before clinical infection. The wise physican will obviously not rely upon antibiotics in lieu of good wound toilet.

The choice of empiric therapeutic or prophylactic antibiotics is the same, since cultures of the wound at the time of first care reflect only poorly the pathologic organisms cultured from infections. Recent studies with dicloxacillin, penicillin, or cephalexin have failed to show any strong advantages of one drug over the others.[13,31] The combination drug of amoxicillin and clavulanate potassium has been reported to be efficacious for initial empiric therapy.[32]

Between 18 and 50% of *Pasteurella multocida* species are resistant to the first-gen-

---

*Prophylaxis is appropriate when:*

The type of bite sustained has a high-infection rate.

Cat bites

Human bites

Puncture wounds (not proven effective)

The consequences of the infection in a particular area are likely to be particularly serious.

Bites on the hand (not proven effective, but considered to be the standard of care)

Bites that penetrate body cavities, such as sinuses or the cranial vault.

The cost and relative toxicity of the antibiotic agent are low.

Penicillin V, semisynthetic penicillins, many cephalosporins

---

*Antibiotic Therapy for Bite Wounds*

Recommended Oral Antibiotics

Dicloxacillin 500 mg 4 times per day for 5 days

Children—50 to 100 mg/kg/day in 4 doses

Amoxicillin 500 mg with clavulanate potassium 3 times per day for 5 days

Children—50 to 100 mg/kg/day in 4 doses

Cephalexin 500 mg 4 times per day for 5 days

Children—50 to 100 mg/kg/day in 4 doses

Erythromycin 500 mg 4 times per day for 5 days*

Children—30 to 50 mg/kg/day in 4 doses

Infection that develops within 24 hours of the bite

Penicillin V 500 mg 4 times per day for 5 days

Cat bites (somewhat controversial)

Penicillin V 500 mg 4 times per day for 5 days

Recommended Intravenous Antibiotics

Cefazolin—25 to 50 mg/kg/day IV in 3 to 4 divided doses plus

Gentamicin 3 to 7.5 mg/kg/day IV in 3 doses (assuming renal function is normal)

---

*For patients allergic to penicillin and cephalosporins

---

eration cephalosporins and the semisynthetic penicillins.[33] With the peculiar spectrum of sensitivity of *Pasteurella multocida*, penicillin G or ampicillin is the best antibiotic for the infection that develops rapidly (within 12 to 24 hours after the bite) (see right).

In the human bite, *Eikenella corrodens* is often found and is resistant to the semisynthetic penicillins, such as methacillin. It is sensitive to penicillin, ampicillin, and some of the cephalosporins. A logical choice may be the combination of amoxicillin and clavulanic acid. The addition of the latter improves the drug's action against staphylococcal species.

Erythromycin may be suitable for those patients who are allergic to both the penicillins and the cephalosporins but has poor activity against *P. multocida*. If erythromycin is used in the allergic patient, close monitoring of the wound is essential. Tetracyclines are logical choices by virtue of their spectrum of activity but are contraindicated in children and pregnant or breastfeeding women.

For an established infection, a penicillinase-resistant penicillin or second- or third-generation cephalosporin would be the most reasonable choice. In these patients, intravenous administration of antibiotics and close monitoring of the wound is essential. This is best accomplished by hospitalization in almost all cases.

In all cases, tetanus prophylaxis should be current. Hyperimmune serum should be used in the standard dosages for those who have never been immunized. These wounds should be treated as high tetanus potential, and tetanus immunization should be renewed if more than five years have elapsed since the last immunization.

## RABIES

Rabies is a viral infection caused by a member of the rhabdovirus group, with an affinity for the nervous system and salivary glands of mammals. About 50% of patients who are bitten by a rabid animal will develop rabies if untreated.

Clear understanding of the relationship between the bite of a mad dog and the human infection has been attributed to Celsus as early as 100 A.D. Celsus described hydrophobia and recommended local cautery to the bite wound in an attempt to prevent the disease in humans.[34] As a particular note, rabies is the first human disease for which a successful vaccine was developed by Louis Pasteur in 1881.

## Incidence

In the United States, the incidence of rabies in humans has declined dramatically over the past 35 years from 23 cases in 1952 to no more than two or three cases per year since 1960. During the 20-year period from 1962 to 1983, there were only 37 cases of human rabies reported in this country. Dogs have been the source of at least 38% of human rabies since 1962. This should underline the importance of continued use of rabies vaccine in domestic pets.

The incidence outside of the United States is strikingly different. Worldwide, the most common vector for rabies is the dog, because of the lack of adequate canine vaccination programs. Human rabies is common in India, Brazil, and the Philippines. Nearly 15,000 deaths occur annually from rabies in India.[35] In Europe, the major vectors are the fox and the dog. Australia and New Zealand are free of rabies.

## Domestic Animal Vectors

As noted earlier, the dog bite is the most frequent animal bite that presents to the emergency department. Fortunately, most of these patients are bitten by angry animals and not "mad dogs." Dogs trained as guard animals are more likely to attack than other animals.

Cats are also a source of rabies. Since 1981, the incidence of rabies in cats has exceeded that found in dogs. Fortunately, however, there has been only one confirmed case of human rabies transmitted by a cat since 1962, and the risk of rabies transmission by a domestic cat is fairly small.

## Wild Animal Vectors

Since the 1960s, the reported incidence of rabies in the wild animal population has exceeded the incidence of rabies in domestic animals. Most cases of human rabies now appear to be transmitted from an infected wild animal.[36] Skunks, raccoons, foxes, and bats are now the major wildlife species that comprise the host population for rabies.[37] Skunks are the largest reservoir accounting for about 40% of all reported cases.[38] Rodents, such as squirrels, rats, mice, rabbits, and hares are rarely infected, although isolated instances have been reported.

---

*Risk of Rabies Transmission*

High Risk
  Bats
  Skunks
  Foxes
  Coyotes
  Raccoons
  Bobcats
  Other carnivores
Low Risk
  Rodents
    Chipmunks
    Gerbils
    Hamsters
    Mice
    Rats
    Squirrels
    Guinea pigs
  Rabbits and hares
  Domestic and farm animals in the United
    States

---

## Clinical Course

The rabies virus invades the peripheral nervous system and moves slowly toward the spinal cord and brain. The virus cannot penetrate intact skin and, except for rare cases of infection via inhalation or corneal transplant, requires a skin break or mucous membrane contact in order to establish an infection.[39,40] After reaching the CNS, it again travels peripherally to the salivary glands where it multiplies explosively. Many cases may initially present as an ascending neuritis or as an acute psychiatric illness.[41] The differential diagnosis of rabies includes tetanus, delirium tremens, other viral encephalitides, and hysteria.

## INCUBATION PERIOD

The average interval between exposure and clinical disease in humans is 1 to 2 months. This incubation period may vary from 2 weeks to 2 years and is one of the longest incubation periods found in human infections.[36] A peripheral bite, for instance, one on a hand or a foot, results in a longer incubation period and a bite on the head results in a shorter one.[42] Generally, 18 to 60 days is the accepted incubation period, although a substantial variance can occur based upon the location of the injury. The victim is usually asymptomatic during this time. During the incubation period, the virus progresses to the CNS by axoplasmic flow at the rate of about 3 mm per hour.

## PRODROME PHASE

The next clinical stage is the prodrome, which is often indistinguishable from a generalized viral syndrome, with headache, malaise, anorexia, lethargy, and perhaps fever. About 50% of the victims will note pain or paresthesias at the site of the wound. This paresthesia or pain may be the first symptom that is specific for rabies. The prodrome lasts about 2 to 10 days.

## ACUTE PHASE

The first signs of the acute phase are often mental status changes, beginning with anxiety and agitation and progressing to confusion, hallucinations, and bizzare hyperactive behavior. The bizzare hyperactive behavior is frequently intermittent and punctuated with periods of calm and lucidity.

At this stage, victims of "classic" rabies will experience pharyngeal spasms with gagging or choking when trying to swallow. These symptoms may be precipitated by water or even by seeing water or feeling an air current on the face, hence giving rise to the well-known hydrophobia or aerophobia. During this phase, other signs of encephalitis will present, including fever, nuchal rigidity, weakness or paralysis, or seizures.

The victim becomes comatose about 4 to 10 days after the acute onset of symptoms. The coma is shortly followed by a respiratory arrest and death if not supported. In the patient with life support, further neurologic involvement causes multisystem failure.

Other victims of paralytic rabies will experience pain, paresis, and flaccid paralysis that develops in the bitten extremity and progresses centrally. As the paralysis ascends, the muscles of respiration become involved. Hydrophobia is unusual and the differential diagnosis includes Guillain-Barre syndrome, polio, postvaccine encephalopathy, other viral encephalopathy, and acute transverse myelitis. Death occurs about 12 days after the onset of symptoms.[43]

The diagnosis and treatment of rabies is difficult and rarely successful. There are no clinical tests available to diagnose the disease prior to the onset of symptoms. After the onset of symptoms, the laboratory is of little help, and the course is inexorable. The only known survivors have received either pre- or postexposure prophylaxis before the onset of the clinical disease.[44] The nature of rabies is such that only prevention is the appropriate management.

## Treatment

## LOCAL TREATMENT

Local treatment of the wound as described earlier is appropriate in all cases. The virus does not survive well outside the human body and cleansing with soap and water or benzalkonium chloride solution is adequate to clean both equipment and humans.

---

*Rabies Prophylaxis*
The decision to immunize against rabies depends upon several factors:
1. The species of the biting animal
2. The circumstances of the attack (provoked or not)
3. The type of exposure (bite or not)
4. Whether the animal is available for observation
5. The vaccination status of the animal
6. The local prevalence of rabies

---

## The Species of Biting Animal, Custody, and Vaccination Status

Carnivorous animals—particularly skunks, raccoons, coyotes, and bobcats—should be captured if at all possible, sacrificed without damage to the head, and the head sent to the state health department or other reference laboratory for testing. Treatment decisions can be made on the basis of this testing. Since the incubation period in these animals is variable, and the virus can appear in the saliva prior to the onset of illness, they should not be held for observation. If the animal cannot be captured, the decision must be made on consideration of the species and local incidence. The only vaccines available are for dogs and cats. Vaccines for wild animals are not available.

When the animal is a dog or cat, an attempt should be made to capture the animal. If it is caught and is behaving abnormally or appears ill, it should be immediately sacrificed. If it is behaving normally, it may be isolated and observed for 10 days. If the animal cannot be captured, information gathered from the victim must be correlated with the health department reports of local infection rates in that species.

## Circumstances of the Attack

A rabid animal is more likely than a healthy animal to attack without provocation. The victim should generally not be asked, "Did you provoke the animal?" but, rather, "Were you feeding, petting, or otherwise handling the animal?" Any effort to feed, pet, or handle a wild animal should be considered provocation.

## Type of Exposure

The critical issue in exposure is the transmission of the virus from the saliva of the animal into open cuts or wounds. Most often this occurs with a biting injury, but any open wound contaminated by saliva or nervous tissue from a rabid animal should be considered an exposure. Casual contacts, including petting an animal, do not constitute exposure and are not an indication for treatment.

## The Local Species-specific Prevalence of Rabies

The local incidence and prevalence of rabies in a particular species of animal can be obtained from the state or local public health service. Generally, the risk of exposure is known well in advance of any bite for most species, such as bats, raccoons, or skunks and should be common knowledge in the emergency departments in the area.

## Pre-exposure Prophylaxis

Rabies research lab workers, vaccine production workers, spelunkers, veterinarians, and animal control workers have a significantly higher risk of exposure than average. Diagnostic and research lab personnel and vaccine production workers should have the antibody titer determined every 6 months. Those persons with continuing risk of exposure should have a booster dose of vaccine every 2 years.

## Post-exposure Prophylaxis

Human diploid cell vaccine (HDCV) has completely supplanted the use of the older duck embryo vaccine for both pre- and postexposure prophylaxis in this country. Use of this vaccine produces an active immune response in 7 to 10 days from the initial injection. The usual method is to give five doses, one each on day 0, 3, 7, 14, and 28. This regimen provides an excellent antibody response, and serum titers to check the response are generally considered unnecessary and expensive. Although extensive studies have not yet been performed, the vaccine is considered safe for use during pregnancy.[45]

HDCV is a live virus vaccine. Caution should be exercised before immunizing patients who have immunosuppressive disease or those taking steroids or immunosuppressive drugs. If at all possible, these agents should be discontinued during therapy, and these patients should have serum antibody titers checked after the regimen is complete to ensure that they have mounted an adequate immune response. Rabies has occurred in patients who have been given only HDCV, so the immunization should be supplanted with passive immunization.[46]

Passive immunization should be provided immediately with RIG (rabies immune globulin), which is administered once on the first day of prophylaxis. This is a concentrated product that is made from human serum and is given in a dose equal to 20 IU/kg. Half of the dose is infiltrated locally into the wound site, and the other half given intramuscularly. Low-grade fever and local wound pain frequently follow its use.

If RIG is not available, antirabies serum (ARS) should be used instead. This drug often produces serum sickness and may cause anaphylaxis in persons who are sensitive to horse serum. A dose of 40 IU/kg is given after testing for hypersensitivity.

Interferon has been demonstrated to offer protection against viral challenges and is being investigated as a possible therapy for rabies. It is still experimental and quite costly.[47,41]

## SUMMARY

Animal bites may cause direct trauma, inoculation of local infections, and inoculation of systemic diseases. Repair of the trauma and prevention of the local infection should proceed hand in hand with careful wound toilet, gentle copious irrigation, and delayed primary closure in high-risk areas. High incidence of wound infections are seen with hand injuries and with cat and human bite wounds. The role of antibiotics is uncertain, but prophylactic antibiotics are probably reasonable for high-risk groups. Hospitalization and intravenous administration of antibiotics is essential for late infections, infections that do not respond to oral antibiotics, and infections in high-risk areas, such as facial and hand wounds. There is no single antibiotic or group of antibiotics that is consistently effective.

Prevention of rabies infection is essential as there is no cure. Although rabies is rarely found in domestic animals in the United States, wild animals, particularly skunks and bats, are frequent carriers. In other countries, this disease is far more frequent in both the domestic and wild animal populations.

## References

1. Moore RM Jr, Zehmer RB, Moulthrop JI, et al. Surveillance of animal bite cases in the United States, 1971–1972. Arch Environ Health 1977;32:267–270.
2. Callaham ML. Human and animal bites. Top Emerg Med 1982;4:1–15.
3. Edlich RF, Morgan RF, Mayer NE, Rodeheaver GT. Mammalian bites. Cur Concepts Wound Care 1986;Summer;15–22.
4. Heller MB. Management of bites: dog, cat, human, and snake. Res Staff Phys 1982; Feb:75–84.
5. Karlson TA The incidence of facial injuries from dog bites. JAMA 1984;251:3265–3267.
6. Kizer KW. Epidemiologic and clinical aspects of animal bite injuries. JACEP 1979;8:134–141.
7. Goldstein EJC, Richwald GA. Human and animal bite wounds. Am Fam Phys 1987;36:101–109.
8. Callaham M. Human and animal bites. Top Emerg Med 1982;4:1–15.
9. Boenning DA, Fleisher GR, Campos JM. Dog bites in children: epidemiology, microbiology, and penicillin prophylactic therapy. Am J Emerg Med 1983;1:17–21.
10. Callaham ML. Treatment of common dog bites: infection risk factors. JACEP 1978;7:83–87.
11. Spencer RC, Matta H, Ferguson DG, et al. Routine culture of dog bites [letter]. Ann Emerg Med 1987;16:730.
12. Ordog GJ. The bacteriology of dog bite wounds on initial presentation. Ann Emerg Med 1986;15:1324–1329.
13. Rosen RA. The use of antibiotics in the initial management of recent dog-bite wounds. Am J Emerg Med 1985;3:19–23.
14. Brown CG, Ashton JJ. Dog bites: the controversy continues [editorial]. Am J Emerg Med 1985;3:83–84.
15. Aghababian RV, Conte JE. Mammalian bite wounds. Ann Emerg Med 1980;9(s):79–83.
16. Francis DP, Holmes A, Brandon G. *Pasteurella multocida* infections after domestic animal bites and scratches. JAMA 1975;233:42–45.
17. Bilos ZJ, Kuchararchuk A, Metzger W. *Eikenella corrodens* in human bites. Clin Orthop 1978;134:320–324.
18. Rest JG, Goldstein EJC. Management of human and animal bite wounds. Emerg Med Clin North Am 1985;3:117–126.
19. Taylor GA. Management of human bite injuries of the hand. Can Med Assoc J 1985;133:191–192.
20. Clarke J: Man is the prey. London: Andre Deutsch Ltd, 1969.
21. Consul BN, Sharma DP, Sharma RG. Orbital fracture due to camel bite. J All India Ophthalmol Soc 1968;16:245–248.
22. Winkler WG. Rodent rabies in the United States. J Infect Dis 1972;126:565–567.
23. Ordog GJ, Balasubramanium S, Wasserberger J. Rat bites: fifty cases. Ann Emerg Med 1985;14:126–130.
24. WHO Expert Committee on Rabies. Fifth Report, WHO Technical Rep Ser No 321, 1966.
25. Centers for Disease Control: Recommendation of the Immunization Practices Advisory Committee. Rabies Prevention. MMWR 1982;31:685–695.
26. Humphrey GL. Rabies: suggested indications for treatment of exposed persons. Calif Med 1967;107:363–377.
27. Hopman L, Stewart CE. Rabies. Emerg Med Serv 1986;May:22G–22J.
28. Lehman WL Jr, Jones WW, Allo MD, Johnston RM. Human bite infections of the hand: adjunct treatment with hyperbaric oxygen. Infect Surg 1985;4:460.

29. Callaham M. Human and animal bites. Top Emerg Med 1982;4:1–15.
30. Wounds and injuries of the soft tissues. In: Emergency War Surgery First Unites States Revision of Emergency War Surgery NATO Handbook. Washington, DC: US Government Printing Office, 1975.
31. Elenbaas RM, McNabney WK, Robinson WA. Prophylactic oxacillin in dog bite wounds. Ann Emerg Med 1982;248–51.
32. Goldstein EJ, Reinhardt JF, Murray PM, Finegold SM. Outpatient therapy of bite wounds: demographic data, bacteriology and a prospective randomized trial of amoxicillin/ clavulanic acid versus penicillin +/− diclox-acillin. Int J Dermatol 1987;26:123–127.
33. Stevens DL, Higbee JW, Oberhofer TR, Everett ED. Antibiotic susceptibilities of human isolates of *Pasteurella multocida*. Antimicrob Agents Chemother 1979;16:322–324.
34. Winkler WG. Clinical rabies—humans. In: Wenkler WG, ed. Rabies concepts for medical professionals. Lyon: Merieux Institute, Inc., 1983:45.
35. Millser A, Nathanson R. Rabies: recent advances in pathogenesis and control. Ann Neurol 1977;2:511.
36. Kauffman FH, Goldmann BJ. Rabies. Am J Emerg Med 1986;4:525–531.
37. Burridge MJ. Wildlife rabies in the United States. Avian/Exotic Practice 1984;1:17–22.
38. Centers for Disease Control. Rabies surveillance. Annual summary 1984. Issued December 1985.
39. Kaplan MD, Koprowski H. Rabies. Sci Am 1980;240:120.
40. Hough SA, Burton RC, Wilson RW, et al. Human to human transmission of rabies virus by corneal transplant. N Engl J Med 1979;300:603–604.
41. Meislin HW, Libby J. Human rabies. Ann Emerg Med 1983;12:217–220.
42. Flanigan TJ, Rippert EJ, Niesman GE. Rabies therapy for animal bites in the head and neck region. J Oral Maxillofac Surg 1985;43:704.
43. Warrell D. The clinical picture of rabies in man. Trans R Soc Trop Med Hyg 1976;70:188.
44. Porras C, Barboza J, Fuenzalida E, et al. Recovery from rabies in man. Ann Intern Med 1976;85:44.
45. Varner MW, McGuiness GA, Galask RP. Rabies vaccination in pregnancy. Am J Obstet Gynecol 1982;143:717–718.
46. CDC. Rabies prevention: United States, 1984. MMWR 1984;33:393–402.
47. Hilfenhaus J, Weinmann E, Majer M, et al. Administration of human interferon to rabies virus infected monkeys after exposure. J Infect Dis 1977;155:846–849.

# Part 3
# Marine Animal Injuries

## INTRODUCTION

The marine environment holds evolutionary memories for all of us. Our babies are nurtured for 9 months in an analogue of the sea, and the fetus develops gills reminiscent of sea creatures during embryonic growth in the uterus. Part of the popularity of swimming in the ocean, diving, and underwater activities may relate to this environmental heritage of ages. The awesome beauty of the underwater environment lures other people to explore it. For others, the call of the last unexplored wilderness on earth is a beacon that cannot be ignored.

Within this wilderness dwell four fifths of all living organisms. This same marine environment has shaped some of the most majestic and deadly organisms on earth. This chapter will discuss the more common animal hazards humans may encounter in the marine environment, along with the mechanisms and treatment of these injuries.

Encounters with hazardous marine animals are usually accidental and can be categorized into four general types.

Trauma
Stings
Bites
Ingestions

## TRAUMA

Marine animals usually attack humans in self-defense, in defense of young or territory, or to provide food. One should constantly remember that the patient who has been bitten by a marine animal may have other associated injuries, such as near drowning, dysbaric accidents, decompression sickness, or aspiration of sea water. These injuries frequently result during a hasty surfacing or rescue attempt.

The wounds sustained in the sea are also to be considered dirty wounds. Recent research has shown that myriad potentially dangerous bacterial contaminants are found in sea water. These bacteria form the basis for complex tissue infections. All wounds should be cultured prior to cleaning or administering antibiotics.

## Sharks

Sharks are a successful predatory evolutionary pathway that have survived unchanged for nearly 100 million years. There are an estimated 250 to 350 different species of sharks, most of which are sea water dwellers. Most sharks are found in the relatively shallow waters off the major continents or around islands in the temperate and tropical zones. Usually, sharks are thought of as fierce predators, such as the great white shark, but they may also be unobtrusive filter feeders like the whale sharks. Of the 30 to 35 species that have been noted to attack humans, only a few of these species (great white sharks, mako sharks, hammerhead sharks, and the bull and reef sharks) are responsible for most of the attacks (see Fig. 7.23).

The media has portrayed the predatory shark as a savage man-hunting beast. Movies and headlines depict multiple unprovoked shark attacks in the search for themes to attract audiences. Seafarers, divers, and fishermen have helped to perpetuate the mythical conception of these legendary ravages. In actual fact, only 30 to 100 shark bites are reported annually (despite millions of bathers and divers).[1,2] The rarity of this event is attested by Welch and Martini, who noted that only 50 reported shark attacks have occurred in the more than 100 years of records for Hawaii, which has one of the most heavily used marine environments in the world.[3] (Of course, solitary missing swimmers may have drowned or may have succumbed to shark attacks.) A shark attack is a terrifying experience, with mutilation, amputation, or death common.[4] The severity of injury adds credence to the legends and stimulates excessive media coverage.

It is amazing that, despite a wealth of folklore and myth, relatively few true studies of the interaction of shark and humans have been performed. The best and most authoritative source of information is the shark attack file at the Mote Marine Laboratory in Sarasota, Florida.

Most shark attacks occur in the warmer climates between 40 degrees north and south latitudes, with the greatest prevalence in water temperatures above 70°F (20°C).

Natural shark habitats, such as deep channels, coastal estuaries, or areas where animal products or sewage are dumped, experience an increased incidence of attack. Shark attacks are also more common where

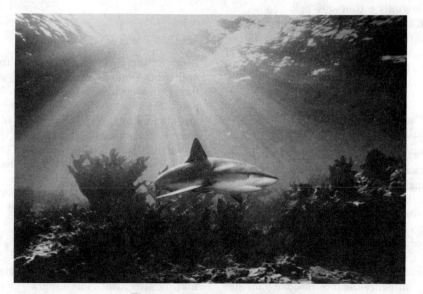

**Figure 7.23.**  Black-finned shark.

there are more people at risk, whether due to an increase in commotion or an increase in the number of targets of opportunity for the shark. Attacks are more likely during the late afternoon and evening hours, both because of an increase in the number of bathers and because this is the shark's natural feeding period.

Sharks are able to detect contrasts well and appear to have a predilection for bright, contrasting, and reflective objects. A shark's visual acuity is not high, but moving objects that contrast with the background may be easily detected in low light conditions.

Substances such as fresh blood are detectable in minute quantities (parts per billion) by a keen sense of smell. Decaying blood, such as that found in menstrual flow, is not as easily detectable. Sharks rely on their sense of smell because their ability to taste is poor. The hearing sense is equally well developed, especially in the lower frequency sounds. A specialized set of organs—the lateral lines and ampullae of Lorenzini—enable them to detect and localize these low-frequency sounds and pressure vibrations from miles away.

Whether the motivation to attack humans is hunger, territorial invasion, or violation of courtship patterns or is purely anomalous is open to question.[5] Probably elements of all of these cause some attacks at various times. It is difficult to assume that hunger is the motivation in all attacks, since at least 70% of victims are only bitten once or twice.[6]

Shark attacks take four different patterns. These patterns are identifiable by the nature of the injuries sustained and the behavior of the animals. These patterns are grouped into three feeding patterns and a defense against territorial invasion.

## CONTACT

Sharks in a feeding pattern tend to circle the prey, gradually increasing the speed and tightening the circle. As the circles become smaller, the shark starts to cross the circle and produce a contact or "bump" injury. With this contact, the rasp-like dentinate skin may produce an extensive abrasion. It is thought that the information gained by the contact and the blood released from the abrasion may influence the likelihood of a further attack.

## BITING

The shark bites with a horizontal or slightly upward direction. The head is tilted slightly back, projecting the lower teeth slightly forward. This position causes the mouth to gape open widely and displays the teeth (see Fig. 7.24). The biting force of the jaws in this position is estimated from 7 to 18 tons per square inch.[7] The shark then grips the prey and will tear a section of flesh with a sideways motion or will sever the limb. Wounds made in this manner are large and gaping.

There appears to be no species of sharks that exhibits a preference for human flesh, despite the media hype to the contrary. A shark feeding on fish may accidently bite a swimmer's leg or the swimmer, in motion, may resemble the shark's normal prey. A surfer on a contrasting board may mimic the motions of a seal and the shark may attack. Spilled fish or human blood may induce the shark to feed, particularly if there is a commotion present. Divers are strongly advised not to tether fish near their bodies for this reason.

Anatomic lesions of the shark's feeding bite are readily identifiable. The crescent shape of the jaw will be reflected in the shape of the wound, with a separate laceration made by each tooth. There are frequently both crush injuries and avulsions of various parts of the body. Arterial bleeding is frequent and severe.

## FEEDING FRENZY

If more than two or three sharks are in the area where blood is released, they may reflexly respond in a "feeding frenzy."[8] At this point, the sharks will attack any moving object, including prey, other fish, and other sharks. The subsequent carnage is quite impressive. Sharks that are attacked or hooked while swimming together may evoke this feeding frenzy in companions. Humans in this circumstance may be grievously wounded or killed.

## AGONISTIC ATTACKS

The shark that is defending its territory or mating area attacks in a markedly different manner than the feeding shark.[9] The shark

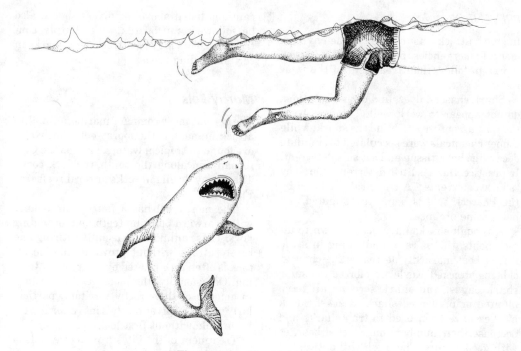

**Figure 7.24.** Shark's biting position.

exaggerates the lateral motion, uses the upper teeth, and arches the spine. It is a more awkward posturing manner than the smooth and fluid feeding attack. If the intruder vacates the area, the shark resumes normal swimming, and a confrontation will be avoided. If the swimmer does not leave, then a solitary upper tooth slash may be inflicted by the shark. Divers provoking sharks may suffer this type of bite.

## TREATMENT

Treatment of the shark's attack is management of the trauma inflicted by the bite. Shark bites may result in deep complex wounds involving all layers of tissue including nerves, tendons, bones, and even viscera. The immediate threat in most cases is that of exsanguination and subsequent hypovolemia. Rarely, airway compromise or pulmonary injury may be found. If bleeding can be controlled, most victims brought ashore alive will survive.

Amputation and subsequent or concurrent major vessel disruption may necessitate tourniquet management of hemorrhage, but this should be reserved for truly exsanguinating injuries. Direct wound pressure will usually suffice for control of bleeding. Replacement of blood loss with crystalloid and blood products should be started as soon as feasible.

Of longer term importance in the care of these injuries is their high level of contamination. The shark's teeth are replaced by outward growth of new teeth; consequently shark's teeth are frequently left imbedded in the tissue. Sand, algae, clothes, and other foreign matter may also be present. The high level of pathogenic bacteria noted in sea water increases the risk of infection. The wounds should be copiously irrigated, and all foreign bodies removed. A radiograph of the area will help locate hidden foreign objects such as shark teeth.

---

*Shark Attack DONT'S*
Swim with open wounds
Swim with dead or dying fish near your
  body
Swim in areas of low visibility
Swim near sewage outflow tracts
Urinate in the water
Swim near deep channels or dropoffs
Play with or provoke sharks

---

## PREVENTION

In shark attacks, as in many of the environmental emergencies, prevention is an easier course to follow than treatment of the injuries.

Shark chasers, dyes, and copper solutions do not appear to work well. The dyes were thought to confuse and blind the shark, while copper chemicals were speculated to simulate decaying shark tissue and act as a deterrent. In practice, there is little deterrent offered by "shark deterrents." A chemical produced by the Peacock sole is being investigated and holds some promise.

Although sharks have been known to attack boats, this is rare, and riding in a life raft or boat markedly decreases the chances of being attacked. Kevlar-reinforced wet suits, shark cages, and shark screens all have blunted or prevented shark attacks. Shark meshes have been used to trap sharks and decrease their numbers on selected beaches with good results. The mesh will entrap the larger sharks, stopping forward motion. Since the shark requires forward motion to push water through the gills, they then die of "drowning."

Divers are advised not to tether dead or dying fish near their body. They should not swim in water with low visibility, near sewage outflow tracts, or around other locales where animal products are dumped. Sharks favor dropoffs and deep channels, and they are most active during the late afternoon hours. Use of underwater explosives and electrical devices may attract sharks to the area. When planning excursions into the underwater world, these factors should be considered. Divers, as always, should swim with a buddy. (Some divers claim that this alone will reduce the chances of a shark's attack by 50%, but this is entirely anecdotal.)

The diver should descend to the bottom or against a reef or cliff, in order to slow or break the shark's normal feeding patterns and thus avoid an attack. Some people feel that a poke or punch to the shark's snout will deflect the attack, but playing with or provoking the shark will often provoke an attack with disastrous consequences.

Swimmers should be advised not to urinate in the water or swim with open wounds. The myth that menstrual blood flow will attract sharks is unproven. All of the other precautions listed above for divers should also be followed. Surfboards with sharply contrasting colors may be attractive to sharks in certain feeding areas.

### Moray Eels

The second most common marine animal to attack humans is the moray eel. Moray eels are found in tropical waters, such as the Caribbean and along the southern U. S. coast. The moray dwells in rocks or coral reefs (see Fig. 7.25).

The moray eel has a fierce countenance with rearward pointing teeth and forbidding jaws. These animals are usually retiring and rarely attack without provocation. The attack is often precipitated by injury or by teasing. Occasionally, the moray eel will attack in defense of their rocky territory, particularly when the diver reaches into a coral crevice or hole without first looking.

Treatment of the bites from moray eels is straightforward management of the trauma involved. Since the moray is smaller than the shark, there is usually no major vessel injury or amputation. The rearward pointing teeth make extrication of the patient from the fish difficult at times, which complicates the management. Infection of the area is common, and the wound should be routinely cultured prior to cleansing.

### Groupers

Groupers are familiar tropical fish with over 30 different species. These fish may attain lengths of 3 to 4 m (10 to 12 feet) and may weigh as much as 500 lbs (200 kg). Humans are usually injured when they pet or feed the smaller groupers and run out of food before the grouper runs out of appetite. Fingers and ears are the usual targets for this pugnacious creature. The grouper usually causes a crush injury from its powerful jaws.

### Barracuda

The most dangerous of the approximately 20 species of barracuda is probably the Sphyraena barracuda. This large fish may exceed 100 pounds and lengths of over 6 feet (see Fig. 7.26). The barracuda are generally inquisitive and attracted to bright shining ob-

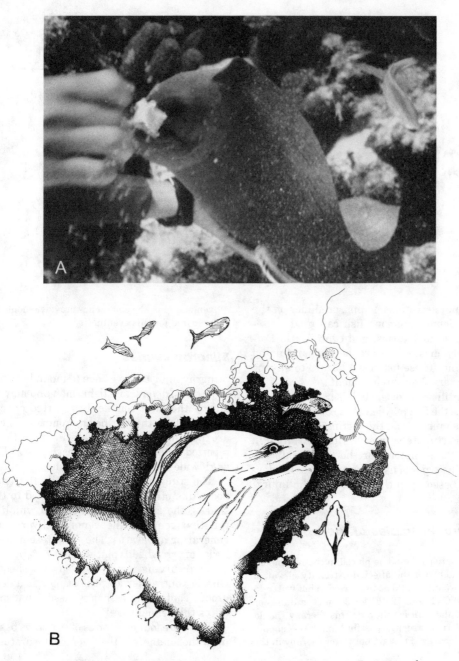

**Figure 7.25.** **A**, green moray eel (courtesy of Bob Koester); **B**, moray eel.

jects. The result is usually a significant laceration for the unwary diver.

Treatment of the bite is usually straightforward management of the trauma. As in the bite of the moray eel, major vessel injury and amputation usually are not found. Barracuda bites are marked by v-shaped or parallel lacerations. The wounds should be cul-tured and infections treated on the basis of the culture.

## STINGS

There are many fish that are equipped with defensive venomous spines that can penetrate human skin. The venom may be from

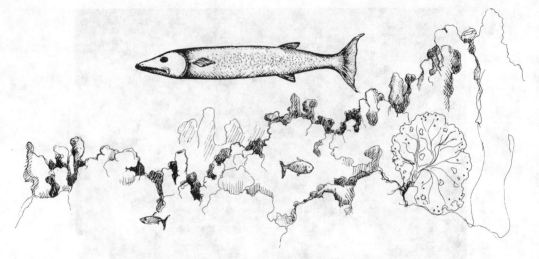

**Figure 7.26.** Barracuda.

glandular secretions, foams, or slimes on the spine. Some venomous fish can produce serious painful injuries, and even death. Fortunately, most stings are merely painful and irritating. These fish are a hazard to anyone who enters their environment.

Identification of the fish is not always possible, as the fish may leave the area, the water may be murky, and the victim is usually excited. Fortunately, there is little variation in either the symptoms or the treatment. The offending types of fish can sometimes be identified, based upon the location of the injury.

### General Principles of Therapy

The patient should be placed in the recumbent position with the affected extremity elevated. The wound should be immersed in hot water 45 to 50°C (113 to 122°F) for 30 to 90 minutes or until the pain is relieved. This therapy should be started as soon as possible, and EMTs should be encouraged to start hot water therapy in the field.

The area should be cleansed and copiously irrigated with normal saline solution. Obvious fragments of spines or surrounding sheaths should be removed if easily accomplished.

Symptomatic therapy for the intense pain is often needed. If hot water therapy does not work, local infiltration of the wound with lidocaine or systemic analgesics may be required.

Therapy for hypotension, shock, and respiratory depression may be needed in severe en-

venomations; the emergency provider should be prepared for this eventuality.

### Stingray Injuries

Stingray injuries have been found in bathers, swimmers, divers, and fishermen and may be among the most commonly reported envenomations from the marine environment. There are thought to be about 1500 stingray attacks reported in the United States each year.[10] The worldwide incidence is unknown.

The stingray has a horizontally flattened body, like other rays. Closely related to the sharks, the stingray has a barbed whiplike tail that contains the venom delivery and generating apparatus. The sting resembles a series of arrowheads placed point to tail, with sharp recurving teeth enclosed in a sheath. On the ventral surface, the sting has a deep groove containing a spongy tissue that produces the venom (see Fig 7.27).

There are four categories of stingrays based upon the anatomy of their venom apparatus[11]:

The gymnuriad has a small 2.5 cm spine located close to the base of a small caudal appendage. The sting is a small, poorly developed striking weapon. The butterfly ray is typical of this category (*Gymnura* sp.).

The urolophid has a short muscular caudal appendage and a 4 cm spine or sting in the adult. The round stingrays (*Urolophus* sp.) are examples of this type.

The mylobatid, or eagle ray (*Aetobatus* sp., *Myliobatis* sp., and *Rhinoptera* sp.), has a long

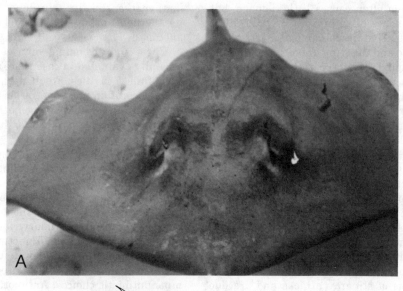

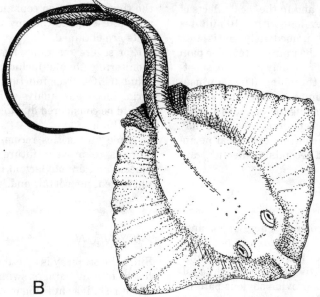

**Figure 7.27.** **A**, southern stingray (courtesy of Bob Koester); **B**, stingray.

whiplike tail and a moderate dual sting of up to 12 cm located at the base of the tail.

The dasyatid type, or true stingray, has a large sting of up to 37 cm at the base of a long whiplike tail. This sting is located farther from the base of the tail and is an effective striking organ.

Stingrays are bottom feeders and are often found buried or lying on the bottom. The usual attack occurs when the unwary person steps on the buried ray.[12] The attack as such is strictly defensive and occurs on the leg or ankle. Rarely, the ray may lash out as a swimmer or diver passes. In these victims, the spine may penetrate a body cavity such as the abdomen or chest, causing potentially fatal injuries.[13-15]

## VENOMOUS EFFECTS

When the sting enters the body, it may cause either a laceration or a puncture wound. The penetration often causes little damage, but serrated edges often prevent withdrawal or cause extensive tissue damage. Parts of the sheathing and the sting are often left behind in the wound. The force of the sting may be sufficient even to penetrate shoes.

Stingray venom contains toxic, high molecular weight proteins: seratonin, 5-nucleotidase, and phosphodiesterase. It appears to be heat labile and has an $LD_{50}$ of about 28 mg/kg. Generalized symptoms include nausea, vomiting, and diarrhea. Envenomations are associated with variable atrioventricular conduction blocks, bradycardia, hypotension, and signs of cardiac ischemia. A variable amount of respiratory depression is noted with large amounts of venom.[16] Rarely reported are paralysis, arrhythmias, or death.[17]

The local symptoms usually predominate in victims of stingray attacks and are due both to the trauma and to the local effects of the venom. Pain develops within 10 minutes of the attack, usually immediately, and is often out of proportion to the injury noted. The pain has been described variously as sharp, shooting, spasmodic, or throbbing. The pain usually peaks by 90 minutes and may last as long as 48 hours. Surrounding the wound is a dusky hemorrhagic and edematous area that may extend for several centimeters. Local necrosis, ulceration, and secondary infections are common sequelae.

## TREATMENT

Treatment is supportive. There is no antivenom. Submersion of the area in hot water (42 to 45°C (107.6 to 113°F) for 30 to 90 minutes will likely inactivate the heat-labile soluble toxin and does provide obvious pain relief. This heat treatment should be started as soon as possible, preferably before the ambulance is called, and should be maintained until either 90 minutes has elapsed or the pain has completely resolved. Use of other solutions, such as papaine, potassium permanganate, and meat tenderizer, is anecdotal and unproven. Potentially more trauma may result from these solutions than from the poison.

Local infiltration of lidocaine without epinephrine may provide pain relief. Some authorities also advocate encouragement of bleeding from the site of the sting and a proximal venoconstrictive tourniquet. These latter therapies are essentially unstudied and anecdotal.

Chest and abdominal injuries should be carefully evaluated in case there is penetration of these cavities. Frequently, the effects of the laceration and penetration injury will outweigh any possible envenomation in these locations. Rapid treatment for hypotension and hypovolemia is essential.

The wound should be debrided carefully and irrigated copiously. Sheathing should be removed if possible. X-ray or xeroradiography may detect parts of the stinger, allowing for easier removal. Wounds should generally be closed by delayed primary closure rather than primary suturing. Puncture wounds should not be sutured. The wound should be cultured and culture results used to determine antibiotic choices. Antibiotics, such as the third-generation cephalosporins, are appropriate empiric therapy until culture results are obtained.

For severe reactions, baseline laboratory monitoring should include complete blood count (CBC), liver function testing, and arterial blood gas analysis. ECG monitoring should be considered due to the possibility of arrhythmias.

Some authorities recommend the use of steroids to prevent future granuloma formation and anaphylactoid reactions. This is unstudied, anecdotal, and, as usual, controversial.

## PREVENTION

Since the stingray is a bottom feeder in shallow waters, all bathers, swimmers, and divers are at risk. If a shuffling motion is used while walking, the stingray will be alerted and have time to move before being stepped on.

### Sharks

There are two known species of venomous sharks (*Heterodontus franscisci* and *Heterodontus portusjacksoni* and the dogfish shark *Squalus acanthius*). These sharks have spines anterior to the two dorsal fins. The clinical syndrome is similar to that induced by the stingray. Generally, treatment should be similar to the stings of the stingray.

## Catfish

Fish stings in fresh water are most often caused by catfish. The incidence is unknown, and most stings are probably not reported. Because catfish stings occur when the animal is handled or excited, they often involve the hands and arms.

Catfish are found in both fresh and salty waters. There are over 1000 species of catfish, most of which are freshwater varieties.[18] The name catfish comes from the "whiskers" or sensory barbels found about the mouth that are thought to represent the whiskers of a cat. These barbels are not the dangerous part of the fish.

The venom apparatus is located in the anterior portion of the dorsal fin and the two pectoral fins, on a single spine in each location.[19] These spines are sharp, may have retroserrated teeth, and are fixed in the extended position when the fins are erected. Like the stingray's sting, these spines are enveloped with a sheath that encloses glandular toxin-producing tissues.

As the sting enters the skin, the enveloping sheath is ruptured. The venom-producing tissue is exposed and releases venom into the wound. The marine catfish is thought to have a more serious sting than the freshwater catfish, but this may be merely a factor of size.

One species, an electric catfish, can discharge electric current through the water to kill prey and defend itself.

### VENOMOUS EFFECTS

The effects of catfish stings are comparable to a mild stingray envenomation. Variously described as stinging, burning, or throbbing, the pain is out of proportion to the small puncture wound usually found. The pain peaks in about 30 minutes, and small species may cause effects lasting only 2 to 3 hours. Large tropical animals, such as *Plotusus* sp., may cause discomfort for up to 48 hours. The wound generally has an ischemic, dusky margin that gradually resolves and progresses to a hyperemic reactive area about the site of the sting. Those species with recurved teeth may inflict significant lacerations.

Systemic effects include nausea, muscle spasm, sweating, and muscle fasciculations.

Radicular pain in the affected limb is not uncommon. Rarely, and generally only with saltwater catfish stings, syncope, hypotension, respiratory distress, and death have been noted.[10,20] Secondary infections are common and lymphedema, lymphadenopathy, and lymphangitis may all be found. Localized necrosis due to infection may be seen in inadequately treated stings.

### TREATMENT

Treatment of the catfish sting should be exactly as that given to a victim of a stingray sting. Hot water will inactivate the heat-labile toxin and will afford significant pain relief.

Local infiltration of lidocaine without epinephrine may provide pain relief. Some authorities also advocate encouragement of bleeding from the site of the sting and a proximal venoconstrictive tourniquet. These latter therapies are essentially unstudied and anecdotal.

Radiographic identification and surgical exploration may be needed for spine and investing sheath fragments. Primary closure of the wound is not recommended. Delayed primary closure may afford the best cosmetic and surgical results.

## Scorpion Fish

Among the venomous fish of the world, the *Scropaenidae* family is considered to be most dangerous, both in the severity and the number of injuries produced.[21] These fish range from ornately colored to drably camouflaged. Most species are colored to blend in with their environment. They inhabit shallow waters and tidepool areas in the tropics and warm temperate areas.

This tropical fish group has several hundred species that are generally divided into three large groups on the basis of the venom delivery apparatus:

Zebrafish (*Pterois*, which includes the turkey-fish, lionfish, and butterfly cod) have long slender spines with a thin sheath and small venom glands. These fish probably have the least noxious venom in the entire group. Zebrafish are among the most beautiful and ornate fish found in coral reefs. They are shallow-water fish often found in crevices. Lionfish are imported in large numbers for aquariums and commercial fish collections because of their coloration.

Scorpionfish (*Scorpaena*, which includes the sculpin and the bullrout) have long heavy spines, a thick investing sheath, and a moderate-sized venom gland associated with each of the spines. These fish dwell in bottom water about bays, rocky coastlines, sandy beaches, or coral reefs. They dwell from tidewater to the 50 m level.

Stonefish (*Synanceja*, including the nohu, and the warty ghoul) have a very thick covering sheath, large, well-developed venom glands, and short, thick spines. These fish are generally considered to have the most dangerous venom in the entire group. Indeed, stonefish venom is thought to be similar to cobra venom in neurotoxicity. Stonefish are shallow water dwellers found in tidepools, shoal reefs, and holes or buried in mud or sand.

Although species characteristics differ, their general makeup of the venom delivery apparatus is similar. There are between 12 and 13 spines located in the dorsal area, 2 pelvic spines, and 3 anal spines for a total of 18 spines. The pectoral spines do not have venom glands. Each spine is covered with an investing sheath and has two anterolateral grooves for venom to travel from the paired venom glands at the spine's base. The venom is injected by puncture through the skin. The skin tears the investing sheath and may break the spine. The venom is released directly into the wounds.

When the fish are disturbed or stepped upon, the dorsal spines are erected. The clinical presentation is usually one of two scenarios. Either the unknowledgeable marine aquarist handles an imported tropical lionfish in a home aquarium or a bather, fisherman, or diver steps on one of the buried species. Thus, the envenomation may occur either on the foot or hand.

## TOXIC EFFECTS

The severity of the envenomation will depend upon the number of stings, amount of venom instilled, species, and underlying health of the victim. As noted earlier, stonefish venom is the most dangerous, with lionfish venom being least dangerous. The zebrafish *Pterois volitans* and the California scorpionfish *Scorpaena guttata* are thought to be capable of producing envenomation similar to that produced by the stonefish.[18] Symptoms produced by the various species are similar, varying only in degree rather than in quality.

The major toxic component is thought to be a high molecular weight protein that is heat labile.[22] In experimental animals, this venom will produce hypotension, vasodilation, and both muscular and respiratory paralysis.[23,24] The venom is thought to remain fully potent for up to 48 hours after death, so dead fish are to be considered equally dangerous.

Following the puncture wound, the immediate symptom is intense pain with a central radiation from the wound. The pain reaches greatest intensity in about 60 to 90 minutes and may persist as long as 6 to 12 hours. Stonefish venom may cause pain for several days. The pain is often described as intense, sharp, shooting, or throbbing.

The wound edges becomes cyanotic, with a surrounding erythema and swelling. Wound sloughing and secondary infections may follow this local damage. Wounds are indolent and may take weeks or months to heal, leaving granulomas and tissue defects in their wake.

In *Synanceja* stings, symptoms are more serious. Wounds produced by *Synanceja* may be markedly painful. The victims may scream, thrash about, and finally lose consciousness. The wound and surrounding area may become numb. These paresthesias may persist for weeks. Further from the wound, the skin may become painful to touch.

Infrequently noted distant symptoms may include nausea, vomiting, diaphoresis, convulsions, respiratory distress, cardiac failure, and death.[10,25,26] Paralysis, respiratory failure, tachycardia, bradycardia, and ischemic electrocardiographic changes are also seen. Death in humans generally occurs within the first 6 to 8 hours.

## TREATMENT

Since the venom is a heat-labile protein, the wound should be immediately immersed in hot water—45°C (113°F). The protein is also inactivated by extremes of pH, hydrogen peroxide, iodine, and potassium permanganate.[27,28] (Unfortunately, these extreme pH changes and other substances are tissue toxic.) It is problematic whether more tissue damage is done by these substances or by the venom. Although multiple authors have advocated addition of papaine, meat tenderizer, or other substances to the hot water, these are entirely anecdotal reports and without substantiating evidence.

Local infiltration of lidocaine without epinephrine may provide pain relief and allow better debridement of the spines. Some authorities also advocate encouragement of bleeding from the sting site and a proximal venoconstrictive tourniquet. The efficiency of these latter therapies is essentially unstudied and anecdotal.

A stonefish antivenom is manufactured by the Commonwealth Serum Laboratories in Melbourne, Australia. It is manufactured from horse serum and has the usual risks and contraindications as discussed in Part 4.[29] Stonefish antivenom is indicated when the patient has no pain relief following heat treatment, local injection of anesthetic, or intravenous analgesics. It should also be used if substantial systemic symptoms are present. Relief is usually obtained within 20 minutes after intravenous injection of antivenom.[30]

The antivenom should be given intravenously in a dose of 1 or 2 ampule. (One ampule is thought to be effective neutralization for two significant punctures.) Stonefish antivenom is available in the United States from the Health Services Department of Sea World (California: 619-222-6363 ext. 2201 or Ohio: 216-562-8101). Local poison control centers may have additional information.

Wounds should be appropriately examined for spine fragments with the aid of radiography or xeroradiography. Copious irrigation of the wound should be done in all cases. Debridement of spine and investing sheath fragments will prevent wound infections and late granuloma formation. Debridement will also decrease the amount of venom absorbed. Care should be taken during debridement to remove any pieces of the investing sheath of the spine as well as the calcific spines.

Serious systemic symptoms should be treated appropriately. Cardiac monitoring is appropriate in view of the electrocardiographic changes and dysrhythmias occasionally seen. Other measures will depend upon the specific symptoms seen.

## Weeverfish

Weeverfish (*Trachinus* species) are the temperate-water analogues of the scorpionfish. They are found in the Mediterranean Sea, the Eastern Atlantic regions, and the European coastal areas from Norway to the Baltic, including the British Isles.

A short and stout fish, the weeverfish also buries itself in the mud or sand while waiting for prey. When the unsuspecting bather steps on the fish, dorsal spines pierce the foot and release venom. Another set of spines is located on the gill covers in these fish. When the weeverfish is provoked, the gill covers are expanded with their spines and the dorsal spines erected. The spines are covered with an investing sheath that contains venom, which is similar to the stingray's sting. Weeverfish spines rarely break off in tissues.

Weeverfish stings produce intense pain, usually described as burning or stabbing and occasionally as crushing. The pain is normally confined to the area of the wound and the affected limb. Peaking within 30 to 60 minutes, it may last as long as 24 hours at peak intensity and then gradually subside. The victim may thrash about, scream, or lose consciousness due to the intensity of the pain. Rare systemic symptoms include bradycardia, convulsions, respiratory failure, and death.[31]

The wounds may blanch, followed by erythema, heat, ecchymosis, and swelling. Local wound infections are common and gangrene has been reported. Marked limb edema is not uncommon and may persist for weeks after the sting.

### TREATMENT

Treatment should be the same as for a stingray sting. The venom appears to respond well to hot water therapy if started immediately.[32] Local and systemic analgesia are appropriate therapies for those patients where hot water has not been used immediately or has been ineffective. Lidocaine infiltration into the wound may effectively relieve the pain and allow local wound exploration.[33]

Puncture wounds should not be sutured. The wounds should be copiously irrigated and explored for spine and sheath fragments. Antibiotics are controversial and should probably be based upon culture results.

### Starfish

The only starfish known to be poisonous is the crown-of-thorns, found in the Indo-Pacific area. This is a large animal, as much as 60 cm in diameter, with between 13 and 16 rays. The dorsal surface is studded with sharp, poisonous spines.

The local effects include the effects of the puncture wound and localized swelling and intense pain. The spines contain a reddish pigment that stains the tissues. Systemic effects include nausea and vomiting, which often occur hours after the injury. Some authors also ascribe paralysis and numbness to envenomations from this animal.

Treatment is symptomatic with removal of the spines, followed by thorough wound cleansing. Anesthesia may be necessary and radiologic examination may assist in ensuring that all spines are removed. Immediate pain relief may usually be obtained by immersion of the area in hot water although, for some patients, parenteral analgesics may be necessary.

Infections are common in these puncture wounds with cellulitis, granuloma formation, lymphangitis, and rarely sepsis. Wounds should be cultured and treatment based upon the organisms isolated from the culture. Late granuloma formation may be treated as appropriate.

### Sea Urchins

Sea urchins are elongated or globular echinoderms that have a thin calcified shell, long spines, and/or triple-jawed pedicellariae. The spines are brittle and may impale the unwary diver or swimmer, breaking off during the process. The pedicellariae are small, seizing organs attached to stalks that are scattered among the spines.

Some species of sea urchins have venom sacs on the tips of the spines. Alternatively, the pedicellariae may attach and inject venom from large venom glands on the jaws. Once the pedicellarium attaches to the victim, it will continue to inject venom until it is removed or the venom sac is empty. Sea urchin venom includes cholinergic substances, serotonin, proteases, and hemolysins.

The sea urchin is a nocturnal creature and injuries often occur during night dives or dark waters. Sea caves or shallow turbulent waters also pose increased risks. Tidepool explorers may also encounter sea urchins. The most common injury is a puncture wound from the spines, when the victim steps on, handles, or brushes against the sea urchin.

Symptoms of the envenomation include severe burning pain and discoloration. Pain is related to the number of spines in the wound. Systemic symptoms are uncommon, unless infection supravenes. Delayed secondary infections and indolent ulcerations are common following punctures. In those species with pedicellariae, systemic symptoms are more common and may include malaise, weakness, paresthesias, hyposthesias, paralysis, arthralgias, aphonia, and, rarely, respiratory distress, hypotension, or death. In most cases, the pain will subside somewhat in 1 to 2 hours, and localized muscle weakness may persist for 4 to 6 hours if present.

Secondary granuloma formation may occur 2 or more months after the original injury. A more diffuse inflammatory process is often found in finger or toe lesions. Actual fusiform swelling and discoloration of the affected digit are noted.

### TREATMENT

Treatment of sea urchin spine injuries is controversial. There are two significant injuries to consider in treatment of sea urchin stings: puncture wounds and envenomation due to either spine or pedicellariae.

### Puncture wounds

Embedded spines may be removed if accessible. Radiographic localization of the spines should be accomplished before removal if possible. Use of operating microscopes and bloodless fields will greatly aid the removal process.

Some local authorities may recommend pounding the affected areas to break up the unremoved spines. This should be condemned as it increases the chances for foreign body reaction and infections. Subsequent removal of the spine fragments is far more difficult. A chronic inflammatory process resulting from the spine fragments in either hand or foot is disastrous.

Although the use of vinegar or other organic solvents to dissolve spines is an attractive option, it is also ineffective. The vinegar does not penetrate into the tissues and may enhance the toxicity of the spine.

Sea urchin spine puncture wounds can also cause secondary infection and purely mechanical injuries to nerves or joints. If the spine has entered a joint cavity or is in close proximity to neurovascular structures, an operating microscope will facilitate removal.

Secondary granuloma formations should generally be excised, since there are few that heal spontaneously. Steroids injected into the granuloma are often recommended, but evidence is entirely anecdotal. Systemic steroids have even less useful evidence of efficacy.

## Envenomation

It is clear that hot water (110 to 115°F or 43 to 46°C for 30 to 90 minutes) will relieve the pain of the toxin. This therapy will inactivate heat-labile components of the venom and may reverse vasospasm from the toxin. Thorough cleansing of the wound is likewise beneficial in all cases. Any detached pedicellariae may be removed by shaving foam and a razor.

## Cone Shells

The cone shell is an attractive multicolored mollusk, common about Hawaii, Mexico, and California. Cone shells can be found in shallow waters, reefs, and tidepools. The alluring colors of these univalve shells tempt both children and adults to pick them up, with disastrous results. Practically all reported envenomations by cone shells have been collectors or children (see Fig. 7.28).

Cone shells are nocturnal predators that kill their prey with a neurotoxin. The venom interferes with neuromuscular transmission in a manner similar to curare and is otherwise poorly investigated.

The cone shell delivers its venom with a long proboscus extendible from the narrow end of the shell. The proboscus carries from 1 to 20 rasplike "teeth" that are previously inoculated with venom.[34] These harpoon-like teeth penetrate and inject the venom into the prey. Of the 400 or so species of cone shells, 18 have caused human envenomation. Cone shells that feed upon fish or other mollusks appear to be more dangerous than the other species.

Initial symptoms of cone shell intoxication include stinging or burning sensation at the site of the sting. This initial pain is often followed by a localized ischemia, cyanosis, and numbness about the wound. The numbness and tingling sensation will spread to the rest of the body with prominent circumoral involvement. Dysphagia and dysphonia are noted first and then generalized skeletal muscle paralysis ensues. Blurry vision, diplopia, pruritis, and nausea may also be noted. The paralysis may be incomplete, with the patient describing only weakness, or may include respiratory paralysis. Respiratory paralysis may cause apnea, unconsciousness, and death.[35] These changes take place in about 10 to 30 minutes after the sting. Infrequently, a coagulopathy has been noted following this intoxication, but this is not well described.

Treatment is entirely supportive. There is no antidote. Marine first aid texts may recommend ligature and removal of the venom by sucking. This technique is unproven and may be dangerous to the first responder. The Australian technique of circumferential pressure dressings has also been advocated and likewise is unproven. It is logical to presume that slowed absorption of the venom may allow the victim to reach competent help. Certainly, wrapping the extremity will cause no long-term harm to either the rescuer or victim. Hot water is thought to provide some pain relief and may inactivate some of the heat-labile toxin.[36] Use of hot water is unproven but should cause no harm, provided care is taken not to burn the victim.

Treatment of the puncture site should be the same as for any other puncture wound. The wound should be cleansed and debrided. Radiographic examination may disclose radular teeth in the wound, but the teeth are frequently not found. Tetanus prophylaxis should be provided as for any dirty wound.

Intubation may be required for airway support in severe cases. Local anesthetics may provide pain relief about the sting. Respiratory stimulants and neuromuscular-blockade reversing agents are not useful in treatment of this poisoning.

If the patient survives the respiratory arrest, recovery is apparent within 24 hours. Minor sequelae at the site of the sting may persist for 2 to 3 weeks after the sting.

Contrary to myth, the "large" end of the cone shell is not safe. The proboscus may be able to reach all parts of the shell and inject venom. Collectors should use forceps and a

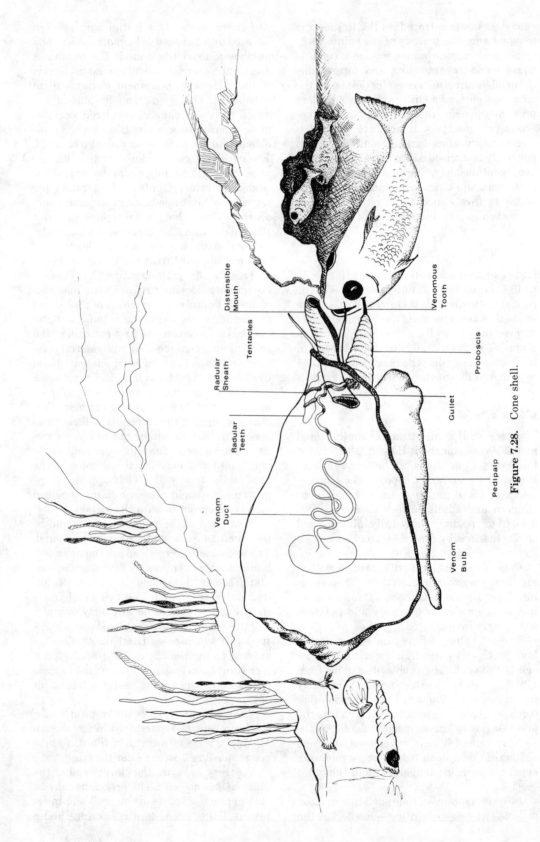

Distensible Mouth

Venomous Tooth

Tentacles

Proboscis

Radular Sheath

Gullet

Radular Teeth

Pedipalp

Venom Duct

Venom Bulb

**Figure 7.28.** Cone shell.

hard bucket to gather these shells. Children should be advised not to pick up these pretty

---

*Recommended Treatment of*
*Cone Shell Stings*

1. Apply circumferential elastic bandages to the area.
2. If available, immerse the area in 45°C water during transport to medical facility.
3. Provide appropriate airway and respiration support.
4. Continue to reassure the patient.
5. Give pain medication as appropriate.
6. Intubation may be needed for respiratory arrest.

---

## CNIDARIA

The *Coelenterata* (also termed *Cnidaria*) are considered to be an organized colonial animal, with specialized smaller animals grouped together to benefit the entire colony, but each cell replicates independently. The phylum is subdivided into three classes. The first, *Hydrozoa*, includes the Portuguese man-of-war, fire coral, and hydroids. The fresh water hydra belongs to this class. Jellyfish comprise the second class, *Scyphozoa*. These are all marine animals. Though of larger size than the *Hydrozoans*, they are less complex. The third class, the *Anthozoa*, includes the sea anemones and the true corals. The latter are the most complex of the marine *Coelenterata*. There are a few fresh water *coelenterates*, but none are capable of injuring humans.

In the ocean, much of life revolves around the *coelenterates*. Tidepools contain anemones and bright hydroids. The shallows contain huge, brightly colored polyps shaped like flowers, massive banks of reef-building corals, and colonial polyps. These banks of coral cover every square inch of bottom area and climb toward the surface, much as the trees dominate the forest.

The term *coelenterate* means hollow tube, which describes the general organization of these animals into an inner digestive and circulatory layer of cells and an outer specialized layer of cells. Two general forms of *Coelenterata* exist, a hydroid form and a medusae form. In the reproductive cycle of some *Coelenterata*, they may change from one form to the other (see Fig. 7.29).

The medusae is a free-floating inverted bag or dome-shaped organism with tentacles about margins of the open inverted end. The mouth is the open end. The medusae forms are frequently generically called jellyfish, even though they may come from several classes within the *Coelenterata* family. These animals propel themselves by rhythmic pulsations of the dome, expelling water through the mouth.

The hydroid or polyp form is generally attached to a surface at the caudal or arboral end and has a mouth and tentacles on the free end. Biology students are familiar with the shape of the fresh water hydra, typical of the hydroid form of the coelenterates. Other typical polyp forms are the fire corals (*Hydrozoa* class), stinging hydroids, feather hydroids, sea anemones, and sea corals (*Anthrozoana* class). Generally, the *Scyphozoa* or jellyfish do not assume this form or assume it only during early stages of reproduction. *Anthozoans* have no medusa stage and exist only in the more complex hydroid form. Reproduction may be either asexual or sexual.

Despite many structural differences, all *Cnidaria* have similar nematocysts that they use to incapacitate their prey while they envelop, kill, and digest it. The *Coelenterata* phylum contains more venomous species than any other invertebrates. Fortunately, of the 9000 members of the *Coelenterata*, only about 70 have the ability to penetrate human skin and cause toxicity.[37] The *Coelenterata* and related *Siponophores* are responsible for more stings in North American waters than any other animals.

### NEMATOCYSTS

There are two types of nematocyst. One type produces a sticky substance used for immobilization of the prey, while the other delivers venom through a barbed stinger. The nematocysts are found in greatest numbers on the long filamentlike tentacles and about the mouth. The long, entangling tentacles tend to perpetuate the stings until removed.

The venomous nematocyst is contained within a capsule or cnidoblast to which is attached a pointed trigger, the cnidocil. Within the cnidoblast is a sharply pointed, coiled thin tube, sitting within a pool of venom. Stimulation of the cnidocil—either by osmotic pressure changes or direct pressure—allows the operculum or opening to release the coiled thread explosively outwards. The pointed thread extends to between 200 and 400 microns and is said to penetrate even a surgical glove.[38] The viscous venom is adherent to the thread and is carried along as the point penetrates into the upper dermis and injected through the body of the hollow tubule. Only those nematocysts stimulated respond by discharging their venom.

The severity of the coelenterate envenomation is related to the toxicity of the venom, the dose of venom delivered, and the condition of the victim. The dose of venom delivered is governed by the number of nematocysts that have discharged into the victim. Jellyfish nematocyst venom has not been completely analyzed and is a complex mixture of toxic and antigenic polypeptides and enzymes. Physical reactions to nematocyst venom range from a mild dermatitis with some jellyfish to rapid death in the cases of Australia's famous Chironex or "box jellyfish." The reactions can be toxic or allergic or a combination of the two. Allergic reactions are not unlike those found with insect envenomation and are treated in a similar manner. The toxic reactions can be further subdivided into systemic reactions and local reactions.

The most common syndrome resulting from contact with a coelenterate sting is that of a painful, linear, urticarial reaction at the site of the contact with the tentacles. The medusae forms may wrap the tentacles about the body and cause extensive lesions. The hydroid forms tend to have smaller lesions. The eruption starts as a linear, blanched area that progresses to urticaria and erythema. Following envenomation, the area involved will become bright red, followed by a brownish-purple coloration, corresponding to the areas of "tentacle prints." The skin rash will persist for as long as 7 days.

Other lesions noted include vesicular, hemorrhagic necrotizing, or ulcerative areas of varying duration.[39] Lymphadenopathy, peripheral nerve lesions, renal failure, fatty atrophy, contractures, vasospasm, and limb ischemia all have been seen after these stings.[40-44] If the nematocysts strike the eyes, corneal ulcerations and conjunctivitis are common.[45]

Because the pain occurs rapidly and is not associated with immunity production after repeated contact, it is felt that the sting's pain is a local toxic reaction. This pain may be due to kininlike substances found in the venom.

Rarely, the cutaneous reaction may recur months or years after the event.[46] These recurrent episodes are apparently associated more frequently with oceanic *Physalia* species.[47] The etiology is thought to be an immunologic response triggered by a sequestered antigen or by exposure to a similar cross-reacting venom.

Systemic reactions may include paresthesias, headache, abdominal cramps, nausea, vomiting, chills, fever, and weakness. In severe envenomations, pallor and cyanosis may precede respiratory distress, cardiovascular collapse, hypotension, shock, and sudden death. The latter is particularly common in envenomation from *Cubomedusae* or sea wasp, also better called the *Chironex* species. This coelenterate has caused death within moments of envenomation.

## SPECIFIC COELENTERATES

Toxicologic research on coelenterates has concentrated on only a few species. These include the Portuguese man-of-war, the sea nettle, and the sea wasp.

### Portuguese Man-of-War

Siphonophores are free-floating creatures with a small, inflated crest that allows them mobility in the winds. The pale blue or pink and bluish-violet crest is filled with carbon monoxide and nitrogen. Typical in this group of animals are the Portuguese man-of-war, *Physalia physalis* (thought to resemble a Portuguese admiral's hat). The Atlantic Portuguese man-of-war is about three to four times larger than the Pacific species (3 to 5 inches versus 12 to 16 inches of body length [8 to 13 cm vs 30 to 40 cm]). The tentacles of the Atlantic species have been measured to be as long as 100 feet (30 m). The tentacles are usually contracted and form folds known as stinging batteries. As the animal moves in the water, the tentacles contract and relax as they sample the water for potential prey. The smaller Pacific version, *Physalia utriculus*, or "blue bottle jellyfish," usually has only a single fishing tentacle of up to 15 feet (5 m).

Unfortunately, the inflated crest also enables these animals to be blown onto shores during storms. Since the jellyfish is a fragile creature, the surf tends to break them up into

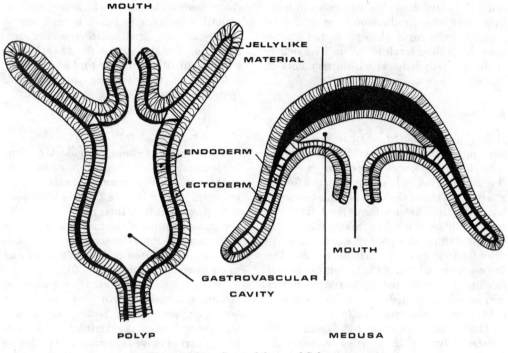

**Figure 7.29.** General forms of Colentera.

smaller pieces. The pieces retain their sting-ing abilities for hours after being washed up, adding to the problems. Children and beach-combers should be advised not to handle the beached jellyfish.

The venom from these animals is toxic to humans and causes frequent and severe sys-temic reactions. Rare deaths are thought to be due to massive envenomations (usually in children) or allergic reactions.

### True Jellyfish (Scyphozoa)

The true jellyfish may be armed with some of the most potent venom available on earth. Fortunately, most species are simply unable to penetrate human dermis. The jellyfish ranges in size from a small jellyfish of a few millimeters to the giant jellyfish (*Cyanea capillata*) of greater than 2 m in width across the bell, with tentacles of up to 120 feet (40 m). The most dangerous of these, the box or cuboid jellyfish, is discussed separately be-low. Lesser species such as *Chrysora quin-quecirrha*, the sea nettle, are still capable of a severe sting (see Fig. 7.29).

Recent research focusing on the sea nettle has shown the venom to contain at least seven different enzymes, histamine, prostaglan-dins, serotonin, and kininlike factors. The en-zymes include at least one cardiotoxic, neu-rotoxic, and dermatotoxic component.[48] With all but the box jellyfish, death is exceedingly rare after envenomation

### Box Jellyfish

The box jellyfish, variously known as *Chi-ronex fleckeri*, sea wasp, box jellyfish, or fire medusae, is one of the most toxic animals in the sea and can kill a healthy adult human. *Chironex fleckeri* is found along the northern shores of Australia and in the western Indo-Pacific area. A cousin, *Chiropsalmus quad-rigatus*, is also found in the same area and has been held responsible for numerous fa-talities. These two jellyfish have been re-sponsible for one or more fatalities per year since 1900. A close morphologic and antigenic relationship exists between these two species; consequently it is difficult to separate one clinical envenomation from the other.

Box jellyfish venom has direct cardiotox-icity and weak hemolytic properties and is a powerful local necrotic agent.[49,50] CNS tox-icity has also been noted in animals.[51] Because the jellyfish applies its venom in multiple injections simultaneously over a wide area, there is rapid absorption and subsequent high blood levels of venom. The venom of the box jellyfish acts within moments of contact.

## Fire Coral

Widely distributed in warmer waters, the stinging corals or hydrocorals are not true corals but are also members of the group *Anthozoa*. These animals are found in two forms, a large branching skeleton of limestone or a low encrusting skeleton form. The latter form is generally harmless. The infamous fire coral of the Atlantic, *Millepora alcicornis*, is a hydrocoral. In the western Atlantic regions, the fire corals may be major contributors to reef formation. Unprotected divers and swimmers may handle or walk about on these reefs with subsequent unpleasant results.

The fire coral possesses two different specialized polyps. A large polyp with a wide mouth serves as a feeding structure for the colony, while a smaller polyp contains the nematocysts and has no digestive function. Both protrude from numerous minute gastropores in the animal's surface.

Symptoms of fire coral envenomation include immediate pain, which is often described as similar to being burned with a "white-hot" iron. Small, raised, reddened areas appear on the skin at the site of each sting within 1 to 10 hours after contact. The pain is localized to the sting and usually persists from 1 to 4 days.

## Sea Anemones

Sea anemones are sessile, cnidarian carnivores usually found attached to rocks or the sea bottom. Most anemones will extrude their tentacles, giving them a flower-like appearance. Anemones have their nematocysts about the inner margins of the mouth and the tentacles, and the tentacles serve to incapacitate the various fish and invertebrates the anemone preys upon (see Fig. 7.30).

Most sea anemone stings occur when swimmers brush against them in shallow water, but, occasionally, facial injuries result when an individual is examining an anemone and a current moves anemone and bather together. The sting is similar to all other forms of coelenterate envenomations with linear lesions where the tentacle nematocysts fire. Because of the anemone's smaller body, the lesions are generally smaller. Sea anemone stings are usually milder and more localized

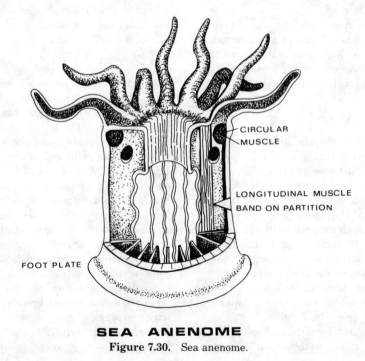

CIRCULAR MUSCLE

LONGITUDINAL MUSCLE BAND ON PARTITION

FOOT PLATE

**SEA ANENOME**
**Figure 7.30.** Sea anenome.

in their effects than the jellyfish stings. Systemic signs are rarely found following anemone stings.[52]

## CORAL

True stony coral exists in colonies that have a calcified outer skeleton, frequently with sharp edges. Envenomation from coral is usually insignificant and, normally, coral produces a cut or abrasion as the swimmer brushes against it. Small animals and flakes of calcium will frequently break off into the wound. The resulting "coral poisoning" is an indolent wound that may take a while to heal. The initial presentation is a red, indurated, pruritic area about the abrasion. This frequently progresses into a local cellulitis.

Coral cuts must be debrided of all pieces of calcium and coral tissue. Vigorous scrubbing with soap and water, followed by jet pressure irrigation, is recommended for these lesions. All major wounds should be cultured and treated with dilute antiseptics such as povidone-iodine or bacitracin. Improperly cleansed wounds may progress into an ulcerated tissue slough.

## TREATMENT

Though the severity of a coelenterate envenomation is primarily determined by the species encountered, it is also dependent upon a host of other factors. The number of nematocysts activated also influences the intensity of the response. Even skin contact with the tentacles may cause only a few of the nematocysts to initially discharge. Mechanical or other stimuli may cause subsequent envenomation as the tentacle contracts, the victim moves, or the first aider attempts to remove the tentacle. Since the number of discharged nematocysts governs the severity of the reaction to a given species, first aid strategies should also focus on first defusing the remaining nematocysts.

Various folk remedies, including ethanol in varying concentrations and forms, meat tenderizer (papain), acetic acid, sodium bicarbonate, formalin, urine, various fruit juices, and boric acid, have been tried with equally varying degrees of success. The problem is compounded in that the agent that causes defusing of one species' nematocysts will cause discharge of another species. This has made

evaluation of these first aid remedies dependent upon proper identification of the offending animal.

For the box jellyfish and Portuguese man-of-war elegant experiments definitively showed that vinegar deactivates the nematocysts rapidly and irreversibly.[53,54] These experimenters simply took pieces of live tentacles of the jellyfish and dipped them in various solutions. They found that most acids and alcohol would cause massive and immediate discharge of the nematocysts. When the tentacle was subsequently applied to volunteers, both pain and reaction were noted and found to be less with vinegar than with other agents. Formalin was also found to be effective but it is too toxic for routine use. In similar experiments, a slurry of baking soda has been found to best inactivate the nematocysts of the sea nettle, *Chrysaora quinquecirrha*.[55,56]

Alcohol in varying forms is often proposed for first aid therapy to defuse the jellyfish nematocysts. The ready availability of alcoholic solutions on populated beaches combined with the need to "do something" has undoubtedly contributed to its popularity as a first aid agent. Evidence for its efficacy in the early treatment of jellyfish stings is anecdotal and rebutted by at least two controlled studies.[53,54] Since alcohol provokes immediate discharge of all nematocysts, it will ultimately defuse these species, but only at the expense of possible increased toxicity to the patient. For this reason, alcohol is inferior to vinegar as immediate therapy for treatment of these jellyfish stings. Part of the supposed pain relief for these agents may be due to the normal lessening of painful stimuli with time.

Other topical agents and drugs proposed have included ammonium hydroxide, urine, papain meat tenderizer, and sodium bicarbonate. These have not been subjected to close experimental scrutiny and should be viewed as anecdotal therapy only. A commercial aqueous solution of aluminum sulfate and surfactant (Stingose) has also been proposed, and its use is controversial. The one well-controlled study by Turner and his associates noted earlier found Stingose to be much less effective than the far cheaper vinegar solution.[54]

No systemic drugs are useful for detoxification of most common coelenterate stings.

Epinephrine and antihistamines are useful for patients with significant allergic components to the reaction. Intravenous verapamil has been proposed for use in severe systemic reactions from selected jellyfish stings, but there is no human clinical experience.[57,58] Nonsteroidal anti-inflammatory drugs have also been proposed and seem quite logical, but no controlled clinical study has been made using these agents.

For treatment of the potentially lethal box jellyfish stings, Commonwealth Serum Laboratories has produced an antivenom, CSL sea wasp antivenom, which has been effective against this particular coelenterate.[59] As with all serum antivenoms, delayed immune reactions are common. Monoclonal antibody preparations have been proposed. These preparations may allow the development of a single protective antivenin or vaccine for all jellyfish stings.

Once the wound has been soaked with the appropriate agents, the remaining nematocysts should be removed. Various methods have been proposed, including scraping and shaving the area with shaving cream or pastes of baking soda, flour, talc or soap.

Aggressive respiratory support may be necessary in some envenomations. As noted earlier, the toxins of both the box jellyfish and the man-of-war are respiratory depressants. The clinician must be prepared to manage this with intubation and artificial ventilation as needed.

Small children have been known to pick up tentacle fragments and suck on them, resulting in rapid and severe oral swelling. Subsequent airway obstruction may result and should be aggressively managed with early intubation before swelling mandates a surgical procedure. Use of intraoral vinegar can inactivate remnants of the tentacle. Airway control should be established before the use of this agent if the patient has any respiratory distress or is not alert.

Allergic responses may cause either airway swelling or bronchospasm. These are managed in the usual fashion with epinephrine, antihistamines, and bronchodilators. Intubation may be needed.

Hypotension may result from the sting, particularly at the extremes of age. In these cases, aggressive fluid replacement with a crystalloid is indicated. Fluid replacement in the elderly should be carefully monitored to ensure that they are not overloaded.

---

*Treatment for Coelenterate Stings*

1. **Protect Yourself!** Rescuer injuries are common.
Inactivate nematocysts if possible. Lifeguards and rescue personnel should carry quantities of species-specific inactivating agents and should know the current species about the local beaches. Rinsing the area with seawater may remove the tentacles and allow you to proceed safely.

2. **Assess airway, breathing, and circulation.**
Respiratory arrest appears to be common and responds to appropriate resuscitation efforts. These signs of systemic decompensation should be aggressively managed in the usual fashion. It should be obvious that this aggressive airway and circulatory support should be done simultaneously with limiting further inoculation of venom by inactivation of the nematocysts and continued until the patient is stabilized.

3. **Inactivate the nematocysts!**
Box jellyfish and man-of-war stings should be inactivated with vinegar or dilute acetic acid. Sea nettle stings should be inactivated with baking soda. Dilute solutions of ammonia, alcohols, and meat tenderizer pastes are poor second choices.

4. **Remove the tentacles.** Do not use your hands. A drying agent, such as baking soda, sand, or talc, may help in removal of the sticky tentacles. Shaving cream and a razor have also been used successfully.

5. **Control pain.** Topical anesthetic ointments or sprays may be useful after control of the nematocysts. Antihistamine creams or corticosteroid lotions are soothing and recommended by some. In severe envenomations, narcotics may be administered. Calcium gluconate or diazepam may be given intravenously for control of severe muscle spasm.

## Electric Rays

Electric rays (electric eels) are found in tropical and temperate waters. The animal feeds in relatively shallow depths and often is found submerged in sand or mud.

The size of the animal determines how much voltage the thick electric organs are able to deliver. The voltage may vary from 8 to as much as 200 volts and is delivered from the electronegative ventral side to the electropositive dorsal side. Tactile stimulation will provoke an involuntary discharge. Repeated discharges are weaker until a latent period is achieved.

Since water is a conductive medium, it is not necessary to be in contact with the electric ray. The shock can cause the distant effects of low voltage electric current, but most important for a diver is the potential for loss of conciousness while underwater. Drowning may result as a consequence. Since the diver is surrounded by water, thermal and arc effects are not seen.

Treatment is not usually required for those who have not lost consciousness. Recovery is most often uneventful, and the ray is usually considered a nuisance, rather than life threatening.

## BITES

### Sea Snakes

Sea snakes (family *Hydrophiidae*) are air-breathing reptiles that have adapted to the marine environment. They may be the most abundant reptiles in the world.[60] Sea snakes are found in the tropical and warm temperate Pacific and Indian oceans. There have been no sea snakes yet found in the Atlantic ocean or the Caribbean seas. The water about the southern tips of Africa and South America are too cold for survival of these reptiles. Sea snakes are only rarely found in fresh water.[61]

Sea snakes can be distinguished from eels by the their scales, nostrils, and lungs. In their adaptation to the ocean, the sea snake has developed two lungs, one of which extends the entire length of the snake's body. This elongated lung provides not only flotation for the snake but allows the snake to submerge for extended periods of time. The tail is flattened and paddle shaped and serves to propel the snake effectively through the water. These snakes are usually less than a meter long and are often brightly colored.

All sea snakes are venomous but are not aggressive and will usually bite only if provoked. Sea snake venom is a potent neurotoxin that causes muscle paralysis and respiratory failure that may lead to death. A second component to the venom may also cause myonecrosis. Recent studies have shown that the sea snake venoms are similar in structure and action to those of the elapid snakes, including the cobra.[62,63] Although the venom is quite toxic, only a small amount of venom is delivered.[64] Only about 20% of those who are bitten will develop symptoms, but of those who are symptomatic, the mortality is about 50% without treatment![64,65]

The venom delivery apparatus consists of two short, fixed fangs, venom ducts, and venom glands. The short fangs often are unable to penetrate a neoprene wetsuit. Bites are an occupational hazard for fishermen and a lesser risk to divers and swimmers in the Pacific and Indian oceans.

The clinical picture of sea snake envenomation is one of paralysis progressing to respiratory failure in the same manner as elapid venom. Myoglobinuria and hyperkalemia may be found in severe cases. Trismus, muscle spasms, ptosis, diplopia, and blurred vision are also noted in severe cases.[66-68] Cardiac arrhythmias due to hyperkalemia and hypoxia are not uncommon. Until hypoxia intervenes, there is no change in the level of consciousness.

Local reaction is variable but most often mild. In some cases, the patient may not note the bite. Muscle pains, first near the bite then at distant sites, are common within 2 hours of envenomation.

The only commercially available sea snake antivenin is manufactured by Commonwealth Serum Laboratories in Australia. This antivenom is manufactured from *Enhydrina schistosa* venom but is effective for *E. schistosa, Pelamis platurus, Hydrophis cyanocinctus, H. spiralis, Lapimis hardwickii, Praescuta viperina, Laticauda laticaudata,* and *Laticauda semifasciata* venoms. A usual starting dose for symptomatic patients is 2 to 4 ampules (2000 to 4000 units). Nonsymptomatic, but suspicious bites should prompt administration of 1 ampule intravenously and observation of the patient for 8 hours.

There is considerable cross-reactivity between sea snake venom and elapid venoms. Sea snake antivenom is also effective against the cobra (*Naja naja*) and other elapid snake venoms. Some antivenin for elapid snake bites is likewise effective for sea snake poisoning.[69] Tiger-snake antivenin is recommended by most Australian authorities if sea snake antinvenin is not available.[70] The usual starting dose is 4 ampules intravenously.[71] Antivenin is then titrated to relieve the paralysis. Symptoms should be relieved within 30 to 60 minutes.

**Preventative Measures for Sea Snake Bites**
1. In high-risk areas, wear protective clothing (such as neoprene wet suits).
2. Do not tease or play with sea snakes.

**First Aid Measures**
1. Immobilize the bitten extremity.
2. Apply a firm pressure dressing over the site.
3. Transport the patient to the hospital.

**Definitive Care Measures**
1. Give 3 to 4 ampules of antivenin IV.
2. Provide respiratory support as needed.
3. Monitor urinary output.
4. Monitor electrolytes and creatinine.
5. Observe patient for 8 hours.
6. In critical patients, consider hemodialysis.

### Blue-Ringed Octopus

Octopi belong to the same class of mollusks as squid and cuttlefish (*Cephalopoda*). Legends about giant octopi or squid and divers or sailor's deaths abound. Despite these horror stories, octopi and squid are shy, retiring creatures that pose little threat to humans (see Fig. 7.31).

Certain species of octopus will bite when trod upon or when picked up. The bite is inflicted by a hard, chitinous, parrotlike beak located in the central ventral surface of the animal. This beak extends out of the mouth for feeding and biting.

In most cases, the symptoms of an octopus bite are transient and mild. Redness, swelling, and itching are most commonly found. Some patients will develop local paresthesias and numbness. Systemic symptoms are noted only after a bite of the blue-ringed octopus (*Hapalochlaena maculosa*) and its close cousin (*H. lunulata*).

The blue-ringed octopus will show brilliant iridescent blue rings on an otherwise tan-yellow body when it is disturbed. It is a small octopus ranging only about 10 to 20 cm from outstretched arm to outstretched arm in the fully grown adult. All reported cases of envenomation by the blue-ringed octopus have occurred in Australian waters. The octopus does not attack humans and the only reported cases of envenomation occur when the octopus has been picked up or stepped upon.

The initial manifestations of the blue-ringed octopus' bite are two small puncture wounds. In many cases, the victim is unaware of the bite or notes only minimal local irritation.[72] The salivary secretions of this octopus contain the same tetrodotoxin found in pufferfish.[73,74] Edema, pain, and erythema occur locally but spread along the entire extremity.

Symptoms of severe envenomations include paresthesias, ataxia, nausea, emesis, dysphagia, dysphonia, hypotension, dyspnea,

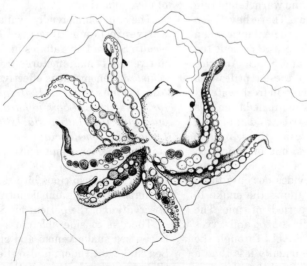

**Figure 7.31.** Blue-ringed octopus.

and paralysis. Progressive paralysis leads to respiratory embarrassment and subsequent death. The duration of paralysis is only about 4 to 12 hours, but weakness may persist for 24 to 36 more hours. Some victims have died from hypotension despite adequate respiratory support.

Australian literature tends to emphasize the use of a compression immobilization dressing to the affected limb. This must be applied immediately to be effective. The bandage should not be removed until airway maintenance equipment is at hand. As in its use in land animal envenomations, this first aid therapy has not been carefully studied and should be considered as anecdotal therapy.

Treatment of *H. maculosa* bites is symptomatic and supportive. Details of treatment may be found in the section on pufferfish intoxication, since the toxins are the same. Some authors have proposed immediate excision of the site of the bite, but there are no controlled studies that support this disfiguring procedure. It should be emphasized that good respiratory support will suffice for most victims.

## INGESTIONS

Ingestion of fish and other seafoods may present serious hazards, particularly to the unwary. Not all of the sea's animals and plants are appetizing or even edible. Some, indeed, are quite lethal.

Many coastal communities rely heavily on seafood in their diets. With air freight, well-traveled consumers, and modern refrigeration, even the most inland of physicians may be exposed to the vagaries of the diagnosis and treatment of ingestion of marine toxins. To those who work about the coasts, are associated with marine medicine in its many forms, or even just spend leisure time near the sea, knowledge of marine toxins is essential.

### Ciguatera Poisoning

Ciguatera poisoning is the most common form of fish poisoning. In 1787, Don Antonio Parra of Cuba gave this name to the symptoms he noted following ingestion of the "cigua" or the turban shellfish.[77] More than half of the outbreaks of fish-related foodborne disease are attributed to ciguatera toxicity. Ciguatera toxicity is not a reportable disease, but the CDC notes it as the most common foodborne illness due to a chemical toxin.[78]

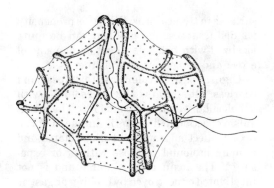

**Figure 7.32.** Gambierdiscus toxicus (ciguatera) dinoflagellate.

Ciguatera toxicity is associated with the consumption of fish that have been contaminated with ciguatera toxin. This toxin is produced by the dinoflagellate *Gambierdiscus toxicus* and is moved up the food chain by carnivores (see Fig. 7.32). At each level of the food chain, it becomes more concentrated, collecting primarily in the visceral organs, especially the liver and gonads, of the fish it contaminates. Humans appear to be the only part of the normal food chain that suffer ill effects from ingestion of ciguatera toxin.

A complete list of all species that can cause ciguatera poisoning is probably not possible, since any predatory fish has the potential to cause the toxicity. It may commonly be linked with such predators as barracuda, grouper, snapper, amberjack, and sea bass. Larger fish seem to have concentrated more toxin and commonly cause more intense and frequent symptoms in humans. The risks appear to be largest with large, bottom-feeding fish that have been caught in shallow waters.

Outbreaks are common in fish around coral reefs from 35 degrees North to 35 degrees South. Ciguatera toxicity is sporadic and seasonal with patchy distribution in most parts of the world, occurring primarily in the tropical and subtropical regions of the world. In the United States, most cases occur in Florida, Hawaii, Puerto Rico, and the U.S. Virgin Islands. An incidence as high as 75 cases per 10,000 population is noted in the U.S. Virgin Islands, dropping off to about 5 cases per 10,000 in southern Florida.[79,80]

Increases in the dinoflagellate population have been linked with disturbances of the waters about the reefs, from such activities as storms or clearing of boat passages. It has been postulated that the growth of the dinoflagellate is greatest about new or denuded surfaces in tropical seas. With this propensity for disturbances, the problem can be quite localized with fish safe to eat on one side of a reef and dangerous on the other.

Ciguratoxin is colorless, tasteless, and odorless.[81] It appears to be lipid soluble, with a molecular weight of about 1100. The mechanism of action in humans is unknown.[82] The toxin's effect appears to be dose related and is more profound in those with prior exposure.[83] The toxin is heat stable and is not inactivated or destroyed by cooking or gastric acids. It is also not removed by preservation methods such as drying, salting, or smoking.

The toxin manifests itself by a sudden onset of abdominal cramps, watery diarrhea, and vomiting, 1 to 6 hours after ingestion. Most patients also complain of diaphoresis, fever, arthralgias, and myalgias. Patients often develop a metallic taste in their mouths.

Soon after the gastrointestinal symptoms unfold, the patient may also develop neurologic symptoms. The unique symptom of ciguatera poisoning is temperature reversal, where hot objects appear cold and cold objects hot to touch. This syndrome is highly suggestive of ciguatera intoxication. Other common neurologic manifestations include perioral numbness, headaches, pruritis, transient blurred vision, or photophobia. Cranial nerve palsies and transient blindness have also been uncommonly reported.

Very rarely, death occurs from either convulsions or respiratory paralysis. Most deaths occur from dehydration due to the vomiting and diarrhea or from respiratory failure. Mortality rates are less than one per 10,000 cases. Other rare manifestations include nonspecific and reversible T-wave changes on ECG and bullous or desquamating rashes.

The pattern of signs or symptoms may differ from one geographic region to another, as well as with the apparent ingested dose. There appears to be some sensitization that occurs with ingestion, so subsequent exposures have more severe symptoms than the first. Also, symptoms are usually worse after ingestion of alcohol.

The acute illness lasts from 1 to 2 days and often resolves within a few weeks. Most cases of ciguatera intoxication are limited, and supportive care is sufficient.

Intravenous fluids may be needed for the patient with severe emesis or diarrhea and subsequent dehydration. Appropriate hydration should be ensured before use of sympathomimetics in patients with hypotension. Those with severe respiratory depression may require supplemental ventilation and intubation. Dopamine in usual doses may be useful for patients with hypotension.

Pruritis may be partially relieved by cold showers. Common antipruritic agents are of limited use in this disease.

In some patients, symptoms may "flashback" during periods of intense stress, recurrent illnesses, or alcoholism. Return of pruritis following alcohol ingestion is suggestive of a flashback.

Since many of the symptoms are anticholinergic in appearance, atropine is often advocated for treatment of the syndrome. Atropine is not consistently useful but can decrease some of the gastrointestinal and cardiovascular manifestations. It is particularly useful in the presence of symptomatic bradycardia.

Protamide has been anecdotally used in the Grand Bahama Islands for treatment of ciguratura intoxication, but this is not a controlled study and needs further investigation. Likewise, vitamin B complex and a high ascorbic acid, high-protein diet are also advocated in anecdotal reports.[82] Histamine antagonists are also promoted by these authors for treatment of the pruritis. Calcium gluconate, pralidoxime, and vitamin $B_6$ are all favored without good evidence of efficacy.

Amitriptyline may be useful for treatment of both pruritis and dysesthesias. Doses of 25 mg twice per day have been found effective in multiple anecdotal studies.[84,85] Certainly, controlled studies would be helpful in establishing the efficacy of amytriptyline and identifying other useful tricyclics and related agents.

Prevention is best achieved by avoidance of carnivorous fish caught in endemic areas. Since liver and roe preferentially concentrate the toxin, these parts of all fish should be avoided. Larger fish may have more toxin than smaller fish and should be likewise avoided.[86,87]

There is no logical or scientific method to predict which species or locale is contaminated. There is simply no way of detecting by inspection, taste, smell, or texture which fish are affected.

Laboratory identification by radioimmunoassay and immunoassays have been developed and found to be specific, sensitive, and relatively inexpensive The tests are just too expensive to screen individual fish before consumption, however.

## Tetrodotoxication (Puffer Fish)

The order *tetraodontiformes* contains a number of fish that lack true scales and have a fused bony headplate. Among these fish are the most poisonous fish found. Although pufferfish and relatives are decidedly toxic, they are considered a delicacy in parts of the world.[89] Puffer fish (fugu) is served in specially licensed restaurants and prepared by chefs trained to recognize the species and to be aware of seasonal variations in toxicity. High tribute is paid to the chef that can retain just enough toxin in the fish to cause numbness of the mouth without generalized poisoning! Even with precautions, an average of 20 deaths per year occur from consuming these fish.

In Japan, despite the extensive experience in management of this intoxication, mortality remains at about 60% in over 6000 cases reported over the past 78 years.[90] Death may occur in as little as 17 to 20 minutes.[91] It should be noted carefully that many of these deaths predate effective tools for respiratory support and that current mortality is much lower.

Tetrodotoxin is a small nonprotein molecule that is found in a variety of animals including the pufferfish and blue-ringed octopus. Land animals that contain the toxin include the South African poison dart frog and the California newt. Structurally, tetrodotoxin resembles morphine.[92] Tetrodotoxin is, perhaps, the most toxic nonprotein substance known. It produces anesthesia, emesis, hypothermia, hypotension, and respiratory depression as primary clinical effects. Tetrodotoxin is readily absorbed by either ingestion or injection.

Puffer fish of the family *Tetraodontidae* are widespread with distribution throughout the warm and temperate waters of the world. Species are found in New Jersey and Long Island in the United States. Pufferfish and newts that are bred in captivity do not acquire the toxin.[93] The tetrodotoxin is concentrated in the liver, intestines, gonads, and skin. The fish appear to be more toxic near spawning.

The first signs of tetrodotoxin poisoning is often tingling of the lips as noted above. Sweating, vomiting, muscular weakness, paralysis, and respiratory arrest follow in short order if sufficient toxin is ingested.

Tetrodotoxin blocks the sodium channel without affecting the potassium channel. It, thus, blocks the preganglionic cholinergic, motor, sensory, and sympathetic nerves in all parts of the central, peripheral, and autonomic nervous systems. Tetrodotoxin produces respiratory depression by direct effect on the respiratory centers and by blockade of the nerves of the muscles of respiration. At high bodily concentrations of tetrodotoxin, there are effects on both skeletal and cardiac muscles. Emesis is also caused by direct action on the brainstem emesis trigger zone. It has been suggested that cerebellar signs may occur with doses insufficient to affect the neuromuscular system.[94] There appears to be no direct action on the myocardium or brain, and consciousness is retained until hypoxia intervenes.

In high doses, tetrodotoxin blocks the central autonomic regulatory systems. The resulting vasodilation causes hypotension that may parallel or precede the respiratory depression.[73,95]

## TREATMENT

There is no known antidote to tetrodotoxin, and the treatment of poisoning from these and related fish is entirely supportive and symptomatic. The toxin appears to be short-acting, with few long-term effects if supportive measures are carried out quickly. Effective maintenance of respirations should be instituted immediately. Intubation will allow effective suctioning of secretions and vomitus. If cerebral anoxia is avoided, the patient is likely to make a complete recovery.

Activated charcoal has been reported to adsorb the toxin. The clinical use of charcoal is open to question in patients who present with hyperemesis and diarrhea or with symptoms delayed after ingestion.

Tetrodotoxin is decomposed rapidly by bicarbonate. Gastric lavage using a 2% solution of sodium bicarbonate is thought to be effective in limiting further absorption if used within the first hour of symptoms.[96] Unfortunately, there is no human experimental support for the use of bicarbonate, but little harm should come from proper lavage with this solution.

Emetics are considered helpful, but emesis is often part of the clinical picture of tetrodotoxin poisoning. Emetics may be quite beneficial in the patient who has only minimal symptoms, but there is little justification for use of emetics in the paralyzed patient. Lavage as described above is more logical in this case.

Atropine and temporary cardiac pacing are often recommended for treatment of transient bradycardia or heart block. Atropinization at 0.01 to 0.02 mg per kg every 5 minutes until heart rate responds is the usual recommended dose. Other dysrhythmias should be treated with usual protocols and usual drugs.

Hypotension should be treated with volume replacement and peripherally acting vasoconstrictors. In various experiments, phenylephrine and noradrenaline appeared most effective in counteracting hypotensive effects, but this research has not been applied to humans.[73] In these animal studies, dopamine and adrenaline were found to be ineffective.

Since the patient is often awake during the entire resuscitation, diazepam or lorazepam in appropriate tranquilizing doses is appropriate. The patient should be continuously reassured, despite the absence of physical responses. Particular attention should be spent on eye and mouth toilet, as in all paralyzed patients.

Because the tetrodotoxin molecule is similar to morphine, use of naloxone and cogeners to reverse the effects of the toxin is logical.[97] For patients with hyperemesis, apomorphine paradoxically appears to be the most effective drug.[98] It is possible that a cogener of apomorphine or nalorphine would provide relief from other effects of the toxin. A large-scale, prospective study of the manifestations and various therapies proposed would answer this and other questions.

## Paralytic Shellfish Poisoning

Paralytic shellfish poisoning results from the ingestion of certain species of mollusks and crustaceans. It has been known for hundreds of years and was long thought to be associated with the "red tide" or "water bloom"—discolorations of the sea due to vast quantities of dinoflagellates. One of the earliest descriptions is by Vancouver as he explored British Columbia in 1793. He described several of his sailors falling sick within the hour after a breakfast of roasted mussels. One of his seamen died within 5 hours. Outbreaks have been reported from both the Pacific and Atlantic coasts of North America, Japan, the Atlantic coast of Europe, South Africa, South America, New Zealand, and Australia. The worldwide incidence is estimated at about 2000 cases per year with possibly 300 deaths.[93]

In the United States, paralytic shellfish poisoning is most likely to be a problem in Maine and Massachusetts on the East Coast and along the entire Pacific West Coast from Alaska to California. Less active toxins may produce a related disease—neurotoxic shellfish poisoning. This latter form of poisoning most often occurs after eating bivalve mollusks from the Gulf Coast and along the Atlantic Coast of Florida.

Paralytic shellfish poisoning is caused by a toxin produced by the dinoflagellate *Gonyaulax catenella* and the related *G. tamarensis*. The phytoplankton is filtered from the water by the shellfish and passed up the food chain. The toxin affects other animals and can be fatal to birds. This toxin, saxitoxin, is related to tetrodotoxin and has similar effects.

### CLINICAL FEATURES

Like ciguatera and pufferfish poisoning, the clinical picture is that of acute neurotoxicity. Paresthesias, ataxia, and muscular weakness are common. In paralytic shellfish poisoning, objects appear paradoxically light and the patients often feel as if they could fly. In severe cases, respiratory paralysis may cause death. Abdominal complaints of nausea, vomiting, tenesmus, and diarrhea are common.

### TREATMENT

Treatment of paralytic shellfish poisoning is similar to that of pufferfish poisoning.

### PREVENTION

High-performance liquid chromatography can be used to monitor these toxins and some others with slightly different structures and toxicities. When the toxin level gets above 80 μg per 100 gm of shellfish, shellfish should not be harvested.

## Hallucinatory Fish Poisoning

An uncommon type of fish poisoning follows the eating of any of about 10 Pacific fish. These include the rock cod, grey mullet, drumfish, rudderfish, damselfish, and surgeonfish.[99]

Initial symptoms are incoordination and dizziness followed by hallucinations and depression. Nightmares may also be noted by the patient. Some patients may also note paresthesias and abdominal complaints.

Treatment of these intoxications is entirely supportive. The agent responsible for the effects is not known.

## Scombrotoxin

Ingestion of poorly preserved, canned, or refrigerated members of the scombroid family (tuna, bonita, swordfish, mackerel, and related species) may result in scrombroid fish poisoning. This syndrome is a histaminelike reaction that is caused by a bacterial enzyme's reaction on the fish' skeletal muscles.[100] Scombroid fish poisoning is associated with fish of tropical and temperate waters, but because of the widespread distribution of these fish, the syndrome may be noted far from the coasts.

The fish, normally safe, become poisonous when left in the sun or unrefrigerated for several hours. Under these conditions, the histadine in the muscle is changed into saurine, a substance like histamine. The enzymes of *Proteus morgagni*, *Klebsiella*, *E. Coli*, *Salmonella*, and *Shigella* species may all cause this conversion of the dark-meat muscle histadine.[101–103]

Since other fish may have the dark-meat muscle, the disease is not confined to tuna and relatives but may be infrequently found in other species.[104,105] Very rarely, scombroid poisoning has been caused by aged cheeses and other foods.[106] The diagnosis may be confirmed, often in retrospect, by a finding of a high histamine level in the implicated fish or food.[107]

The first manifestations of an attack may occur within minutes to hours after the ingestion of the tainted fish. The fish may be reported to have a sharp or peppery taste but often looks and tastes normal.[108] Clinically, the patients develop the features of a histamine reaction with erythema of the face, neck, trunk, and extremities. Diarrhea, vomiting, tenesmus, headache, and palpitations are also commonly noted. In very severe cases, bronchospasm and respiratory distress may complicate the picture. Reactions are more severe in patients who are taking isoniazid. These patients may be at increased risk of a reaction.[109] Although the symptoms may resemble an acute allergic reaction, it is not an allergy but a toxidrome.

Treatment should include administration of antihistamines and possibly intravenous cimetidine. Antihistamines have been reported to shorten the course of the illness, this effect is variable. Cimetidine has been used with a prompt effect on a series of four patients.[110] This study was without controls or protocols, and further study is suggested. An appropriate dose of cimetidine for an adult appears to be 300 mg intravenously over 30 minutes.

Intravenous fluids and oxygen may also be required for severely affected patients.

### PREVENTION

Identification of spoiled fish is difficult. There are no color or smell changes in the fish that are characteristic of early decomposition. Physical appearance of the spoiled fish is not remarkable. Even bacterial counts are difficult to ascertain and difficult to associate with contamination.

Prevention is impossible once the decomposition of the fish begins, so prevention must be directed to proper preservation of the fish. The toxins are heat stable and are not affected by freezing, smoking, cooking, marinating, or drying. The most important step in prevention of scombroid fish poisoning appears to be rapid refrigeration of the fish to 0°C (32°F) or below.[111]

## DISEASES OF INGESTION

Clams, scallops, oysters, and mussels feed on plankton by filtering them from the water.

Often other organisms, contaminants, and toxic chemicals may be absorbed as well during this filter-feeding process. These contaminants would be concentrated in the visceral organs of the animals. Those who ingest raw shellfish do so at their own peril.

The disease of major epidemiologic importance that is linked to shellfish ingestion is hepatitis. Hepatitis A is more frequently found than any other type, although there are varying reports of non-A, non-B hepatitis infections that are traceable to shellfish. Hepatitis B is not commonly found associated with shellfish. Steaming is not sufficient to destroy hepatitis A virus in clams.

In the past, typhoid fever has been associated with the ingestion of shellfish, particularly clams and oysters. Fortunately, this does not appear to be a problem in the United States, due to intensive public health and water treatment programs.

*Vibrio parahemolyticus* ingestion may produce a profound gastroenteritis after a 12 to 24 hour incubation period. The syndrome is characterized by 24 to 48 hours of explosive watery diarrhea, nausea, and tenesmus. Although self-limiting, intravenous rehydration may be required due to significant hypovolemia. *V. parahemolyticus* is sensitive to chloramphenicol, gentamicin, and the tetracyclines. Prior to initiation of antibiotic therapy in suspected cases, stool and blood cultures should be obtained. Raw clams appear to be more dangerous than oysters, because the clam can migrate somewhat to new environments.

Patients with shellfish-borne gastroenteritis should receive hepatitis immune serum globulin initially and again in 1 month as prophylaxis against hepatitis A.

Norwalk virus, polio, echovirus, enteroviruses, and reoviruses have all been found in shellfish about U.S. coastal cities. These causes of human diseases have not been clinically associated with proven human infections.

## References

1. Davies DH, Campbell GD. The aetiology, clinical pathology, and treatment of shark attack. J R Nav Serv 1962;3:110–136.
2. Gilbert PW, Schultz LP, Springer S. Shark attacks during 1959. Science 1960;132:323–326.
3. Welch K, Martinin FH. Non-fatal shark attack on Maui. Hawaii Med J 1981;40:95–96.
4. Kizer KW. Shark attack: remember the basics. Emerg Med Serv 1986;15:31–34.
5. Baldridge HD Jr, Williams J: Shark attack: feeding or fighting? Milit Med 1969;134:130–133.
6. White JAM. Shark attack in Natal. Injury. Br J Accident Surg 1974;6:187–194.
7. Auerbach PS. Hazardous marine animals. Emerg Med Clin North Am 1984;2(3):531–544.
8. Myrberg AA. Behavior of sharks: a continuing enigma. Nav Res Rev 1976;29:1–11.
9. Johnson RH, Nelson DR. Agonistic display in the gray reef shark *Carcharinus menisorrah* and its relationship to attacks on man. Copeia 1973;1:76–84.
10. Halstead BW, Vinci JM. Venomous fish stings (Ichthyoacanthotoxicoses). Clin Dermatol 1987;5(3):29–35.
11. Grainger CR. Multiple injuries due to sting rays. J R Soc Health 1987;107:100.
12. Russell FE. Stingray injuries. Pub Health Rep 1959;74:855–859.
13. McCall J, Sugrue W. An unusual diving injury [letter]. NZ Med J 1986;March:205.
14. Cross TB. An unusual stingray injury: the skindiver at risk. Med J Aust 1976;2:947–948.
15. Ronka EKF, Roe WF. Cardiac wound caused by the sting of the stingray (suborder masticura). Milit Surg 1945;97:135–137.
16. Grainger CR. Sting ray injuries. Trans R Soc Trop Med Hyg 1985;79:443–444.
17. Russell FE, Panos C, Kang LW, et al. Studies on the mechanism of death from stingray venom: a report of two fatal cases. Am J Med Sci 1958;235:566–584.
18. Shultz KE. Hazardous marine life. Emerg Med Serv 1985;14:62–75.
19. Scoggin CH. Catfish stings. JAMA 1975;231:176–177.
20. Ratzan RM Correia CJ, Cardoni AA. Poisoning by marine life: recognizing and treating water-related stings and bites. Consultant 1983;Aug:29–41.
21. Kizer KW. Marine envenomations. J Toxicol Clin Toxicol 1984;21:527–555.
22. Saunders PR, Taylor PB. Venom of the lionfish *Pterois volitans*. Am J Physiol 1959;197:437–440.
23. Weiner S. Observations on the venom of the stonefish (*Synanceja trachynis*). Med J Aust 1959;2:620–627.
24. Caots JA, Pattabhiraman TR, Russell FE, et al. Some physiopharmacologic properties of scorpionfish venom. Proc West Pharmacol Soc 1980;23:113–115.
25. Halstead BW. Injurious effects from the sting

of the scorpionfish *Scorpaena guttata*. Calif Med 1951;74:395–396.

26. Smith JLB. Two rapid fatalities from stonefish stabs. Copeia 1957;3:249.

27. Weiner S. Stonefish sting and its treatment. Med J Aust 1958;2:219–222.

28. Weiner S. Fish sting treatment [letter]. Med J Aust 1984;2:801–802.

29. Weiner S. The production and assay of stonefish antivenene. Med J Aust 1959;2:715–719.

30. Weiner S. A case of stonefish sting treated with antivenene. Med J Aust 1965;1:191.

31. Cain D. Weever fish sting: an unusual problem. Br J Med (Clin Res) 1983;287:406–407.

32. Russell FE. Weever fish sting: the last word [letter]. Br J Med (Clin Res) 1983;287;981–982.

33. Gonzaga RAF. Venomous fish stings on the European seashore. Postgrad Med 1985;77:146–148.

34. Hinegardner RT. The venom apparatus of the Cone Shell. Hawaii Med J 1958;17:533–536.

35. Rice RD, Halstead BW. Report of fatal cone shell sting by *Conus geographus* (*Linnaeus*). Toxicon 1968;5:223–224

36. Kizer KW. Marine Envenomations. J Toxicol Clin Toxicol 1983–4;21:527–555.

37. Lee T. The invertebrate corner. Marine Fish Monthly 1987;2(4):8–24.

38. Auerbach PS. Hazardous marine animals. Emerg Med Clin North Am 1984;2(3):531–544.

39. Ioannides G, Davis JH. Portugese man-of-war stinging. Arch Dermatol 1965;91:448–451.

40. Drury JK, Noonan JD, Pollack JG, Reid WH. Jellyfish sting with serious hand complications. Injury 12:66–68.

41. Filling-Katz MR. Mononeuritis multiplex following jellyfish stings. Ann Neurol 1984;15:213.

42. Chand RP, Selliah K. Reversible parasympathetic dysautonomia following stinging attributed to the box jelly fish (*Chironex fleckeri*). Aust NZ J Med 1984;14:673–675.

43. Adiga KV. Brachial artery spasm as a result of a sting. Med J Aust 1984;Feb 4:181–182.

44. Spielman FJ, Bowe EA, Watson CB, Klein EF Jr. Acute renal failure as a result of *Physalia physalis* sting. South Med J 1982;75:1425–1426.

45. Wong SK, Matoba A. Jellyfish sting of the cornea [letter]. Am J Ophthamol 1985;100(5):739–740.

46. Reed KM, Bronstein BR, Baden HP. Delayed and persistent cutaneous reactions to coelenterates. J Am Acad Dermatol 1984;10:462–466.

47. Burnett JW, Calton CJ. Jellyfish envenom-ation syndromes updated. Ann Emerg Med 1987;16:1000–1005.

48. Burnett JW, Calton GJ, Burnett HW. Jellyfish envenomation syndromes. J Am Acad Dermatol 1986;14:100–106.

49. Williamson JA, Callanan VI, Hartwick RF. Serious envenomation by the Northern Australian box-jellyfish (*Chironex fleckeri*). Med J Aust 1980;1:13–15.

50. Burnett JW, Calton GJ. Review article: the chemistry and toxicology of some venomous plagic coelenterates. Toxicon 1977;15:177–196.

51. Freeman SE, Turner RJ. A pharmacological study of the toxin of a Cnidarian, *Chironex fleckeri Southcott*. Br J Pharmacol 1969;35:510.

52. Maretic Z, Russell FE. Stings by the sea anemone *Anemonia sulcata* in the Adriatic Sea. Am J Trop Med Hyg 1983;32:891–896.

53. Hartwick R, Callanan V, Williamson J. Disarming the box jellyfish: nematocyst inhibition in *Chironex fleckeri*. Med J Aust 1980;1:15–20.

54. Turner B, Sullivan P, Pennefather J. Disarming the bluebottle: treatment of *Physalia envenomation*. Med J Aust 1980;Oct 4:394–395.

55. Burnett JW, Rubenstein H, Calton GJ. First aid for jellyfish envenomation. South Med J 1983;76:870–872.

56. Burnett JW, Calton GJ. Jellyfish envenomation syndromes updated. Ann Emerg Med 1987;16:1000–1005

57. Burnett JW, Calton GJ. Response of the box jellyfish (*Chironex fleckeri*) cardiotoxin to intravenous administration of verapamil. Med J Aust 1983;2:192–194.

58. Burnett JE, Gean CJ, Warnick JE, et al. The effect of verapamil on the cardiotoxin of the Portuguese man-of-war (*Physalia physalis*) and the sea nettle (*Chrysaora quinquecirrha*). Toxicon 1985;23:681–689.

59. Sutherland SK. Response to Chironex antivenom [letter]. Med J Aust 1979;Dec 15:653.

60. Halstead BW, Engen P, Tu A. The venom and venom apparatus of the sea snake *Lapemis hardwicki* (Gray). Zool J Linn Soc 1978;63:371–396.

61. Watt G, Theakston RD. Seasnake bites in a freshwater lake. Am J Trop Med Hyg 1985;34:770–773.

62. Tu A. Biotoxicology of sea snake venoms. Ann Emerg Med 1987;16:1023–1208.

63. Mori N, Tue AT. Isolation and primary structure of the major toxin from sea snake, *Acalyptophis peronii*, venom. Arch Biochem Biophys 1988;260:10–17.

64. Reid HA. Poisoning due to snake bite. In: Vale JA, Meredith TJ, eds. Poisoning diagnosis and treatment. London: Update Books, 1981.

65. Fulde GW, Smith F. Sea snake envenomation at Biondi. Med J Aust 1984;141:44–45.

66. Audley I. A case of sea-snake envenomation [letter]. Med J Aust 1985;143:532.
67. Acott CJ. Sea-snake envenomation [letter]. Med J Aust 1986;144:448.
68. Dobb GJ. Sea-snake envenomation [letter]. Med J Aust 1986;144:112.
69. Coulter AR, Harris Rd, Sutherland SK. Enzyme immunoassay and radioimmunoassay: their use in the study of Australian and exotic snake venoms. Proc Melbourne Herpetological Symp 1981;39–43.
70. Baxter EH, Gallichio HA. Cross-neutralisation by tiger snakes (Notechis scutatus) antivenene and sea snake (Enhydrina schistosa) antivenene against several sea snake venoms. Toxicon 1974;12:273.
71. Sutherland S. Australian animal toxins: the creatures, their toxins, and care of the poisoned patient. Melbourne: Oxford University Press, 1983;158–184.
72. Williamson JA. The blue-ringed octopus bite and envenomation syndrome. Clin Dermatol 1987;5:127–133.
73. Flachsenberger WA. Respiratory failure and lethal hypotension due to blue-ringed octopus and tetrodotoxin envenomation observed and counteracted in animal models. Clin Toxicol 1987;24:485–502.
74. Sheumack DD, Howden MEH, Spence I, et al. A neurotoxin from the venom glands of the octopus Hapalochlaena maculosa identified as tetrodotoxin. Science 1978;199:188–189.
75. Williamson JA. The blue ringed octopus. Med J Aust 1984;140:308–309.
76. Rosce MD. Cutaneous manifestations of marine animal injuries, including diagnosis and treatment. Cutis 1977;19:507–510.
77. Halstead BW. Poisonous and venomous marine animals of the world. Vol I. Invertebrates. Washington DC: US Government Printing Office, 1965:59–61.
78. Lange WR. Ciguatera toxicity. Am Fam Phys;1987;35:177–182.
79. Lawrence DN, Enriquez MB, Lumish RM, Maceo A. Ciguatera fish poisoning in Miami. JAMA 1980;244:254–258.
80. Morris JG Jr, Lewin P, Smith CW, et al. Ciguatera fish poisoning: epidemiology of the disease in St. Thomas, US Virgin Islands. Am J Trop Med Hyg 1982;31:574–578.
81. Ho AMH, Fraser IM, Todd ECD. Ciguratera poisoning: a report of three cases. Ann Emerg Med 1986;15:1225–1228.
82. Ragelis EP. Ciuatera seafood poisoning—overview. In: Ragelis EP, ed. Seafood toxins. ACS Symposium Series, 262, Washington, DC: American Chemical Society, 1984:25–36.
83. Bagnis R, Kuberskin T, Laugier S. Clinical observations on 3009 cases of ciguatera (fish poisoning) in the South Pacific. Am J Trop Med Hyg 1979;28:2067–2073.
84. Bowman PB. Amitriptyline and ciguatera [letter]. Med J Aust 1984;140:802.
85. Davis RT, Villar LA. Symptomatic improvement with amitriptyline in ciguatera fish poisoning [letter]. N Engl J Med 1986;315:65.
86. Hessel DW, Halstead BW, Peckham NH. Marine biotoxins. I. Ciguatera toxin: some biological and chemical aspects. Ann NY Acad Sci 1960;90:788–797.
87. Craig CP. It's always the big ones that should get away [editorial]. JAMA 1980;244:272–273.
88. Hokama Y. A rapid, simplified enzyme immunoassay stick test for the detection of ciguatoxin and related polyethers from fish tissues. Toxicon 1985;23:939–946.
89. World Health Organization: Aquatic (marine and freshwater) biotoxins. (Environmental Health Criteria 37), Geneva: WHO, 1984:15.
90. Halstead BW. Poisonous and venomous marine animals of the world. Volume 2. Washington, DC: US Government Printing Office, 1967:679–901.
91. Halstead BW. Poisonous and venomous marine animals of the world. Princeton, NJ: Darwin Press, 1978:437–548.
92. Sims JK, Ostman DC. Pufferfish poisoning: emergency diagnosis and management of mild human tetrodotoxication. Ann Emerg Med 1986;15:1094–1098.
93. Mills AR, Passmore R. Pelagic paralysis. Lancet 1988:Jan 23:161–164.
94. Schultz J. Unusual symptoms after octopus bite. Med J Aust 1969;1:146.
95. Kao CY. Tetrodotoxin, saxitoxin and their significance in the study of the excitation phenomena. Pharmacol Rev 1966;18:997–1049.
96. Yokoo A: Chemical studies on tetrodotoxin. Report III. Isolation of spheroidine. J Chem Soc Japan 1950;71:591–592.
97. Sims JK. A theoretical discourse on the pharmacology of toxic marine ingestions. Ann Emerg Med 1987;16:1006–1015.
98. Fukada T, Tani I: Records of puffer poisoning. Report I. Kyushu University Medical News 1937;11:7–13.
99. Southcott RV. Australian venomous and poisonous fishes. Clin Toxicol 1977;10:291–325.
100. Lange WR. Scombroid poisoning. Am Fam Phys 1988;37:163–168.
101. Arnold SH, Brown WD. Histamine(?) toxicity from fish products. Adv Food Res 1978;24:113–54.
102. Niven CF Jr, Jeffrey MB, Corlett DA Jr. Differential plating medium for quantitative detection of histamine-producing bacteria. Appl Environ Microbiol 1981;41:321–322.
103. Lerke PA, Werner SB, Taylor SL, Guthertz

LS. Scombroid poisoning. report of an outbreak. West J Med 1978;129:381–386.

104. Prescott BD Jr. "Scombroid poisoning" and bluefish: the Connecticut connection. Conn Med 1984;48:105–110

105. Etkind P, Wilson ME, Gallagher K, Cournoyer J. Bluefish associated scombroid poisoning: an example of the expanding spectrum of food poisoning from seafood. JAMA 1987;258:3409–3410.

106. Taylor SL. Histamine food poising: toxicology and clinical aspects. CRC Crit Rev Toxicol 1986;61:91–128

107. Henion JD, Nosanchuk JS, Bilder BM. Capillary gas chromatographic-mass spectrometric determination of histamine in tuna fish causing scombroid poisoning. J Chromatogr 1981;213:475–480.

108. Pugno PA, Kaufman D, Feder HM Jr. Bluefish: a newly discovered cause of scombroid fish poisoning. J Fam Pract 1983;17:1071–2, 1081.

109. Uragoda CG. Histamine poisoning in tuberculous patients after ingestion of tuna fish. Am Rev Respir Dis 1980;121;157–190.

110. Blakesly ML. Scombroid poisoning: prompt resolution of symptoms with cimetidine. Ann Emerg Med 1983;12:104–106.

111. Behling AR, Taylor SL. Bacterial histamine production as a function of temperature and time of incubation. J Food Sci 1982;47:1311–1314

---

# Part 4
# Venomous Land Animals

---

## INTRODUCTION

The bite of a snake is a toxicologic emergency that has electrifying social and historical implications. Whether the Judeo-Christian religious concepts of the snake as ultimate villain, the visions of Cleopatra's asp, or the tales of cobras and kraits have caused these implications in our modern culture is uncertain. Because the patient, the family, the situation, and often the medical providers themselves are so emotionally charged, the medical provider may lose perspective and use dangerous folk and medical remedies.

There is scant consensus within the medical community on prehospital care for the victim of a venomous reptile bite and uncer-

tainty about the hospital management. This, of course, makes the treatment of the victim more difficult and the emergency prehospital provider less sure of the proper therapy. Because the consensus is lacking, and data to support any viewpoint skimpy, the following distillation of the literature may be subject to both current controversy and revision upon the arrival of newer data. Controversy is clearly noted where it exists.

## Demographics

On the average, 45,000 snakebites are thought to occur each year throughout the world. Only 6,000 to 8,000 snakebites are reported annually in the United States. Of course, many snakebites may be left untreated because they are viewed as not serious, because of conflict with religious beliefs, or because of some macho mystique of self-treatment. Of the snakebites that occur, only 5 to 15 deaths result each year in the United States.

These fatalities are usually associated with delay in treatment, underlying diseases, or true intravenous injection of venom.[1] Most of these fatalities are due to rattlesnake bites.[2] The overall mortality rate is lower than that caused by allergic reactions to insect stings. Unfortunately, while mortality is uncommon, serious disability and deformity is not. A patient with a snakebite should be taken seriously but not hysterically.

Snakes hibernate during the winter and are most active during the spring and summer. Logically, most bites are therefore between April and October. The victims are most often male (10:1) and usually between 10 and 19 years of age. Hikers, backpackers, and gardeners are often bitten. An increasing number of snakebites are suffered by amateur herpetologists who frequently will have imported exotic snakes for pets. Most bites occur on the extremities, usually on the upper extremities during handling of the snake.

## Epidemiology

Snakes and lizards belong to the vertebrate class *Reptilia* in the order *Squamata*. There are only two families of dangerous snakes: the *Viperidae*, which includes the *Crotalidae* or pit vipers, and the *Elapidae* or coral snake and cobra family, which pose a substantial threat to humans. A third family, the *Columbrids*, are also venomous but have fixed posterior fangs that rarely cause human envenomation.[3,4] The fourth and last family, the *Boidae*, which includes the boa constrictors, anacondas, and pythons, has no venom and kills by crushing. About 95% of North American snakebites are due to the pit vipers, about 2% from elapids, and the rest from exotic imports and the rare poisonous lizards (3%).[5] There are two venomous lizards, the Gila monster and the Mexican beaded lizard. A few reptiles have evolved poisonous skin secretions or the deposition of toxins in internal organs or in the skin. Sea snakes were discussed in Part 3. See Table 7.4 for a listing of venomous animals.

## OTHER POISONOUS REPTILES

Some poisonous reptiles secrete a toxin within part of their bodies or on their skin that serves as a fatal defense warning to other species, as opposed to the venom delivery system of the Gila monster and the snakes. There are three major known species of reptile in North America that have toxic effects when ingested: the Colorado River toad, the Columbian poison-dart frog, and several species of newt.

### Newts and Salamanders

The internal organs and skin of several species of newt possess a neurotoxin that is similar to that of the pufferfish. An Oregon rough-skinned newt (*Taricha granulosa*) has caused cardiorespiratory arrest when consumed by an inebriated camper.[6] The camper swallowed a 20 cm newt and died from cardiac arrest 8 hours later. The patient complained of numbness of his lips and progressive numbness and weakness in his extremities 10 minutes after the ingestion.

Eastern species of newt (*Neopthalmidae*) appear to be somewhat less toxic that the West Coast varieties.[7] There are no published reports of human poisoning from eastern newts. It can be assumed, however, that if they are consumed, the results would be similar to the experiences of the intoxicated camper.

Treatment is not well defined, because there

**Table 7.2.**
**Nomenclature of Venomous Animals**

| Snakes |
| --- |

***Columbrids***
*Boomslang*
    *Dispholidus typhus*
    Toxic (Africa)
*California lyre snake*
    *Trimorphodon vandengurghi*
    Possibly toxic (USA)
*European montpelier*
    *Malpolon monspessulanus*
    Toxic, no fatalities
*Mexican Vine Snake*
    *Oxybelis aneus auratus*
    Possibly toxic (North America)
*Mole or burrowing adders*
    *Atractaspis engaddensis*
    *Atractaspis irregularis*
    *Atractaspis microlepidota*
    Toxic
*Night snake*
    *Hypsiglena toquata*
    Possibly toxic (USA)
*Sonoran lyre snakes*
    *Trimorphodon lambda*
    Possibly toxic (USA)
*Southeast Asian red-necked keelback*
    *Rhabdophis subminatus*
    Toxic, no fatalities
*Vine Snake*
    *Thelotornis kirtlandii*
    Toxic (Africa)
*Yamakagashi*
    *Rhabdophis tigrinis*
    Toxic (Japan)
**Vipers and Crotalids (all toxic)**
*Asp (European asp) (asp viper)*
    *Vipera aspis* (Europe)
    *Vipera berus* (Europe)
*Long-nosed viper*
    *Vipera ammodytes*
*Berg viper*
    *Bitis atropos*
*Bushmaster*
    *Lachesis muta*
*Canebrake rattlesnake*
    *Crotalus horridus articuadatus* (North America)
*Cascabel (Central American rattlesnake)*
    *Crotalus durissus*
*Copperhead*
    *Agkistrodon contortrix* (North America)
*Cottonmouth (water moccasin)*
    *Agkistrodon piscivorus* (North America)
*Eastern diamondback rattlesnake*
    *Crotalus adamanteus* (North America)

**Table 7.2. (*cont.*)**
### Snakes

*Eyelash viper*
  *Bothrops schleglii*
*Massasauga*
  *Sistrurus catenatus* (North America)
*Mojave rattlesnake*
  *Crotalus scutalatus* (North America)
*Pygmy rattlesnake*
  *Sistrus milarius* (North America)
*Sidewinder*
  *Crotalus cerastes* (North America)
*Timber rattlesnake*
  *Crotalus horridus horridus* (North America)
*Western diamondback rattlesnake*
  *Crotalus atrox* (North America)
*Western rattlesnake*
  *Crotalus viridis* (North America)
  Also called
    Southern Pacific rattlesnake
    Prairie rattlesnake
    Hopi rattlesnake
    Grand Canyon rattlesnake
*Lancehead*
  *Bothrops lasbergii* (American tropics)
*Cantril*
  *Agkistrodon bilineatus* (North America)
*Malayan pit viper*
  *Agkistrodon rhodostoma* (Asia)
*Mamushi*
  *Agkistrodon halys* (Asia)
*Russell's viper*
  *Vipera russelli* (Africa, Asia)
*Fer-de-lance*
  *Bothrops asper* (American tropics)
  *Bothrops atrox* (American tropics)
*Gaboon viper*
  *Bitis gabonica* (Africa)
*Jararaca*
  *Bitis jararaca* (Central America)
*Tommygoff or "jumping viper"*
  *Bothrops nummifera* (South America)
*Death adder*
  *Acanthophis artarticus* (Australian)
*Tiger snake*
  *Notechis scutatus* (Australian)
**Elapids (all toxic)**
*Arizona or Sonoran coral snake*
  *Microides euryxanthus* (Western North
    America)
*Eastern coral snake*
  *Micrurus fulvius* (North America)
*Banded krait*
  *Bungarus fasciatus* (Asia)
*Fire coral snake*
  *Millepora sp.* (North America)
*Indian krait*
  *Bungarus caeruleus* (Asia)

**Table 7.2. (*cont.*)**
### Snakes

*Egyptian cobra*
  *Naja haje* (Africa, Asia)
*Indian or Asian cobra*
  *Naja naja* (Asia)
*King cobra*
  *Ophiophagus hannah* (Asia)
*Malayan krait*
  *Bungarus candidis* (Asia)
*Spitting cobra*
  *Naja nigricollis* (Asia)
**Poisonous Reptiles**
*Gila monster*
  *Heloderma suspectum* (North America)
*Mexican beaded lizard*
  *Heloderma horridum* (North America)
*Miscellaneous poisonous lizards*
  *Columbian dart frog* (Central America)
  *Colorado river toad* (Western USA)
  *Oregon roughskinned newt* (Western USA)

are so few people who eat newts. The neurotoxin causes hypotension and respiratory paralysis. The patient should be observed for 24 hours. If respiratory depression or hypotension develops, these signs may be treated symptomatically. Gut decontamination with emetics, cathartics, and charcoal is recommended.

## Colombian Poison-Dart Frogs

Skin secretions of the Columbian poison-dart frog contain one of the most potent toxins known to humans—batachotoxin.[8] The Choco Indians of Western Columbia discovered that roasting the frog over a fire caused the frog to secrete this poison. The Indians then used the toxin for their blowpipe darts. A single frog secretes enough poison to load over 30 darts, with each dart having a lethal dose for a fully grown man. At least three species from Central America (*Phyllobates terribilis, P. bicolor*, and *P. aurotaenia*) possess this poison in the skin secretions.

The poison has an action similar to the calcium channel blockers but affects a separate and distinct site from that of the calcium channel blockers. The effects seem to be irreversible, and there is no known antidote. There is no known effective first aid or medical therapy.

## Toads

Thera are 18 different species of the genus *Bufo*, which contains at least two toads that are poisonous when ingested. All toads secrete a poison from the parotid glands as a defensive protection. If the secretion is ingested or rubbed into the eyes, it can cause stinging or burning sensations. In severe cases, it can cause temporary blindness. The Colorado River toad, *Bufo alvarius*, is the most toxic toad in North America. Simply placing one of these toads in the mouth of a 5-year-old boy caused prolonged seizures, left-sided hemiparesis, and slurred speech within 15 minutes.[9] *B. marinus*, another extremely toxic toad, has caused many cat and dog deaths but no reported human poisonings.

Toad toxins contain cardioreactive steroids that are similar to the digitalis compounds (bufogenins). Treatment is supportive. Seizures were controlled with the standard anticonvulsants diazepam and phenobarbital, and steroids were used with good effect in the one case mentioned.

## Venomous Lizards

As noted above, there are only two venomous lizards in the world, both of which are found in the southwestern United States and western Mexico. The Gila monster is pinkish with attractive black spots and may attain a half meter in length. It is a relatively sluggish thick lizard, normally not aggressive except when aroused. It may live as long as 25 years and has few natural predators. The animal is a nocturnal recluse and most bites occur when handling the animal in captivity. Its diet of small mammals is thought to help keep the desert rodent population under control (see Fig. 7.33).

The Gila monster (*Heloderma suspectum*) and the Mexican beaded lizard (*H. horridum*) both deliver venom by chewing and biting with the grooved teeth of the lower jaw. There appear to be no substantial differences in delivery, action, or treatment between the bites of the two lizards and their subspecies. A modified salivary gland delivers the venom to the grooves in the teeth where it dribbles into the wound during chewing. While this venom delivery apparatus is more primitive than that of the venomous snakes, it is effective for defense. The lizard is tenacious

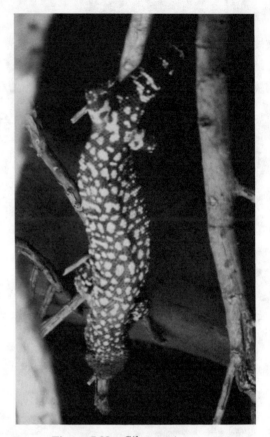

**Figure 7.33.** Gila monster.

and the jaw is quite strong, so the patient may be brought to the emergency provider with the animal still attached. The lizard's teeth are loosely attached and often break off during the chewing instillation of venom.

The Gila monster's venom is a complex of enzymes, vasoactive substances, and neurotoxins. Milking the venom glands yields about 17 mg of dried venom each 2 to 3 months, but the yield from a bite is not known.[10] There are no known deaths from envenomation by the Gila monster or relatives. Determination of the human $LD_{50}$ is, therefore, unknown and, hopefully, unknowable.

### LOCAL EFFECTS

If envenomation occurs, local tissue swelling and pain occur within 5 minutes. The edema is usually much less severe than that following rattlesnake bites.[10] The pain is severe and may involve the entire extremity bitten. Radiation of the pain into the affected extremity is common in severe envenomations. Maceration and crush injuries are common findings due to the method of envenomation and the tenacity of the creature.

## SYSTEMIC EFFECTS

Systemic reactions include increased perspiration, fever, nausea, and vomiting in some. Gila monster bites may also cause weakness, dizziness, hypotension, and tachycardia. In severe envenomations, hypotension is common. The mechanism of this hypotension is not known. Anaphylaxis has been reported as a complication of envenomation in a patient without known prior exposure to the venom.[11]

## FIRST AID AND SCENE CARE

There are no proven first aid measures for bites of the Gila monster. The only known help is to disengage the animal as soon as possible. This usually may be accomplished by use of a stick or crowbar between the jaws. Another method proposed has been to use a flame on the undersurface of the lizard's lower jaw. If these methods do not work, the muscles of the jaw may be cut, freeing the lower jaw. Since the venom is dribbled into the wound, not injected, the cut-and-suck method of venom removal is not a logical first aid measure.

## HOSPITAL CARE

Local therapy consists of wound care, with copious irrigation of the puncture wounds and careful debridement of the crush injuries. The wounds should be explored with a blunt probe for broken teeth. Lidocaine has been used for anesthesia for both debridement and exploration without problems. Tetanus immunization should be managed as usual.

Severe hypotension has been controlled with intravenous fluids and low-dose dopamine.[12] No commercially available antiserum exists for the venom; however, an unlicensed experimental antivenom has been developed by Findley Russell. Pain can be controlled with narcotics or nonsteroidal anti-inflammatory drugs. There is no evidence that corticosteroids, ice packs, heat packs, or constricting bandages have any efficacy.[13]

## POISONOUS SNAKES

The evolution of the signs and symptoms of snake envenomation depends upon the type of snake, the nature of the venom injected, the amount of venom injected, and the site of injection. Venomous snakes frequently do not inject venom with every bite, with as many as 20% of crotalids and 50% of elapids in North America failing to envenomate with a strike. The reasons for this are uncertain.

## Venom

Venom reactions may be roughly divided into cytotoxic or proteolytic with local tissue damage, neurotoxic with CNS damage, and hemotoxic with destruction of the coagulation system by various means. It should be emphasized that snake venom is a complex mixture of toxins and that multiple effects may be found from the bite of any snake. Which effect will predominate may be roughly predicted by species, but in any snakebite, other effects may also be found. Species-dependent effects of venom will be discussed later with that species.

## Crotalidae

The North American pit vipers or crotalids consist of five subspecies of copperheads (*Agkistrodon contortrix*), three subspecies of cottonmouth or water moccasins (*A. piscivorous*), three subspecies of massasauga (*S. catanatus*), three subspecies of pygmy rattlesnakes (*S. miliaris*), and at least 26 species of true "rattlers" (*Crotalus* sp). Over 95% of U. S. envenomations are from crotalid snake species.

## RECOGNITION

Pit vipers of the *Crotalidae* group have movable anterior fangs, triangular-shaped heads, and a thermoreceptor pit on each side of the face—hence, the name pit vipers.[14] The thermoreceptive pits are located between the eyes and the nostrils and are exquisitely sensitive to infrared radiation, allowing the snake to strike at prey even at night. Pit vipers have a good sense of smell but see poorly, sensing only motion.

## Cottonmouth

Cottonmouths, or water moccasins as they are often called, have a characteristic whitish color to the buccal mucosa, a flat broad head, a heavy thick body, and a darkish color. They inhabit the marshy, swampy environment about lakes, river valleys, or swamps from the Mississipi Valley, stretching from southern Virginia to Florida and west to eastern Texas. They are found as far north as Illinois and Indiana. These animals are more aggressive than rattlesnakes, but the venom is considered less toxic.

## Copperhead

The copperhead is identified by a copper-tinged head and buff, pink, or hazel body color. The body markings are described as hourglass or dumbbell like in shape. Copperheads are moderate-sized animals with adult lengths up to a meter and a half. The copperhead is found in the eastern half of the country, from Massachusetts to Florida and as far west as Texas. Copperheads are responsible for about two thirds of the poisonous envenomations in the United States, because they are willing to share human environments.

The copperhead is considered to have a very mild venom and most authorities recommend a conservative treatment for verified copperhead bites. Antivenom may be indicated in the very young, old, or infirm.

## Pygmy Rattlesnakes and Massasauga Rattlesnakes

These small, phylogenetically early rattlesnakes are both found in swamps and other moist areas. They both grow to a maximum length of a meter but are usually less than two thirds meters long.

The massasauga has the typical rattles, fangs, and venom glands of the pit vipers. The venom is thought to be more toxic than that of the water moccasin or the copperhead but less toxic than the rest of the rattlesnake family.

The pygmy rattlesnake likewise has the typical features of a pit viper in a frame that is only a half meter long. The venom of the pygmy rattlesnake is thought to be somewhat less toxic than that of its cousin, the mas-

sasauga. The small size and short fangs mean that bites are always superficial.

## Rattlesnakes

True rattlesnakes are distributed throughout most of the United States with the exception of Maine, Wisconsin, Michigan, Minnesota, North Dakota, Oregon, and Washington.[15] They range in size from 1.5 m to nearly 3 m in length, but most specimens are somewhat less than 2 m in length. There are at least 15 separate species of rattlesnakes in North America, with the eastern and the western diamondback rattlesnakes considered the largest and most dangerous snakes.

The tail rattle is the appendage that has captured the fancy of generations of visitors and settlers. It appears to be both unique in function and development. Although other animals may use signals or sounds for mating calls or as a warning for other members of the group, this snake rattles its tail to drive away other creatures that may harm it. It sounds when the snake is molested or alarmed. Unfortunately, many rattlesnake bites occur without warning.

The rattle is the caudal appendage of the rattlesnake and consists of one or more attached, interlocking segments of the tail. The rattle is vibrated at rates from 21 to about 100 cycles per second, depending upon the temperature, age, disposition, and species of the snake. The sound is produced by the action of all interlocking pieces of the tail and is more of a hiss than a rattle.

## SIGNS

The signs, symptoms, and magnitude of pit viper envenomation depend upon multiple factors. The size and species of the snake and the amount of venom injected will influence the degree of the reaction. The age of the patient, presence of underlying disease, and time from envenomation to therapy are also important.

One of the more frequently touted signs of pit viper envenomation is the presence of fang marks. Although the classic description is of two fang marks, this is not always the case. A glancing blow may leave only one fang mark, or the pit viper may have new growing reserve fangs that make secondary or even tertiary marks. Even two puncture wounds do not imply envenomation, as the snake does not always inject venom when it strikes. About one third to one half of snakebites, depending upon the species, end in nonenvenomation. For signs of envenomation, it is better to depend upon the presence of local swelling, pain, or ecchymosis.

---

*Emergency Evaluation of Crotalid Envenomation*

Evaluate ABCs.

Grade the envenomation (must be repeated q 15 min for 4 hours).

Ensure intravenous lifeline in unbitten extremity.

Obtain laboratory evaluation below.

Give antivenin as needed.

Monitor cardiac function.

If shock is present, consider fresh frozen plasma or packed red blood cells.

Cleanse wound with soap and water.

Monitor compartment pressures as appropriate.

Observe all patients at least for 4 hours.

Consider Swan-Ganz or CVP monitoring in unstable patients.

Consider broad-spectrum antibiotics.

---

## CROTALID VENOM

Rattlesnakes are classically thought to have venom with both proteolytic and hemotoxic activity, but rattlesnake venom may also cause neurotoxic effects. One species, the Mojave rattlesnake, has gained a wide reputation for such neurotoxicity.

### Proteolytic Effects

The enzymatic or digestive proteins contained in crotalid venom include proteases, phospholipases, and hyaluronidases. The proteases primarily cause tissue necrosis at the site of injection of venom. The hyaluronidases help to spread the venom by breaking down cell-cell junctions. The phospholipases break down cell wall membranes and capillary membranes. This last action allows serum proteins and plasma to leak into the interstitial tissues and is thought to be responsible for the local edema.

### Hemotoxic Effects

Both an anticoagulant and a hemorrhagic factor may be found in crotalid venom, although these effects may be variable and unpredictable.[16] The anticoagulant enzymes are found in the venom of many of the North American crotalid species, including the eastern diamondback, Pacific, black-tailed, and timber rattlesnakes.[17] The hemorrhagic factors are found in many species of both the Asiatic and New World pit vipers. In the United States, the eastern diamondback, timber rattlesnake, cottonmouth, and copperhead are commonly associated with hemorrhagic factors.[18,19] Another fraction of the timber rattlesnake's venom has been shown to aggregate platelets.[17]

Snake venom procoagulant esterases, similar to thrombin in structure, convert fibrinogen to fibrin more rapidly than thrombin and split off fibrin fragments. Unlike thrombin, procoagulant esterases do not cause activation of the factor XII chain. They also do not activate the extrinsic clotting system. Procoagulant esterases are not inhibited or inactivated by heparin.

### Local Effects

If envenomation from a pit viper does occur, pain or numbness at the site ensues rapidly. The pain may be localized or may radiate to the trunk from the bitten extremity. The pain appears to be most severe after the eastern and western diamondback rattlesnake bites and somewhat less severe after the other viridis rattlesnakes.[20] It is least severe after copperhead, pygmy rattlesnake, and massasauga envenomations.

Edema rapidly follows the envenomation and is progressive up the extremity as the venom flows along the lymphatic channels. Subsequent tissue swelling is often frightening with a local ecchymosis and bluish hue to the extremity. This extravasation of blood and fluid may contribute to the early hypotension seen with pit viper bites. Because this swelling may be truly massive, extremity circumferences should be obtained and a flow chart kept of the measurements.

Bleb formation may be seen in more severe envenomations. These blebs usually develop within 24 hours and infrequently migrate up the extremity from the site of the bite. Bleb formation is more common when the patient has had no antivenin for 12 hours or more, regardless of subsequent therapy. Lymphangitis is freqently found after 24 hours.

## SYSTEMIC SIGNS

Systemic signs are first marked by the appearance of a metallic taste in the mouth or by perioral paresthesias. Paresthesias may extend to the scalp, fingers, and toes and about the wound. Weakness, sweating, nausea, and faintness are common. Other neurologic findings are reputed to occur with the Mojave rattlesnakes and those vipers not indigenous to the United States.

This overall picture is that of an edematous, painful, ecchymotic, and dusky-appearing extremity. The reaction appears within hours and progresses up the extremity. It is small wonder that the lay person is driven to heroic lengths to prevent further damage.

## COMPLICATIONS

### Hematologic Complications

Hematologic complications are frequent in severe crotalid envenomations. The potential for coagulopathy exists in most, if not all, of the venoms from North American pit vipers. Petechiae, conjunctival hemorrhage, wound bleeding, and hypotension not responsive to fluid administration all may mark the onset of coagulopathy. True disseminated intravascular coagulopathies are rare, but alteration of clotting studies is common.[21] Hypofibrinogenemia, thrombocytopenia, fibrinolysis, and prolongation of both PT and

---

*Laboratory Evaluation of Crotalid Envenomation*
CBC and platelet counts
Serum electrolytes
Coagulation screen (PT, PTT, fibrinogen levels)
Urinalysis
Draw blood for type and crossmatch (before antivenin)
Creatinine phosphokinase
BUN and creatinine
ECG for patients over 40
Draw serial coagulation screens on patients with severe envenomation

---

PTT are seen.[22] Rarely, intravascular hemolysis may be noted. Disorders of coagulation should be treated with platelets, fresh frozen plasma, or cryoprecipitate as available.

### Shock

Shock is a common complication, often due to hypovolemia, although there may be multiple causes. The hypovolemia is frequently postulated on the basis of third space (edema) sequestration of fluid and pooling in splanchnic and pulmonary circulations. This appears to be an incomplete answer and the pit viper's venoms may trigger the release of vasoactive substances in the victim.[23] Bradykinin may cause the early transient hypotension seen in many severe envenomations. The capillaries become more permeable to protein and red blood cells, increasing fluid losses.

Low molecular weight proteins found in the venom of the eastern diamondback and canebrake rattlesnakes have been shown to be cardiotoxic. Administration of the cardiotoxic factor induces a dose-related myocardial failure that can be measured by cardiac output, left ventricular systolic and mean pressures, and pulmonary wedge pressures.[24]

### Renal Failure

Envenomated patients may develop renal failure due to the precipitation of red cell debris, hemoglobin and hemoglobin fragments, and myoglobin from muscle destruction. Hypotension may contribute to the onset of renal failure. Fortunately, renal failure from snakebite responds favorably to dialysis and does not usually present a long-term problem.[5]

## Elapidae

Elapids are responsible for thousands of deaths in the world each year. The order contains the cobras, the kraits, the mambas, and all of the snakes of Australia and New Guinea (perhaps the most poisonous snakes in the world).

### ELAPID VENOM

The more neurotoxic elapid venoms may be divided into two groups according to the mechanisms of action. The first group binds to the postsynaptic acetylcholine receptors and causes a nondepolarizing neuromuscular blockade with a progressively decreased reduction of the postsynaptic potentials. This blockade may be reversed by cholinesterase inhibitors.[25] The second group causes an augmentation of the acetylcholine release followed by a presynaptic depletion of acetylcholine. This latter toxin cannot be reversed by cholinesterase inhibitors or antivenom. Venom may also contain cholinesterase and acetylcholine, but this appears to contribute little to the toxicity of the venom.[26]

Cobra venom contains hemolysins and cardiotoxins in addition to the neurotoxins. In a review of 46 cases of elapid bites, the following symptoms were noted[27]:

**Signs and Symptoms of Cobra Envenomation**
Neurotoxicity          42/46 patients
  Ptosis 86%
  Respiratory paralysis 81%
  Ophthalmoplegia 43%
  Coma 26%
  Palatal paralysis 38%
  Pharyngeal paralysis 38%
  Limb paralysis 26%
  Convulsions 19%
Cardiotoxicity         4/46 patients

Cardiotoxicity from bites of these Asian elapids was associated with 100% mortality. The interval between the bite and cardiotoxic symptoms was 12 to 30 minutes.[28] Fortunately, in the United States, this is a distinctly uncommon emergency. For example, there are only two reports in the literature of cobra bites in the United States.[29]

None of the elapid venoms appear to cross the blood-brain barrier.[30] Cerebral symptoms, such as seizures or lethargy, may also be noted from hypoxia induced by respiratory insufficiency.[31,32] In at least one study of coral snakes, no cardiac failure or arrhythmias were noted.[33] There appear to be no permanent sequelae although some patients may require months before recovery from major paralysis.

## CORAL SNAKES

There are three species of coral snakes in the United States; the eastern coral snake or harlequin snake (*Micrurus fulvius fulvius*), the Texas coral snake (*M. fulvius tenere*), and a smaller Sonoron coral snake (*Micuroides euryxanthus euryxanthus*). The eastern coral

snake is found throughout the southern United States from North Carolina through Florida and west to Mississippi. The Texas coral snake is found in the Mississippi valley and westerly into mid Texas. The Sonoran or Arizona coral snake is found in Arizona and western New Mexico.[1] There are eight species of tropical coral snakes that are larger and not always brightly banded. In Mexico, coral snakes are called Coralilla or the "20-minute snake," suggestive of the lethal nature of the toxin.[34]

### Recognition

The coral snake has a black nose and bright-colored bands of red and yellow or white and black. The maxim "red with black, venom lack; red on yellow, kill a fellow" well described the placement of red bands between yellow and white in the coral snake. The coral snake's colored bands also completely encircle the abdominal portion of the snake. The eastern and Texas coral snakes are fairly large and may exceed a meter in length. The Sonoran coral snake is small and is usually less than one half meter in length.[35]

### Local Signs

The native North American elapids have small, fixed anterior maxillary fangs. When they bite, they use a series of chewing motions, resulting in multiple tiny puncture wounds. Coral snakes are reclusive and most bites result when the snake is handled. The bite wounds are minimally painful and cause little or no local reaction. Some minimal redness and swelling is noted in about half the cases. A higher risk of envenomation is noted when the reptile "hangs on" after biting.[33]

---

*Emergency Treatment of Elapid Envenomation*
Treatment of coral snake envenomation includes the use of 3 to 5 vials of *Micrurus fulvius* antivenin in all cases with puncture wounds. If the patient becomes symptomatic despite this therapy, 3 to 5 more vials of antivenin should be given.
Treatment is otherwise supportive.
Be prepared to intubate the patient and give respiratory support with a ventilator.

## Systemic Signs

Systemic manifestations of coral snakes include drowsiness, nausea and vomiting, dysphagia, diplopia, paralysis of extremities, and, lastly, respiratory paralysis. Symptomatic evidence of envenomation is often delayed for several hours, with the first symptom being reported as euphoria.[36] Paresthesias around the bite may occur within several hours. Salivation, weakness, ptosis, tremors, and loss of taste or other sensations may also be noted. Antivenin, if given early, will prevent the paralysis but will usually not reverse it.

---

*Signs and Symptoms in Coral*
*Snake Envenomation*
Fang marks 85%
Local swelling 40%
Paresthesias 35%
Nausea 30%
Vomiting 25%
Euphoria 15%
Weakness 15%
Dizziness 10%
Diplopia 10%
Dyspnea 10%
Diaphoresis 10%
Muscle tenderness 10%
Fasciculations 5%
Confusion 5%

---

## OTHER ELAPIDS

Other elapids have varying amounts of neurotoxins, cardiotoxins, hemotoxins, or vasculotoxins in their venom. The primary effect found in many of the elapid toxins appears to be from the neurotoxins or the cardiotoxins with a small variable degree of localized damage. An exception to this is the greater degree of local reaction noted with some species of cobra.[37] Treatment must be aimed at effects from these components and differs substantially from treatment of the crotalid envenomations. Consultation with an experienced medical herpetologist is essential in management of patients suffering from bites of these exotic species.

## Columbridae

The family *Columbridae*, a large family of usually nonvenomous snakes, contains the medically important boomslang and the vine snake, both from Africa. In North America, this family is normally considered nonvenomous. About 12% of this family do have rear grooved fangs and venom glands and are capable of envenomation of a human.

## PREHOSPITAL CARE

There appears to be little doubt that the emphasis that has been placed on rapid first aid of a snake bite is misplaced. Certainly, much of the first aid that has been proposed in the past has been found to be ineffective and contradictory. This leads to confusion about the proper field treatment for a snake bite. The decision to "do something" in this highly charged situation should be based upon a knowledge of toxicology, anatomy, and the field situation. It makes little sense to use a highly controversial field treatment when the patient is only a few minutes away from help, the hospital, or rapid aeromedical transportation. The situation is arguably different when faced with a 2-day evacuation through hostile territory with worsening weather patterns. The physician faced with this situation should recall that, at least in the United States, disability from improperly applied "treatments" exceeds the number of deaths from snake bites. At least one authority notes that "If you don't do anything, you haven't done anything wrong."[38]

---

*Prehospital Care*
Retreat out of striking distance (usually 3 or more paces).
Encourage the victim to remain calm.
Splint the affected extremity.
Elevate the affected extremity to just below heart level.
Remove rings and other constrictive items.
Give appropriate reassurance.
Evacuate the patient, minimizing activity if possible. The patient should be a litter patient, if at all possible.

---

Probably the single most important principle of first aid in handling the victim of a snake bite is to ensure that you do not become a victim yourself. Retreat out of the range of the snake, at least two to three full strides from the snake, if possible. It is unlikely that a snake will strike more than one half of its body length, and they certainly do not pursue humans.

Identification of the snake is helpful, but the snake should not be approached by untrained personnel. Some authors recommend killing and bringing the dead animal in for identification, but this does not seem wise, when even preserved heads have caused symptomatic envenomation.[39,40] The emergency provider should record a verbal description of the snake, a description of the initial wounds, the progress of the injury, and the signs and symptoms of systemic envenomation.

## Initial Therapy

Encourage the victim to remain calm and avoid any unnecessary movements. A person in the backcountry with an envenomated bite should not walk but should be carried out. At least one study has shown increased mortality in those animals who were exercised, compared with resting animals.[41,42] McCullough and Gennaro also noted that patients who were immobilized had a generally milder course than those who had moderate to extreme activity following the snakebite.[42] Immobility will reduce lymphatic flow and decrease systemic absorption of venom.

Often, splinting has been proposed in the treatment of snakebite. No studies exist that adequately support it, but the pain relief afforded by splinting would recommend it in any case. Certainly, decreasing the mobility of the extremity will cause no further damage and may offer some delay in absorption of the venom. A splint that has been secured too tightly may, of course, cause distal vascular compromise.

## Unsubstantiated Therapies

### CUT AND SUCK

Placement of incisions and then suction removal of the venom has been used for years. The presumed purpose of this method of first aid is to remove the venom before it has a chance to produce toxic symptoms. The cut and suction of venom has been popularized by scores of Hollywood films and appeals to the lay person but is unlikely to help most patients.

Local incisions and suction (the cut-and-suck method) are more likely to introduce infection, damage underlying structures, and cause bleeding than to remove significant amounts of venom. In one Indian study of viper bites, 94% of patients who had had an incision developed an infection.[43] In personal experience, enthusiastic incisions to the dorsum of the hand have caused lacerations to the extensor tendons. Certainly, the untrained or inexperienced individual should not use this technique because it can damage tendons, nerves, and blood vessels as well as compromise local wound healing.

The cut-and-suck method is effective only if started within the first half hour of the bite and then only at the site of the venom deposition.[44] Incisions and suction have been shown to remove some of the venom from the wound, and some victims have been reported to have a less severe reaction to the bite.[45-47] It is difficult to evaluate this latter contention since in 20% of snakebites there is no injection of venom and no possible way to determine which snake has caused venom deposition.

Incisions should be made no deeper than about ¼ to ½ inch. The cut should not go blindly and deeply into muscle or fat. To avoid damage to underlying structures, incisions should be linear and along the longitudinal axis of the limb. The hand, wrist, foot, ankle, face, and neck contain superfical, underlying structures that are easily damaged and incisions should not be made about this area. Incisions should only be made at the site of the bite.

Suction should then be applied with a suction cup or suction device. Although there is little danger from aspirated venom, human oral bacteria are particularly prone to cause destructive infections, so oral suction should be avoided. Suction should be continued for about 30 minutes and then stopped.

A technique that may be expected to have few harmful effects is suction without incision. Suction alone may have a place in field treatment, as it avoids both the infectious and disfiguring surgical complications of incision. A commercial suction device (Sawyer's extractor) has removed as much as 34% of venom without the use of incisions and may be quite useful.[48] Certainly, further studies with this relatively innocuous device are indicated.

The Wilderness Medical Society feels that the cut and suction technique no longer has a place in emergency care of snake bites.[49]

The authors advocate the use of suction and incisions only by well-trained and qualified providers, cognizant of the anatomy, and only if there is to be a greater than 6-hour evacuation time before antivenin is available. If an appropriate suction device such as the Sawyer extractor is available, this alone would be the preferred technique.

## EN BLOC EXCISION

A hospital-based variant of the cut-and-suck technique, en bloc excision of tissue, has also been proposed.[50,51] The rationale is to remove the section of tissue with the venom in it in order to reduce both local and systemic illness. This technique seems particularly likely to damage structures even if used by a physician, unless the physician has surgical training, appropriate instruments, and the lighting of an operating suite. Due to relatively rapid spread of the venom, it is unlikely to be effective later than 30 minutes after the bite. En bloc dissection may have a place when the bite is less than 30 minutes old, the patient is showing significant signs of toxicity, and the patient has a significant allergic reaction to the antivenin. In less trying circumstances, it is not recommended. Few emergency departments will ever see the patient who has been bitten by a snake, presents and is diagnosed, and is then transferred to the operating room for en bloc dissection—all in under 30 minutes.

## THE AUSTRALIAN METHOD

In Australia, highly toxic bites are more common than in the United States. It should be noted that most of these snakebites are from elapids, not from the viper family.

Sutherland and his colleagues in Australia have developed a method of decreasing the spread of venom of these very toxic Australian snakes until antivenom is available.[52,53] Sutherland's method has the approval and recommendation of both the Australian Resuscitation Council and the National Health and Medical Research Council. Sutherland clearly outlines the compression method as a *first-aid* technique to slow absorption of venom until proper antivenin is available. It is not intended to replace antivenom therapy in any way.

The method consists of compression and immobilization with an Ace wrap (crepe bandage). The extremity is compressed with the Ace wrap from distal to proximal, and the wrap is loose enough to be comfortable.[54] This method has been shown clearly to retard venom uptake systemically in both the Sydney funnel-web spider and Australian snakes.[55,56] This delay of uptake is supposed to allow a more leisurely administration of antivenom and allow the patient to be transported to an appropriate medical facility.

At this point, whether or not to use the "Australian method" is speculative for North American snakebites. There may be some application in the treatment of coral snakebites, which are the only elapid snakes in the United States. Animal studies with crotalid venom have shown no advantage to compression.[57] Even the advocates of the Australian compressive method note that there are unusual complications attributed to the long-term effects of large amounts of localized venom, however. In the more locally destructive crotalid venoms, this may markedly aggravate the wound. The question that needs to be answered is, simply, will sequestration of a venom with locally toxic effects harm or help the patient? That question remains to be answered in either the Australian or the American literature.

In absolute fairness to the Australians, Australian snakes have venom with rapid systemic toxicity and high chances of mortality. Delay of uptake of this venom may literally be lifesaving until antivenom can be obtained. This is not the case with the relatively innocuous North American crotalid snakes, and critics of the compressive method should be clearly aware of this toxicologic and clinical difference between the continents' venomous animals. The Australians are quite certain that this is a lifesaving technique in their clinical practice. It may have a place in the treatment of elapid envenomations in the United States.

## LIGATURE (TOURNIQUETS, CONSTRICTING BANDS, ETC.)

Standard first-aid recommendations for poisonous snakebites call for the patient to have a "constricting band" applied to retard lymph flow. In the past, a common recommendation was to place a tourniquet that impeded arterial flow. This therapy resulted in substantial ischemic damage and has been abandoned. The present recommendations represent, therefore, a "softening" of earlier first-aid therapy.

The lymph constrictor should properly be applied so that one finger can pass beneath the ligature. Unfortunately, in the heat of the moment, many lay workers simply apply a tourniquet, with potential loss of the limb. Worse still, the lay person may apply the ligature just tight enough to retard the venous outflow and not impede the arterial inflow. This leads to rapid engorgement of the extremity and increase in the local tissue damage.

The purpose of this measure is to retard the spread of venom and thereby to minimize the systemic effects of the venom until antivenin can be given. Depending upon the species of snake and the systemic symptoms, this may make some sense.

As noted earlier, it does not seem appropriate to sequester locally toxic venom and increase the local morbidity, unless there is systemic benefit in doing so. No such clear systemic benefit has been demonstrated in the literature in treatment of crotalid envenomation in the United States. At least one animal study has shown sequestration to be of no benefit.[42]

It does seem appropriate to sequester a systemic toxin until appropriate antivenin is available. The toxins of this nature are found in bites of the elapids and possibly the Mojave rattlesnake. With the complications and difficulty of applying a true constrictive band, perhaps the compression dressing of the Australian method may make more sense. This is a clinical decision that needs more research and should be based in part on the time until antivenin is available. There are too few documented North American elapid envenomations to adequately recommend for or against this maneuver at this time. Good multicenter data collection is needed in the case of elapid and Mojave rattlesnake envenomation before unequivocal recommendation can be made.

At present, despite multiple, unsubstantiated recommendations, no clear case can be made for the use of ligature in the treatment of crotalid envenomation. The major morbidity is loss of tissue and scarring, resulting in crippling deformities. Misapplication with subsequent worsening of the injury is common. Ligature of any fashion by lay persons is, therefore, not recommended for crotalid envenomation. Trained emergency responders should consider the entire picture of local tissue damage, degree of difficulty in extrication of the patient from the wilderness, duration of the evacuation, and availability of antivenom before application of an unproven and potentially harmful therapy.

## Worthless Therapies

### COLD TREATMENT

For many years, emergency providers and physicians were told to cool the area of the bite. Indeed, some "authorities" went so far as to issue instructions to pack the limb in ice. Cold packs were advocated in all snakebite kits. It was thought that the cold would reduce the amount of swelling, inactivate the enzymatic venom, and retard systemic absorption of the venom. These practices have all been abandoned as dangerous.

There are no studies that support the contention that application of cold will improve the overall outcome of a snakebite. Ya and Perry found that a combination of arterial ligature and ice therapy would increase survival in dogs who had delayed administration of antivenin but only at the cost of extensive damage to the limbs.[58] These same authors also found that cryotherapy did not reduce the mortality of the venom to the same levels as early administration of antivenom. There are indications that cold may worsen the effects of the snake's venom and that it does not inactivate the toxins as previously speculated.[59] Since only part of the venom's effect is due to enzymes, cooling would be expected to slow these enzymatic effects only minimally.

It is obvious that long-term application of ice directly to skin already compromised by swelling, direct effects of the venom, and stasis will result in a severe cold injury. There are multiple instances of frostbite causing limb loss after a snakebite that support this contention. McCullough and Gennaro found that, in children, 75% of amputations associated with snakebite were preceded by cryotherapy, while Russell and his associates noted that no amputations were seen as a result of snake venom poisoning while 26 were performed for cold injury due to cryrotherapy.[22,60]

The message given by these authors about the efficacy of cold therapy in the treatment of snakebite seems quite clear. Cryotherapy is a dangerous practice and should not be used. It is mentioned only in condemnation.

## ELECTRIC SHOCK

Recent literature has attested to the use of electric shock in the treatment of various snakebites.[61] Russell notes that there is nothing new about the use of electric shock for treatment of snakebite since it has been used since at least 1887 — without substantial success at that time.[62] It is unlikely that it would work any better on the new and improved human species developed since then. Electric shock is mentioned only as a folk remedy that may delay use of appropriate therapy.

## HOSPITAL TREATMENT

The in-hospital therapy of snakebite is in some dispute between a surgical faction and an internal medicine and emergency medicine faction. The champion of the surgical faction is Dr. Thomas Glass, Jr., from Texas. The emergency and internal medicine group is more numerous and well represented by Dr. Findley Russell, from California. The heart of the dispute centers around two decisions —whether to use antivenin, and whether to perform fasciotomy. As in all controversies, there is probably some exaggeration from both factions, with the truth lying somewhere in between.

### Initial Therapy and Evaluation

The initial evaluation and assessment should include a brief history to evaluate the possibility of a nonvenomous injury, such as plant thorn injuries or other animal bites. A medical history should also include past illnesses, such as diabetes mellitus, hypertension, or other cardiopulmonary problems, medication allergies, and medications taken by the patient on a daily basis.

The envenomation should be graded and the distal neurovascular status evaluated. Reevaluation of neurovascular status and gradation of envenomation should be continued and regular as the status may change over time. Limb circumference should be repeatedly measured at multiple sites.

An intravenous line should be started with normal saline for both administration of fluids and antivenin. If there is serious envenomation, then a second line should also be started. The intravenous cannula should never be placed in a bitten extremity as both local bleeding and swelling may progress.

Wound care with saline or saline and a dilute solution of povidone-iodine should be started. Blebs should be left intact. Tetanus prophylaxis should be routinely given to patients who are not up to date on their immunizations.

## GRADING OF THE ENVENOMATION

Grading of the envenomation is useful for bites of the North American crotalids and may be useful for other vipers. It is not useful for patients who have been bitten by the elapids, as their toxins are more subtle and delayed in effects.

| Categories of Envenomation | |
|---|---|
| Degree of Envenomation | Signs and Symptoms |
| None | No local or systemic symptoms |
| Minimal | Local swelling only |
| Moderate | Edema progressing beyond the area of the bite, systemic reactions and laboratory abnormalities found |
| Severe | Marked local reaction, severe systemic signs and symptoms, multiple significant laboratory abnormalities |

### No envenomation

No pain or swelling is found at the site of the "envenomation" at least 4 hours after the bite. Laboratory data are essentially normal. No systemic symptoms are present for 4 or more hours after the strike. For crotalid envenomations, no further therapy is indicated.

### Minimal envenomation

Minimal edema exists at the site of the bite. Perioral paresthesias, metallic tastes, or nausea may be present but without other systemic symptoms. Laboratory data are essentially normal.

## Moderate envenomation

Signs of envenomation extend beyond the bite site but do not involve the entire extremity. Laboratory data show moderate coagulation or other abnormalities. Significant systemic symptoms are present.

## Severe envenomation

The entire extremity is involved with swelling, ecchymosis, or petechiae. Serious systemic signs or symptoms are present. Laboratory data reflect serious coagulation or other abnormalities.

## LABORATORY DATA

Baseline laboratory data should include a CBC, electrolytes, BUN, creatinine, platelet count, and urinalysis. With the high frequency of coagulopathies noted in cases of snakebite, it is appropriate to obtain prothrombin times, bleeding and clotting times, fibrinogen, and fibrin split products. Any patient who is hypotensive should have blood typed and crossed. Myoglobin measurements are indicated in patients with a severe reaction.

In severe cases, insert a Foley catheter and, if vomiting is persistent, insert a nasogastric tube. Analgesics can be administered, but in these patients, as in all critically ill patients, should be given by intravenous routes.

## Antivenin

Antivenin (antivenom) is prepared from the serum of animals that have been hyperimmunized against the venom of a specific species of animals. The first antivenin was prepared against the venom of the king cobra by Calmette in 1890. Currently, horses are the only animals used in the preparation of antivenin, and the technique is essentially unchanged from that developed by Calmette.

Due to the foreign protein contents of all of the antivenins, both acute hypersensitivity reactions and delayed serum sickness reactions can occur after administration. A history of allergies to horse serum, hay fever, urticaria, or prior history of horse serum injections may place the patient at some increased risk of a hypersensitivity reaction and certainly increases the odds of a delayed reaction. Skin testing with a 1:10 dilution of the horse serum is recommended 30 minutes prior to administration of the antivenin. In cases of severe envenomations, this grace period is not always possible.

Antivenin therapy is the treatment of choice for all seriously envenomated persons. As noted earlier, not every snakebite will have deposition of significant amounts of venom. Small children often require more antivenin than adults, because a larger amount of venom per kilogram is involved.

## SPECIFIC SPECIES

### Crotalids

The decision to administer antivenin in the case of pit viper bites, which includes the rattlesnakes, copperheads, massasaugas, and water moccasins, must be made by clinical observation. Bites are classified by the local and systemic signs that develop following envenomation into four groups as noted earlier. While this classification is useful for almost all of the pit vipers found in the United States, it should not be used for coral snakes and exotic snakes. It may not completely apply in the case of the Mojave rattlesnakes.

| Crotalid Envenomation | Starting Dose of Antivenin |
|---|---|
| Mild | None to 5 vials |
| Moderate | 5 to 15 vials |
| Severe | 15 to 20 vials or more |

The antivenin should be titrated against symptoms and signs of envenomation. If enough antivenin is given, the symptoms should start to resolve. If antivenin is given too rapidly, urticaria and hypotension may occur.

### Elapid Envenomation

Elapid envenomations are quite different from crotalid bites. The signs and symptoms of an elapid bite are often delayed for hours, and fang marks may not be seen. The pain of a coral snake envenomation is mild and local with only minimum swelling. Local symptoms are not reliable in predicting the presence of systemic symptoms. If the snake is positively identified as a coral snake, envenomation must be presumed and the patient treated with antivenin. Since cardiovascular and respiratory collapse occur as late symptoms, these patients must be given antivenin on the suspicion of a coral snake bite. The usual dose is 3 to 6 vials of Micrurus fulvus antivenin, which should neutralize the maximum dose of venom that a coral snake can deliver. It should be remembered that antivenin is unlikely to reverse the paralysis of a coral snakebite.

Endotracheal intubation is recommended if there are any signs of bulbar paralysis, such as slurred speech or diplopia. Respiratory support with a ventilator is needed in these cases.

### Exotic Snake Envenomation

Cross-reactivity with domestic antivenins is possible but unlikely with exotic snakes. The best advice, when dealing with an exotic snakebite, is to contact the Antivenin Index at the Arizona Poison Control Center (602-626-6016). A listing of all available antivenins that can be used for that species is available, together with the location of the antivenin and the contact person who will be able to obtain the antivenin.

In most cases, envenomation by an exotic snake may not be graded as is done with the pit vipers. There is a significant incidence of life-threatening late systemic effects after these snakebites and local symptoms may be absent. Species-specific antivenin is advised if there is any possibility of envenomation, unless otherwise contraindicated, or specific advice is obtained from a medical herpetologist who is familiar with the species.

### ADMINISTRATION

Antivenin should be diluted with 50 to 100 cc of normal saline or Ringer's lactate and given intravenously. Under no circumstances should the antivenin be injected into the wound. Not only is it poorly absorbed from the wound, but it only distends the tissues and decreases the blood flow. Intramuscular injections of antivenin have been used in the past, but in any seriously ill patient decreased blood flow to the muscles will retard medication uptake. Antivenin is no exception to this rule. The very person who has hypo-

tension and needs the medication most will be the one with the least uptake!

### COMPLICATIONS

A major problem arises when the patient either has a history of allergies to horse serum, develops a positive reaction to the skin test, or has an allergic reaction during the first few vials of antivenin. The problem is simply resolved if the patient is severely envenomated, and in the clinical judgment of the physician, would die without antivenin. In the moderately envenomated patient, the problem is not easily resolved, however. The clinician should remember that these patients will likely not die from crotalid envenomation but may have a major disability from the tissue destruction. The chance of a reaction must be weighed against the odds of amputation or death. It is not an easy decision, and the clinician would be well advised in this case to consult with a poison control center or a specialist in management of venomous animal bites.

Some authorities advocate the use of intravenous antihistamines, large doses of corticosteroids, and dilution of the antivenin if the patient has a high likelihood of allergic reaction or great necessity despite known allergies. Dilution of the antivenin may be made at 1:100, 1:1000, or 1:10,000, depending upon the need and ability of the patient to tolerate the fluid challange. Oxygen, suction, intubation equipment, and resuscitation medications should be available at the bedside if the decision is made to give antivenin. A second intravenous line should be started in an unbitten extremity.

The use of steroids in snakebite patients is controversial, and some authors feel they may be harmful.[63-65] Steroids are certainly advocated in other diseases when antibiotics are indicated despite allergic reactions, or when a patient develops an anaphylactic reaction, and may have similar utility in the patient with a serious immediate reaction to antivenin. Steroids are not helpful in the routine treatment of snakebite, however.[66]

If the patient receives more than 5 vials of antivenin, serum sickness becomes likely in 5 to 15 days after administration of the antivenin. The incidence of serum sickness has varied between 50 and 75% of those who have received greater than 5 vials of antivenin.[67] A 5- to 7-day course of oral prednisone, together with antihistamines will likely relieve the patient's symptoms. In refractory or severe cases, intravenous corticosteroids and hospitalization may become necessary.[68]

## SOURCES

Currently available antivenins in the United States include polyvalent antivenin for Crotalids and monovalent antivenin for coral snakes. Both of these antivenins are produced by Wyeth laboratories and are commercially available. Black widow spider venom is also commercially available and was discussed previously.

Experimental antivenins are available for many other species of venomous animal but are not commerically produced in the United States. A listing of antivenins available in the United States under Investigational and New Drug permits may be obtained by calling the Arizona Poison Control Center at 602-626-6016, 24 hours a day. The Antivenin Index can determine the correct antivenin if the type of snake is known either by its common or scientific name. The location of the nearest supply of antivenin will be given, but it is up to the physician to arrange for delivery. Zoos and herpetologists usually have registered their supply of antivenin with the Antivenin Index but may be checked first. If the bite occurred in the local zoo, antivenin will frequently be available from the herpetologist immediately. The author can personally vouch for the efficacy of the Antivenin Index in locating a supply of antivenin when he had to treat an amateur herpetologist who had been bitten by a king cobra. Antivenin manufacturers are listed in Table 7.5.

If the treating physician or patient does not know the species of snake, then the snake must be identified before treatment can be obtained.

## The Controversy

It is this high incidence of serum sickness following the administration of antivenin that sparks the controversy. Some surgical authorities feel strongly that the use of antivenin is dangerous and that the patient is better treated with high doses of steroids and

**Table 7.5.**
**Manufacturers of Antivenin**

Behringwerke AG, Poatfach 167, D-355 Marburg-Lahn, Federal Republic of Germany
*European, Middle Eastern, and most African snakes*
Central Research Institute, Kasauli, Punjab, India
*Most Indian and Southeast Asian snakes*
Commonwealth Serum Laboratories, 45 Popular road, Parkville, Victoria 3052, Australia
*Australian snakes, spiders, jellyfish, stonefish, and ticks*
Instituto Butantan, Caixa Postal 65, Sao Paulo, Brazil
*South American vipers, Loxosceles, and Phoneutria spiders*
Institute Pasteur Annexe de Garches, 92 (Hauts de Seine), Paris, France
*European, Middle Eastern, and African snakes*
Laboratorios MYN, S.A., Avenue Coyoacan 1707, Mexico City 12, D.F. Mexico
*Mexican crotalids, scorpions, and most other American crotalids*
Laboratory of Chemotherapy and Serum Therapy, 1 Furukyomachi, Kumamoto City, Kyushu, Japan
*Habu and Mamushi*
Merck, Sharp, and Dohme, West Point, PA 19486, USA
*Black widow spiders*
National Institute of Preventive Medicine, 161 Kun-Yang, Nan-Kang, Taipei, Taiwan
*Cobras, Southeast Asian kraits, vipers, and habu*
Queen Saovabha Memorial Institute, Rama IV Street, Bangkok, Thailand
*Southeast Asian cobras, kraits, and vipers*
The South African Institute for Medical Research, Hospital Street, PO Box 1038, Johannesburg 2000, Republic of South Africa
*African snakes*
Universidad de Costa Rica, Instituto Clordormiro Picado, Cuidad Universitaria, Costa Rica
*North and South American vipers and coral snakes*
Wyeth Laboratories, Box 8299, Philadelphia PA 19101, USA
*North American pit vipers and coral snakes*

surgical decompression. The medical authorities point to the ease of treatment of the serum sickness and the disfigurement involved in surgical decompression as major drawbacks.

Of one fact there can be no doubt. The only effective therapy for the venom of a venomous snake is antivenin. This should indicate that administration of antivenin should be a non-issue in the treatment of a snakebite.

Since the mortality of snakebite in the United States is low, the patient may well survive without it in most cases. This would make for a fine series of "survivals" without the use of antivenin.

### The Solution (New Developments)

There are three promising developments that may spell an end to the controversy about antivenin's toxicity vs. its benefits. The first two developments increase the specificity of the antivenin for the snake toxins, and the third decreases the indecision about use of available antivenin. The first involves purification of the antivenin by immunosorbent affinity chromatography. In this method, IgG(T) is purified, eliminating much of the extraneous protein that causes reactions and making a much more effective antivenin.[69-71] The second technique also improves the specificity of the venom by the use of FAB fragments (fractional antibody fragments of the IgG(T) specific for single species of snake venom).[72] It is thought that renal clearance of the venom will be increased by the use of the smaller FAB fragments. In addition, the FAB fragments are much less immunogenic than are whole antibodies.

The final technique, ELISA antibody detection, may decrease the use of antivenin, particularly in exotic and elapid species.[73] Enzyme-linked immunoassays can detect small quantities of specific snake venom in wound, serum, or urine. When employing this test, only patients with envenomation will be treated with antivenin, and potentially antivenin can be titrated against active remaining venom. At the time of publication, all of these techniques are experimental.

### Fasciotomy

The findings of a rattlesnake bite are very similar to those of a compartment syndrome.[74] The crux of the controversy about fasciotomy centers on the development of a compartment syndrome and the effects thereof. This controversy has sparked intense debates about the need for surgical intervention in a snakebite, with zealots on both sides. The following discussion applies to crotalid snake-

bites only as the elapid's venom does not usually cause local tissue damage.

### SUBFASCIAL VS. SUBCUTANEOUS ENVENOMATION

The first point to make is that subfascial snake envenomation is not common and may occur in only 5% or less of crotalid strikes. The crotalids have fangs that are ½ inch (1.2 cm) in length. The average strike will penetrate a maximum of ½ inch, which is very unlikely to deposit venom in the fascial compartments. Multiple authors have shown experimentally that subcutaneous injections of venom do not produce compartment syndromes.[75]

### PREVENTION VS. TREATMENT

The nonsurgical camp feels that the tissue necrosis is produced by the venom and not by the internal pressure in the compartment. They also note that surgery within the first 8 hours of envenomation often leads to excessive bleeding due to the transient coagulopathy induced by crotalid venom. This leads to a strong advocacy of early use of antivenin to reverse the effects of tissue destruction. This is logical, indeed. There is compelling evidence that the *early and proper* use of species-specific antivenin is the single best preventive factor for compartment syndrome in snakebites. Prevention is not quite the same as treatment, however. There is no evidence that antivenin will reduce compartment pressures or will reverse the tissue damage found after delays in treatment.

### COMPARTMENT SYNDROME

Compartment syndrome is a condition in which the perfusion and function of the tissues within an anatomic space bounded by fascia or bone is compromised by increased pressure within that space. Increased pressure leads to increased local venous pressure and reduced local arteriovenous gradient. Since the veins are collapsible tubes, an increased external pressure will cause decreased blood flow. This leads to further tissue necrosis and a vicious cycle of increasing damage.

The most common etiologies of compartment syndrome are fractures, crush injuries, and burns. Snakebite is a distinctly uncommon cause of compartment syndrome. Since compartment syndrome is caused primarily by orthopedic trauma, we must turn to the orthopedic literature for advice on diagnosis and treatment. A change in two-point discrimination is often the earliest clinical finding of a compartment syndrome. Muscle weakness is a late sign. Capillary fill and arterial pulse are routinely present in bona fide compartment syndromes and should not be used as diagnostic criteria.[76] Acceptable techniques of pressure measurements in the compartments include the wick catheter technique, the slit catheter technique, and the manometry catheter technique.[77,78] These techniques are well described and details available in many emergency and surgical references.

In clinical studies of patients at risk for compartment syndrome, the pressure tolerance has varied from 30 to 55 mm Hg, as determined by correlating direct pressure measurements with clinical findings.[79,80] The duration of the pressure elevation is fully as important as the magnitude of pressure elevation, however.[81] A pressure within the compartmental space that is tolerated for a few hours may be detrimental if allowed to persist for longer periods of time. Unfortunately, as has been amply shown in other causes of compartment syndrome, not all damage is produced by local tissue destruction.

## TECHNIQUE

The technique for fasciotomy is likewise well described in the surgical literature and need not be repeated here. It is important that the procedure be skillfully performed, as immense damage may be done in structures distorted from the usual anatomy. The administration of mannitol has reduced compartment pressures to tolerable levels in one patient, who did not need subsequent surgery (personal communication, JB Sullivan). This possible alternative method bears further investigation. It should also be remembered that surgical incisions may become sites for life-threatening hemorrhage should a coagulopathy occur.

## RECOMMENDATIONS

The middle road, then, is the rapid and proper use of antivenin, combined with frequent neurovascular evaluations and compartment pressure measurements in affected compartments. It would be appropriate to perform a fasciotomy for the accepted indications of rising compartment pressure, compartment pressures above 30 mm Hg on two or more measurements, or evidence of neurovascular damage. Even in the surgical literature, this occurs in less than 1 of every 20 serious snakebites.[82] *A routine fasciotomy is not indicated.*

To paraphrase Dr. Findley Russell, the jury will be highly critical of the physician or expert who states that he "knows from past experience that a compartment syndrome must be present" in the absence of valid and objective measurements and past experiences with adequate controls.[83] Likewise, it is certain that the jury will be equally intolerant of the physician who blindly assumes that all tissue damage will be due to the effects of the venom and that fasciotomy is never indicated. It behooves the physician to make proper pressure measurements of the internal fascia-bounded compartments that may be affected and evaluations of the neurovascular status and to act upon these measurements and evaluations appropriately.

It should be remembered that there are zealots in both the surgical and nonsurgical camps who are ready to defend or attack all who stray from the middle road. It will be difficult indeed for a physician to defend the suit for footdrop after two compartment pressure measurements of 70 mm Hg without a surgical consultation. It should be equally difficult to defend the care of the serious envenomation that proceeds without measurements of the compartment pressure. Routine compartment pressure measurements and neurovascular evaluations are always indicated; fasciotomy without compelling evidence is most certainly not indicated. The controversial issue of fasciotomy should not be an issue at all if these recommendations are followed.

## Adjunctive Therapy
### TETANUS IMMUNIZATION

With the large amount of tissue damage and an open wound, a snake bite is considered a high-risk injury for tetanus. All patients should be appropriately immunized against tetanus. The usual protocols should be followed.

## ANTIBIOTICS

Although snake venom itself is sterile, the snake's mouth is not, and all venoms cause enough local damage to facilitate an infection. An appropriate broad-spectrum antibiotic such as one of the cephalosporins is indicated. In higher level envenomations, the wound should be cultured and antibiotics given on the basis of the cultures.

## HEPARIN

Although heparin is not effective in treatment of the bleeding diathesis associated with snake envenomation, it may be useful after 24 to 48 hours after envenomation. At least one author describes phlebitis after severe envenomation.[84]

## PREVENTION

The ideal treatment for snakebite is, of course, not to be bitten at all. To accomplish this, first avoid all known snake habitats. Snakes are cold blooded and nocturnal hunters. Avoid places where they may sun themselves and avoid travel in snake-infested areas after night. Do not handle poisonous snakes, even when "dead."

Do not put hands or feet into places that you cannot look into. Make no sudden movements around rock piles, wood piles, or cracks or crevices.

Protective clothing, such as jeans and boots, should be worn. Snakes rarely strike higher than ankle high and boots that cover the ankles will prevent or deflect many bites. It is particularly important to wear footgear at night.

Avoid solo hiking in areas that are known to be infested with snakes or at night. If solo, ensure that both route and expected time of return are registered with either park rangers or responsible friends.

## SUMMARY

The treatment of snake venom poisoning in the United States is controversial, despite an overall low mortality. Morbidity and disability are, unfortunately, not unusual in the treatment of snakebites. Other poisonous land animals are not common and do not cause significant problems in humans.

Recognition of a snakebite is usually simple, and, in the United States, identification is equally simple. Exotic species imported by amateur herpetologists may complicate both identification and treatment of snakebites. In North America, crotalid envenomations predominate, and all emergency departments should be prepared to manage envenomations by these animals.

Treatment both in the field and in the emergency department is controversial, but this controversy is sparked less by facts than by opinions. Few controlled studies are available to support immediate surgical therapy, and few appropriately controlled studies have evaluated compartment pressures in patients with serious envenomations. Other procedures, such as cryotherapy, ligature, and en bloc excision have little or no place in therapy.

Snakebite is a medical emergency requiring immediate attention and medical judgment. The effects of snake venom are time dependent, and delay in therapy will increase patient morbidity. If the physician has any question, advice should be sought from the nearest major poison control center or a physician experienced in the care of snakebites.

## References

1. Kunkel DB, Curry SC, Vance MV, Ryan PJ. Reptile envenomations. J Toxicol Clin Toxicol 1983;21:503–526.
2. Russell FE. Snake venom poisoning in the United States. Ann Rev Med 1980;37:247–259.
3. Hayes WK, Hayes FE. Human envenomation from the bite of the Eastern garter snake. Toxicon 1985;23:719–721.
4. Minton, SA. Beware: non-poisonous snakes. Clin Toxicol 1979;15:259–265.
5. Wingert WA, Sullivan JB. Snakebite management: which approach to use. Emerg Med Rep 1984;5:37–44.
6. Bradley SG, Klika LJ. A fatal poisoning from the Oregon roughskinned newt (*Taricha granulosa*). JAMA 1981246:247.
7. Brodie ED Jr. Investigations of the skin toxins of the adult rough skinned newt *Taricha granulosa*. Copeia 1968;1:306–313.
8. Daly JW. Biologically active alkaloids from poison frogs (*Dendrobatidae*) J Toxicol Toxin Rev 1982;1:33–86.

9. Hitt M, Ettinger DD. Toad toxicity. N Engl J Med 1986;314:1517.

10. Russel FE, Bogert CM. Gila monster: its biology, venom, and bite—a review. Toxicon 1981;19:341–359.

11. Piacentine J, Curry SC, Ryan PJ. Life-threatening anaphylaxis following Gila monster bite. Ann Emerg Med 1986;15:959–961.

12. Streiffer RH. Bite of the venomous lizard, the Gila monster. Postgrad Med 1986;79:297–302.

13. Burnett JW, Calton GJ, Morgan RJ. Gila monster bites. Cutis 1985;35:333.

14. Kunkel DB. Bites of venomous reptiles. Emerg Med Clin North Am 1984;2:563–577.

15. Klauber LM. Rattlesnakes (abridged edition). Berkeley: University of California, 1982.

16. Russell FE, ed. Snake venom poisoning. Great Neck, NY: Scholium International. 1983; 168,169, 198, 213, 334.

17. Curry SC, Kunkel DB. Death from a rattlesnake bite. Am J Emerg Med 1985;3:227–235.

18. Watt CJ, Cennaro JF. Pit vipers in south Georgia and north Florida. Trans South Surg Assoc 1966;77:378.

19. Homma M, Tu AT: Morphology of local tissue damage in experimental snake envenomation. Br J Exp Pathol 1971;52:538.

20. Russell FE, Carlson RW, Wainschel J, and Osborne AH. Snake venom poisoning in the United States: experience with 550 cases. JAMA 1975;233:341–344.

21. Hasiba U, Rosenbach LM, Rockwell D, et al. DIC-like syndrome after envenomation by the snake *Crotalus horridus* horridus. N Engl J Med 1975;292:505.

22. Budzynski AZ, Pandya BV, Rubin RN, et al. Fibrinogenolytic afibrinogenemia after envenomation by eestern diamondback rattlesnake (*Crotalus atrox*). Blood 1984;63:1–14.

23. Clement JF, Pietrusko RG. Pit viper snakebite envenomation in the United States. J Fam Pract 1978;6:269–279.

24. Bonilla CA, Rammel OJ. Comparative biochemistry and pharmacology of salivary gland secretions. III. Chromotographic analysis of a myocardial depressor protein from the venom of *Crotalus atrox*. J Chromatogr 1976;124:303.

25. Naphade RW, Shetti RN. Use of neostigmine after snake bite. Br J Anaesth 1977;49:1065–1068.

26. Jimenes-Porras JM. Biochemistry of snake venoms. Clin Toxicol 1970;3:389–431.

27. Banerjee RN, Saharir AL, Siddiqui ZA. Advances in the treatment of snake venom poisoning. Toxicon [suppl] 1978;1:447–455.

28. Bannerjee RN, Siddiqui ZA. Epidemiological study of snakebite in India. Toxicon [suppl] 1978;1:439–446.

29. Stuevan H, Aprahamian C, Thompson B, et al. Cobra envenomation: an uncommon emergency. Ann Emerg Med 1983;12:636–638.

30. Pettigrew LC, Glass JP. Neurologic complications of a coral snake bite. Neurology 1985; 35:589–592.

31. Swift TR. Disorders of neuromuscular transmission other than myasthenia gravis. Muscle Nerve 1981;4:334–353.

32. Willson P. Snake poisoning in the United States: a study based on analysis of 740 cases. Arch Intern Med 1908;1:516–570.

33. Kitchens CS, Van Mierop LHS. Envenomation by the Eastern Coral Snake (*Micrurus fulvius fulvius*). JAMA 1987;258:1615–1618.

34. Levy CK. A field guide to dangerous animals of North America. Brattleboro, VT: The Stephan Greene Press, 1983.

35. Zim HS, Smith HM: Reptiles and amphibians. New York: Golden Press, 1956.

36. Talpers SS, Bergin JJ. Snakebite: first aid and hospital management. Kansas Med 1985;May:1155–1167.

37. Kunkel DB. Bites of venomous reptiles. Emerg Med Clin North Am 1984;2:3.

38. Russell FE [participant]. In: Snakebite: a round table. Phys Sports Med 1980;8:30–48.

39. Stark DR, Kenney JG, Morgan RF, et al. Emergency treatment of snake venom poisoning. Curr Concepts Trauma Care 1986;Spring: 16–21.

40. Griffen D, Donovan JW. Significant envenomation from a preserved rattlesnake head (In a patient with a history of immediate hypersensitivity to antivenin). Ann Emerg Med 1986;15:955–958.

41. Leopold RS, Huber GS, Kathan RH. An evaluation of the mechanical treatment of snakebite. Milit Med 1957;120:414–416.

42. McCullough NC, Gennaro JF Jr. Evaluation of venomous snakebite in the southern United States from parallel clinical and laboratory investigations: development of treatment. J Fla Med Assoc 1963;49:959–967.

43. Bhat RN. Viperine snake bite poisoning in Jammu. J Indian Med Assoc 1974;63:383.

44. Russell FE, Sullivan JB, Egen NB, Rumack BR. Negative pressure suction in field treatment of rattlesnake bite. Vet Hum Toxicol 1985;28:297.

45. Winneberger TR, Allison EJ, Mitchell JM, et al. Snakebite treatment in the 80's. North Carolina Med J 1985;46:572–573.

46. Jackson D. Treatment of snakebite. South Med J 1929;22:605–608.

47. Jackson D, Harrison WT. Mechanical treatment of experimental rattlesnake venom poisoning. JAMA 1928;90:1928–1929.

48. Bronstein AC, Russell FE, Sullivan JB. Negative pressure suction in the field treatment of rattlesnake bite victims. Vet Hum Toxicol 1986;28:485.

49. Wilderness Medical Society. Position statements. Wilderness Med 1987;4:4.

50. Huang TT, Blackwell SJ, Lewid SR. Tissue necrosis in snakebite. JAMA 1981;77:53–58.

51. Glass TG. Early debridement in pit viper bites. JAMA 1976;235:2513–2516.

52. Sutherland SK, Coulter AR, Harris RD. Studies on the movement and effects of tiger snake venom in monkeys (*M. fascicularis*). In Proceedings of the Australian Society of Clinical and Experimental Pharmacologists. Monash University, December 4–6, 1978.

53. Sutherland SK, Coulter AR, Harris RD. The rationalisation of first aid measures for elapid snakebite. Lancet 1979:1:183–186.

54. Sutherland SK. When do you remove first aid measures form an envenomed limb. Med J Australia 1981:May 16:542.

55. Pearn J, Morrison J, Charles N, Muir V. First-aid for snakebite. Med J Aust 1981;Sept 19: 293–295.

56. Murrell G. The effectiveness of the pressure/immobilization first aid technique in the case of a tiger snake bite. Med J Aust 1981;Sept 19:295.

57. Russell FE. Pressure and immobilization for snakebite remains speculative [letter]. Ann Emerg Med 1982;11:701.

58. Ya PM, Perry JF Jr. Experimental evaluation of methods for the early treatment of snake bite. Surgery 1960;47:975–981.

59. Gill KA Jr. The evaluation of cryotherapy in the treatment of snake enveomization. South Med J 1968;63:552–556.

60. McCullough ND, Gennaro JR. Evolution of venomous snakebite in the Southern United States. J Fla Med Assoc 1963;40:959–967.

61. Herzog R. Shocks for snakebites. Outdoor Life 1987;June:55.

62. Russell FE. A letter on electroshock for snakebite. Vet Hum Toxicol 1987;29:320–321.

63. Cunningham, ER, Sabback MS, Smith RM, et al. Snakebite: role of corticosteroids as immediate therapy in an animal model. Am Surg 1979;45:757–759.

64. Russell FE. Snake venom poisoning in the United States. Ann Rev Med 1980;31:247–259.

65. Garfin SR. Rattlesnake bites: current hospital therapy. West J Med 1982;137:411–412.

66. Russell FE. Snake venom poisoning. Philadelphia: JB Lippincott, 1980.

67. Sullivan JB The managment of snake envenomations. In: Bayer MJ, Rumack BH, Wanke LA, eds. Toxicologic Emergencies, Bowie MD: RJ Brady Company, 1984.

68. Otten EJ. Antivenin therapy in the emergency department. Am J Emerg Med 1983;1:83–93.

69. Bar-Or D, Sullivan JB, Black E. Neutralization of crotalidae venom-induced platelet aggregation by affinity chromatography isolated IgG to *Crotalus viridis helleri* venom. Clin Toxicol 1984;22:1–9.

70. Sullivan JB. Immunotherapy in the poisoned patient: overview of present applications and future trends. Med Toxicol 1986;1:47–60.

71. Russell FE, Sullivan JB, Egen NB, et al. Preparation of a new antivenin by affinity chromatography. Am J Trop Med 1985;34:141–150.

72. Sullivan JB. Past, present, and future immunotherapy of snake venom poisoning. Ann Emerg Med 1987;16:938–944.

73. Minton SA. Present tests for detection of snake venom: clinical applications. Ann Emerg Med 1987;16:932–937.

74. Garfin SR, Murbarak SJ, Evans KL, et al. Rattlesnake bites: current concepts. Clin Orthop 1979;140:50–57.

75. Bailey WJ. Fasciotomy for snakebite? Emerg Med 1983;15:11–12.

76. Hayden JW. Compartment syndromes. early recognition and treatment. Postgrad Med 1983;74:191–202.

77. Whitesides TE Jr. Harada H, Morimoto K. Compartment syndromes and the role of fasciotomy. Its parameters and techniques. In: The American Academy of Orthopaedic Surgeons Instructional Course Lectures (Vol 24). St. Louis: CV Mosby, 1975;179–96.

78. Murbarak SJ, Hargens AR. Compartment syndromes and Volkmann's contracture. Philadelphia: WB Saunders, 1981:1–4.

79. Matsen FA III. Compartmental syndromes. Hosp Practice 1980;113–117.

80. Matsen FA III, Winquist RA, Krugmire RB. Diagnosis and management of compartmental syndromes. J Bone Joint Surg 1980;62A:286–291.

81. Hargens AR, Romine JR, Sipe JC, et al. Peripheral nerve conduction block by high muscle compartment pressure. Trans Orthop Res Soc 1979;4:18.

82. Murbarak SJ, Hargens AR. Acute compartment syndromes. Surg Clin North Am 1983;63:539–565.

83. Russell FE. Fasciotomy for snakebite? [letter]. Emerg Med 1983;15:11–12.

84. Watt CH. Poisonous snakebite treatment in the United States. JAMA 1978;240:654–656.

# CHAPTER 8

# Plants That Poison

## INTRODUCTION

Plant poisonings are one of the most common reasons for a call to a poison center, yet, fortunately, serious poisoning from plants is unlikely.[1] Toxic exposures to plants may be either topical or internal. The variety of symptoms caused by plant exposures may extend beyond the limits of the treating physician's medical knowledge and, perhaps, even beyond the ability of the toxicologist or biologist. Multiple organ systems may be simultaneously affected, and different parts of the plant may concentrate different active toxins, depending upon weather, season, soil, and gender of the plant. The clinical response may be, therefore, unpredictable.

Lay advocates of the back-to-the-earth philosophy may take Bradford Angier's, Euell Gibbon's, and similar authors' collections of edible plants to heart. Articles on the use of herbs and wild plants are also easily found in literature akin to *The Mother Earth News*. Warnings about artificial sweeteners, food additives, and force-fed growth of animals has encouraged such movements. While these articles, literature, and thoughts are not in error, the dishes or principles described may be applied, cooked, or prepared in error, or in haste, by someone who has incompletely read the instructions, descriptions, or just does not know what is safe and what is not.

Likewise, the plant may be ingested strictly for "pleasureable" purposes with hallucinogenic or mind-altering intent. Smoked, ingested, and injected plants may have different effects based upon the route of application. Significant morbidity may be encountered when children ingest these substances, rather than the intended adult who is more knowledgeable about the "appropriate" dose.

Alternative medical providers may prescribe herbal preparations for common conditions, in addition to, or as alternatives to, medical prescriptions. The herbalist, particularly, may alter, dilute, or concentrate active principles of plant products. Astute clinicians in past times have provided us with some of the most powerful of our current pharmacopia, from atropine to curare to digitalis. Many of the newer herbalists do not have the experience, judgment or botanical knowledge and pharmacognosy to accurately identify or measure the active ingredients found in the plants that are prescribed.

Dermatologic effects account for a substantial morbidity among trekkers, climbers, campers, and workers in forested areas. Although a self-limited and nonfatal disease, the morbidity of rhus dermatitis alone is a major factor among outdoorsmen at both work and play. Other plants, far too numerous to mention, have been reported to cause various kinds of skin reactions of various types.[2]

This chapter does not discuss the teratogenic and carcinogenic effects of plants. Likewise, the antimetabolic, antivitamin, and enzyme inhibition or mimicking effects of some plant products are not discussed. It is felt that these effects are experienced when the plant

260 / ENVIRONMENTAL EMERGENCIES

is consumed for long periods of time or is a substantial component of the diet, rather than as an emergency experience.

## GENERAL PRINCIPLES FOR INGESTIONS

The following discussion of plant ingestions is not intended to be exhaustive or worldwide but, rather, to discuss common problems treated in emergency departments and to avert potential tragedies among those using the out of doors.

Emergency medical aid for plant ingestions is usually sought when an adult notes a child chewing on a plant part or when an amateur naturalist makes a meal of a field "find."

The toxicology of plant ingestions is poorly studied in medicine. Although 25% of our drugs and pharmaceuticals are made from plants, the effects of ingestion of many plants is simply uncertain. Many of the toxic factors are not well identified and even less well understood. To further add to the complexity, a plant may elaborate toxins only into a certain part or during a specific part of the life cycle. This means that parts of a plant may be quite safe to eat, while other parts are noxious or even toxic, and these parts may change during the year. In subsistence economies, some local authorities can vouch for the safety or danger of many plants for ingestion but cannot tell why or what toxin is present.

Unfortunately, we have also lost some of the skills of identification of plants as we have moved into cities and become more civilized and less dependent directly upon fruits and products of the earth. The problem is compounded by nomenclature changes, variance of local names, and inaccurate or misleading drawings in identification texts. Listings of toxic plants may give active principles or toxic chemicals present, but the true concentration, presence, or even effect of the chemicals present in the plant is often unknown and, after cooking and ingesting, may be unknowable.

For the physician treating a person who has ingested an unknown plant, the task is impossible. For the practitioner who is treating a known ingestion, it is often difficult to predict whether or not toxic symptoms will occur.

Fortunately, most of the ingestions appear to occur with children, and the menu seems to be rather small. In multiple studies, 45 to 55% of ingestions were of only 12 "feature" items.[3-5] The magnitude of the problem is also, fortunately, small. In these same studies, less than 3% of the ingestions were associated with symptoms, and in over 1500 cases, only one person required admission.

### Frequent Plant Ingestions[3]

Philodendron†
Jade plant†
Nightshade
Swedish ivy†
Poinsettia†
African violet†
Yew
Pokeweed
Spider plant†
Schefflera†
Wandering Jew†
Rubber tree†

### Symptomatic cases of plant ingestion[3]

| | |
|---|---|
| Jimsonweed | 2 |
| Dieffenbachia† | 2 |
| Unknown berries | 2 |
| Chickory | 1 |
| Chili pepper | 1 |
| Caladium† | 1 |
| Unknown leaves | 1 (of 325 children) |

†Houseplants

### Important Historical Data

The factors that affect the toxicity of a particular ingestion include the amount of active principle ingested, the duration of exposure to the toxin, interactions between other ingested plants or drugs, and preparation of the ingested material. The part of the plant, such as leaf, berry, root, fruiting body, or stem, also affects the amount of toxin ingested as plants may sequester different concentrations of toxin in varying parts of the plant. This data must be ascertained in history from all suspected ingestions.

Another factor that is prominent in toxic ingestions is improper identification of an edible species, with consumption of a similar toxic plant. Deaths have frequently occurred when mushrooms are improperly identified or when fool's parsley or water hemlock is consumed in lieu of their nontoxic look-alikes.

Whenever possible, every effort should be made to obtain as much of the original plant or plants as possible. Expert identification should be made of the remains if it is not possible to provide samples of the whole plant.

## DOSE

As with all drugs, the amount of a plant ingested or absorbed is directly related to the effects and actions of the toxin. If possible, the amount of a plant ingested should be ascertained. An individual's body weight often influences the severity of symptoms. A smaller individual will feel the effects of a particular dose sooner or more seriously than a heavier person. The specific part of the plant eaten should also be noted, as toxin concentrations differ markedly within the plant.

## DURATION

A herb or plant that is ingested may have little or no immediate effects, yet may cause marked effects if ingested over a long period. A prime example of this is tobacco. Nicotine, ingested acutely, can cause the cholinergic effects of salivation, lacrimation, urination, defecation, and emesis—the SLUDE syndrome. Nicotine products ingested over long periods of time have been implicated in cancers, teratogenesis, heart disease, and obstructive lung disease. As noted earlier, these longer term mutagenic and carcinogenic effects are not covered in this discussion of emergency therapy.

The time of ingestion, onset of first symptoms, and number of people who ingested the plant should be obtained. Note that not every person who ingested a plant may currently be symptomatic.

## COEXISTING DISEASES

Coexisting diseases, age, and general health may markedly influence the outcome of an ingestion. Obvious results are found in patients with heart disease who can poorly tolerate extended bouts of diarrhea or emesis. Less obvious reactions, such as the thiaminase activity of horsetails and subsequent exacerbation of the thiamine depletion found in chronic alcoholics, may also occur.[6] Genetic factors may also protect or adversely influence the effects of a toxin.

Past medical illnesses and current medications should be noted for all patients. Nonprescription ingestions, such as alcohol, cannabis, aspirin, and acetaminophen, should also be noted.

## INTERACTIONS WITH OTHER AGENTS

Since plants contain biologically and pharmacologically active agents, it is logical that these agents may interact with drugs and medications taken by the patient. The most obvious interaction is when the inky cap mushroom interacts with alcohol and results in a disulfiram-like syndrome.

## PREPARATION

The preparation of a plant species may be all-important in determination of the toxicity of the plant. Certain toxins are heat labile or easily vaporized. When heated, plants containing these toxins become safe to eat. Other toxins are easily leached out with water, and when the plant is boiled with multiple changes of water, they become harmless. Pokeweed is an example of the latter type of plant. Other plants may be toxic in stems or roots and not toxic in berries or fruit. The potato, for example, is quite toxic except for the tubers.

The method of preparation should be noted, whether it is boiling, stewing, frying, or whether it is dried, raw, or cooked with other foods. Common preparations that are often overlooked include teas and infusions, ingestions of ornamental plant seeds, such as jequirty peas, and inclusion of plant leaves and fungi in salads.

## Physical Examination

When examining a patient, the presence of coexisting trauma or other medical problems should be noted and treated. This will ensure that the symptoms are not the result of other correctable conditions.

Often, there is no specific pattern or toxidrome that separates the symptoms of one toxic plant ingestion from another. Gastrointesinal (GI) symptoms are a common complaint, but this does not provide data as to the potential severity of the ingestion. Patients need to be carefully evaluated for the common toxidromes, such as anticholinergic crisis caused by atropine-like alkaloids, cholinergic symptoms caused by muscarinic mushrooms, or digitalis overdose caused by foxglove and its cousins.

## General Management

As in all toxicology, the patient should be first evaluated for Airway, Breathing, and Circulation (ABCs). Since many plant ingestions cause emesis or diarrhea, special attention must be paid to rehydration. The most frequent cause of death in children following a toxic plant ingestion is dehydration.[7] Fluid intake and output should be carefully watched in children and those over 65 years of age.

In symptomatic patients, baseline laboratory testing should include complete blood count (CBC), urinalysis, and one of the sequential multiphasic analysis profiles (SMA). If the SMA is not available, a more expensive alternative is separate electrolytes, blood urea nitrogen (BUN), creatinine, and liver function studies. If an *Amanita*-type toxin is suspected, baseline coagulation profiles may help in predicting the course of the illness. For *Cortinarius* mushroom ingestions, serial renal function studies are appropriate. Cardiac glycosides, such as those found in foxglove (digitalis), oleander, and yew, should mandate serial electrocardiograms.

Evacuation of the stomach with either ipecac or lavage may be helpful in those patients who are either not already vomiting or who have not had substantial delay in seeking therapy. Evacuation of the stomach should follow standard principles of care, with appropriate airway protection for those patients who are not fully conscious. Following evacuation of the stomach, the patient should be given activated charcoal in liberal doses (1 gm per kg of body weight). Repeat doses of charcoal should be considered for any toxin that enters the enterohepatic circulation or is secreted into the gut and then reabsorbed. Cathartics may be useful in the patient that does not already have diarrhea.

Further attempts at removal of toxin should be carefully considered, with the advice of a poison control center or consultant knowledgeable in the particular toxin ingested. Hemodialysis and charcoal hemoperfusion are advocated by some authorities for certain fungal toxins. Dialysis may be needed for both care of renal failure and removal of circulating toxins. Plasmapherisis is thought to be useful in some ingestions, but this is controversial and not well substantiated.[8]

## Active Agents

The principle active agents of most plants can be grouped into one of seven categories: volatile oils, fixed oils, resins, alkaloids, glycosides, phytotoxins, and tannins. Oxalates and other crystals may also be included but cause a more mechanical trauma than true poisoning.

### VOLATILE OILS

The volatile oils are short chain fatty acids and alcohols that can evaporate at room temperature. Some examples of volatile oils include the rose oils, clove oils, and citrus oils, used for flavoring and perfume. Herbal remedies include pennyroyal oil, eucalyptus oil, and catnip.

Volatile oils (such as those found in mustards and horseradish) act as mucous membrane irritants and spasmolytics. When taken in excess, volatile oils can also act as central nervous system (CNS) stimulants or depressants. Seizures and coma are common symptoms associated with volatile oil ingestions.

Pennyroyal oil is also used as an over-the-counter abortifacient and may cause hepatic necrosis, disseminated intravascular coagulation, and death.[9]

### FIXED OILS

Fixed oils are the longer chain fatty acids and alcohol complexes. Examples include the seed oils, such as castor oil, linseed oil, and coconut oil. These agents often form emollients and laxatives in herbal medicine. Generally, they are relatively inactive agents, with cramping and catharsis as major symptoms.

### RESINS

Resins are amorphous complex combinations of acids, alcohols, esters, resenes, alkaloids, and acid resins. Physically, they often form hardened, transluscent, or transparent masses that melt readily with minimal heat. Examples of resins include opium resis, pitch, and rosins. Since they are so complex, the effects are often not easily predictable. Volatile oils may be found in combination with resins and are used as salves and linaments.

## ALKALOIDS

Alkaloids are organic nitrogen-based ring structures. They are not otherwise homogenous in either chemical structure or physiologic or biologic activity. Some of the most potent pharmacologic and toxic substances known are alkaloids. All alkaloids have some biologic activitiy if administered in sufficient amounts. There are 10 classes of alkaloids, based upon the structure of the ring. These ten groups include pyridine-piperidines, tropane, quinidine, isoquinoline, indole, imidazole, steroid, lupinone, alkaloidal amines, and purine. The effects of the alkaloids are generally predictable by the ring and surrounding structure.

Most of the plants containing substantial quantities of alkaloids are well-known poisons, including nicotine and atropine. Others are hallucinogenic agents of abuse. Opium and related narcotic agents are found in the isoquinoline and quinoline groups of alkaloids.

## GLYCOSIDES

Glycosides are sugar and ether combinations where the sugar portion is the glycone and the nonsugar portion is an aglycone. The aglycone portion often accounts for the major toxic effects of this group. Glycoside distribution is ubiquitous in plants and may be divided into 11 major categories. These categories include phenols, alcohols, aldehydes, lactones, cardioactives, saponins, clavanols, anthraquinones, cyanophores, isothiocyanates, and other neutral agents.

The dangers of at least one glycoside, digitalis, are well known to all medical providers. Surprisingly enough, closely related plants, such as the lily of the valley, are used as herbal medicines and have quite similar activity. Saponins are also noted to be common causes of poisoning. Other glycosides yield hydrocyanic acid upon hydrolysis. The most important of these cyanogenic glycosides is amygdalin, found in pits of cherries, apricots, plums, and peaches and in the seeds of apples.

## PHYTOTOXINS

Phytotoxins are perhaps the most toxic substances of the plant kingdom. They are composed of large proteins and resemble the toxins of bacteria in both structure and antigenic character.[10] The mechanism of action of phytotoxins is not completely understood. Phytotoxins are readily absorbed from the GI tract.

Phytotoxins are found in the *Fabacae* and *Euphorbiaceae* families. Representative examples include the jequirty seed and castor bean, both of which are described later.

## TANNINS

Tannins are a large group of complex colloidal solutions that are noncrystallizable. Tannins are widely distributed in leaves, bark, roots, and stems. The concentration of tannins varies by part of the plant, the season of the year, and the local growing conditions. Tannins are acids that precipitate alkaloids and proteins. They are most famous in precipitation of the proteins of leather and hides (tanning) from which the name derives. Medically, the protein precipitation causes an "astringent" action.

Ingestion of the tannins can produce GI symptoms, such as nausea, vomiting, diarrhea, and tenesmus. They are not well absorbed and do not usually cause other than GI symptoms. Rarely, hepatic and renal damage may be noted with large ingestions and significant absorption.

## HOUSE PLANTS

### Caladium (Caladium) and Other Arum *Plants*

#### PART OF PLANT AND ACTIVE PRINCIPLE

Members of these widely scattered house and field plants have calcium oxalate crystals in the leaves and roots. The tiny needle-sharp crystals called raphides produce intense pain and swelling upon contact with the soft mucosal tissues of the mouth and throat.

#### OTHER ARUM PLANTS

Dumbcane (*Dieffenbachia sequine*)
Philodendron (*Philodendron scandens* and other species)

Elephant's ear (*Colocasia antiquorum*)
Jack-in-the-pulpit (*Arisaema triphyllum*)
Rhubarb leaves (*Rheum rhaponticum*)

## CLINICAL PICTURE

*Arum* ingestion is not usually a problem in diagnosis. A child takes a bite of leaf and almost instantly will cry out in pain. The calcium oxalate will cause intense burning of the oral mucosa and the tongue almost immediately. Swelling may cause airway obstruction in severe cases. Nausea, vomiting, and diarrhea are common when these plants are ingested. Cases of renal failure have been reported with rhubarb leaf ingestion, possibly due to the deposition of oxalate crystals in the kidney. Serious oxalate poisoning is generally found when a gastronome uses rhubarb leaves in a salad or as cooked greens. Rarely, bulbs of the jack-in-the-pulpit may be served by mistake as edible roots.

The leaves of the rhubarb plant cause the same symptoms when ingested as the other *arum* plants. Only the stalks are edible.

In the past, poinsetta plants (*Euphorbia pulcherrima*) have been variously described as poisonous and fatal if ingested. Large quantities of poinsetta leaves have been fed to rats without systemic or local toxicity. Recent evidence leads one to believe that there may be some local toxicity, similar to the arum plants, but no significant systemic toxicity.[11]

## TREATMENT

Gastric emptying with either lavage or emesis is appropriate. Milk or milk of magnesia may sooth the oral irritation by combining with the oxalic acid. Ice or cool solutions may also help. Popsicles or ice cream will provide both cooling and soothing of the lesion. Diphenhydramine may decrease the reaction somewhat. Most children can easily be managed at home, after this ingestion. Only rarely will airway problems develop and then tissue swelling will be gradual in onset. The child's course should be checked hourly at home by a family member.

The pain and edema will often persist for hours to days and then recede slowly without further therapy. Some areas of superficial necrosis may appear and require appropriate therapy.

In severe ingestions, calcium gluconate may be administered intravenously. The calcium will combine with oxalic acid to form soluble calcium oxalate. Intravenous fluids should be increased so that the calcium oxalate does not precipitate in the kidney.

## Castor Bean (Ricinus communis)

### PART OF PLANT AND ACTIVE PRINCIPLE

The leaves and seeds contain ricin, a phytotoxin that may be one of the more potent toxins known. The estimated lethal dose for humans is about 1.0 mg/kg.[12] Ricin is a glycoprotein that is composed of two peptide chains with a disulfide bond between them. The smaller peptide chain is a cellular toxin that interferes with protein synthesis.[13] Castor oil, a nontoxic cathartic, is made by pressing the beans while cold (less than 50°F).

### CLINICAL PICTURE

Chewing the beans releases the ricin from the seed, and swallowing the seeds whole is thought to be not as dangerous as chewing the seeds due to a hard shell on the outside. The seeds are thought to be highly allergenic and may cause skin rash, urticaria, and systemic allergic responses from contact alone.

Ricin causes burning of the mouth and throat, nausea, vomiting, abdominal pain, and protracted diarrhea, sometimes with tenesmus. Development of the symptoms may be delayed as long as 24 hours after ingestion, perhaps due to the hard shell surrounding the seeds. Gastrointestinal symptoms may be protracted and are prominent. Headache, malaise, loss of consciousness, convulsions, thirst, hypotension, tachycardia, and uremia have also been reported following castor bean ingestion. Terminal liver failure may be noted.

Many of the reported systemic signs and symptoms following castor bean ingestion appear to be the result of dehydration due to these GI effects. Death from "uremia" has followed ingestion of as few as four to eight seeds for an adult, and only two to three beans for a child. In other cases, the elevated BUN and decreased urinary output has improved following fluid administration.

## TREATMENT

Rapid gastric emptying is essential in treating castor bean poisoning. Either lavage or emesis with ipecac has been effective. The use of cathartics may not be necessary due to profound diarrhea. Alkalinization of the urine with sodium bicarbonate may prevent precipitation of hemoglobin in the renal tubules.

Careful monitoring of the patient is essential for dehydration is common. Vital signs should be assessed frequently, and laboratory data should include both hematologic screens, urinalysis, and renal function studies such as BUN and creatinine. With persistent vomiting and diarrhea, parenteral alimentation may be needed.[14]

## JEQUIRTY BEAN (JEQUIRTY PEA, ABRUS PRECATORIUS)

The jequirty bean or rosary pea is used frequently for ornaments and decorations, such as necklaces and bracelets, because of the shiny black coloring. These ornamental beans contain a deadly phytotoxin. If chewed, the phytotoxin is released. If the beans are swallowed whole, the beans may pass through the GI tract without harm to the patient (see Fig. 8.1).

Effects from the phytotoxins of jequirty beans are similar to those of ricin contained in castor beans. Treatment is supportive and similar to that described for castor beans. There is no antidote.

## Latana (Latana camara)

Latana or red sage is a highly poisonous plant found in flower gardens and as a perennial

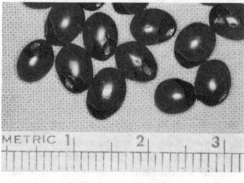

METRIC

**Figure 8.1.** Rosary pea.

potted plant throughout the southern United States. In the deep South, it has become naturalized and grows wild. Latana is also known as red sage, bunch berry, or wild sage.

## PART OF PLANT AND ACTIVE PRINCIPLE

The toxic principles of latana red sage are lantadene A and B, which are found in all parts of the plant. They are concentrated in the unripe green berries, and ingestion of only four or five of these berries may constitute a lethal dose.

## CLINICAL PICTURE

The toxic triterpenoid compounds, lantadene A and B, cause vomiting, diarrhea, and abdominal pain when ingested. Acute effects may resemble toxicity from atropine. Muscle weakness, lethargy, visual disturbances, and respiratory depression have also been reported. Occasional patients may have photosensitivity. Rarely, cardiovascular collapse will be found. Symptoms are delayed as much as 24 hours after ingestion.

## TREATMENT

Treatment of ingestion of lantadene is symptomatic. Any child with ingestion of the bunchberry should be observed for 24 to 48 hours for development of delayed symptoms. If ingestion is recent, gastric emptying, activated charcoal, and cathartics are recommended in the usual doses.

## Mountain Laurel (Kalmia latifolia)

Also known as the mountain ivy or ivy bush, this flowering evergreen grows to a height of 35 feet in the Appalachain mountains. The related azeleas and rhododendrons are also found on the West Coast.

## RELATED PLANTS

Azelea
Rhododendron (*Rhododendron* species)
Rosebay
Pieris (*Pieris* species)
Laurels (*Kalmia* species)

## PART OF PLANT AND ACTIVE PRINCIPLE

In the laurel, azalea, and rhododendron family, the entire plant is poisonous. The leaves, flowers, and twigs contain andromedotoxin.

## CLINICAL PICTURE

This toxic resinoid produces lacrimation, salivation, bradycardia, hypotension, convulsions, progressive paralysis, and death. Honey made from the laurel blossoms is said to be toxic but is also, fortunately, bitter and astringent. Shoots of mountain laurel have been mistaken for wintergreen and teas have been made from the leaves with unfortunate results.

## TREATMENT

Treatment for laurel ingestion consists of gastric emptying if the patient is alert, lavage with a protected airway if the patient is unconsious or paralyzed, and administering activated charcoal. Cathartics may also be indicated. Appropriate supportive measures should be used for the other signs and symptoms.

## Yellow Jessamine (Gelsemium sempervirens)

The yellow jessamine or Carolina jessamine is found throughout the southeastern United States. It is a tall, showy, high-climbing vine that is native to lowland areas, and it flowers in the early spring. This vine is often cultivated for decoration.

## PART OF PLANT AND ACTIVE PRINCIPLE

All parts of the plant contain three alkaloids: gelsemine, gelseminine, and gelsemoidine. The greatest concentration is in the roots, but children have been poisoned by sucking or eating the blossoms. Honey bees have been poisoned by the nectar and have made poisonous honey.

## CLINICAL PICTURE

The symptoms of gelsemine (and cogeners) alkaloid poisoning include profuse sweating, muscular weakness, dilated pupils, diplopia, convulsions, paralysis, and respiratory failure. The strychnine-like poison paralyzes motor nerve endings resulting ultimately in respiratory arrest.

## TREATMENT

The usual gastric emptying procedures should be followed. If paralysis or coma is present, the airway should be protected with an endotracheal tube before lavage. Airway and respiratory support should be used as indicated. Atropine is thought to help with the secretions and other symptoms.

## VEGETABLES

### Potato (Solanum tuberosum)

All parts of the lowly potato, except the ripened potato tuber, are highly toxic. The potato is closely related to the deadly nightshade family and the clinical picture and management of toxic ingestions are abundantly discussed in that section.

## PART OF PLANT AND ACTIVE PRINCIPLE

Solanine, a glycoalkaloid, is distributed throughout the entire potato plant, with the highest concentrations found in the unripened tubers. Sprouts and the sun-greened skin of the potato have particularly high concentrations of solanine. Greened potatoes should be discarded or pared to remove all green tissue before use. Cooking in water tends to leach out the solanine and may destroy what is left.

## CLINICAL PICTURE

Ingestion of potato leaves or stems can cause nausea, vomiting, diarrhea, and crampy abdominal pains. Dilated pupils, clammy skin, hypothermia, confusion, convulsions, and circulatory and respiratory depression have all been noted. Death has been reported following ingestion of this plant.

## RELATED PLANTS

Eggplant (Solanum melongena) is related to the potato. Eggplant leaves and vines have substantial concentrations of solanine and should never be consumed. The fruit is safe to consume.

## TREATMENT

See treatment for nightshade family.

### GARDEN FLOWERS
#### Foxglove (Digitalis purpurea)

This flowering biennial herb is well known to medical personnel as a source of digitalis. It is ubiquitous in the Pacific Western United States and is grown in flower gardens throughout the United States (see Fig. 8.2).

### SIMILAR PLANTS
#### Oleander (Nerium oleander)

This plant is often grown as an ornamental shrub or houseplant. It grows up to 25 feet in height and is found in the south and in California.

#### Lilly of the Valley (Convallaria majalis)

Lilies of the valley are common garden flowers throughout the United States, and the plant grows wild in many eastern states.

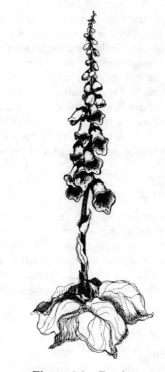

**Figure 8.2.** Foxglove.

#### Star-of-Bethlehem (Ornithogalum umbellatum)

This low plant with white, starlike flowers is found in gardens in the northern United States from New York to Ohio.

### PART OF PLANT AND ACTIVE PRINCIPLE

The action of the cardiac glycosides are well known to all emergency providers and do not need extensive repetition here. Foxglove contains about a dozen different cardiac glycosides scattered through the entire plant. The leaves and seeds are particularly toxic and children have also been reported to poison themselves by sucking on the tubers.

At one time, yellow oleander was used as a cardiac glycoside, similar to digitalis. It was abandoned because of increased toxic effects compared to digitalis.[15] Oleander's cardiac glycoside is said to be particularly toxic, and people have been poisoned by cooking meat skewered on its branches. Water from a vase containing oleander boughs has been noted to produce toxicity in children, and ingestion of a single leaf has killed an adult. Honey made from oleander blossoms is said to be toxic. In one case of oleander poisoning, digoxin radioimmunoassays were used to confirm the presence of digoxin-like glycosides.

Lily of the valley contains the cardiac glycosides, convallarin and convallamarin, in the leaves, roots, fruit, and the bell-shaped flowers. Star-of-Bethlehem and lily of the valley are thought to be somewhat less toxic than digitalis.

### CLINICAL PICTURE

The clinical picture of toxic ingestion of any of these plants is that of a digitalis overdose. Early symptoms may include abdominal pain, nausea, and diarrhea. After a few hours, irregular heart rates, dysrhythmias, and possibly convulsions will predominate.

### TREATMENT

Early treatment is the usual emesis or lavage, followed by charcoal and cathartics. If there are any signs of dysrhythmias, the patient must be hospitalized and monitored. Pharmacologic treatment should be as for a digitalis overdose.

Phenytoin sodium and propranolol both

have been used in managing digitalis-induced tachyarrhythmias with success. Symptomatic bradycardia can be treated with atropine, isoproterenol, or electric pacing. Magnesium sulfate has helped some tachyarrhythmias. Fractional antibody (FAB) fragments have been proposed for treatment of these other cardiac glycoside overdoses.[16] There is no data to support or refute their clinical utility in any but digitalis overdoses.

### Larkspur (Delphinium)

There are about 200 species of this relative of the buttercup or crowfoot family. The wild varieties are a major cause of death among range cattle in the western United States. The tall, flowering plants can be lethal to humans if consumed in large quantities.

#### RELATED PLANTS

Larkspur
Monkshood (*Aconitum napellus*)
Aconinte
Wolfsbane
Staggerweed
Buttercup
Marsh marigold (*Caltha palustris*)

#### PART OF PLANT AND ACTIVE PRINCIPLE

The toxic alkaloids delphinine, delphineidine and ajacin are found concentrated in the seeds and young plants. As the plant ages, the toxicity decreases. The related marsh marigold or cowslip contains protoanemonin, a vesicant. Protoanemonin is apparently neutralized by cooking, as some foragers boil the young leaves and shoots for greens. Raw leaves and stems are severely irritating, however.

#### CLINICAL PICTURE

Symptoms of larkspur or monkshood poisoning appear promptly, often within minutes, and include tingling or burning sensations, restlessness, bradycardia, and muscular weakness. Delphinium is less toxic than monkshood and larger quantities must be consumed for serious effects. Later symptoms include vomiting, diarrhea, convulsions, respiratory failure, and death. Death can occur within hours after ingestion. Field gastro-nomes have mistaken the roots of monkshood for wild horseradish, with tragic results. The marsh marigold can cause irritation of the mouth, oropharynx, esophagus, and stomach. Severe poisonings from marsh marigold may cause respiratory depression, hypotension, and convulsions.

#### TREATMENT

Lavage or emesis should be performed as appropriate. Because the marsh marigold contains a vesicant, removal of even small swallowed portions of the ingested plant is important. Hospitalize these patients immediately. Monitor all patients who ingest the delphinium and its relatives for signs of respiratory and cardiac depression. Atropine in the usual doses may be helpful for bradycardia.

### Narcissus (Narcissus)

#### RELATED PLANTS

Jonquil
Daffodil
Hyacinth (*Hyacinthus orientalis*)
Iris (*Iris versicolor*)

#### PART OF PLANT AND ACTIVE PRINCIPLE

The bulbs or roots of these flowers contain an unidentified alkaloid that can be dangerous if large amounts are consumed. The leaves and flowers have also been reported to cause symptoms.

#### CLINICAL PICTURE

The alkaloid causes nausea, vomiting, diarrhea, convulsions, and, rarely, death. The usual presentation is a severe gastric upset appearing within 30 minutes or so.

#### TREATMENT

Treatment should include the usual lavage or emesis. If only a bite has been consumed, milk and close observation may be appropriate. If vomiting is protracted, the patient should be hospitalized and intravenous fluids started. In the rare case where an entire bulb has been consumed, the patient should be monitored closely.

## Periwinkle (*Vinca* species)

Periwinkle was once the herbalist's cure for diabetes and now is often used as an anti-inflammatory ointment and brewed as a tea for treatment of pharangitis.

### PART OF PLANT AND ACTIVE PRINCIPLE

Periwinkle contains the vinca alkaloids that form the basis for several of our most potent oncologic chemotherapy agents (vinblastine and vincristine).

### CLINICAL PICTURE

The alkaloid causes hepatotoxicity. Excessive use of periwinkle tea can cause nausea, vomiting, and, rarely, convulsions.

### TREATMENT

Treatment should include the usual lavage or emesis. If only a bite has been consumed, milk and close observation may be appropriate. If vomiting is protracted, the patient should be hospitalized and intravenous fluids started. In the rare case where an entire bulb has been consumed, the patient should be monitored closely.

## FIELD PLANTS

### Nightshade (*Solanum* species)

Black nightshade and deadly nightshade are weeds or shrubs found throughout the United States. The black nightshade, also called the wonderberry or garden huckleberry, produces a black ripe berry that is sometimes eaten in pies. The woody nightshade is found in the eastern, north central United States and along the Pacific Coast. Woody nightshade may be one of the more commonly ingested plants, because of the translucent red berries seen as it grows on trellises, fences, and hedges.

### RELATED PLANTS

Potato (discussed earlier)
Black nightshade (*Solanum nigrum*)
Blue nightshade (*Solanum dulcamara*) (also called the woody nightshade)
Deadly nightshade (*Atropa belladonna*)
Jimsonweed (*Datura stramonium*)
Jerusalem cherry (*Solanum pseudocapsicum*)

### PART OF PLANT AND ACTIVE PRINCIPLE

All of these species contain solanine, a glycoalkaloid, with the highest concentrations in the unripened fruit. Solanine is very poisonous, and small amounts can be lethal. Deadly nightshade contains between 0.25 and 0.5% atropine and related alkaloids. A single berry from the deadly nightshade contains a lethal amount of atropine.

### CLINICAL PICTURE

These plants contain the same toxic alkaloids in differing amounts. The symptoms of deadly nightshade are usually those of a massive overdose of atropine, where in the other plants, the solanine alkaloids may predominate. The woody nightshade (solanine) rarely produces more than abdominal pain, constipation, or diarrhea with small ingestions. Large ingestions may produce muscle weakness, drowsiness, and paralysis. Black nightshade (solanine and atropine) can produce abdominal pain, dilated pupils, hyperthermia, vomiting, diarrhea, and circulatory and respiratory depression. Deadly nightshade (atropine) may induce dry mouth, blurred vision, hallucinations and convulsions, fever, hot and dry skin: ("Dry as a bone, blind as a bat, crazy as a loon, and hot as hell.").

Solanine ingestion usually causes GI effects of nausea, vomiting, and diarrhea. Fortunately, these effects start decontamination of the GI tract and decrease the subsequent absorbed dose. In severe cases, diarrhea, abdominal pain, and even bloody diarrhea may be seen. Unlike the atropine alkaloids, solanine causes prominent salivation and sweating. CNS, respiratory, and cardiovascular depression follow ingestion of larger doses. Muscle weakness, paralysis, and renal failure may be seen uncommonly.

### TREATMENT

Early treatment of ingestions of the nightshade family should include the usual emesis or lavage. Aggressive decontamination is recommended by some and is probably appropriate, considering the toxicity of these plants.[17] Charcoal and cathartics may be of some use.

The cholinesterase inhibitor, physostigmine, may be useful for treatment of seizures, hallucinations, or coma due to the ingestion of anticholinergic agents. Relative indications may include hypertension and arrhythmias. Physostigmine will also decrease fever and reduce agitation, but should not be used solely for these indications, as safer therapies exist. In severely affected pediatric patients, physostigmine may be tried in 0.5 mg doses in 5-minute intervals until toxic effects or a maximum of 2 mg has been given. Adult patients may require 1 to 2 mg doses at 5-minute intervals to control life-threatening symptoms. Physostigmine is titrated at the *lowest* effective dose possible (at no more than 1 mg per minute) to achieve symptomatic relief of arrhythmias, hypertension, convulsions, severe hallucinations, or coma.

Contraindications for use of physostigmine include mechanical obstruction of GI and urinary tracts and asthma. These contraindications should be considered relative to the clinical picture of the intoxication. Physostigmine may also produce either bradycardia or tachycardia and either hypotension or hypertension.[18] For these reasons, physostigmine use is controversial.

## False Hellebore (Veratrum viride)

A member of the lily family, false hellebore is also known as hellebore or Indian poke. These plants are widespread throughout the United States in swampy meadows and wet pastures.

### PART OF PLANT AND ACTIVE PRINCIPLE

The roots, seeds, and leaves of this plant all contain a variety of alkaloids, including veratrin. Root extracts have had teratogenic effects. The effects are similar to that of the death camas. The taste is said to be bitter and stinging and ingestions are fortunately rare.

### CLINICAL PICTURE

These alkaloids cause salivation, vomiting, diarrhea, and crampy abdominal pains. Large ingestions may be marked by paralysis, hypothermia, hypotension, bradycardia, convulsions, and respiratory paralysis.

### TREATMENT

Treatment is entirely supportive. Emesis should be induced or lavage performed at the earliest opportunity as appropriate. Catharsis and charcoal are also helpful. The patient should be admitted and carefully monitored.

## Jimsonweed (Datura stramonium)

Originally called Jamestown weed, the name has been corrupted to jimsonweed. This ground plant became notorious in 1676 when a party of British Regulars who were sent to Jamestown, Virginia dined on this weed and were unable to participate in Bacon's Rebellion.[19] More recently, jimsonweed has served as a hallucinogenic for those seeking such experiences.[20,21] Because of this wide experience, this plant's toxic effects are now well detailed (see Fig. 8.3).

### PART OF PLANT AND ACTIVE PRINCIPLE

Jimsonweed contains anticholinergic alkaloids, and all parts of the plant have been used as hallucinogenics. Children under 5 are most likely to ingest the leaves of the plant, while adults and adolescents are more likely to smoke them. Young children have also been poisoned by eating the fruits or by drinking

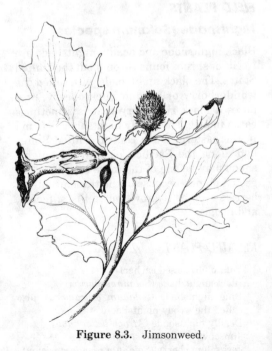

**Figure 8.3.** Jimsonweed.

the flower's nectar. Intravenous use of a "tea" has also been described. The seeds are particularly laden with toxin.

The toxin of the jimsonweed includes hyosycamine, atropine, and scopalamine. All act in a similar fashion as anticholinergic agents by blocking the receptor sites at cholinergic nerve endings.

## CLINICAL PICTURE

Jimsonweed intoxication can be readily identified by the widely dilated pupils, tachycardia, flushed facies, and dry, hot skin. Large ingestions may present with hallucinations, trancelike states, seizures, decerebrate posturing, or coma. As in all atropinelike overdoses, tachycardia, tachypnea, thirst, hypertension, and urinary retention are common at even modest doses. In warmer climates, heatstroke may be precipitated by the fever and inability to sweat.

## TREATMENT

Treatment of jimsonweed includes induction of emesis and administration of activated charcoal for early cases. Cases discovered later may benefit from gastric lavage and charcoal. Therapy is symptomatic and aimed at reducing the atropinic effects. Management of the ABCs should take the usual priority.

Further therapy is detailed in the section on nightshade.

## Pokeweed (Phytolacca americana)

Pokeweed is also called pokeberry, poke, inkberry, or pigeonberry. It is commonly found in the east, ranging from Maine to the Gulf. The plant measures about 3 to 10 feet high from a large root system. Dark-purple to black pokeweed berries contain a reddish juice that was once used as a coloring agent.[22] Children frequently discover this property and make pokeberry ink, hence the common name inkberry. The plant has been used for folk medicine as an emetic, purgative, rheumatism salve, and for itching.[23]

## PART OF PLANT AND ACTIVE PRINCIPLE

Pokeweed is considered edible, but the plant must be properly prepared by boiling the leaves, shoots, or roots, discarding the water,

and repeating the process at least once more. Boiled pokeweed leaves prepared in this manner are commercially available. Any or all plant parts contain the glycoside saponins and a pokeweed mitogen.[24] Toxins are most concentrated in the immature berries and the roots. The cooked mature berries are thought to be nontoxic, but symptomatic cases have been reported following ingestion of 10 or more raw ripe berries. The saponins are mucous membrane and skin irritants. Saponin glycosides are not generally considered cardiotoxic. The pokeweed mitogen causes the division of white blood cells and the production of interferon.

## CLINICAL PICTURE

The usual clinical presentation of pokeweed intoxication is an oral burning sensation, sore throat, diaphoresis, nausea, diarrhea, and vomiting. Abdominal cramps may be prominent and generally occur 2 to 4 hours after ingestion. Those with severe intoxications may present with hematemesis, melena, hypotension, and tachycardia. Lethargy, convulsions, and coma have also been reported in severe poisonings. Occasional amblyopia and transient blindness have been noted. Symptoms normally resolve over 24 to 48 hours, and those that last longer are ominous.[25]

Long-term use may cause gastroenteritis similar to the effects of the chronic use of nonsteroidal anti-inflammatory agents. Some herbalists recommend the use of one dried berry 4 times daily for treatment of arthritis.[26]

## TREATMENT

The usual principles of gastric emptying by either lavage or emesis as appropriate should be closely adhered to. Dehydration and hypotension should be treated with adequate doses of intravenous fluids. All symptomatic patients should be admitted and observed.

## Hemlock (Conium maculatum)

This tall weed is famous for the fatal concoction used to execute Socrates and still lives up to its reputation. The plant resembles Queen Anne's lace and wild carrots and is a member of the carrot family. Also known as the poison fool's parsley, it is found in the East, the Rocky Mountains, and along the Pacific Coast. The plant is most frequently consumed by mistake because its leaves resemble parsley, its root resembles the wild carrot, and the seeds look like anise. Fortunately, the taste is unpleasant and only small quantities are usually ingested.

## RELATED PLANTS

### Water Hemlock (Cicuta maculata)

The water hemlock, also known as spotted water hemlock, cowbane, spotted cowbane, poison parsnip, and wild parsnip, is found along wet marshy areas and stream beds. As can be seen from the common names, the plant is mistaken for wild parsnips or, rarely, wild carrots or artichokes with unfortunate results.[27] Water hemlock apparently is not unpleasant tasting.

## PART OF PLANT AND ACTIVE PRINCIPLE

The roots of the hemlock plants contain a yellowish oil that smells like carrots. The oil contains cicurtoxin, a poison so toxic that a single mouthful of roots may kill an adult in 15 minutes. Poison hemlock is not as toxic as water hemlock. The entire hemlock is toxic, not just the roots, and children are reported to have been poisoned by peashooters and whistles made from the stems. Whenever a forager develops a paroxysmal illness, water hemlock poisoning should be suspected.

## CLINICAL PICTURE

Cicutoxin is a CNS stimulant, producing excitement, convulsions, and death. As with most plant ingestions, abdominal pain, nausea, and vomiting may precede the more serious symptoms.

## TREATMENT

Vomiting must be induced immediately, if the patient is not comatose or convulsing. Convulsions should be controlled with diazepam or barbiturates. Further treatment is symptomatic.

## Tobacco (Nicotina tabacum)

Tocacco and related plants were first noted by Columbus in his explorations of the West Indies. Indeed, in the early years of exploration, more Spaniards were converted to smoking than Indians converted to Christianity.[28]

Nicotine and the related pyridine and piperidine groups of alkaloids are found in many plants, including the nightshade family, jimsonweed, petunias, potatoes, and tomatoes. The most classic of these is, of course, tobacco, known for smoking, chewing, and snuff.

## RELATED PLANTS

Wild tobacco (*Nicotinia rustica*)
Tree tobacco (*Nicotinia glauca*)
Desert tobacco (*Nicotinia trigonphylla*)
Coyote tocacco (*Nicotinia attenuata*)

## PART OF PLANT AND ACTIVE PRINCIPLE

Tobacco contains nicotine, nornicotine, anabatine, and anabasine alkaloids. All parts of the plants contain these alkaloids. The nicotine alkaloid is primarily found in the leaves of the plants, with the other alkaloids being concentrated in the roots. Common tobacco has lesser concentrations of these alkaloids than some of the wild tobaccos, particularly tree tobacco.

Nicotine is well absorbed from the skin, buccal membranes, lungs, and rectum. It is poorly absorbed from the stomach, due to an alkaline pKa. Nicotine is water soluble and may be readily absorbed through the skin. This leads to "green tobacco sickness," which develops from handling leaves or applying poultices of tobacco plants. The serum half-life is only about 30 to 60 minutes, with the bulk of detoxification occurring in the liver, lungs, and kidneys. Nicotine in the form of tobacco and many other related plants has been smoked, chewed, dipped, snuffed, and used rectally. Inadvertent ingestion occurs when the leaves of the wild tobaccos (particularly tree tobacco) are confused with edible salad greens.

Nicotine is often used as an insecticide in either spray, liquid, or fumigant form. One of the best known insecticide preparations is Black Leaf 40 garden spray. Nicotine has also been used in the past as a paralyzing agent for control of animals but is no longer available for this purpose.

## CLINICAL PICTURE

The basic action of nicotine is a stimulation of the parasympathetic and sympathetic ganglions by an action analogous to that of acetylcholine. This initial stimulation is followed by a ganglionic blockade at sympathetic, parasympathetic, and neuromuscular junctions. This causes an initial tachycardia and hypertension, followed by bradycardia and hypotension. In small doses, this stimulation causes the pleasant effects of smoking tobacco. Larger doses are less pleasant and show the truly poisonous effects of tobacco. Late effects of large doses include a complete neuromuscular blockade, resulting in paralysis of both voluntary and respiratory muscles and death. Direct effects on the CNS include initial stimulation with tremors and convulsions followed by profound CNS depression with coma and death. Vomiting is common early in the course of effects and may save children from an otherwise lethal dose. Increased bronchial secretions, salivation, and sweating are also noted early in the course of an ingestion.

Nicotine is addictive, with a typical withdrawal pattern in those who attempt to quit. The initial ganglionic stimulation and direct CNS stimulation noted in smaller doses probably contributes to the addiction. Nicotine was used as a mind-altering agent in pre-Columbian Indian rituals. Confirmed addicts (chronic smokers) will note that the drug gives an increased ability to concentrate and a decreased appetite. A paradoxical calming effect is noted by many smokers.

The associated health hazards of smoking and other forms of chronic nicotine use have been well documented in other literature and do not need repetition here.

## TREATMENT

As in all noncaustic ingestions, gut decontamination is recommended. Use of emetics may not be necessary due to the emetic effects of nicotine. Gastric lavage and activated charcoal should be considered in all patients with history of significant ingestion.

Supportive care should be given for all symptoms, including airway toilet to remove secretions, ventilation if paralysis intervenes, treatment of bradycardia, and treatment of hypotension if it develops. Seizures may be treated in the customary fashion. Atropine may be used for treatment of hypersecretions. If the acute stimulation phase has significant hypertension, nitroprusside may be used to safely and temporarily lower the blood pressure. When the patient becomes hypotensive, nitroprusside is rapidly cleared and reversed. Hypotension will usually respond to fluids and dopamine, which likewise can be titrated to achieve proper control.

## Baneberry (Actaea)

Baneberry is also known as snakeberry, coralberry, doll's eyes, and white cohosh and grows wild throughout much of the country. The chalk-white or red berries are said to resemble a doll's eyes in appearance.

## PART OF PLANT AND ACTIVE PRINCIPLE

All parts of the plant, sap, and berries contain a cardiotoxic glycoside. The sap is also a vesicant, causing severe irritation of the mucous membranes.

## CLINICAL PICTURE

As few as six berries can cause severe abdominal symptoms with nausea, vomiting, diarrhea, and crampy abdominal pain. Larger ingestions may show the cardiotoxic effects and exhibit tachycardia and circulatory failure.

## TREATMENT

Treatment of ingestion of the baneberry is supportive. Emesis or lavage is indicated to remove even small amounts of ingested plant. Intravenous fluids should be given for protracted vomiting or diarrhea.

## TREES AND SHRUBS
### Elderberry (Sambucus canadensis)

The black elder shrub is found from Canada to the Gulf coast, and west to Arizona. The scarlet elder (*S. pubens*) is found in the Rockies and the Appalachians and along the Pacific coast.

## PART OF PLANT AND ACTIVE PRINCIPLE

The elderberry is unusual in that the flowers and ripe fruit are completely nontoxic. Indeed, elderberry wine, pies, and jellies are consumed with gusto. Unfortunately, the elder shrub's shoots, leaves, and stems contain sambunigrin, an amygdalin or cyanide derivative.

## CLINICAL PICTURE

Occasional children who use elderberry shrubs as a whistle, flute, or peashooter may develop abdominal cramps, nausea, or vomiting. Cyanide toxicity is distinctly unusual and would require ingestion of large amounts of stems and shoots.

## TREATMENT

In the rare case of large ingestions, lavage or ipecac is indicated. Standard treatment for cyanide toxicity should be given if confirmed by symptoms. In most cases, observation alone will suffice.

## Black Locust (Robinia pseudoacacia)

Black locust, a small tree that is found in the eastern United States and along the west coast, is rarely implicated in poisonings.

## CLINICAL PICTURE

The inner bark, young leaves, and seed pods contain robin, a phytotoxin, and robitin, a glycoside. These poisons cause abdominal pains, nausea, vomiting, and CNS depression. Hypotension has been noted, but the bad reputation of the black locust appears to be somewhat exaggerated.

## TREATMENT

Treatment is entirely symptomatic. There has not been enough experience with black locust poisoning to make other appropriate recommendations.

## Horse Chestnut (Aesculus hippocastanum)

### CLINICAL PICTURE

Ingestion of the brown nuts of the horse chestnut can produce nausea, vomiting, and abdominal pain. Ingestion of large quantities can produce coma, but such large ingestions are not common as the nuts are quite bitter.

### TREATMENT

Since the fruit is so bitter, there are few ingestions that need therapy. Therapy should be supportive. If substantial quantities are thought to be ingested, gastric emptying should suffice.

## Mistletoe (Phoradendron species)

The American mistletoe is sold commercially as a Christmas decoration. It has been also recommended as an infusion (tea) for hypertension and as an antispasmodic and calmative agent. These herbal remedies have caused fatalities. Rarely, ingestion of quanties of these Christmas decorations causes toxic symptoms in children.

### CLINICAL PICTURE

Ingestion of only a few berries or leaves of the American mistletoe appears unlikely to cause significant symptoms. In one study, no serious symptoms were noted in any of 141 patients.[29] A number of potential toxins have been identified in both berries and leaves, but in view of the paucity of serious symptoms, it is unlikely that a child will require other than gastric emptying and supportive therapy. Fatalities have been described in patients who have ingested teas brewed from these plants. One patient developed respiratory distress, abdominal pain, and cardiovascular collapse.[30] The active agent is thought to be peptide toxin that causes bradycardia, hypotension, and myocardial depression.

### TREATMENT

Since ingestion of only a small quantity of the mistletoe causes little toxicity, only observation and gastric emptying is indicated. Caution should be used in administration of ipecac, as seizures have been reported with mistletoe ingestion. Hypotension should be treated with intravenous fluids and pressor agents as needed. Seizures should be controlled with intravenous diazepam.

## MUSHROOM POISONING

The true incidence of mushroom poisoning, like other plant ingestions, is probably both unknown and unknowable. Many poisonings are not severe enough to prompt the victim to seek help at an emergency department. Even when the victim does seek help, few public health agencies require reporting of reactions. Statistics of calls to poison control centers do not always help, because competent physicians may not need the help offered by the center, and unknowledgeable physicians may not seek the help they need.

Younger patients may come from the ranks of those seeking "higher" planes through the use of hallucinogens. The seekers of such enlightenment may run into trouble in one of two ways: either they consume a merely toxic mushroom when a psychedelic variety was sought, or they consume too many of the psychedelic variety and suffer toxic symptoms.

The matter becomes worse when a child ingests a mushroom, sometimes thinking, like Alice in Wonderland, that a bite may confer magical properties. The child's curiosity, lack of appropriate training, and appetite all conspire to increase the incidence of severe mushroom poisoning. Needless to say, the bright colors of some of the more poisonous varieties help ensure their consumption.

People of recent European origin are often surprised (occasionally, fatally!) to find that not only are there more mushrooms and fungi in North America but that more of these are toxic. Exposures are most frequently seen in the northeast and northwest parts of the United States.

Equally surprising is the finding by some that the folktales about toxicity are usually unfounded. Mushrooms do not darken a silver coin or spoon. Peeling the cap may remove some of the toxin, but much more may remain. Color changes are not meaningful in determination of toxicity. Animals may be able to detoxify ingestions lethal to humans.

## Diagnosis

In the typical patient with mushroom poisoning, the patient presents with nausea, vomiting, GI cramps, and, occasionally, diarrhea. There is usually a history of ingestion of mushrooms, although the history may be difficult to elicit. (The amateur "expert" may insist that there were no poisonous varieties consumed and, indeed, may have so convinced the rest of the family and guests that no one proffers the history.) Mushrooms may be consumed with soups, stews, or salads and only the cook knows for certain the origin of the flavorings used. Unfortunately, many other toxic agents produce the same or similar picture.

If possible, the mushrooms must be collected and preserved for proper identification. Unfortunately, cooking or storing at room temperature may destroy the mushroom or render accurate identification impossible. The judgment of amateur mycologists varies greatly and accurate identification should be left to those who are truly professional. Identification of mushrooms from spores, stems, or pieces should best be left to a very experienced mycologist. Even the most experienced mycologist may have difficulty with macerated specimens or specimens retrieved from gastric aspirate.

Compounding the clinical picture is a variance in toxic effects among individuals. The severity of the poisoning also depends upon the season, the degree of maturation of the mushrooms, the part of the mushroom consumed, and the number of the mushrooms eaten by the victim. Unhappily, it is often uncertain whether the amature mushroom picker has ingested only 1 toxic mushroom and 20 nontoxic similar varieties or has ingested all toxic mushrooms. The method of preparation of the mushroom also may destroy or change the toxic products of the mushrooms.

Toxins in mushrooms can be divided into seven different groups that affect various organ systems. Each group has a different clinical picture and requires a different specific therapy.

A general rule of thumb is that if the symptoms develop quickly after ingestion (within 6 hours), **usually**, the ingestion will not cause serious illness. Mushroom ingestions that develop symptoms after more than 6 to 8 hours will frequently be associated with serious systemic problems and may cause death. Groups I and III are most often deadly ingestions, while *Cortinus* species (group IA) has been recently identified as causing late renal damage. It is important to remember that multiple species of mushrooms with both rapid and delayed onset toxins may be simultaneously ingested.

A second question to answer: "What were the initial symptoms?" Mushroom intoxications with rapid onset can be divided into primarily gastrointestinal distress symptoms with nausea and vomiting (group VIII), primarily sweating (group IV), inebriation and hallucinations without drowsiness (group VI), or inebriation or delirium associated with drowsiness or coma (group II). Those with delayed onset can be grouped into: abdominal fullness and headache after about 6 hours (group III), emesis and diarrhea noted about 12 hours after ingestion (group I), and polyuria or oliguria noted about 3 days after the meal (group IA).

## Group Principle Toxin and Typical Mushrooms

| | | |
|---|---|---|
| I | Cyclopeptides | —*Amanita phalloides* |
| IA | Cortinarius | —*Cortinarius* species |
| II | Muscimol, ibotenic acid | —*Amanita muscaria* |
| III | Monomethylhydrazine | —*Gyromitra* |
| IV | Muscarine | —*Boletus, Clitocybe, Inocybe* |
| V | Coparine | —*Coprinus atramentarius* |
| VI | Indoles (psilocybin) | —*Psilocybe, Gymnopilus* |
| VII | Miscellaneous GI irritants | —"Little brown mushrooms" |

## GROUP I: CYTOTOXINS (CYCLOPEPTIDES)—Delayed Onset

The symptoms of the cyclopeptide toxins develop late after ingestion and are among the most potent and well known of the mushroom poisonings. Eating a single mushroom cap of the *Amanita phalloides* (the European Death Cap) can kill a healthy adult. Amanita has been implicated in many of the mushroom-related fatalities in both the United States and in Europe. Mortality of documented *Amanita* mushroom intoxication is about 50% in patients under 10 years and about 15% in patients over 10 years old.[31] The overall mortality is 1 in 5.

Amatoxin is a collective name for a number of 8-membered cyclic peptide ring compounds with a weight of about 900 daltons.[32,33] Amatoxins do not bind to protein or albumin. When ingested, the amatoxin inhibits ribonucleic acid polymerase II in the victim's cells and interferes with protein synthesis. This causes the delayed damage to cell walls, nuclei, and organelles within the cells. Hepatic, gastrointestinal, and renal tubule cells seem particularly sensitive since they are relatively rapidly multiplying tissues. Amatoxins are exceptionally toxic, with a le-thal dose of less than 0.1 mg/kg body weight. Death is due to liver or kidney failure or, rarely, to GI hemorrhage.[34]

The other toxin found in *Amanita* species is phallotoxin, which appears to cause the initial nausea and vomiting found following ingestions of these mushrooms. Phallotoxin is a heptapeptide that may be unstable and easily destroyed by cooking or digestive enzymes. This toxin appears to act within 6 to 8 hours.[35]

Amatoxins and phallotoxins may be detected by radioimmunoassay in biologic fluids or by thin layer chromatography.[36,37] A rough approximation test for amatoxins may be performed by placing a drop of juice squeezed from the mushroom on newspaper. The area should then be dried away from sun or excessive heat. A drop of concentrated hydrochloric acid should cause a blue-green color to form. The subsequent reaction depends upon lignin set free by the strong acid aldehydes and is not yet completely understood but was well described by Weiland in 1949.[38] Filter paper does not contain lignin and will not work. Some forms of newspaper have been shown to have a false positive, which can be shown with a drop of acid on a juicefree portion of the newspaper. The test will not work

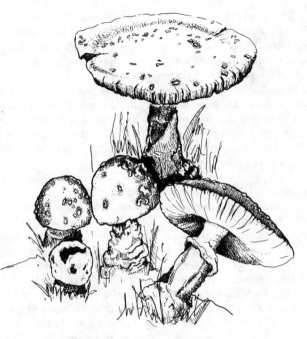

**Figure 8.4.** *Amanita* mushroom.

on fragments obtained from the stomach and may have false positives from mushrooms containing terpenes, psilocybin, or bufotenin.

These cytotoxins are found in some species of the genera *Amanita* and *Galerina*. Common names for these toxic mushrooms include the fly agaric (*Amanita muscaria*), the death cup (*Amanita phalloides*), and the destroying angels (*Amanita virosa and verna*) (see Fig. 8.4).

## Clinical Picture

The Amanita is probably more dangerous due to the delayed onset of symptoms. About 6 to 24 hours after eating the mushroom, symptoms start to appear. The average delay appears to be about 10 hours and is characteristic enough to be a hallmark of amatoxin poisoning. The delay causes the mushroom to be completely digested and the toxin to be completely absorbed.

Some folks may lose the connection between their symptoms now and the meal that they had hours or days ago. This lapse of memory may be particularly true of those who are "completely confident" that they know how to identify dangerous mushrooms—even after admission for ingestion of a poisonous mushroom.

There is some variability in individual susceptibility, both in time of onset and in severity of symptoms. Members of a group may eat a meal with toxic mushrooms and not every member will develop symptoms. This may be partly explained by a variance in quantity of mushrooms ingested. It would be assumed that the concentration of toxin in mushrooms picked in a similar location would be comparable, despite known variances with season or state of maturation. If one person in a group has developed symptoms after ingestion of mushrooms, the others should be presumed to have had a similar dose and treated aggressively.

A second reason that the *Amanita* is so dangerous is that the symptoms occur in a biphasic pattern with an apparent "recovery" stage between the 2 phases. The first phase, after the initial delay, is that of gastrointestinal disturbance with vomiting, diarrhea, and abdominal cramping. The diarrhea is often profound and may be "rice water" in nature. This phase lasts as long as 24 hours. After this initial insult, the patient appears to completely recover. Uninformed medical providers may actually discharge the patient from the hospital at this point. The remission of symptoms lasts about 24 to 36 hours and is followed by signs and symptoms of both renal and hepatic damage. The renal damage is most obvious by the third day after ingestion and the hepatic damage after the fourth.

The liver disease is manifested by the usual elevation of the transaminases to 2 or 3 times the normal levels. Bilirubin is often normal or only minimally elevated. The serum ammonia is usually elevated and the prothrombin time is often 2 to 3 standard deviations above the mean. This laboratory picture, of course, is also found in many other causes of liver failure.

One third of the patients ingesting *Amanita* species will die, if untreated. Immediate admission to a hospital is appropriate, even when there is "only a low risk" of potential ingestion. These patients must be treated aggressively and rapidly in order to lower the mortality. By the time renal and hepatic damage is manifest, the liver damage is significant and it is too late for detoxification.

## Treatment

Treatment of *Amanita* poisoning is a therapeutic challange. With few controlled studies and little knowledge about the phamacologic properties of the amatoxins, all proposed therapy is controversial. The following discussion presents the salient known points applicable to all patients and discusses those therapies that may have beneficial effects.

Supportive therapy with continuous monitoring of vital signs and correction of water and electrolyte imbalances is inarguably important in the management of these overdoses. Diarrhea and vomiting may rapidly cause profound dehydration. Early volume replacement to correct the hypovolemia caused by this GI phase of toxicity is an essential element in treatment of this intoxication. Reduced renal excretion due to hypovolemia may contribute to the effects of the toxin, both on the hepatocytes and on the renal tubular cells. Indeed, some authors advocate forced diuresis as a form of detoxification in the management of the suspected *Amanita* toxicity. This latter contention seems appropriate, but renal failure may cause rapid fluid overload and the clinician needs to monitor the patient quite carefully.

Gastric lavage and drainage of gastroduodenal fluids are advocated by some authorities. These authors argue that the toxin may be recirculated in the entero-hepatic-bi-lary system and that gastroduodenal drainage may remove some of the toxin. Toxins have been found in duodenal aspirates as long as 36 hours after ingestion, so delayed gastric emptying may yet be beneficial.[39] Certainly, gastric lavage will remove any remaining mushroom pieces, perhaps allowing identification. Unfortunately, due to the late development of symptoms, gastric emptying is usually not used when it would be most beneficial.

Since duodenal drainage is not particularly difficult, expensive, or dangerous, it should be accepted until a well-controlled study validates or disproves it. Endoscopic biliary diversion has been proposed to enhance the elimination of hepatically recirculated toxin.[40,41] Cathartics are not usually needed because diarrhea is a prominent part of the clinical picture.

Multiple doses of activated charcoal may serve a similar purpose and deserve similar consideration. Certainly, repeated doses of activated charcoal are innocuous and should be used even if they only *may* be beneficial. The adult patient may be given 50 to 100 gm of charcoal every 2 hours for 24 to 36 hours for this purpose.

Probably the most controversial part of therapy for the *Amanita* toxins centers about the multiple drug regimes proposed to detoxify the patient. Some of the therapies advocated have included thioctic acid, penicillin G, cimetidine, vitamin C, sylimarine, steroids, and neomycin. No controlled studies for any of these drugs exist for human patients and all should be viewed as strictly experimental therapies. At the present time, there is not any proven successful therapy for *Amanita* intoxication.

Thioctic acid has been proposed despite ineffectiveness in animal studies and an unclear proposed mechanism of action.[42-44] It should probably not be used in the therapy of *Amanita* ingestions until good controlled clinical studies are available.

Penicillin may reduce the liver uptake of amatoxins and may be appropriate to include in therapy. Certainly, the proposed dose of penicillin G [250 mg every 4 hours] is innocuous and may be safely given to all patients not allergic to the drug. Silymarin, a drug extracted from Mediterranean milk thistle is alleged to have similar effects as penicillin, but is not available in the United States. Silymarin has been shown to have protective effects in animals given it prior to amatoxin, but curative actions are uncertain.[45,46] It is thought to act as either a free-radical scavenger or by displacing amatoxin from cell wall binding sites. Vitamin C has been proposed as a similar free-radical scavenger. Cimetidine has been proposed but also has not studies that validate its use. Further clinical experience is needed before any recommendations can be made about these agents.

Neomycin is advocated on the same theoretical basis as in all patients with fulminant hepatitis or hepatic coma. It is not considered specific therapy for the ingestion but, rather, is general therapy for the patient with potential hepatic necrosis.

Different forms of extracorporeal removal of amatoxin have also been employed with varying success. Since amatoxins have a high affinity to charcoal, charcoal hemoperfusion has had some anecdotal success, but no quantitative data are available for this costly and time-consuming method. Plasmapheresis makes no logical sense since amatoxin does not bind to albumin. Peritoneal and hemodialysis have been used and are recommended for reducing the serum toxin load. Since the molecule is small, hemodialysis is logical and should be effective. No large series exists that proves or refutes this contention, however.

Perhaps the ultimate in therapy is liver transplantation, which has been used for at least one case of *Amanita* poisoning.[47] This therapy was associated with a stormy postoperative course and should not be recommended. Neurologic findings, possibly attributable to *Amanita* toxins, were noted but could not be distinguished from similar findings noted with hepatic failure.

The following treatment guidelines are recommended in summary:

1. Immediate and vigorous fluid replacement
2. Gastroduodenal lavage and aspiration of fluids or, alternatively, endoscopically placed biliary diversion (controversial)
3. Instillation of activated charcoal orally every 2 hours for 36 hours
4. Forced diuresis or hemodialysis for serious (symptomatic cases); alternatively, charcoal hemoperfusion (controversial)
5. Administration of 250 mg of penicillin G every 4 hours (controversial)
6. Consider administration of neomycin and other therapy for hepatic failure

Immediate admission to the intensive care unit, aggressive detoxification as outlined above, and close monitoring of the liver status is appropriate even when poisoning is suspected but not proven. It seems meaningless to identify low-risk subjects when any delay in therapy may mean serious hepatic involvement. Hepatic necrosis is an inelegant and preventable way to prove that the patient ingested *Amanita*. Needless to say, those companions who shared the meal with symptomatic patients should be treated just as aggressively.

## GROUP IA: CORTINARIUS—DELAYED ONSET

The largest group of mushrooms in Europe consists of species of *Cortinarius*. Of these mushrooms, several are known to be toxic and others suspected to be so, based upon recent evidence. The toxin appears to cause an irreversible renal damage that occurs after an unusually long incubation period of 3 to 20 days. With the extreme length of the latent period, it is likely that other cases have escaped correlation with the ingestion (see Fig 8.5).

Symptoms of intoxication include intense thirst, vomiting, and persistent headaches. In serious cases, renal function defects were noted followed by oliguria and, in particularly severe cases, anuria. Autopsy and biopsy data show lesions characteristic of a toxic interstitial nephritis.[48]

Toxicologic studies have identified 2 separate toxins, both orellanines, each with a capacity to cause renal damage. The toxins are thought to act at sites similar to vasopressin, but unlike the hormone, with an extremely long half-life. Structural similarities to vasopressin support this contention.[48]

### Treatment

Treatment for intoxication with *Cortinarius* species mushrooms is problematical. Patients treated early after intoxication with a combination of hemodialysis and hemoperfusion have regained kidney function.[49] Those patients treated after long intervals have not. Unfortunately, the extremely long delay before symptoms means that many patients will not be appropriately diagnosed and will not respond to therapy. Until other, more effec-

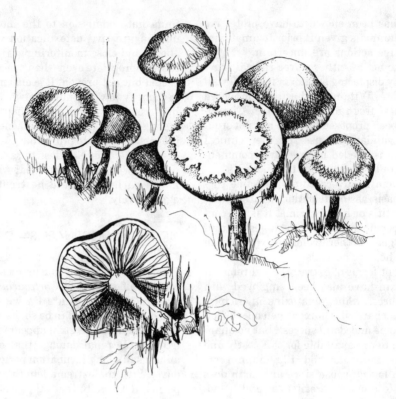

**Figure 8.5.** *Cortinarius.*

tive therapy is found, supportive therapy and hemodialysis are recommended.

## GROUP II: MUSCIMOL, IBOTENIC ACID—IMMEDIATE ONSET

Although the first mushroom toxin to be identified was muscarine from the fly agaric (*Amanita muscaria*), it actually has far more muscimol and related ibotenic acid than muscarine. *Amanita pantherina* also contains the same 2 toxins in somewhat larger amounts, although both mushrooms are very variable in toxicity. Unfortunately, the "panther" is pretty and often used as a model for pictures, illustrations, and as a decoration. These mushrooms are often picked by children who recognize them from children's books and other illustrations. Adults will sometimes eat them because they look good. These fungi apparently taste delicious.

Inebriation, manic behavior, delirium, and visual distortions have all been reported by those who have ingested mushrooms containing ibotenic acid or muscimol. These fungi have been used as a popular inebriant by the Siberians, who also noted that voices may be heard, visions seen, and perception altered while under the influence. It apparently may have been a status drug similiar to cocaine today. Particularly common is an alteration in the sense of the size of things and the sense of time. Following the intoxication, drowsiness and dizziness develop, and the subject usually falls asleep. Alternation of drowsiness and manic behavior may be noted in some patients. Small children may have complex neurologic signs, convulsions, or coma persisting for as long as 12 hours.

Ibotenic acid is decomposed by the body into muscimol, which is the active toxin. Muscimol appears to act as a false neurotransmitter, mimicking the action of gamma-aminobutyric acid (GABA). The toxic threshold is about 6 mg of muscimol. Either *Amanita muscaria* or *pantherina* may have that much toxin in a single mushroom.[50] The effects start about an hour after the meal and continue about 3 to 4 hours. Rarely, some residual effects may be seen 10 hours after ingestion.

In small children, supportive care to include respiratory support may be necessary. Most patients will need only protection against harm during the manic phases. Other therapy is not usually needed. Providers should be cautioned that even small doses of diazepam have been reported to cause paralysis in cases of ingestion of *A. muscaria*.

The differential diagnosis of ingestion of *Amanita muscaria* includes ingestion of antihistamines, parasympatholytics, cocaine, amphetamines, alcohols and ether. Infections, such as *Clostridium botulinum* may also present with similar symptoms. Clostridia may be suspected when ocular muscle palsies are noted and the patient is drowsy but clear of sensorium.

## GROUP III: MONOMETHYLHYDRAZINE— DELAYED ONSET

All mushrooms of the *Gyromitra* species contain gyromantin, which is hydrolyzed in the body to produce monomethylhydrazine. Monomethylhydrazine then inactivates pyradoxine. This produces an initial GI disturbance with nausea, vomiting, diarrhea, tenesmus, and abdominal cramps. More serious poisonings may be marked by both hepatic failure and CNS symptoms. Acidosis and convulsions may be prominent.

The most common ingestion of *Gyromitra* occur when the false morel (*Gyromitra esculanta*) is mistakenly identified as the true succulent morel. The toxin may be removed by boiling the mushrooms and then discarding the water, but the inhaled vapors can be absorbed. This means that the cook may become intoxicated by smelling the fumes of the cooking mushrooms. All raw and sauteed *Gyromitra* mushrooms are poisonous, and all that are cooked and served with broth are also potentially fatal. Because the toxin is volatile and water-soluble, air-dried *Gyromitra* mushrooms are completely edible (see Fig. 8.6).

Symptoms generally appear within 4 to 8 hours and both severity and timing depend upon an individual ability to acylate gyromantin to monomethylhydrazine. In some individuals, symptoms may appear in as little as 2 hours and but as much as 24 hours delay has been reported in others. Patients with G-6-PD deficiency may have a marked reaction to this fungus. Gastrointestinal symptoms are generally preceded by a feeling of bloating,

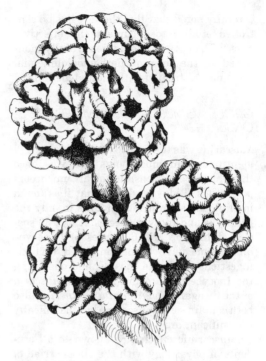

**Figure 8.6.** *Gyromitra esculenta* mushroom.

followed by the nausea, vomiting, and abdominal cramping pains. The patient who ingests *Gyromitra* is said to present with headache and emesis without diarrhea, while those who ingest *Amanita* are thought to not have headache and to have marked diarrhea. Visual differentiation of the 2 species is easy; *Amanita* has gills, while *Gyromitria* does not.

The delay in symptoms means that, as in the *Amanita* mushroom intoxication, the individual may lose sight of the cause and effect relationship and the toxic dose has a greater chance of being absorbed. The result is clear; the mortality of *Gyromitra* mushroom intoxication approaches 50%. Fortunately, intoxication from this mushroom is relatively rare and only some 20 or 30 cases have been reported in North America since 1900. Whether this is because the variation in individual susceptibility is great, or the cooking process is more effective in removing gyromantin than appreciated, is uncertain.

Proposed specific therapy for this toxin is high-dose pyridoxine hydrochloride (25 mg/kg) administered as an intravenous infusion over 15 to 30 minutes. This dose can be repeated to control the neurologic symptoms. The maximum total daily dose necessary may be as high as 15 to 20 grams.[51] It should be carefully noted that this therapy has no controlled studies to document the effectiveness.[37] The patient should be carefully monitored for the onset of methemoglobinemia. This may be treated with methylene blue.

## GROUP IV: MUSCARINE—IMMEDIATE ONSET

Muscarine was the first toxin to be positively identified from mushrooms and was once thought to be responsible for all mushroom poisonings. Today we know that it is found in clinically significant amounts in only the Clitocybe and Inocybe species. About 30 species of Inocybe and 6 species of Clitocybe mushrooms have been implicated in toxic ingestions, with the most dangerous being the Inocybe mushrooms. *Amanita muscaria* or the fly agaric and *Amanita pantherina* also both contain some muscarine but in clinically insignificant amounts.

Muscarinic effects are known to all students of physiology with the classic triad of salivation, lacrimation, and perspiration. This cholinergic syndrome is also seen in poisonings by anticholinesterase inhibitors (nerve gases and some pesticides). Ingestions of small amounts of muscarine may cause only abdominal discomfort and sweating. Larger amounts may produce gastric discomfort, abdominal pain, nausea and vomiting, and blurred vision.

Since the effects are those of anticholinergic agents, administration of atropine is both logical and effective. If severe discomfort is noted by the patient, atropine should be titrated until the patient experiences a dry mouth. Unfortunately, atropine may worsen symptoms from muscimol or ibotenic acid. Muscarine intoxication usually improves within 2 to 3 hours.

## GROUP V: COPARINE—IMMEDIATE ONSET

The *Coprinus* mushrooms cause poisonings only when consumed with or just before alcohol. The toxin is found in the otherwise delicious inky cap (*Coprinus atramentarius*) and related species (*C. micaceus*, *C. insignis*, and *C. fuscescens*). A related toxin found in *Clitocybe clavipes* may cause symptoms in some people (see Fig. 8.7).

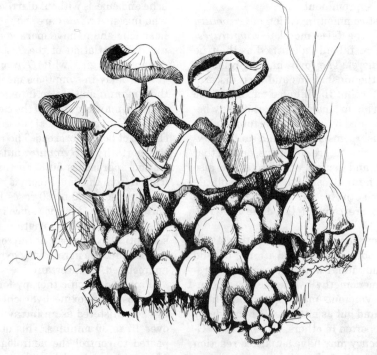

**Figure 8.7.** Inky caps.

Coparine inhibits the breakdown of acetaldehyde in a manner similar to disulfiram, resulting in tachycardia, flushed facies, anxiety, nausea, vomiting, and headaches. The intensity of the reaction depends both on the amount of alcohol consumed and the timing of the alcohol consumption. Some patients have had reactions as late as 4 or 5 days after eating the inky cap, but most symptoms occur when the mushroom and alcohol are consumed within 30 minutes.

Propranolol has been shown to decrease the excitement state of this intoxication. Propranolol may be given in a dose of 10 to 15 mg orally. The patient should be instructed to avoid alcohol in all forms for at least 72 hours after the reaction to avoid precipitation of another reaction.

## GROUP VI: INDOLES—IMMEDIATE ONSET

This group of mushrooms is also called the hallucinogenic or psychoactive fungi. Ott has listed 21 species of psychoactive fungi, all of which produce the hallucinogens psilocin and psilocybin.[52] Certain species of *Psilocybe, Paneolus, Gymnopilus*, and *Conocybe* mushrooms contain these hallucinogens. These mushrooms are common throughout the world as "little brown mushrooms" that grow on dung (see Fig. 8.8). Hallucinogenic mushrooms have been used in religious worship in many primitive societies—"the flesh of the gods" of the Aztecs.[53]

Psilocybin is a relative of LSD and has similar effects on humans.[54] Mood elevations and hallucinations are the sought for effects and appear within 20 to 30 minutes after ingestion of the fungus. These hallucinations are often accompanied by reports of alterations in sensation, such as brighter colors, sharper outlines, or colored patterns. In addition to the hallucinations, some patients will become ataxic, exhibit hyperkinetic activity, or muscle weakness. Incoherent or inappropriate speech is often seen during the hallucinations. Following the hallucinations, a period of drowsiness is common.

Physicians seldom see those who ingest hallucinogenic mushrooms for 2 valid reasons: first, in many states of the United States,

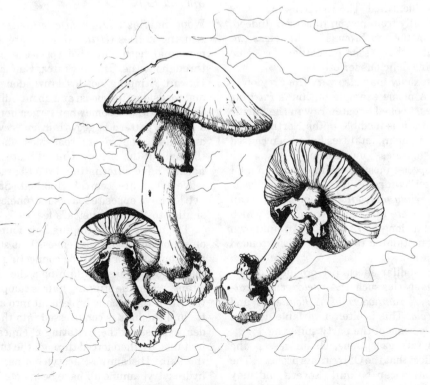

**Figure 8.8.** Psilocybin mushroom.

it is illegal, and, second, few truly "bad trips" or severe reactions are obnoxious enough to present for medical care. Most will weather the mind storms at home with friends and seem to prefer this therapy. Treatment for those who do present includes reassurance and benzodiazepine if symptoms are severe. Recovery is usually within 6 hours.

Small children who have ingested large amounts of these fungi may have convulsions, hyperthermia, or coma. Hyperthermia will require cooling and respiratory therapy. Convulsions may require lorazepam or diazepam for control.

### GROUP VII: MISCELLANEOUS GASTROINTESTINAL—SYMPTOMS IMMEDIATE ONSET

GI irritation is the only common denominator of the largest group of toxic mushrooms. The GI irritants produce abdominal discomfort, nausea, vomiting, and diarrhea in a variable pattern but usually within 3 hours of ingestion. Little is known of the pharmocology or chemistry of the mushrooms that produce these effects, and, in many cases, the toxins have yet to be identified. The reactions may vary substantially from person to person. Indeed, several of the mushrooms of this class are powerful cathartics or purgatives for some people and delicious for others.

The toxicity may also vary from region to region. A prime example of this is *Paxillus involutus*. Cooked or eaten raw in the Pacific Northwest, it is inedible in the Northeast. In Europe or Japan, fatalities have been caused by this "harmless" mushroom.

The species most often implicated in a GI irritation syndrome in North America is *Chlorophylum molybdites*. *C. molybdites* can produce severe and repetitive emesis, which may last as long as 72 hours.[55] An unknown toxin is postulated to produce this extended GI irritation.

Other similar effects are produced by the *Agaricus* species such as *A. meleagris, A. californicus, A. xanthodermus, A. hondensis,* and *A. silvicola.* This is often a variable distress with only some of the party suffering.

With rare exceptions, GI distress is the worst effect that the GI irritants produce. The GI irritation can be quite severe and may pose a threat to the old, infirm, or to young children. Symptomatic relief may include intravenous rehydration for these patients.

## SKIN EXPOSURES

Plant-induced dermatitis can account for as many as 5 to 10% of visits to dermatology clinics.[56] This dermatitis is best known with the members of the *Rhus* and nettle families but may be seen from the fine hairs and bristles of other plants that can cause microtrauma to the skin. Direct skin contact with low molecular weight acids, proteolytic enzymes, and crystals may also cause skin irritation.

### Irritant Chemical Injury

Many plants have irritant saps or plant juices. The chemicals affect almost all and are not related to an allergic response but, rather, are due to a direct irritant effect of the plant's sap. The lesion is limited to the exposed area, and the response is usually quite prompt, in contrast to the allergic contact dermatitis.

### STINGING NETTLES

Wood nettles (*Laportea canadensis*) and stinging nettles (*Urtica dioicia*) are similar perennial herbs. Related species are found throughout the United States, Canada, and Hawaii. Stinging nettles grow along trails and roadsides, in woods, and about buildings. Wood nettle is a somewhat larger herb with a similar pattern of growth in moist wooded areas and about rivers, roadsides, and trails throughout the eastern United States. Wood nettles have alternating broad-based oval leaves that are coarsely toothed. Stinging nettles have opposite leaves morphologically similar to the wood nettle's leaves.

The nettle has a stinging hair found both on stems and about the leaves. This stinging hair consists of a fine tube connecting with a bladder at the base containing a chemical irritant. When the stinging hair is compressed, the tip of the tube is broken off into a sharp tip and the hair is compressed into the bladder, expressing the irritating chemical. The irritants are then forced through the tube into the skin. Histamines, acetylcholine, and 5-hydroxytryptamine all have been noted in the irritant juices.

The typical response to nettles is a rapid, intense burning sensation at the site of the injection. Following the immediate reaction, the area may itch for several hours. No systemic effects are usually noted. This reaction could be predicted from the histamines and acetylcholine contained in the irritant. The response is not allergic and, therefore, no prior exposure is needed.

Treatment is symptomatic. Antihistamines may be used as indicated and will be somewhat helpful. The duration of the reaction is measured in hours, rather than days, so little but symptomatic therapy is usually needed.

## SPURGES

The largest family of direct contact irritants are the spurges. These plants contain a diterpentene, with the best known diterpentene being croton oil from the seeds of the croton plant (*Croton tiglium*). When the stem is broken, the plants release a milky sap in copious amounts. This fluid causes a direct contact irritation ranging from mild erythema to bullous lesions, depending upon dose and contact time on the skin. Interestingly enough, this sap can be polymerized into rubber.

Included in this group of plants are the crown of thorns, snow on the mountain, and milk weeds. These plants are found in a wide variety of soils and conditions both as ornamentals, weeds, and in the wild.

Another group of irritant plants includes the buttercups (*Ranunculaceae*) and mustard seed plants (*Brassicaceae*). These plants tend to produce large bullous lesions rather than urticaria. In buttercups, the irritant may be a glycoside.[57] Buttercups are found in fields, meadows, and low-lying wet areas.

## TREATMENT

Cleanse the area with soap and water. Corticosteroids are recommended by some but have not been found to have significant benefit and will not shorten the course of illness. Since the mechanism is direct chemical trauma and not an allergic reaction, corticosteroids would not be expected to offer significant relief. Conservative therapy with soaks and compresses is probably beneficial. Antihis-

tamines have relatively little effect but may be helpful. The dermatitis is self-limited and will heal in a short time if no complications ensue or if there is no secondary infection or significant tissue damage.

## Plant-Induced Trauma

The myriads of visits for abrasions, scratches, and puncture wounds caused by plants are poorly documented and completely untallied. The perils of roses, brambles, briars, and cacti are well known and documented in abundant folk literature. Branches cause uncounted numbers of corneal abrasions and other lacerations of hands and face annually.

Best recorded in the literature is the trauma resulting from the spines of cacti. These plants are ubiquitous in the southwest, as many a "dude" has found during a fall. Cacti are also found as ornamental plants throughout cities, gardens, and houses as ornamental plants. The typical patient will give a history of a fall from a ledge, horse, cross-country motorcycle, or all-terrain vehicle. Many patients will show up shortly after the fall, literally bristling with spines. Others will delay 7 to 10 days and present with multiple grouped pustular lesions, typically on the buttocks or lower extremities. Penetrations of thorns, spines, and cacti can lead later to an imbedded foreign body with subsequent foreign body granuloma.[58] These plant-induced granulomas must be differentiated from other causes of granulomatous disease by biopsy.

## TREATMENT

Usually, spines can be easily, but tediously, removed with forceps. Some physicians feel that these spines will be easier to remove a few days after the initial trauma, when a local reaction is present and the spines are more readily identified. For spines that are too fine to remove with forceps or splinter tweezers, apply rubber cement to the area. Then immediately apply paper to the rubber cement. When the cement has hardened, the paper can be peeled off together with the spines.

Steroids will provide little relief for the foreign body reaction, as long as the foreign body remains imbedded. Antibiotics should be reserved for areas of obvious infection.

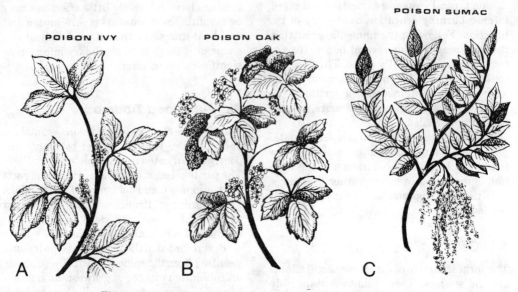

**Figure 8.9.** **A**, Poison ivy; **B**, poison oak, and **C**, poison sumac.

## Contact Dermatitis

Dermatitis is a major clinical problem associated with exposure to plant toxins or direct contact with irritant plant products. In California, for example, over 50% of workmen's compensation claims are related to the dermatitis produced by *Rhus* species.[59] Numerous other plants have been reported as causing skin reactions, either following ingestion, as an allergen, or by direct toxic effects.

*Rhus Dermatitis.* Rashes in outdoorsmen and women are most likely due to the members of the *Rhus* (or the more recent name *Toxicodendron*) genus: poison ivy, poison oak, and poison sumac. The stems and leaves of these plants contain an immunogenic resin that can cause a profound allergic dermatitis in exposed and sensitized skin. Exposure to the resin results when the stems or leaves are broken, crushed, or burned.

Although the 3 common varieties of the *Toxicodendron* genus are well known, there are actually 4 members: poison ivy (*Rhus radicans*), poison oak (*Rhus toxicodendron*), Western poison oak (*Rhus diversilobum*), and poison elder or sumac (*Rhus vernix*). These closely related plants are found throughout the United States.

Poison ivy, the hallmark plant, is a small woody shrub or vine that grows along the ground, low fences, and about woody areas.

The characteristic 3 leaflets are hairless or only slightly hair. The fruit is small and yellowish-white and found in hanging clusters.

Poison oak is found throughout southern Canada and the United States. It is common about paths, the edges of wooded areas, about stream banks, and along fences and buildings.

Both poison oak and poison ivy are extremely variable in their morphology.[60,61] They can occur as ground vines, shrubs, small individual plants, or climbing vines. The leaves vary greatly in size, texture, and margin shapes, throughout the country. Victims who can recognize poison oak or poison ivy in one part of the country are often confused by the variances in the same plant elsewhere and may not be able to identify the plant (see Fig. 8.9).

The antigenic resin is similar in all species and is collectively known as urishiol. Contact with urishiol results in a complete antigen formation as the urishiol binds with skin proteins. Since the allergen is the same among poison ivy, poison oak, and poison sumac, exposure to one plant sensitizes the victim to all of the species. The resulting antigen is very active and over 50% of the U. S. population is thought to be sensitized. Only one exposure is needed to sensitize the victim, and the next exposure will cause an intense reaction. The sensitization persists for years.

Nearly 10% of Forest Service field employees are incapacitated by exposure to various *Rhus* species each year.

A genetic, antigen-specific tolerance for the sensitizing allergen of *Rhus* species is found in 15 to 30% of the population. This tolerance is not predictable by age, race, or sex.

The resin is deposited when the stems or leaves are broken or crushed. Danger of poisoning is greatest during the spring and early summer, when the sap is running freely, and the plant is easily bruised. Burning the dried leaves or stems may also release the antigen in the smoke. Urushiols are not volatile but particles may be carried on pollen or ash. The resin may be carried about on the clothing and on animal fur for long periods of time. The author has had at least one patient who sustained typical lesions in the spring after putting on outdoor clothing that had been unwashed and last used during a fall cleanup.

Since the leaves may be crushed by brushing up against them, the classic lesion of *Rhus* dermatitis are parallel lines of small, reddened, edematous vesicles where the victim brushes against the plant. The initial symptoms of itching, redness, and burning may appear within a few hours or may develop within 72 hours, depending upon the individual's allergic sensitivity. Erythema, vesicles, and vesiculobullous eruption forms may all be noted. Urticaria may be found both about the original lesions and in distant locations. Smoke may cause diffuse skin, facial, and respiratory distribution of lesions. A particularly nasty form of inoculation is found in children and "greenhorns" who unknowingly use the plants to cleanse themselves after defecation.

Treatment of *Rhus* dermatitis is directed towards minimizing further exposure and defusing the current exposure. Most exposures are mild and may be successfully treated on an outpatient basis, although the patient may be exceptionally uncomfortable. Severe dermatitis may have large confluent bullae formation and local swelling. These severe cases may benefit from hospitalization.

Since the resin is oily, immediate washing of the skin with soap and water will both deactivate and remove it. Clothes may be washed in commercial detergents in a washing machine with good results. Animals should be bathed, and the operator should wear long sleeves and gloves for the first few steps. Furniture and car seats can be decontaminated with soap and water solutions as needed.

Unfortunately, the resins bind to the skin within 30 minutes. After about 30 minutes, soap and water will no longer serve to defuse the impending reaction. Treatment then is directed towards classic therapy of a contact dermatitis, after removal of all unbound resins with soap and water. Useful agents have included soothing lotions, such as oatmeal paste and calamine lotions, antihistamines, and, in severe cases, oral corticosteroids. Calamine lotion will help to dry the lesions in all cases, while bland ointments and oatmeal pastes will decrease the pruritis. Soothing, cool baths have been used for centuries as a home remedy with good effect. Antihistamines will not reverse the current lesions but will decrease the itching and decrease the response of further lesions.

Steroids are employed by many practitioners with varying effects. No well-controlled series exist that show unequivocal results, but abundant anecdotal testimony is supportive. For widespread dermatitis, oral steroids in a dose equivalent to 60 mg of prednisone for a 3 to 5 day course may be useful. Intramuscular or intravenous steroids should be reserved for those patients with disabling exposure, such as greater than 25% of the body surface or extensive facial or genital lesions. Early (within 6 hours of exposure) application of topical steroids may also be beneficial but usually is not considered, due to the delay in symptoms.

Secondary infections may occur when the bullae are excoriated and weeping. Children, in particular, are prone to generalized excoriations with subsequent secondary infections. Persistent symptoms and apparent spreading should be considered due to new contact with the plants or spread of the irritant from previous areas of contamination. The vesicular fluid is not known to contain urushiols, but the allergen can be spready by scratching. This spread underscores the importance of immediate washing of the area and potentially contaminated clothing following a suspected exposure.

Prevention of further reactions in susceptible individuals by oral desensitization has not proven particularly efficacious. A suspension of activated charcoal, clay and linoleic acid salts has been recently shown to be useful in binding and inactivation of the urishiol resins. This suspension may have utility in sunscreens and preventative lotions.

Further preventative efforts include removal of the plants with herbicides, by burning, or by turning the ground. Needless to say, proper protective clothing should be worn and the plants should not be burned near housing areas. The allergen can be removed from clothing or contaminated equipment with soap and water.

Allergic contact dermatitis is also noted from other plants in addition to *Rhus*. These plants usually have lesser effects and require far more extensive exposure for sensitization. Liverworts, tulips, and lillies (*Juulaceae, Orchidaceae* and *Liliaceae*) in particular have been implicated.

### Selected Extended Reading

Lincoff G, Mitchell DH, eds. Toxic and hallucinogenic mushroom poisoning. New York: Van Nostrand Reinhold Co., 1977.

Rumack BH, Salzman E. Mushroom poisoning: diagnosis and treatment. Cleveland: CRC Press, 1978.

Lampe KE, McCann MA. AMA handbook of poisonous and injurious plants. Chicago: Chicago Review Press, 1985.

Kingsbury JM. Deadly harvest. New York: Holt, Rinehart, and Winston, 1976. [Particularly good for nonphysicians]

### References

1. Kunkel DB. The toxic emergency. Emerg Med 1985;October 15:93–100.
2. Mitchell J, Rook A. Botanical dermatology. Vancouver, Greengrass, 1979.
3. Tilton BR, Ryan ME, Edson LY, Martyak GG. Plant ingestions in children. Penn Med 1985;45–49.
4. Schilling R, Der Marderosian A, Speaker J. Incidence of plant poisonings in Philidelphia noted as poison information calls. Vet Human Toxicol 1980;22:148–150.
5. Fawcett NP. Pediatric facets of poisonous plants. J Fla Med Assn 1978;65:199–204.
6. Saxe TG. Toxicity of medicinal herbal preparations. Am Fam Phys 1987;35:135–142.
7. Geehr E. Common toxic plant ingestions. Emerg Med Clin North Am 1984;2:553–562.
8. Jones JS, Dougherty J. Current status of plasmapherisis in toxicology. Ann Emerg Med 1986;15:474–482.
9. Sullivan T, Rumack B, Thomas H, et al. Pennyroyal oil poisoning and toxicity. JAMA 1979;242:2873–2874.
10. Kingsbury JM. Poisonous plants of the United States and Canada. Englewood Cliffs, NJ: Prentice-Hall, Inc., 1964.
11. Edwards N. Local toxicity from a poinsetta plant: a case report. J Ped 1983;192(3):404–405.
12. Kopferschmitt J, Flesch F, Lugnier A, et al. Acute voluntary intoxication by ricin. Hum Toxicol 1983;2:239–242.
13. Olsnes S, Refsnes K, Pihl A. Mechanism of action of the toxic lectins abrin and ricin. Nature 1974;249:627–631.
14. Wedin GP, Neal JS, Everson GW, Krenzelok EP. Castor bean poisoning. Am J Emerg Med 1986;4:259–261.
15. Arnold HL, Middleton WS, Chen KK. The action of thevetin, a cardiac glycoside and its clinical application. Am J Med Sci 1935;189:193–206.
16. Haynes BE, Bessen HA, Wightman WD. Oleander tea: herbal draught of death. Ann Emerg Med 1985;14:350–353.
17. Ozegewalla CD, Bonfiglio JF, Sigel LT. Common plants and their toxicity. Pediatr Clin North Am 1987;34(6):1557–1598.
18. Levy R. Arrhythmias following physostigmine administration in jimson weed poisoning. JACEP 1977;6:107–108.
19. Jennings PE. Stramonium poisoning. J Pediatr 1935;6:657–664.
20. Levy R. Jimson seed poisoning–a new hallucinogenic on the horizon. JACEP 1977;6:58–61.
21. Klein-Schwartz W, Oderda GM. Jimsonweed intoxication in adolescents and young adults. Am J Dis Child 1984;138:737–739.
22. Roberge R, Brader E, Martin ML, et al. The root of evil—pokeweed intoxication. Ann Emerg Med 1986;15:470–473.
23. Jaeckle KA, Freemon FR. Pokeweed poisoning. South Med J 1982;74:639–640.
24. Lewis WH, Smith PR. Poke root herbal tea poisoning. JAMA 1979;242:2759–2760.
25. Haddad LM, Winchester JF. Clinical management of poisoning and drug overdose. Philadelphia: WB Saunders Co., 1983:332.
26. Saxe TG. Toxicity of medicinal herbal preparations. Am Fam Phys 1987;35:135–142.
27. Larkin T. Herbs are often more toxic than magical. HHS publication no. (FDA) 84–1105. Rockville, MD: Department of Health and Human Services, 1984.
28. Kunkel DB. The toxic emergency: Tobacco and friends. Emerg Med 1985;Nov 15:142–158.
29. Hall AH, Spoerke DG, Rumack BH. Assessing mistletoe toxicity. Ann Emerg Med 1986; 15:1320–1323.
30. Moore HW. Mistletoe poisoning. a review of

the available literature and the report of a case of probable fatal poisoning. J S Carolina Med Assoc 1969;59:269–271.

31. Floersheim GL, Weber O, Tschumi P, Ulbrich M. Die Klinische Knollenblatterpilzvergiftung (*Amanita phalloides*). Prongostiche Faktoren und Therapeutische Massnahamen. Schweiz Med Wokenschr 1982; 112:1164–1177.

32. Weiland T. Poisonous principles of mushrooms of the *Amanita* genus. Science 1968;159:946.

33. Litten W. The most poisonous mushrooms. Sci Am 1975;232:90.

34. St. Omer FB, Giannini A, Botti P, et al. *Amanita* poisoning: a clinical-histopathological study of 64 cases of intoxication. Hepatogastroenterology 1985;32:229–331.

35. Frimmer M. What we have learned from phalloidin. Toxicol Lett 1987;35:169–182.

36. Fiume L, Busi C, Campadelli-Fiume G, et al. Production of antibodies to amanitins as a basis for their radioimmunoassay. Experientia 1975;31:1233.

37. Bivens HG, Knopp R. Lammers R. et al. Mushroom ingestion. Ann Emerg Med 1985;14:1099–1104.

38. Weiland T. The toxic peptides from *Amanita* mushrooms. Int J Peptide Protein Res 1983;22:257–276.

39. Basi C, Fiume L, Costantino D, et al. *Amanita* toxins in gastroduodenal fluid of patients poisoned by the mushroom *Amanita phalloides* [letter]. N Engl J Med 1979;300:800.

40. Frank IC, Cummins L. Amanita poisoning treated with endoscopic bilary diversion. J Emerg Nurs 1987;13:132–136.

41. Duffy TJ, Vergeer P. Treatment of mushroom amantin [letter]. West J Med 1986;145:521.

42. Vesconi S, Langer M, Iapichino G, et al. Therapy of cytotoxic mushroom intoxication. Crit Care Med 1985;13:402–406.

43. Olson KR, Pond SM, Seward J, et al. *Amanita phalloides* type mushroom poisoning. West J Med 1982;137:282–289.

44. Hanrahan JP, Mordis GA. Mushroom poisoning, case reports and a review of therapy. JAMA 1984;254:1057–1061.

45. Parrish RC, Doering PL. Treatment of *Amanita* mushroom poisoning: a review. Vet Hum Toxicol 1986;28:318–322.

46. Hruby K, Csomos G, Fuhrmann M, Thaler H.

Chemotherapy of *Amanita phalloides* poisoning with intravenous silibinin. Hum Toxicol 1983;2:183–195.

47. Woodle ES, Moody RR, Cox KL, et al. Orthoptic liver transplantation in a patient with *Amanita* poisoning. JAMA 1985;253:69–70.

48. Tebbett IR, Caddy B. Mushroom toxins of the genus *Cortinarius*. Experientia 1984;40:441–446.

49. Holmdahl J, Mulec H, Ahlmen J. Acute renal failure after intoxication with *Cortinarius* mushrooms. Hum Toxicol 1984;3:309–313.

50. Beug M. Toxins and Hallucinogens. Mushroom 1983–4;*Winter*:8–13.

51. Hanrahan JP, Mordis GA. Mushroom poisoning, case reports and a review of therapy. JAMA 1984;254:1057–1061.

52. Ott J. Recreational use of hallunicogenic mushrooms in the United States. In: Rumack BH, Salzman E., eds. Mushroom poisoning: diagnosis and treatment. Boca Raton, FL: CRC press, 1978:241

53. Wasson RG. The hallucinogenic mushrums of Mexico: an adventure in ethonomycological exploration. Trans NY Acad Sci. 1959;21:325–339.

54. Musha M, Ishii A, Tanaka F, Kusano G. Poisoning by hallucinogenic mushroom Higageshibiretake (Psilocybe argentipes K. Yokoyama) indigenous to Japan. Tokohu J Exp Med 1986;148:73–78.

55. Picchioni AL. Mushroom poisoning. Am J Hosp Pharm 1965;22:634–635.

56. Epstein WL. Plant-induced dermatitis Ann Emerg Med 1987;16:950–955.

57. Benezera C, Ducombs G, Sell Y, et al: Plant Contact Dermatitis. Toronto, Ontario: Decker, Inc,. 1985:211–213.

58. Epstein WL. Plant-induced dermatitis. Ann Emerg Med 1987;16(9):950–955.

59. Lampe KF, McCann MA. AMA handbook of poisonous and injurious plants. Chicago: Chicago Review Press, 1985:188.

60. Kingsbury JM. Deadly harvest: a guide to common poisonous plants. New York: Holt, Rinehart and Winston, 1976.

61. Kingsbury JM. Poisonous plants of the United States and Canada. Englewood Cliffs: Prentice-Hall, 1974.

# CHAPTER 9

# Electrical Injuries

## Part 1
## Commercial Electric
## Current

### *ELECTRICAL BURNS*

Electrical injuries are relatively common. There are about 2000 burn unit admissions and about 1000 deaths per year due to an electrical injury.[1] The people that are most commonly injured by electricity are, of course, those who work with it, such as electricians and construction workers. Others that are commonly involved in an electrical accident are exploratory youths and infants and hobbiests who are working with electrical appliances and devices. About 93% of electrical injury victims are male.[2]

Injuries caused by artificially generated electrical current differ in many aspects from those caused by lightning. In electrical burns, extensive local burns and systemic damage is common, while lightning injuries frequently have little associated permanent damage. Please refer to the second part of this chapter on lightning-induced injuries for further information.

The effects of the passage of electricity on various inorganic substances may be one of the most widely studied phenomenon in science. These effects are unchanged in the organic human model, but since the substances are no longer uniform in composition, the descriptions become more complex.

In the inorganic model, the most important determinants of the extent of damage induced by electrical current are the intensity of the current and the duration of the contact. Intensity of current flow is governed by Ohm's law which states that the electrical current is directly proportional to the voltage difference between two points and inversely proportional to the resistance between these two points.

Ohm's Law: $E_{voltage} = I_{current} * R_{resistance}$

In the organic, human model this law still is applicable, but multiple other factors, such as variability skin or tissue resistance, grounding, and pathway of the current, influence these determinants. Perspiration, low tissue resistance, a small contact area, and high voltage all tend to increase the current density to various organs.

The production of heat by the passage of electrical current is significant, particularly in high tension electrical injury. This heat is generated by the passage of electrical current through a resistance and is expressed by Joule's law.

Joule's Law: $Heat_{(Power)} = 0.24 \, I^2 * R$

High voltage is particularly important because dangerous current passage is more likely as the voltage is increased if all other factors are constant. High voltage is arbitrarily defined as greater than 1000 volts. An equal number of deaths from high and low voltage electrocutions occurred in a study of 220 fatalities.[3]

Very high frequency alternating current tends to flow on the outside of a conductor, rather than through the conductor—the Faraday effect. This means that little deep tissue effects are found with radio frequency electrical currents. This may be the basis for the lesser deep tissue effects associated with lightning injuries.

Four separate tissue effects due to the passage of the current are noted in the electrical burn:

1. Direct tissue heating
2. Contact burns (entry and exit point burns)
3. Arc burns
4. Thermal burns from ignition of clothing

In addition to these tissue effects, distant effects on the body from the effects of the electrical passage are found:the cardiac and respiratory center effects, the neurovascular effects, and the late effects. In addition, mechanical trauma may result from the contractions induced by the current or from a fall caused by loss of consciousness.

## Tissue Heating Effects

As noted earlier, passage of current through the tissues will cause heating of the tissues. This heating can cause vascular spasm and thrombosis, peripheral and central neurologic injury, and muscle necrosis. As the current continues to heat the tissues, it literally cooks the tissues from within. This thermal injury is similar to a crush injury in effects upon the body.

Different tissues have varying resistances to electric current. The least resistance is, of course, encountered in the nervous system, which is designed to carry electric current. Blood vessels and muscles carry electricity well because of their high electrolyte composition. Skin, tendon, fat, and bone are rather resistant to the flow of electricity. Unfortunately, if the voltage is high enough, the current will flow through all resistant structures, and the heating becomes greatest in the most resistant tissues. When the contact is prolonged, fat and tendons will melt. Bone heats, and this may cause inapparent periosteal damage.

Muscle necrosis or rhabdomyolysis due to the electrical injury has potentially serious systemic consequences. Fluid rapidly extravasates from the vessels with increased compartment pressure and decreased vascular volume results. The absorbed myoglobin pigment has detrimental effects upon the renal cortical cells. The exact site of the renal effects of myoglobin is not well understood.

Classically, the diagnosis of rhabdomyolysis is made by the finding of dark urine that is strongly positive for hemoglobin but without red cells or red cell fragments. Such urine should be quantitatively assayed for myoglobin. The finding of creatinine phosphokinase (CPK) levels in excess of 5000 units clinches the diagnosis. In most cases, the CPK is greater than 20,000 units.

## Contact Lesions

The contact lesions (entry and exit) consist of three characteristic areas: a charred, blackened center, a middle zone of grayish white coagulation necrosis, and a periphery of partial tissue damage. These contact lesions are due to the increased current density and subsequent local tissue heating at the points of entry and exit. If the patient has contact with the current source over a wide area, either an exit or entry point may be absent. The classic example is the patient who is standing in a body of water when contacting the current source. Extensive electrothermal damage at the entry and exit points indicates that there is significant current flow and increased chances of subsequent deep tissue damage.

Specific mention must be made of lip burns. These almost uniformly occur in toddlers who bite on an electric cord or suck on an extension cord socket. The electrolytic saliva rapidly bridges the current source and a burn occurs. These injuries are local in nature and have no systemic involvement. They may be associated with lip contractures and delayed bleeding from the labial artery. An electric burn of the lip should be managed by a surgeon familiar with this injury.

## Arc Burns

The second effect is the arc burn, which results from the external passage of high voltage current. This spark consists of ionized, heated plasma with temperatures from 5000 to 20,000°C and arcs about 1 inch for each 10,000 volts. It is the arc burn that causes the charred central portion of the electrical injury. The severity of the surface burns will depend upon the proximity of the skin to the arc. Arc burns may be seen at both entry and exit points if very high voltage is involved.

## Thermal Injuries

Needless to say, the exceedingly hot plasma arc can also ignite flammable materials such as clothing. This creates the third type of local burn effect, the thermal burn. Thermal burns are treated as described in Chapter 2.

## Current Flow Sensation

Humans are very sensitive to the flow of electric current. The most sensitive organ is the tongue where the first sensations are detected at only 45 microamperes. When 60-cycle current is passed through the body, an unpleasant tingling sensation is felt at about 1.1 millamperes current flow. Direct current requires substantially more current to be detected and is felt as increasing warmth.

With increasing flow of alternating current, the unpleasant tingling sensation soon is replaced by muscular contractions. As a sufficiently high level of alternating current is reached, the subject is no longer able to release a grasp on the conductor (the "let go current").

This tetanizing effect on muscles is most pronounced in frequencies from 15 to 150 cycles per second. The strong muscle contractions cause frequent and well-documented fractures and dislocations, particularly bilateral scapular fractures and shoulder dislocations. As the frequency increases above 150 cycles per second, the tetanizing effects fall off and above 500,000 cycles per second are not noted.[4] Direct current does not have a let-go threshold, and produces only heat sensations. The abrupt release of direct current will, however, cause a muscle contraction and often throw the victim back some distance.

## Cardiovascular and Respiratory Effects

As many as a third of patients with significant electrical injury may have some significant cardiac component. The shock produces ventricular fibrillation with alternating current and asystole with direct current. If the respiratory center is involved, a respiratory arrest may be produced. Indeed, early research on cardiopulmonary resuscitation was motivated by the effects of electrical current on the heart and respiratory system and funded by the electrical utility companies.

Ventricular fibrillation is the most common cause of death in both high and low voltage electrical injuries.[5] Many studies on the effects of frequency on the ventricular fibrillation threshold in animals show that the greatest hazard occurs at about 50 to 60 cycles—the power line frequencies.[6] (See chart below.) It should be emphasized that these currents are **surface** currents. With a low-resistance conductor in the heart, alternating current "leakage" into the system would be dangerous in an amount that is a hundred times less than that required to produce fibrillation via surface electrodes. The increased danger of electrodes directly on the heart have been recognized for many years.[7,8]

**Effects of 60 Hz Current Flowing Through the Human Body with 1 Second Contact**

| | |
|---|---|
| 1 mA | Threshold of perception |
| 5 mA | Accepted as maximum harmless current |
| 10 to 20 mA | "Let-go" current |
| 50 mA | Pain, fainting, exhaustion, ? mechanical injury; heart and respiratory function ok |
| 100 to 300 mA | Ventricular fibrillation threshold |
| 6 A | Sustained myocardial contraction followed by a normal cardiac rhythm; respiratory paralysis temporary; burns may result if current density is high |

The respiratory arrest often persists after the patient's ventricular fibrillation has been corrected. Ventilation must be continued until the patient has spontaneous respirations.

Electrocardiogram (ECG) findings are usually that of a diffuse coronary ischemia. The electrical injury often does not correlate well with standard patterns of ischemia, since the injury may not follow the coronary vessels. Posterior myocardial injury is a frequent ECG finding of ischemia, however.

## Central Nervous System Effects

Central nervous system (CNS) dysfunction is a prominent feature of high-tension electrical injuries. Both acute and delayed central and peripheral neurologic effects have been described.

Acute CNS complications include respiratory arrest, seizures, mental status changes, coma, amnesia, quadriplegia, and localized paresis. Motor deficits appear to occur more frequently than sensory losses. If the current passes through the skull, coagulation of the brain paryenchyma, epidural and subdural hematomas, and intraventricular hemorrhages may occur.

Peripheral nerve injury may result from the direct heating effects of the passage of current through the nerves or vascular damage from the current. Compartment syndromes, as discussed below, frequently compress nerves and cause subsequent peripheral neuropathy.

Unusual manifestations of electrical injury are delayed neurologic complications. These delayed complications include ascending paralysis, transverse myelitis, and amyotrophic lateral sclerosis. Mechanisms of these late manifestations are unclear, and the prognosis for recovery after development of late complications is not good.[9]

## Renal Injuries

The renal manifestations found in electrical injuries are expectedly similar to those found in crush injuries. Electrical injuries are associated with a much higher incidence of renal failure than are burns. Myoglobinuria occurs frequently and is proportional to the amount of muscle damaged by the electric current. As a direct toxin to the kidney, myoglobin causes acute renal failure.

## Vascular Injuries

Vascular injuries fall into two broad categories: those due to the passage of the current and those due to the damage to the surrounding tissue.

### COMPARTMENT SYNDROME

The loss of intravascular fluid into a burned extremity results in marked swelling of the contents of the relatively inelastic fascial compartments. The fascial investments limit the amount of swelling with a resultant rising of the interstitial pressure and a consequent reduction of capillary perfusion pressure. The consequences of the decrease in capillary perfusion are tissue hypoxia, resultant increased capillary permeability, and extravasation of further fluid. A vicious cycle is completed by the resulting increased interstitial pressure of the compartment.

Since this is primarily an ischemic phenomenon due to damage to the surrounding tissues, it is potentially a reversible injury. After 6 hours of this cycle, however, the muscle damage is usually irreversible. The compartment syndrome can be recognized by the classic symptoms of peripheral vascular disease: pain, pallor, paresis, and pulselessness. The most consistent finding is deep diffuse pain that is out of proportion to the purported injury. This may be difficult to assess in the electrical injury. Passive movement of the extremity frequently intensifies the pain. Absent pulses, capillary refill, and pallor are most often late signs of a compartment syndrome.

In a flame burn or an electrical burn with a component of thermal injury, these diagnostic signs may be difficult to apply because the leathery eschar may render the skin insensible. The treatment of both flame burns and electrical injuries with potential compartment syndromes is identical. Escharatomy and possibly fasciotomy is indicated early to ensure salvage of the ischemic limb. These techniques are performed as described earlier in the section on thermal burns. Any conservation of tissue in the burned upper extremity is of great significance in reconstruction. Hand and digital escharotomy, in particular, reduces the frequency of phalangeal losses.[10,11]

Another complication of the compartment syndrome is a consequence of the necrosis of muscle by ischemia. The resulting breakdown of muscle releases creatinine phosphokinase and myoglobin. The results are indistinguishable from the muscle injury due to primary electrical burn of the muscle.

### DIRECT VASCULAR TRAUMA

Because blood vessels are basically pipes carrying electrolytes, they, thus, carry electricity efficiently. Electrical energy tends to flow along blood vessels and they typically sustain severe injury. The veins tend to thrombose first, because they are low flow and do not dissipate heat as well as the higher flow arterial pathways. Needless to say, the resulting flow into an extremity without outflow provides a rapid swelling, capillary damage, and subsequent compartment syndrome.

## Other Complications

### CATARACTS

In electric injuries about the head and neck, the delayed development of cataracts is not uncommon. Cataracts caused by electric injury are often 4 to 6 months after the accident and are usually associated with a point of contact near the affected eye. Ophthalmologic referral and long-term follow-up is indicated in all high-voltage injuries of upper chest, neck, and head.

### ABDOMINAL INJURY

A wide spectrum of intra-abdominal complications have been reported following high-voltage electrical injury. These injuries may result from either the passage of electrical current through the abdominal viscera or vessels supplying it or through direct injury to the intra-abdominal structures from an exit or entry point. Nausea, vomiting, and adynamic ileus are seen in up to 25% of electrical injuries. Stress ulcer (Curling's burn ulcer) is frequently reported in conjunction with electrical injuries. Injuries to the pancreas, gallbladder, and intestines have all been reported in association with electrical burns.[12] Bowel injuries are particularly troublesome, because ascertaining viability of tissue is often difficult. Both wound and bowel anastomoses have a high frequency of dehiscence after electrical injuries.[13]

### FRACTURES AND BONE COMPLICATIONS

Patients with an electrical injury must be inspected for fractures and dislocations caused by severe muscle contractions. Falls after the shock may also be associated with fractures.

The high resistance of bone to the passage of the electrical current may result in local bone destruction that is difficult to diagnose at the time of initial debridement of the wound. Long-term complications of bony areas are common and should be suspected.

### INFECTION

Infection secondary to tissue necrosis is a common complication of the electrical injury and may be the most common cause of death in those who survive the initial resuscitation period. With the large amounts of necrotic tissue found in the electrical injury, patients are at increased risk for clostridial infections to include both gas gangrene and tetanus. Topical antibiotics rarely penetrate sufficiently and debridement is preferable. A burn surgeon should be consulted prior to administration of any antibiotics for prophylaxis. Tetanus prophylaxis should not be overlooked.

## PREHOSPITAL MANAGEMENT

The most important factor in the prehospital management of the electrical injury is the safety of the rescuer. If the power line is intact, this is not usually a problem. If the power line is down, there has been an accident, or the current source is still active, then the rescuer needs special equipment and training. If there are circuit breakers that are readily available, these should be shut down.

Numerous techniques have been advocated for removal of downed power lines including brooms, ropes, sticks, and tree branches. All of these techniques are hazardous. Special-purpose electrical gloves, if tested and kept in good condition, will allow handling of the downed power line. Unfortunately, gloves that are not inspected and sealed prior to use may have unacceptably dangerous current leaks. "Hot sticks" and polypropylene throw lines are somewhat safer when dry but conduct well when wet. None of these techniques is safe when dealing with the very high-tension line. The safest technique is to allow the electric utility to remove the downed power line. This may mean leaving a victim until the utility company can respond.

Victims in cars, trains, and buses are a special circumstance. They are actually safe and should be advised to stay where they are, unless there is another reason, such as fire, forcing an evacuation.

As soon as the patient has been removed from the current source, the ABCs assume priority. Oxygenation, cardiopulmonary resuscitation, and intubation remain the mainstays of care. Arrhythmias will respond to the same medications as for any medical emergency. Cervical spine immobilization is indicated if there is any suspicion of cervical injury by either mechanism of injury or findings.

Since cardiac and vascular injuries are so common in the electrical burn, these patients should be carefully monitored in the field. Pulses and capillary refill should be checked in all extremities, documented, and repeated at frequent intervals. Cardiac monitoring is essential.

Fluid requirements in the electrical burn are often far greater than the surface burns would indicate Large-bore intravenous lines should be started in at least two locations. Involved extremities should be avoided from point of contact to point of exit, if possible. Slowly developing vascular thrombosis will render intravenous lines in involved extremities worthless. Either Ringer's lactate or normal saline is appropriate for an intravenous solution.

The electrical burn victim should be transported by the most expeditious means available to the closest facility able to handle the special problems of the electrical injury. Any patient with a serious electrical injury should be sent to a burn center that is much better equipped to handle the major, multiple systems injuries involved. These centers also usually have integral physical and occupational therapy and can manage the patient who may require amputations and subsequent therapy and counseling.

## EMERGENCY DEPARTMENT MANAGEMENT

Hopefully, the diagnosis of an electrical injury will be obvious. In suspected cases, with unconscious patients, a careful examination of the patient's body may show characteristic burns of exit and entry wounds. Kissing burns of the flexor creases at the wrist, elbow, or axilla may help affirm the diagnosis. The palmar surface of the skin and the scalp are the the most likely site for entrance wounds. There is no correlation between the number of exit and entrance wounds, however. In rare cases, a history of finding the patient in a tub or shower with an electric appliance with the patient may give the diagnosis.

Upon arrival at the emergency department, the patient's cardiac and respiratory status should be reassessed and corrected as needed. The estimated voltages involved, contact times, and prior medical illnesses, history, and allergies should all be ascertained. The patient should be carefully examined for other actual and potential injuries.

Because many patients will be persistently apneic, the patient should be ventilated with high-flow oxygen and intubation strongly considered. The cervical spine should be immobilized prior to intubation.

Radiography of the cervical spine and skull is mandatory in those patients who have sustained falls or cranial burns. A chest x-ray is useful as a baseline. Specific other x-rays are indicated in those with complaints or findings of fracture or dislocation.

If not already in place, two large-bore intravenous lines should be started in uninvolved extremities. Extensive injuries will require either a Swan-Ganz catheter or a central venous line. Blood should be drawn for arterial blood gases, complete blood count, electrolytes, blood sugar, creatinine, blood urea nitrogen, creatinine phosphokinase, prothrombin time, partial thromboplastin time, calcium, uric acid, and phosphates at a minimum. A type and crossmatch of blood should be considered in all electrical injuries. A Foley catheter should be inserted and urine sent for analysis and myoglobin determination.

After the ABCs are assured, a complete physical survey to evaluate the extent of injuries should be done. The wounds and associated fractures and dislocations should be managed with usual techniques. Neurologic deficits should be recorded and peripheral pulses confirmed with Doppler flow techniques. Note any findings of intra-abdominal injuries or ileus.

Myoglobinuria can be treated with an initial bolus of 25 gm of mannitol in the adult or 0.5 to 1 gm per kg in the child. This bolus should be followed with a drip of 0.5 gm per kg per hour. Fluid rescusitation MUST be asssured when using this drug. Acidosis should be corrected with bicarbonate and is best guided with arterial blood gases.

Debridement is best done by the burn surgeon who is going to manage the patient on a long-term basis. Muscle debridement is particularly difficult because the current flow is often not uniform and leaves spotty areas of necrosis within muscles. Amputation and repair of damage should be left to the burn specialist.

Remember that the compartment syndrome is far advanced when the examiner waits for signs of pulselessness. Measurement of compartment pressures and prompt fasciotomy for decompression are the mainstays of therapy in this common complication of electrical injuries. Fasciotomy and escharotomy should, however, be performed whenever there is vascular or respiratory compromise, without waiting for a burn surgeon or transfer to a burn unit.

An abnormal neurologic status may result from intracerebral hemorrhage, blunt injury, vascular spasm, hemorrhage, electrical effects, or thermal injury to the brain. Deterioration of the level of consciousness should prompt evaluation of a potential intracranial injury and rapid cranial computerized tomagraphy scanning.

### Fluid Replacement

Fluid replacement is essential and adequate rates are far more difficult to estimate than with the thermal injury. A crystalloid challange of 20 to 40 ml/kg is an appropriate starting point for fluid replenishment. Fluid losses are greatest in the first 24 hours, and urine output and vascular pressure monitoring should be used as a guide for fluid replacements. Urine output should be maintained at about 0.5 to 1.5 ml/kg/hr. Serial measurements of the hematocrit, electrolytes, and osmolality will aid in estimation of the fluid requirements.

As previously noted, hypovolemia, combined with myoglobinuria, will lead quickly to an acute tubular necrosis. Hypovolemia may be quite pronounced in these patients due to the large masses of tissue damaged. Intravenous bicarbonate to alkalinize the urine may be used based upon appropriate urine and blood pH measurements. A blood pH below 7.2 should mandate sodium bicarbonate administration to correct the pH in the electrically injured patient. Intravenous mannitol should be given in an initial adult dose of 25 gm followed by a drip of 12.5 gm per hour to aid in maintaining urine output.

### Tetanus

Tetanus immunization should be ascertained and corrected if needed. Standard tetanus prophylaxis is appropriate.

### Local Therapy

Most authorities advocate mafenide acetate (Sulfmylon) as a topical agent in the electrically injured patient due to its greater penetration. If this is not readily available, silver sulfdiazine may be substituted. Metabolic acidosis is a frequent complication of mafenide acetate. Lip and oral cavity burns should be cleansed and dressed. Splints and tube feedings may be prescribed for some oral electrical burn patients.

### Admission or Transportation Decisions

The electrical burn injury is difficult to treat, with abundant complications and pitfalls. It is, perhaps, the one injury that the emergency physician should consider rapid stabilization and transport to a specialized burn center to be the most approprate therapy, even at a Level I center. Any patient with significant electrical injuries should receive the care offered by trained burn specialists with equally trained supporting staffs. Even Level I hospitals used to caring for thermal burns do not have the resources for the devastating electrical injury.

Transport of these patients may be accomplished with the same guidelines as noted in the section on thermal injuries. Unlike the thermal injury, these patients are quite likely to become hypovolemic early in transport. Although airway edema is not potentially as dangerous in the electrical burn, cardiac dysrhythmias and late apnea are more common.

The minor electrical injury is more problematic. Where there is little argument about the severe high-tension injury and subsequent management, the oral low-voltage electrical burn may be successfully managed by many plastic or oral surgeons. The smaller, lower voltage isolated wound of an extremity may also be successfully managed by orthopedic, general, or plastic surgeons. Guidelines for these minor burns should be arranged in advance to expedite the care and decisions.

Finally, the patient with a low-voltage injury who is asymptomatic may be safely discharged after a short period of observation. These patients should have close follow-up with a cogent surgeon.

### References

1. Cooper MA. Electrical and lightning injuries. Emerg Med Clin North Am 1984;2:489–501.
2. Robinson M, Seward PN. Electrical and lightning injuries in children. Pediatr Emerg Care 1986;2:186.
3. Wright RK, Davis JH. The investigation of electrical deaghts: a report of 220 fatalities. J Forensic Sci 1980;25:514–521.
4. Nichter LS, Bryant CA, Kenny JG, et al. Injuries due to commercial electric current. JBCR 1984;5:124–137
5. Sances A, Larson SJ, Myklebust J, et al. Electrical Injuries. Surg Gynecol Obstet 1979;149:97.
6. Geddes LA, Baker LE. Response to passage of electric current through the body. J Assoc Advancement Med Instr 1971;5:13–18.
7. Zoll PM, Linenthal AJ. Long term electric pacemakers for Stokes-Adams disease. Circulation 1960;22:341–345.
8. Furman S, Schwedel JB, Robinson G, et al. Use of an intracardiac pacemaker in the control of heart block. 1961;49:98.
9. Levine NS, Atkins A, McKeel DW. Spinal cord injury following electrical accidents: case reports. J Trauma 1975;15:549.
10. Salisbury RE, Taylor JW, Levine NS. Evaluation of digital escharotomy in burned hands. Plast Reconstr Surg 1976;58:440–443.
11. Salisbury RE, Hunt JL, Warden GD, Pruitt BA. Management of electrical burns of the upper extremity. Plas Reconstr Surg 1973;51:648–652.
12. Baxter CR. Present concepts in the management of major electrical injury. Surg Clinic North Am 1970;50:1401–1418.
13. Goodwin CW, McManus WB, Mason AD Jr, et al. Management of abdominal wounds in thermally injured patients. J Trauma 1982;22:92–97.

# Part 2
# Lightning Injury

Lightning inspired awe in all primitive societies, and they tried to explain the phenomenon in understandable terms. The Viking's god Thor had his hammer, Moljinar, that slew his enemies, and Jupiter threw thunderbolts to express his wrath. Modern explanations are more mundane and rather more accurate.

The frequency of thunderstorms varies in different parts of the world depending on the local climate. For instance, Florida has about 90 thunderstorms per year, Colorado Springs 60, the midwest plains 45, and the west coast averages just 3 thunderstorms per year. The humid tropics are the source of more storms than any other region of the world; Uganda has an average of 242 thunderstorms per year. Overall, there are about 1800 thunderstorms in progress at any moment on the earth and about 100 lightning strikes hit the earth each second.

Although lightning is most commonly associated with thunderstorms, any phenomenon that increases the energy in the air can provoke lightning. Other sources have included volcanic eruptions, snowstorms, sandstorms, and even rocket launches and nuclear weapons tests.

Lightning is difficult to study because it is one of the fastest of all natural events and one of the most unpredictable. It was only 250 years ago that Benjamin Franklin performed his famous experiment with the kite and the key in a thunderstorm. After storing some of the energy in a Leyden jar, Franklin went on to show that the energy from the storm was identical to his generated electricity. Unfortunately, we have not progressed much further than Franklin did in prediction or prevention of lightning strikes.

Streak lightning is the most common form of lightning and the best understood. Thunderclouds form at the top of large rising air currents. Large water drops fall through the air current and become positively charged. As they fall, they carry the positive charge to the earth. The normally electrically negative earth then becomes positive as the thundercloud moves over it and rain falls. The earth's charge moves beneath the cloud like a shadow, climbing any objects such as steeples and hills. Millions of volts of electrical potential develop between the cloud's base and the ground (see Fig. 9.1).

When the electrical potential becomes so strong that the air no longer acts as a barrier, the current begins to jump. A spark, the stepped leader, proceeds from the cloud to the ground. The stepped leader proceeds about 50

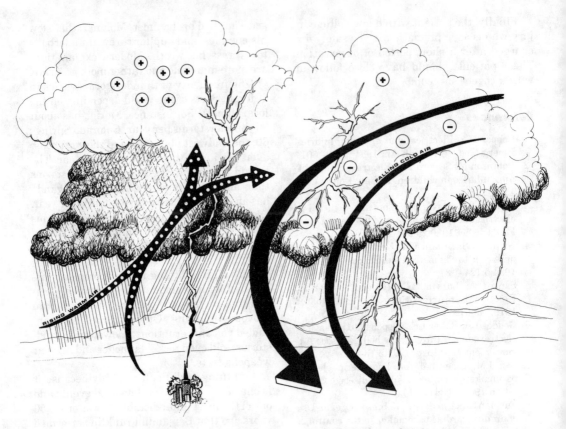

**Figure 9.1.** Thunderhead with lightning formation.

meters every 0.05 milliseconds in a downward branching fashion to the ground. This initial flow of electricity reaches the ground in about 20 milliseconds and often takes side channels and wrong turns on the way down. Within the leader is a current-carrying core about 1 to 2 cm in diameter, and the total diameter of the leader may be as much as a few meters. The tip of the leader stroke is its most luminous portion due to the great amount of energy needed to initially ionize the channel of air.

As the branching stepped leader comes closer to the ground, an upward discharge from the ground meets it at about 50 m above the ground. At this point, the electrical discharge occurs and a luminous return stroke of high current proceeds from the ground to the cloud. Other secondary leader and return strokes may follow in quick succession through the already ionized pathway.

Because the stepped leader is slower than the return stroke, the perception is that lightning travels from cloud to ground. The majority of current flow, however, is from ground to cloud in the return stroke. As much as 10,000 to 200,000 amperes of current may pass in only 0.07 milliseconds during the return stroke. The return stroke may occasionally be visualized as brightening of the pathway but is usually not noted. The massive potential and current flow in the lightning bolt heats the surrounding air up to 50,000°F.

Occasionally, a stroke of lightning may be initiated from the ground to cloud. This happens rarely and only from tall structures or hills. The typical branching pattern is reversed in this ground-to-cloud lightning.

Sheet lightning is a shapeless flash that usually occurs between clouds and is invisible from the ground. Ribbon lightning is formed when rapidly moving winds blow the ionized channel formed by the stepped leader across an area. The successive secondary and return strokes seem to parallel each other. Bead and ball lightning are rare, poorly understood, and unpredictable.

The air heated by the electrical discharge

expands rapidly. So rapidly, in fact, that it produces a shock wave following the course of the lightning stroke. The cylindrical shock wave slows rapidly and decays within meters to merely a sonic boom—the thunderclap. Because the sonic boom occurs along the entire length of the lightning's pathway and then may bounce off of itself and other clouds or objects, the thunder clap is often prolonged and perceived as rumbles, rolls, and peels of thunder.

Observation of the time interval between an observed lightning flash and the thunder from it will permit a rough approximation in either kilometers or miles. Sound travels at about 335 m per second (1100 feet per second), and light travels at $3.00 \times 10^8$ m per second ($1.86 \times 10^5$ miles per second). The time interval divided by 3 is the distance in kilometers; the time interval divided by 5 is the distance in miles.

Because both the voltage and the current intensity is so great, the mechanism of a lightning strike is different from that of commercial electric current. Lightning most often strikes those in outdoor occupations or recreational activities and often injures more than one person.[1] Lightning causes more fatalities in an average year than all other meteorological events combined, including floods, hurricanes, and tornadoes.

There are four modes of contact with the lightning current: direct strike, splash phenomenon, step potential, and flashover phenomenon.

## DIRECT STRIKE

The direct strike, as the name implies, uses the person's body as part of the major pathway for the current flow. Direct strikes are doubly dangerous because of the high electric currents and the secondary heat production of the lightning bolt. Most lightning fatalities and serious injuries are associated with direct strikes. Often, the electric pathway through the body involves the head. Cooper's study noted that victims with cranial burns were two to three times more likely to suffer cardiac arrest and had an overall mortality of 38%.[2]

Direct strikes occur when the victim, who may be carrying a metal object such as a golf club or umbrella, is outside (see Fig. 9.2). Golde

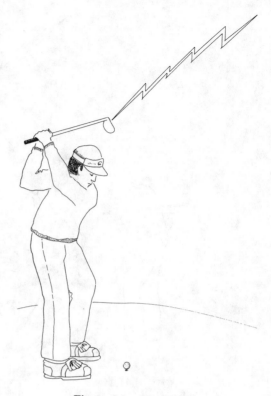

**Figure 9.2.**  Direct strike.

and Lee report that metal worn in the hair increases the chances of a direct strike more than similar quantities of metal worn lower on the body.[3]

## SPLASH PHENOMENON

The most common type of lightning strike is the splash injury that occurs as the lightning strikes another object. This frequently happens as the victim seeks shelter beneath a tree that is subsequently struck by lightning. Lightning can also splash from person to person. Splash effects occur when the person is a better conductor of electricity than the original object struck. For this reason, taking shelter underneath a tall tree in a lightning storm is not a good idea.

## STEP POTENTIAL

When lightning strikes the ground, the electric current spreads throughout the surface layer of the earth. A victim standing with legs spread, near the point of impact of a

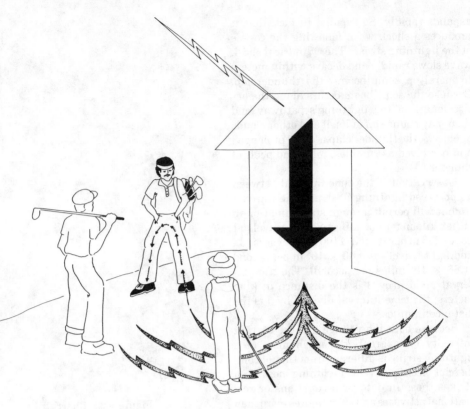

**Figure 9.3.** Step potential.

lightning bolt, may have a significant voltage difference created between his legs, since the resistance to flow of the ground may be greater than through the person. The current flow may then enter one leg and exit through the other. Cooper has noted an increased mortality in patients who have sustained leg burns during lightning strikes and speculates that the step potential may be an important mechanism of injury in these patients.[2] The step potential and the splash phenomenon probably account for the majority of injuries when there are multiple casualties resulting from a single lightning strike (see Fig. 9.3).

### FLASHOVER PHENOMENON

It is well known in physics that a high frequency alternating current will travel on the outside of a conductor. Although lightning is a direct current phenomenon, the rapidity of the pulse may cause it to act like a high-frequency alternating current. Hence, it flows on the outside surface of a victim. The majority of lightning strike victims are caught in the open wearing water-soaked clothing that facilitates the flashover phenomenon. Because of the enormous current, sweat and moisture in clothing and shoes may be vaporized, blowing the clothing or shoes off. This would account for the often-cited finding of the patient's clothing being torn open but not burned.

### BLUNT TRAUMA

Incidental blunt trauma may occur from objects flung by the force of the bolt, by the expansion of the superheated air around the lightning bolt, or as the victim falls. As the current rapidly heats water vapor in trees or rocks, these objects may explode and cause either blunt or penetrating trauma. The shock wave of lightning has been known to blow open 10-foot craters in the ground and split huge boulders in two. Local shock waves from these events may produce blast effects in brain, lungs, bowel, myocardium, or spleen.

## CLINICAL EFFECTS

As lightning follows the route of least electrical resistance between contact points of the human body, almost every organ system is vulnerable. Lightning causes a serious injury or fatality in about one third of the cases, and permanent injury in about two thirds of the survivors.[2] The most common cause of death is an immediate respiratory or cardiac arrest.

---

*Signs of a Lightning Stroke*
Asystole
Respiratory arrest
Paresis or paralysis
Confusion or coma
Trauma from shock wave
Tympanic membrane rupture
Feathery cutaneous burns with punctate
third degree areas
Cataracts (LATE)

---

### Neurologic

The most profound and longest lasting effects of a lightning strike may well be neurologic. These neurologic sequelae may be due to the effects of either direct current or the blunt mechanical trauma.

The immediate effects of the current passage through the CNS may range from an altered level of consciousness to a devastating fatal injury. In the most severe cases, the respiratory centers are paralyzed and the patient ceases to breathe. This is rapidly fatal unless treated. Cooper reported that in her series of 66 cases, 72% of the patients suffered loss of consciousness and 86% experienced retrograde amnesia. Frequently, the victims will have confusion and amnesia for several days— a reaction similar to that following electroshock therapy.[4] Victims may also have seizures from either the hypoxic injury, or from a primary cerebral injury.[5]

Peripheral nervous system effects are almost as common as CNS effects, occurring in the upper extremities in 70% of the patients and in the lower extremities in 30%. Paralysis due to lightning strikes was first described in 1889 by Charcot and continues to be found in the majority of patients with lightning strike in one form or another.[6] Res-

olution of the paralysis occurs in the majority of cases.

Cases of blunt head trauma due to the side effects of a lightning strike may take any form of CNS trauma. These cases should be treated as appropriate for the injury. Such injuries are not within the scope of this text and advice should be sought in the current literature and standard emergency texts.

### Cardiac

Lightning acts as a massive direct current shock, causing atrial and ventricular arrhythmias and direct myocardial injury.[7] This direct current (DC) countershock depolarizes the entire myocardium simultaneously with a variable period of asystole. Ravitch and Safar first proposed that the cardiac activity would usually return slowly, first as a marked bradycardia, then gradually accelerating until normal.[8] There has been no evidence to disprove this theory. Since this is the ultimate "cosmic cardioversion," it is unlikely that primary ventricular fibrillation occurs.

As noted above, Cooper reported in a survey of the literature that victims with cranial burns experience cardiopulmonary arrest two to three times more frequently than those without such head strikes. This is probably due to the current traversing the trunk and heart as it travels to the ground.

If the patient develops respiratory arrest due to the lightning strike, then hypoxia may cause further dysrhythmias, including ventricular fibrillation. Without prompt intervention, hypoxia-induced ventricular fibrillation will deteriorate to a fatal asystole. ECGs of those who recover may show ischemic changes, premature ventricular complexes, and other dysryhthmias. Virtually the entire spectrum of dysrhythmias may occur with the combination of massive electrical shock and hypoxia.[9]

### Peripheral

Lightning may cause injuries to the extremities either by mechanical trauma or by the passage of the electrical current. Damage to the peripheral nervous system by lightning has already been discussed, but the lightning may also cause muscle, bone, and skin injuries.

## SKIN

All of the DC injuries occur because the electric current is converted to heat, just as in a toaster's element. Lightning burns are frequently quite superficial, in contrast to the burns sustained from commercial electric current. Linear "fern-like" flash or "feathering" burns are almost pathognomonic of lightning injuries. This peculiar form of burn is probably due to the flashover phenomenon and the transmission of the electricity about the skin surface in areas of varying resistance.[10] The stigmata consists of reddish markings that do not blanch with pressure, accompanied by other areas that may contain punctate burns, erythema with blistering, or whitish mottling. This stigmata may be a valuable clue for the paramedic or EMT who finds an unconscious victim with no witnesses to the events. The feathery stigmata of a lightning strike fades within 24 to 48 hours and normally causes no permanent changes.

Deeper burns may be due to superheated air or metal objects heated by conduction of electricity. Heated metal objects may also ignite clothing.[11] Arc burns from the intense current may occur from the victim to the ground. Arc temperatures in the range of 3000 to 4000°C will cause full-thickness charring and eschar formation.[12] Lesser temperatures from burning clothing or objects nearby may cause erythema, mottling, or blistering. These deeper burns are not unique and are treated as are other electrical burns.

Linear burns about the axillae or down the chest may also be found. These burns appear to be due to superheated water vapor produced by the flashover phenomenon and occur where sweat or water accumulates.[2]

Unlike commercial electrical current injuries, a lightning strike should not be ruled out by the absence of an exit or entry burn. Lightning injuries rarely have entry and exit points.

## MUSCLE AND BONE

When someone is struck by lightning, the current may produce muscular contractions that may be quite violent and cause fractures, cervical spine injuries, and dislocations. These tetanic muscle contractions may throw the

victim incredible distances and cause further blunt trauma.[6]

There is controversy surrounding the extent of deeper injuries to muscle and bone. Certainly, as noted above, there are numerous reports of fractures and dislocations. Less frequently noted are deeper burns, occurring in only 5% of cases.[13] Indeed, some authors feel that third and fourth degree burns are rare, as are internal damage and myoglobinuria.[14] Others report frequent occurrence of myoglobinuria and postulate rhabdomyolysis on that basis.[6,15]

Peripheral blood vessels may be found in prolonged and intense vasospasm following the lightning strike. This vasospasm may be so severe as to cause loss of pulse, mottled cool extremities, and peripheral arterial thrombosis. Generally, the vasospasm resolves spontaneously after a few hours.[16,2]

## Ophthalmologic

Lightning can also injure the eye and surrounding tissues. The most common intraocular lesions found are cataracts.[15] Lightning-induced cataract formation is not an emergency but should be well recognized by the emergency clinician so that referral may be made. These cataracts are also seen in patients with other high-voltage electrical current injuries.[17] Retinal involvement, to include chorioretinal atrophy, hemorrhage, and retinal detachment have been noted also. The potential of both retinal damage and cataract formation must be considered in the evaluation of the victim of a lightning strike.

Direct trauma to the eye may occur from a blast, with subsequent hyphema and hemorrhage, or by objects flung in the wake of the lightning strike. Ocular and lid burns may also be seen in the patient with a direct lightning strike to the head.

## Otologic

Over 50% of victims sustain a rupture of at least one tympanic membrane.[2] This rupture may be due to either thunderclap shock waves or the electric burn injury. The blast may be so powerful that disruption of the ossicles and mastoid may occur. Although most resolve spontaneously, permanent deafness may occur.[18,19] The damages from the passage of the

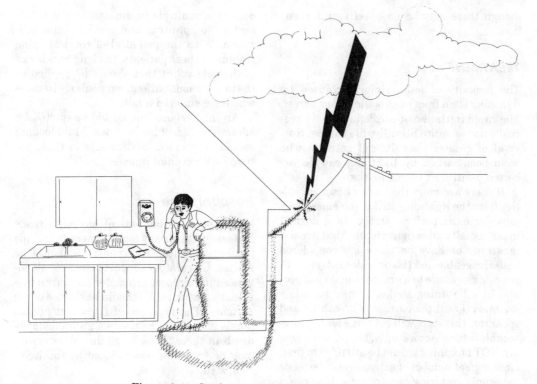

**Figure 9.4.** Conduction of lightning by telephone wires.

electric current may also cause substantial ear damage and these injuries may be difficult to separate from the blast effects. Lightning strike damage of the ear is particularly common when the energy is transmitted through the telephone wiring and the victim is using the telephone.[20,21] Burns of the pinna and ear canal may be noted in these cases. As with any injury to the tympanic membrane, cholesteoma formation may follow months or years later.

### Other Sequelae

Of less pressing interest to the emergency clinician are the later phenomena associated with a lightning strike. Patients and parents, spouses, or other supports should be counseled about these longer term complications, however.

Multiple psychiatric problems may result from being a victim or in the close proximity of a victim of lightning strike. Hysterical "revelations" may occur, an increased sense of subjective probability for lightning strikes may be noted, and abnormalities of mood, af-

fect, and memory may persist for months.[22,23] Children have been noted to have sleep disturbances, separation anxieties, and depression.

Less common, but occasionally noted, include neuritis with a painful neuralgia and a form of atrophic spinal paralysis.[24,25] Ear pain, tinnitus, and hearing abnormalities may be persistent following a lightning strike. Cataract formation after lightning strike is more common than after a commercial high-voltage injury. Follow-up of the lightning strike victim should include ophthalmologic and otolaryngologic surveillance to detect late ocular and otic sequelae.

Fetal death has been reported with lightning strikes in pregnancy, but lightning strike in pregnancy is quite rare, having been reported only 11 times in the literature.[26] Fetal prognosis with cardiopulmonary arrest from any cause is quite poor and lightning provides no exception to this trend. With a lightning strike, the fetal mortality is 50% despite a reported maternal mortality of zero. Close monitoring of the fetus following a lightning strike to the mother is clearly indicated, although there may be no effective intervention.

## TREATMENT

The majority of lethal injuries caused by lightning stem from cardiopulmonary arrest. The rapid initiation of cardiopulmonary rescusitation is, quite literally, life saving. Survival of greater than 70% of patients who have been struck by lightning can be expected, contrary to some myths.

If there are more than one or two casualties from the lightning strike, the emergency provider must perform triage. In a normal mass casualty situation, victims that are not breathing or have no pulse are considered nonsalvageable and the provider moves on to provide more care to a greater number of people. In a lightning strike, it may be safely assumed that if the patient is breathing and speaking, this state will continue for the foreseeable future. Accordingly, the patients who are NOT breathing should be attended to first, since a great number of salvages may be made by simply restoring respirations. It appears that the lightning strike victim with a cardiac or respiratory arrest has a higher chance of survival than the usual trauma arrest and attempts at salvage are justified.

### Immediate Care

The patient who has been struck by lightning should be resuscitated vigorously. As with all other patients, lightning strike victims should have ABCs evaluated and abnormalities corrected before proceeding further. Apnea requires artificial ventilation and intubation if the rescuer is qualified. Pulselessness in the lightning strike victim does not carry an ominous prognosis and immediate CPR will often salvage these younger victims.

First responders and EMTs should be aware that the lightning strike victim is not "charged" like a commercial burn victim who may still be a "live" source of electricity. Unfortunately, however, lightning does strike twice, and the EMT who goes to rescue a victim may be exposing him- or herself to another lightning strike. The victim should be rapidly evacuated to a place of safety, such as the ambulance, if the storm is still in progress.

The lightning strike victim should be handled as a multiple-trauma patient with attention to splinting and cervical immobilization. With the potential of cervical spine trauma in these patients, the long backboard is the sole splint that should be applied in the unconscious patient, particularly in those who have suffered a fall.

An intravenous line should be started for administration of medications. Fluid loading should be avoided, particularly in those patients with cranial injuries.

### Hospital Care

If the nonbreathing patient has not already had adequate airway maintenance to include intubation, these interventions should be started. Circulatory support to include all advanced life support principles and cardiopulmonary rescusitation should be started on all patients. The presence of fixed and dilated pupils should not be used as an indicator of death in these patients, as this abnormality may be transient and induced by the lightning strike.

---

*Laboratory and Studies for Lightning Strike Victims*
Hematocrit/hemoglobin
Electrocardiogram
Urinalysis (include myoglobin)
Electrolytes
BUN
Creatinine
Creatinine phosphokinase with isoenzymes
X-rays as appropriate (include cervical spine)
Consider CT scan with head trauma or head strike

---

Wet clothing should be removed, the rectal temperature taken, and hypothermia treated, if present. The victim should have an ECG, be monitored for both rhythm and vital signs for 24 hours, and have serial cardiac enzyme determinations.[27]

Obvious injuries should be treated as appropriate after the ABCs have been attended to. Little therapy is needed for the vast majority of burns received in a lightning strike. The feathering burns usually fade without therapy in 24 to 48 hours. Small punctate lesions may be dressed as needed but are usually too small for primary excision and grafting. Escharotomy and fasciotomy are usually needed only if there are associated thermal circumferential burns.

Unlike the management of the commercial high-voltage burn, during management of the lightning strike, fluid loading, mannitol, furosemide, and fasciotomy are rarely needed. If myoglobinuria is found, an osmotic diuretic, such as mannitol, may be given in appropriate amounts and bicarbonate used to normalize pH.[28] The main danger of renal failure is from hypoxia due to cardiac arrest, and this failure may be managed in the customary fashion.

The management of tympanic membrane rupture should be conservative, with cleansing of debris and blood from the external canal, systemic antibiotics, and otic drops. Steroid-containing preparations are thought by many otolaryngologists to inhibit healing of the tympanic membrane and should not be used. No drops should be applied if there is a CSF leakage. Long-term care should be the responsibility of an otolaryngologist.

The management of an ocular injury should proceed in the usual fashion with slit lamp and routine examination of the cornea, lens, and retina. Traumatic injuries of the eye should be managed as appropriate with ophthalmological consultation early in the course. With increased incidence of cataracts in those who have had a lightning strike, all patients should be referred to an opthalmologist within 6 months.

## PREVENTION

Many of the precautions that will prevent one from becoming a victim of a bolt from the blue are extrapolations from the physics of the lightning itself. Certainly, the person who stands on the top of a mountain, as the highest point around, will present the greatest risk. Likewise, the mast of the only boat on the lake will be the highest point around. Similarly, if the party seeks shelter under the only tree on the plain, they are seeking trouble. If one carries a golf club, metal umbrella, or tools overhead on the bare golf course, one is duplicating the effect of Mr. Franklin's lightning rods and is at greater risk.

Avoid wide open areas or promontories where the body may be the highest projection. The person at risk should drop golf clubs, umbrellas, and tools. Swimming and boating should cease during thunderstorms. Avoid standing under trees, bridges, or shelters that may be the most likely site of lightning strikes.

Lightning strikes to power lines are usually protected by surge protectors or lightning arrestors in modern buildings, but these are not always provided, nor are they completely effective against the massive surge induced by a nearby lightning strike. During a storm, contact with plumbing and electrical appliances should be avoided. Phone lines usually have a lightning arrestor that will reduce the possibility of propagation to the user. Again, these are not always completely protective and do not modify the loud noise that a local strike may induce in the earpiece. This loud noise may cause severe acoustic trauma. Telephones should not be used during electrical storms.[29] Television antennae are frequently improperly or inadequately protected and may be hazardous.[30]

Automobiles appear to be a safe place during a storm. If a lightning strike occurs, the energy will travel about the outside of the metal vehicle before arcing to the ground. Plastic or fiberglass vehicles theoretically do not offer this protection. Although some authorities cite the rubber tires of a car as "insulation" from the storm's fury, it is ludicrous to believe that a lightning bolt that has just traveled 3 miles to hit the highest point around is going to be stopped by an inch or so of wet rubber.

Of practical significance is the previously cited report that metal worn above the waist may be more significant in lightning strikes. Hair clasps, metal combs, headphones, and large earrings should probably be removed in a storm, particularly if the person is in an area of risk. Small earrings are probably of no significance.

Phenomenon such as St. Elmo's fire or hair that stands on end are good evidence that there is a mounting potential between one's body and the clouds. In this case, one should seek low ground or assume the fetal position on the ground. Placing a rubber or plastic ground cloth on the earth will protect the person from the mud but not from lightning. Again, it is absurd to believe that 1/4 inch of rubber will be an effective "barrier" from a lightning bolt that has traveled 3 miles to the earth. It may protect somewhat against the possibility of a step potential, however.

## SUMMARY

Lightning causes more fatalities than any other meteorologic phenomenon, including hurricanes, floods, and tornadoes. The most important characteristics of lightning injuries are multiple system involvement and widely variable severity of the injury. Victims with head injuries and with leg burns are particularly likely to be fatally injured.

The prognosis for victims of a lightning strike is surprisingly favorable, particularly if CPR is promptly instituted and maintained after the strike. Victims who return to consciousness after a lightning strike are unlikely to die. The victim of a lightning strike should be treated as a multiple trauma patient with appropriate cervical immobilization until evaluation is complete.

Postresuscitation care should include cardiac monitoring, local burn care, and monitoring. The majority of these patients will do well and need only supportive care. Long-term complications include otic, optic, psychologic, and neurologic problems. These complications, quite properly, are not the province of this book.

The best places to be during an electrical storm, in order of preference and descending risk are: home or office, car, grove of trees, and valleys or hollows. Promontories and rises should be particularly avoided. Telephones should not be used during an electrical storm.

### References

1. NOAA, Weigel, EP. Lightning, the underrated killer. NOAA 1976;6:2.
2. Cooper MA. Lightning injuries: Prognostic signs for death. Ann Emerg Med 1980;9:134–138.
3. Golde RH, Lee WR. Death by lightning. Proc Inst Elec Eng 1976;123:1163–1180.
4. Critchley M. Neurological effects of lightning and of electricity. Lancet 1934;1:68–72.
5. McCrady-Kahn UL, Kahn AM. Lightning burns. West J Med 1981;134:215–219.
6. Charcot JM. Des accidents nerveux provoques par la fondre. Bull Med (Paris) 1889;3:1323–1326.
7. Auerbach PS. Lightning strike. Top Emerg Med 1980;2:129–135.
8. Ravitch M, Lane R, Safar P, et al. Lightning stroke: Report of a case with recovery after cardiac massage and prolonged artificial respiration. N Engl J Med 1961;261:136–138.
9. Krantz H, Wasserman M, Valaitis J, et al. Lightning injury: management of a case with a 10 day survival. Am J Dis Child 1977;131:413–415.
10. Bartholome CW, Jacoby D, Ramchard SC. Cutaneous manifestations of lightning injury. Arch Dermatol 1975;111:1466–1468.
11. Myers G, Colgan M, Van Dyke D. Lightning disaster among children. JAMA 1977; 238(10):1045–1046.
12. Rouse R. Dimick A. The treatment of electrical injury compared to burn injury: a review of pathophysiology and comparison of patient management protocols. J Trauma 1978;18:43–47.
13. Amy BW, McManus WF, Goodwin CW, Pruitt BA. Lightning injury with survival of five patients. JAMA 1985;253:243–245.
14. Cooper, MA. Of volts and bolts. Emerg Med 1983;15:99–121.
15. Tribble CG, Persing JA, Morgan RF, et al. Lightning injury. Curr Concepts Trauma Care 1984;Spring:5–10.
16. Taussig H. "Death" from lightning and the possibility of living again. Ann Intern Med 1968;68:1345–1355.
17. Noel LP, Clark WN, Addison D. Ocular complications of lightning. J Pediatr Ophthamal Strabisimus 1980;17:245–246.
18. Bergstrom L, Neblett LM, Sando J, et al. The lightning damaged ear. Arch Otolaryngol 1974;100:117–121.
19. West GB. Lightning as a cause of hearing loss. MD State Med J 1955;4:1350–1354.
20. Poulson P, Knudstrup P. Lightning causing inner ear damage and intracranial haematoma. J Laryngol Otol 1986;100:1067–1070.
21. Plueckhahn VD. Injury and death caused by lightning. Med J Aust 1986;144:673.
22. Kotagal S, Rawlings CA, Chen SC, et al. Neurologic, psychiatric, and cardiovascular complications in children struck by lightning. Pediatrics 1982;70:190–192.
23. Dollinger SJ. Lightning-strike disaster among children. Br J Med Psychol 1985;58:375–383.
24. Beuchner HA, Rothbaum JC. Lightning stroke injury—a report of multiple casualties resulting from a single lightning bolt. Milit Med 1961;126:755–762.
25. Appelberg DB, Masters RW, Robinson DW. Pathophysiology and treatment of lightning injuries. J Trauma 1974;14:453–460.
26. Pierce MR, Henderson RA, Mitchell JM. Cardiopulmonary arrest secondary to lightning injury in a pregnant woman. Ann Emerg Med 1986;15:597–600.
27. Burda CD. Electrocardiographic changes in lightning stroke. Am Heart J 1969;72:56–58.
28. Yost JW, Holmes FF. Myoglobinuria following lightning stroke. JAMA 1974;228:1147–1148.
29. Johnstone BR, Harding DL, Hocking B. Telephone-related lightning injury. Med J Aust 1986;144:706–707.
30. Viemeister PE. The lightning book. Cambridge MA: MIT Press, 1972.

# CHAPTER 10

# Sunburn

## INTRODUCTION

A welcome part of the presence in the wilderness is uninterrupted basking in the sun's rays. The bleached hair and bronzed skin of the ranger or lifeguard signify a commitment to the outdoors in the eyes of observers. The increased free time and higher economic status allow the leisured classes to cultivate their suntanned appearance. In fact, an entirely new industry with tanning "salons" has evolved that caters to those who desire the perceived effects and social status of a suntan throughout the year, regardless of climatic conditions. A person with a pasty white complexion may be shunned and become the butt of snide remarks.

The popularity of a suntan was not always as it is now. The Victorian era considered a suntan to be the mark of those who labored for a living and those who could afford servants would not have such exposure. Most people in that era protected the skin as much as possible from the sun and considered a fair complexion becoming. Indeed, the swarthy complexion denoted a lower class.

Not so highly thought of are the consequences that may result from the exposure to the sun's rays. Sunburn is a common affliction of those who dally too long in the sun. As a consequence of the increase in sun exposure, there has also been an increase in those diseases that are aggravated or caused by the sun's rays. These diseases include premalignant and malignant skin lesions, uneven pigmentation, and more rapid aging of the skin. In addition, the effects of certain drugs and chemicals may be exacerbated by the sunlight.

## PHYSICS OF SUNLIGHT AND RADIANT ENERGY

### Nature of Radiant Energy

Electromagnetic radiation may be described by both a particle (photon) theory and a wave theory. The waves are oscillations that travel through the atmosphere that surrounds us. All electromagnetic radiation travels at the speed of light ($3 \times 10^8$ m per second or $1.86 \times 10^5$ miles per second). Knowing the speed of light, the frequency or wavelength can be determined easily:

$$C = V \times F$$

Where C = the velocity of light

V = the frequency
(vibrations per second)

F = wavelength

Wavelength is customarily measured in angstroms or nanometers (10 angstroms or .000001 cm) for the portion of the spectrum within the visible wavelengths.

The energy in a light wave is directly proportional to the frequency of the radiation, so a high frequency means higher energy. Thus, ultraviolet light has more energy than either visible or infrared light.

Photons are thought to be small particles and represent the smallest identifiable "quanta" of energy in a light beam. These high-energy photons enter the skin and interact to produce the changes that subsequently result in a suntan or sunburn. The target that the photon strikes in the skin is not yet known. The interaction occurs primarily in the epidermis, within 0.1 mm of the skin surface. The blood vessels in the skin are also affected by the ultraviolet A (UVA) portion of the ultraviolet light. UVA penetrates more deeply than ultraviolet B (UVB), with about 50% of the incident UVA transmitted through the epidermis into the dermis. Only a minimal amount of UVB passes through the epidermis (see Fig. 10.1)

### Biologically Active Radiation

Only a small fraction of the radiant energy from the sun causes any biologic effect at the earth's surface. About one third of the radiant energy reaching the earth is either reflected, absorbed, or scattered, allowing only the wavelengths between 2900 and 18,000 angstroms to reach the earth in appreciable quantities. This spectrum consists of the infrared (40%), ultraviolet (30%), and the visible wavelengths (30%).[1] The infrared spectrum is important in that it imparts heat to the skin's surface but has no other known effects.

The ultraviolet spectrum has been rather arbitrarily divided into three major components: the UVA band (UVA 320 to 400 nanometers or 3200 to 4000 angstroms), the UVB band (UVB 2900 to 3200 angstroms), and the ultraviolet C (UVC) band (2000 to 2900 angstroms). The biologically active ultraviolet bands are the UVB and UVA ranges. The only known beneficial effect of solar radiation on human skin is to help metabolize vitamin D in the skin.

The clinical effects of UVA may include initiation of photosensitivity to medications,

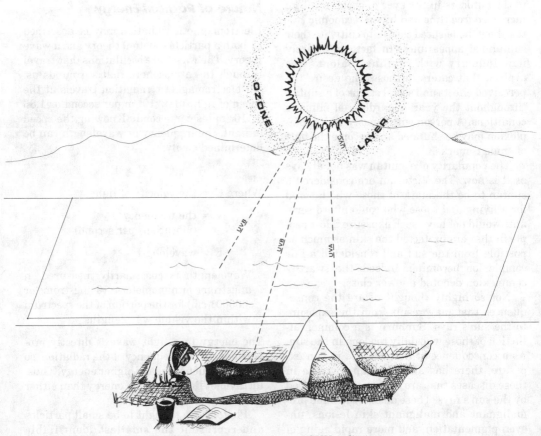

**Figure 10.1.** Penetration of UV radiation.

urticaria, exacerbation of porphyria, aging of the skin, and carcinogenesis.

Recent data indicate that UVA:

1. Augments UVB induced erythema
2. Injures and depletes the Langerhans cells
3. Alters structural proteins and blood vessels in the dermis.
4. Is a co-carcinogen with UVB.

UVB produces suntanning but is also responsible for sunburn and skin cancer. After 60 minutes of exposure, UVA can cause sunburn. UVB contributes significantly to aging of exposed skin. UVB damages DNA in the skin by forming thymine dimers.

The UVC band is almost completely absorbed by the ozone in the stratosphere and does not reach the surface of the earth. Occupational exposure may occur from acetylene torches and germicidal ultraviolet lamps. UVC readily damages cellular DNA and causes erythema (see Chapter 5).

Of the ultraviolet light received on the earth's surface, 99% is UVA. UVB is 1000 times more effective at causing erythyma and sunburn than UVA and comprises the remaining 1% of the received ultraviolet light. Because of the atmospheric filtering of UVB and the lowered sensitivity to UVA, only about 10% of sunburn is thought to be a result of UVA radiation. Window glass, which blocks UVB and passes UVA, provides effective protection from the sun (see Fig. 10.2). Water, because it readily transmits an appreciable fraction of UVB, offers little protection from sunburn.

## Factors Modifying Radiation Intensity

The spectrum and the intensity of the radiation emitted by the sun is relatively constant and varies by only a few tenths of a percent. The intensity of the radiation received by a person on the earth's surface is, therefore, determined by factors other than a variation in the source.

Of these factors, probably the most important are the latitude and altitude of the

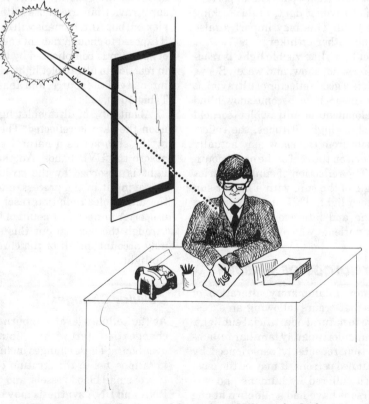

**Figure 10.2.** Reflection and Scattering of Ultraviolet Light

site and the time of the day and season of the year. The longitude has no effect on the amount of radiation impinging upon the earth, since the earth rotates. In general, the most intense radiation occurs between 10 A.M. to 3 P.M., and peaks at 12 noon. During this time, the earth receives two thirds of the radiation that strikes the surface. The most intense part of the year is in June in the northern hemisphere and in December in the southern. Needless to say, the Tropics receive more radiation, with the most radiation at the equator and falling off with the higher latitudes. The time it takes to produce a minimal erythema in June in Florida (24 degrees N latitude) is 10 minutes as compared to 21 minutes in New Jersey (40 degrees N latitude).[2]

For each 1000 foot increase in altitude, there is roughly a 4 to 5% increase in the incident UVB radiation. This means that the backpacker at high altitude (10,000 feet) has about 40% more exposure at midday than the sea level dweller.

Clouds, smog, and fog may reduce the energy received from the sun in proportion to their density. Thin clouds with minimal water vapor or dust may easily pass the important UVB band of ultraviolet light, while blocking some visible light. This may impart a false security to the bather or hiker.

Ultraviolet light, like visible light, is readily reflected by sand, snow, and water. Snow, in particular, is a good reflector of ultraviolet. Many mountaineers have become snow-blind by the development of ultraviolet corneal burns. Indeed, at high altitudes, the reflection on the sun from the snow may actually cause a sunburn on the roof of the open mouth in climbers. The reflection of sunlight varies with the angle of the sun, with a higher sun reflecting more light. This also means that early morning and late evening walks are preferred for patients who are sun-sensitive.

## PATHOPHYSIOLOGY OF SUNBURN

Sunburn is an inflammatory alteration of normal skin that occurs following an excessive exposure to natural or artificial sunlight. Sunburn is an unfortunately familiar inflammatory reaction repeatedly experienced by many fair-skinned persons. It may be the most common burn suffered by humans and virtually all persons have had a sunburn at one

**Table 10.1.**
**Assessment of Risk of Actinic Injury**

| Skin Type | Description | SPF |
|---|---|---|
| I* | Always burns easily (freckles); never tans | 8+ |
| II | Always burns easily; tans minimally | 7-6 |
| III | Burns moderately; tans gradually (lightly) | 5-4 |
| IV | Burns minimally; tans well (moderate brown) | 2-3 |
| V† | Rarely burns; tans profusely (dark brown) | 2(?) |
| VI | Almost never burns (blacks) | NONE |

*Light-skinned, red heads with blue eyes and some with dark brown hair and blue or green eyes
†Darker skinned persons such as Latin Americans, some Asians, and those of Mediterranean descent

time or another. It is produced by UVB radiation and rarely UVA.

The sensitivity of the skin to sunlight is partly determined by the amount of pigment (melanin) that it contains. Darker hued individuals are generally more resistant to the sun's rays than are those with a light complexion, but ALL humans will eventually burn if exposed to enough radiant energy. The study of sunburn is complicated by these variables in reaction to ultraviolet light, skin color, light intensity of the source, and anatomic site (see Table 10.1).

About 10% of ultraviolet light impinging upon the skin is reflected. The oils secreted by the skin act as a natural sunscreen and absorb the UVB bands. Another 70% of the light is absorbed by the stratum corneum, damaging it in the process, and only 20% of the ultraviolet radiation reaches the dermis proper. A miniscule amount of light will pass through the dermis, but this small amount may account for all of the chronic effects of sunlight.

### Cellular Changes

At the cellular level, sunburn is marked by changes that start within minutes and evolve over hours. These changes include vacuolated keratinocytes in the stratum corneum, dilation of small blood vessels, and diffuse edema. RNA and DNA synthesis may be inhibited in the cells that are damaged by UV light. This may also lead to cell death. The basal cells in the dermis may also be affected by the "drip down" of substances in the damaged cells above them.[3] Like other burns, the histologic evidence of damage persists for several days and is accompanied by a lymphocytic infiltration.[4]

The cellular reactions are mediated in part by histamine, seratonins, prostaglandins, and kinins. Increased levels of prostaglandins have been found in sunburned human tissues. As might be expected, prostaglandin inhibitors have been found to delay the onset and severity of sunburn.[5]

After 3 to 4 hours, the skin will start to redden. The redness will intensify over 12 to 24 hours and then fade over a period of 1 to 4 days, depending upon the severity of the sunburn. During the period of maximum inflammation, sweat glands cease to function over the burned area. The area will appear warm or hot, and there will be marked pain and tenderness. The skin acts like other organs with the findings of pain, redness, heat, and loss of function to inflammation. Prolonged exposure to the sun may produce not only pain but pruritis.[6]

Bullae formation (blistering) may be noted with a "second" degree sunburn after a severe exposure, but full-thickness burns are not found. A full-thickness tissue loss is seen only with a secondary infection of the burned area.

Systemic manifestations may occur if a large surface area is involved. These systemic problems include malaise, chills, fever, weakness, and a peripheral leukocytosis. The lay term often used for this complex is sun poisoning although there is no specific toxin involved. Rarely, nausea, vomiting, prostration, or even shock may be seen.

Laboratory manifestations of sunburn may include decreased blood glucose, decreased serum cholesterol, and decreased serum thyroxine.[7]

In mild sunburn, skin vasodilation is noted, and sweating may be partially inhibited. With severe sunburn, the entire thermoregulatory capacity may be lost. If there is a shutdown of the thermoregulatory system due to the inhibition of sweating, heatstroke may occur.

The effects of sunburn are enhanced by wind in the well-known windburn effect.[8] Heat and humidity appear to enhance the effects of ultraviolet radiation on the skin. The reason is not completely understood, but the effect is reproducible. One thought is that the surface oils are stripped away by the action of wind and water, with subsequent decreased skin protection.

Within 7 to 10 days, the skin approaches its original status. The damaged stratum corneum will frequently peel off in sheets of skin after a moderate sunburn. Increased thickness of the stratum corneum and increased melanin production are noted for many weeks after the insult.[2]

## Melanin

Melanin is a complex polymer pigment that is a remarkably effective absorbent of both ultraviolet and visible light. It is formed in the melanocytes of the basal cell layer of the epidermis. Melanin is generally regarded as the body's major defense against the acute and chronic effects of sunlight. Once formed, melanin protects the dermis against subsequent sunburn by absorbing UV light and by acting as a free radical trap.[9] As a free radical trap, melanin will allow other structures damaged by UV light to return to the original state and repair the damage.

## Suntan

A suntan is essentially a temporary melanin increase in the epidermal cells. A more permanent increase is genetically determined by racial characteristics. Suntans fade over time because the melanin-containing epidermal cells slough off the skin at the end of their 28-to-35 day life cycle as the patient washes and wears clothes. An individual who stays tan without exposure to the sun or who is tan in areas that are not exposed to the sun should be carefully evaluated for the presence of Addison's disease. Needless to say, long-term pigmentation changes due to racial characteristics should also be considered.

Suntan is the result of a biphasic increase in melanin production. In the first phase, changes in the cells natural supply of melanin produce an immediate pigment darkening (initial tanning). The second phase has a maximum peak at about 10 to 14 days after the exposure as the total supply of melanin in the skin increases. This is called delayed melanogenesis. Initial tanning is probably the result of exposure to UVA waves, while the delayed melanogenesis is due to the exposure to UVB waves. For this reason, UVA light is sometimes called tanning rays. UVB light has over 1000 times the melanogenic stimulation than UVA light.

The increased melanin in the epidermal layer of suntanned skin protects the skin from further exposure and subsequent sunburn. A gradual suntan provides excellent natural protection against the sun's ultraviolet light. If the patient recieves a sufficient dose of UVB rays, despite the increased melanin layer, a sunburn will occur.

## TREATMENT

Treatment of the patient with sunburn is difficult. Once ultraviolet exposure has occurred, no agent is of proven effectiveness in blocking the sunburn reaction.

For the control of pain of mild-to-moderate sunburn, indomethacin and aspirin are effective and the related nonsteroidal anti-inflammatory (NSAID) agents, such as ibuprofen, may be assumed to be effective.[10] These agents also are effective in reducing the erythema response to UV light. Indomethacin and other NSAIDs topically applied may likewise provide erythema reducing effects as well as preventing some further sunburn.[11,12] A 2.5% solution of indomethacin has an SPF of about 4 if applied early in the course of the sunburn.[13]

For severe sunburn, a short burst of steroids has been anecdotally found by many to be helpful. There is scanty data in the literature about this, however. Usually recommended is prednisone 40 to 60 mg tapered over 3 days. In at least one well-controlled study, oral steroids were found to be completely ineffective, however.[14] No use of oral steroids seems justified by the current evidence available.[15]

Strong fluorinated topical steroids that are applied immediately after the exposure may be slightly protective.[16] If a "Saran wrap" occlusion is used with the steroids, there is somewhat better effect.[17] The overall effect of topically applied steroids in most studies has been less than half as effective as topical indomethacin, however. The lesser steroids are probably not worth the expense or pain

of application to large sunburned areas. A combination of indomethecin and a flourinated steroid may provide better relief than either one alone. There is no study that supports this contention, however.

Also, antihistamines have been shown to be effective early in the course of sunburn in one study.[18] This may be clinically useful, since there is little contraindication or expense to usual antihistamines. Calamine and similar soothing lotions may provide some comfort. The use of silver sulfdiazine cream probably provides no more relief and little more protection for the sunburned patient than other soothing lotions. It certainly costs more than other lotions.

There is no study that provides **comparisons** of the relief afforded by any of the agents mentioned. Anecdotal evidence alone has caused many physicians to prescribe powerful steroids orally or topically, albeit for short periods. A well-controlled study comparing steroids, NSAIDs, antihistamines, and topical agents would be welcomed.

## PREVENTION

There are two basic techniques to prevent sunburn: block the sunburn with a physical agent or absorb the harmful rays with a chemical. Personal physical protection includes hats, shirts, and long sleeve pants. The protection given by these items cannot be underestimated, and they should be available on all expeditions in desert or arid lands. Shelter from the sun may be also achieved by buildings and vehicles, although both of these can also increase heat exposure of the individual.

A standardized testing method for sunburn is needed to compare the various chemical blocking agents. The minimal dose of radiant ultraviolet energy needed for producing erythema (MED) can be measured with relatively noninvasive techniques. This measurement can be then used to calculate how much protection a product gives to the wearer. This calculation is called the sun protection factor (SPF).

$$\frac{\text{MED with sunscreen}}{\text{MED without sunscreen}} = \text{SPF}$$

To determine the SPF for a particular product, volunteers are exposed to natural or artificial light for a period before and after application of the product. Needless to say, the volunteers are selected from several skin types and are screened to ensure that they are not taking medications that would produce an abnormal sunlight response.

The higher the sunscreen number, the greater the protection from the effects of the sun. The higher numbered products will prevent tanning in most people as well as preventing sunburn. The SPF is now printed on the label of the sunscreen products and allows the user to readily compare the effectiveness of the various brands of sunscreen. Unfortunately, the comparision is for the agent as applied in a "standard" test and does not take into account water immersion, sweat, and clothing absorption and abrasion. Some products are now advertising their "substantivity" or ability to resist washoff or ruboff.

Sunscreens may act either physically or chemically to scatter, absorb, or reflect the ultraviolet radiation. Physical sunscreens, such as zinc oxide, will provide an actual barrier to the solar radiation and reflect essentially all of the ultraviolet light. Once considered unacceptable, these agents are now found in a variety of colors. It should also be remembered that a shade is also an excellent physical sunscreen, whether the shade is provided by a tent, a hat, or a building.

Wet, white cotton will transmit UVA light readily, and patients can be sunburned while wearing these clothes. Nylon and white cotton do not block UVA or visible light, and medications that cause photosensitive reactions may be activated through these fabrics.

The chemical agents absorb specific portions of the ultraviolet light spectrum. These chemicals typically contain paraaminobenzoic acid (PABA) or PABA esters, benzophenones, cinnimates, salicilates, or anthranilates[19]. The PABA and PABA esters absorb the UVB radiation with peak absorption at 2780 angstroms but transmit the UVA fraction. Benzophenones block both the UVA and the UVB. The newer sunscreens often contain combinations of these agents.

PABA appears to be absorbed into the stratum corneum and confers increased protection with continued application. Skin moisture at the time of application appears to increase this topical absorption. If the skin is then kept dry for 2 hours after the application, then some protection is present, even when the individual goes swimming or perspires.[20]

The substitution of side chains on the PABA molecule produces other sunscreen chemicals. Many of these agents may be combined to increase their overall effectiveness. All of them protect from UVB and most into the UVA ranges, although they may be washed off somewhat more easily than PABA.

The benzophenones are also frequently used to protect the skin over the entire UV spectrum. The higher the concentration of the benzophenones, the greater the protection.[21] These agents are used in various vehicles to produce the higher numbered (SPF) sunscreens.

As always in medicine, the chemical sunscreen agents are not entirely innocuous. Benzocaine, the thiazide diuretics, sulfanilamides, and several types of hair dye will cross-react with PABA, causing a drug-induced dermatitis in those who are sensitive to either these agents or to PABA. PABA will stain clothing, backpacks, and other gear a yellowish color.[22] A photodermatitis may be provoked by PABA in selected individuals. The preservatives and carrier agents, such as alcohol, that are used in manufacture of the sunscreens may also cause burning and stinging about the eyes or an allergic contact dermatitis. Non-PABA sunscreens are available for these sensitive individuals.

## PHOTOSENSITIVITY

### Phototoxic Reactions

An exaggerated response to sunlight is frequently seen in the phototoxic reaction. This presents as an exaggerated sunburn due to either topical or systemic sensitizing chemicals. The excitation spectrum of ultraviolet light that causes the phototoxic reaction varies for every chemical.[23]

The absorption of the resonant wavelength of light causes the molecule to assume an excited and unstable state. When the molecule returns to the ground state, it releases energy with subsequent damage to the cellular components surrounding it.

Most of the phototoxic drugs are polycyclic, low molecular weight compounds. Al-

**Table 10.2.**
**Causes of Phototoxic Reactions**

| Systemic Chemicals |
| --- |
| Tetracyclines |
| Sulfa drugs |
| Griseofulvin |
| Oral antidiabetics |
| Thiazides |
| Phenothiazines |
| Psoalens |
| Dyes |
| Saccharine |
| Antihistamines |

| Topical Chemicals |
| --- |
| Cosmetics |
| Plants (particularly mustard, celery, parsnip, and carrot) |
| Some fruits (lime, lemon, citron, fig) |
| Coal tar dyes |

most any cyclic compound may be responsible, but the most frequent offenders are:

> Tetracyclines
> Thiazides
> Phenothiazines
> ?? NSAIDS
>
> See also Table 10.2.

It is very difficult to distinguish simple sunburn from a phototoxic reaction. This reaction can occur on the first exposure to the sun and is confined to skin exposed to the sun. The erythema associated with a phototoxic reaction peaks later and lasts longer than simple sunburn. Histologically, a phototoxic eruption is the same as a severe sunburn.

UVA rather than UVB incites this reaction, so unlike true sunburn, phototoxicity can happen through windows and during winter.[24] History of ingestion or exposure to a causative chemical is the most important factor.

## Photoallergic Reactions

Photoallergy is a delayed hypersensitivity to a specific chemical. It requires prior exposure to the chemical and is uncommon. It may manifest as erythema or papules that occur hours after the ultraviolet light exposure. Rarely, bullae formation is seen in very se-

**Table 10.3.**
**Drugs That Can Cause Photoallergic Reactions**

| |
| --- |
| Griseofulvin |
| Some sulfa drugs |
| Thiazide diuretics |
| Cyclamates |
| Saccarine |
| Oral hypoglycemic agents |
| Some phenothiazines |

vere cases. Fortunately, photoallergic reactions are rare.

In this case, the chemical combines with proteins to form an allergen complex. The person must become sensitized to this complex before an allergic reaction can take place, so there is an incubation period. Once the person is sensitized, even a small amount of the chemical can cause a severe allergic reaction. The photoallergic eruption can involve areas that are not exposed to the sun (see Table 10.3).

## *Exacerbation of Systemic Disorders*

**Table 10.4.**
**Differential Diagnosis of Sunburn**

| |
| --- |
| Phototoxic drug reaction |
| Photoallergic drug reaction |
| Contact dermatitis |
| Polymorphous light eruption |
| Exacerbation of underlying disorder |
|     SLE |
|     Protoporphyria |

## *Carcinomas*

The most important results of **chronic** exposure to sunlight are actinic (solar) keratoses, which can develop into squamous cell or basal cell carcinomas. One third of all cancers that occur in the United States are the nonmelanoma skin cancers such as basal and squamous cell carcinomas. Ninty percent of actinic keratoses and nonmelanoma skin cancers occur on areas that are exposed to the sun. The incidence of these cancers is increased in the population centers closer to the equator. Most cases occur in patients greater than 50 years old, but there is an increasing incidence in 20 to 30 year olds.[7]

Regular use of a sunscreen for the first 18 years of life may decrease the incidence of basal and squamous cell carcinomas of the skin by as much as 78%.[25]

## SUMMARY

The most important factor in the prevention of sunburn is the proper protection from the sun. If a group is on a trek, the leader should ensure that appropriate planning is done to prevent sunburn. Clothing, to include light-weight long-sleeve shirts and pants should be carried by all members of the party. Hats will protect the head from the direct rays of the sun. Sunglasses will provide protection from the effects of the sun upon the retina.

Application of a high SPF PABA sunscreen the night before exposure to the sun will provide a longer lasting and effective protection. An alcohol-based PABA sunscreen should be applied nightly after a shower in every person who is regularly exposed to the sun. This regimen will allow maximum penetration of the stratum corneum by the PABA solution. Areas, such as lips and noses, should be protected by an opaque-based ointment if there is significant exposure on a routine basis.

## References

1. Gates D. Spectral distribution of solar radiation at the earth's surface. Science 1966;151: 523–529.
2. Russell S, Stafford JB IV, Edlich RF. Sunburn. Curr Concepts Trauma Care 1982:Summer;14–17.
3. Norins AL. Effects of light on skin. In: Demis DJ, ed. Clinical dermatology. Hagerstown, MD: Harper and Row 1981.
4. Gilchrest BA, Soter NA, Stoff JS, Mihm MC. The human sunburn reaction: biochemical and histologic studies. J Am Acad Dermatol 1981;5:411–422.
5. Snyder DS, Eaglstein WH. Intradermal anti-prostaglandin agents and sunburn. J Invest Dermatol 1974;62:47.
6. Ramsay CA. Solar urticaria. Int J Dermatol 1980;19:233–236.
7. Schreiber MM. Exposure to sunlight: effects on the skin. Compr Ther 1986;12:38–42.
8. Owens, DW, Knox JM, Hudson HT, Troll D. Influence of wind on ultraviolet injury. Arch Dermatol 1974;109:200–201.
9. MacLeod TM, Frain-Bell W. The study of the efficacy of some agents used for the protection of the skin from exposure to light. Br J Dermatol 1971;84:266.
10. Edwards EK, Horwitz SN, Frost P. Reduction of the erythema response to ultraviolet light by non-steroidal antiinflamatory agents. Arch Dermatol Res 1982;272:263–267.
11. Schwarz T, Gschnait F, Greiter F. Photoprotective effect of topical indomethacin: an experimental study. Dermatologica 1985;171:450–458.
12. Tan P, Flowers FP, Araujo OE, Doering P. Effect of topically applied flurbiprofen on ultraviolet-induced erythema. Drug Intel Clin Pharm 1986;20:496–499.
13. Gschnait F, Schwarz TH, Seiser A. Topical indomethacin protects from UVB and UVA irradiation. Arch Dermatol Res 1984;276:131–132.
14. Greewald JS, Parrish JA, Jaemocle KF, Anderson RR. Failure of systemically administered steroids to suppress UVB-induced delayed erythema. J Am Acad Dermatol 1981;5:197–202.
15. Cavallo J, DeLeo VA. Sunburn. Dermatol Clin 1986;4:181–187.
16. Kaidbey KH, Kurban AK. The influence of corticosteroids and topical indomethacin on sunburn erythema. J Invest Dermatol 1976;66:153–156.
17. Sukanto H, Nater JP, Bleumink E. Suppression of ultraviolet erythema by topical corticosteroids. Dermatologica 1980;161:84–86
18. Lowenthal LJA. Tripolidine hydrochloride in the prevention of some solar dermatoses. Br J Dermatol 1963;75:254–256.
19. Forbes MA Jr., Brennen M, King WC. Benzophenone as a sunscreen. South Med J 1966;59:121.
20. Langner A, Kligman AM. Further sunscreen studies of aminobenzoic acid type sunscreen. Arch Dermatol 1972;105:851.
21. Knox JM, Guina J, Cockerell E. Benzophenones: ultraviolet light absorbing agents. J Invest Dermatol 1957;29:435.
22. Rothman S, Henninsen AB. Sunburn and para-aminobenzoic acid. J Invest Dermatol 1942;5:445.
23. Pathak MA. Sunscreens: topical and systemic approaches for protection of human skin against harmful effects of solar radiation. J Am Acad Dermatol 1982;7:285–312.
24. Gilchrest B. Human sunburn reaction: an update. Res Staff Phys 1984;30:72–76.
25. Sunscreens. Med Lett 1988;30:61–63

# CHAPTER 11

# Near-Drowning

## INTRODUCTION

Whether from accident, shipwreck, or as a result of overextension of our abilities, water has claimed lives from those who have explored it since humans ventured from land's shore.

The resuscitation of those who have been submerged and prevention of drowning have been an important part of both medical literature and folklore for ages.[1] Indeed, the ancient Hebrew Talmud teaches us that one of a father's duties is to teach his children to swim. Many of the current techniques of cardiopulmonary resuscitation (CPR) can be traced to the evolution in treatment of the victim of a submersion accident. We have found that the likelihood of recovery is directly related to the rapidity and effectiveness of the initial resuscitation. For those involved in emergency care, knowledge of the pathophysiology and treatment of submersion injury is critical, since they are involved in providing the initial care for most of these casualties.

Of the lethality of submersion accidents there is no doubt. The only confusion is to the exact percentage of the vast numbers of minor submersion incidents and subsequent saves that result in a lethal outcome. A 1977 study in South Carolina reported that at least 15% of school children had had at least one submersion incident over the prior year.[2] With a reported drowning rate of 7.4 per 100,000 in that state, the authors calculated that at least a half million incidents per year oc-

curred that presented a serious risk of drowning in South Carolina alone.

## Demographics

Each year about 6000 to 7000 people die from drowning accidents in the United States.[3] The tragedy is compounded by the age skew of the victims, as most drowning victims are healthy young people under the age of 24. Drowning is the second largest cause of death in people of this age group, and it is the third largest cause of death for 1 to 15 year olds. Males drown three times more frequently than females at all ages. Forty percent of all drownings are children under 4.

People using alcohol and drugs are also at increased risk for drowning. Judgment is impaired and these victims may attempt tasks or stunts that they would recognize as being foolhardy and even dangerous in a sober state. Others may lose either consciousness or ability to balance and fall into the water. Their self-protective reflexes may then be so depressed that they slip quietly below the water's surface without trying to save themselves. Probably one half of drownings are alcohol related, with the incidence being estimated from 20 to 75% by various authors.[4] The number of drownings where "recreational" drugs are involved is not known. The use of illicit drugs is thought to play a relatively major role in drownings, but, again, the true incidence is not known.

Half of all drownings occur in warm weather, during the months from May through

**Table 11.1.**
**Statistical Risk Factors**

Age—Youth (40% under 4 years old)
Location—Home Swimming Pools or bathtubs
Sex—Male 3:1 ratio
Drugs—Particularly alcohol
Trauma—Diving or falls
Predisposing illnesses (particularly epilepsy)
Warm weather months (50% from May to
  August)

Near-drowning may result from an inability to swim, panic, accident or trauma while swimming, or use of alcohol or drugs prior to swimming. Suicide may also present as a near-drowning, either after a leap from a bridge or other high place or as a primary drowning episode.

August. Drownings are a problem in all states, including the desert states.[5] Two thirds of drownings occur in fresh water. The most common sites are home swimming pools, bathtubs, and open bodies of water, the latter may partly explain the summer increase in incidence. About 90% of children who drown do so in swimming pools with the parents nearby. Most drownings occur within 10 feet of safety and two thirds of the victims cannot swim.[6]

Children under 13 years of ages are more likely to drown in home swimming pools or bathtubs, while older children and adults drown more frequently in open bodies of water. Approximately 6% of drownings may represent child abuse or neglect.[7] Suicide and murder may also present as drownings.[8] The water is, of course, a favorite place to "dispose" of an inconvenient body as attested by tales of "cement overcoats" and the like. Probably water has also been used as the murder weapon in countless crimes.

Boating accidents and floods are well-known scenarios of drowning. Another common scenario is enacted by people swimming in unfamiliar waters. They may get caught in rough surf or an undertow, become exhausted, and then drown (see Table 11.1).

## Definitions

The terms used to describe drowning and near-drowning may be confusing and are somewhat controversial. The following terms are frequently used and have been adapted from Modell and others.[9]

## DROWNING

Drowning is suffocation by submersion in a fluid, whether or not the fluid is aspirated into the lungs. This is considered as the cause of death if the death occurs within 24 hours of the insult.

## NEAR-DROWNING

Near-drowning is survival beyond 24 hours after the submersion and implies that recovery has occurred after the insult. This may be termed a submersion injury or submersion incident in some literature.

## SECONDARY DROWNING

Secondary drowning implies that the victim is initially resuscitated, but death occurs minutes to days after the initial resuscitation. This condition is also termed delayed death subsequent to near-drowning. Death is frequently due to the delayed onset of respiratory insufficiency resulting from the submersion incident. A small minority of authors feel that the existence of secondary drowning is questionable, and that established, detectable respiratory insufficiency can be found in these patients upon initial examination.[10]

## IMMERSION SYNDROME

The immersion syndrome is a form of sudden drowning that may be caused by a vagally induced arrhythmia secondary to sudden exposure to cold water ($< 20°C$ or $68°F$). The two most commonly proposed arrhythmias are asystole and ventricular fibrillation.[11,12] Ingestion of alcohol and other intoxicants predisposes an individual to this syndrome.

## IMMERSION HYPOTHERMIA

Drowning can also result from hypothermia due to prolonged immersion. In the water, unconsciousness will set in when the core temperature reaches about 32 to 33°C (89.6 to 91.4°F). At that point, swimming ceases and drowning may occur.

## SAVE

A save refers to a water rescue or removal from the water by anyone who felt that the victim was in danger of a submersion injury.

## PROBLEMS WITH DEFINITIONS

The definitions of near-drowning and drowning are, of course, retrospective. As such, they are of little help to the emergency physician, the paramedic, the emergency medical technician, the lifeguard, or, indeed, even the parents. There is no prognostic import to any of the definitions, except a "save." Clinicians at any level in immediate care should treat ALL patients as near-drowning casualties, unless there is an obvious injury that is incompatible with life. Only after documented submersion times are greater than 1 hour should clinicians consider that the patient is nonresuscitatable.

## Mechanism of Drowning

The sequence of events that follow submersion is different for every case. We can, however, find some similarities in the course of events following submersions. The typical drowning sequence has been abundantly described in animal studies that have provided us with a model of drowning. In Orchard Beach, Long Island, Pia filmed actual drownings during a summer swimming session that confirm some of these animal model simulations.[6]

## STAGE I: PANIC AND STRUGGLE

In most drownings, a period of panic and struggling followed by exhaustion are the initial events. Brouardel in France during the 1890s described this as the "stage of surprise" and described it as lasting about 5 to 10 seconds.[13] Pia noted that this stage lasts about 20 to 60 seconds in humans, with a mean of about 40 seconds. During this stage, the victim will make motions to try to reach or remain at the water's surface. Arm motions may approximate a rapid above-water breast stroke. Frantic hyperventilation occurs as long as the head can be held above water. Other clues that identify potential drowning victims are an open but not vocalizing mouth and a rolled back (far hyperextended) head.

## STAGE II: BREATH HOLDING

Breath-holding apnea begins with submersion and lasts about 60 seconds. The mouth is shut and respirations are voluntarily stopped.

## STAGE IIIA: ASPIRATION

Brouardel then describes a stage where agitation ceases, and the victim may swallow water and begin to vomit. Approximately 90% of drowning victims aspirate the water and vomitus, cough violently, and then gasp involuntarily, flooding the lungs and air passages with water.

## STAGE IIIB: LARYNGOSPASM

The other 10% die of asphyxia thought to be secondary to laryngospasm. No evidence of aspiration is found in these victims. This entity is also called "dry drowning" or "drowning without aspiration." Unfortunately, laryngospasm was not described in the dog experiments. Fluid in the larynx in humans can result in severe and prolonged laryngospasm. This suggests that in humans, breath holding may be followed by laryngospasm of variable duration. Ultimately, of course, asphyxia relaxes the glottis, and the lungs will flood with water. Although only about 15% of victims fit into this category, 90% of the successfully resuscitated patients come from this subset.

## STAGE IV: RESPIRATORY ARREST

Brouardel then described the "second stage of respiratory arrest" where no thoracic movements occurred and the animals became unconscious.

## STAGE V: AGONAL MOVEMENTS AND DEATH

Agonal respiratory movements, cardiac arrest, and death then ensue in both types of drowning.

## EXCEPTIONS TO THE STRUGGLE

Three major exceptions occur to this sequence of events:

**Hypothermia.** In very cold water, as noted previously, hypothermia may rapidly disable a victim, and little or no exhaustion, panic, or struggle may occur before the victim ceases to swim and aspirates water. This is not to assume that hypothermia plays a role in drowning only in frigid waters. From experience with World War II and wrecks at sea, it is clear that even in relatively warm water, the body temperature of victims can be lowered to the point where loss of consciousness ensues with subsequent drowning.

**Unconsciousness.** Events that render the patient unconscious, such as use of drugs or alcohol, seizures, or head trauma, will also prevent a struggle and exhaustion prior to aspiration.[6,14]

**Voluntary Hyperventilation.** Another cause is hyperventilation prior to swimming underwater. By hyperventilation, swimmers can lower their $PaCO_2$ to 20 mm Hg, but the $PaO_2$ will be only modestly increased. As the victim exercises, his $PaCO_2$ will return to between 40 and 47 mm Hg, which is not sufficient to trigger the urge to breathe. Simultaneously, the $PaO_2$ will fall to 30 to 40 mm Hg, which is sufficient to render the victim unconscious, with subsequent drowning.[15,16]

In rapidly moving water, it is unknown whether the same struggles take place. It is conceivable that the force of the moving water and objects struck underwater may cause rapid loss of consciousness due to trauma. Certainly in surf and in mountain streams, both drowning and near-drowning are often associated with evidence of multiple trauma.

As a group, near-drowning victims appear to suffer the same percentages of aspiration and laryngospasm as drowning victims.

## PATHOPHYSIOLOGY

The most important abnormality is profound hypoxemia and its sequelae, but the duration of hypoxia is often unknown and literally unknowable. The immediate effect of asphyxia is a rapidly decreasing arterial $PO_2$ with a concomitant increase in the pCO2 that leads to a combined respiratory and metabolic acidosis.

In wet drowning, there is direct pulmonary damage from fluid aspiration. Pulmonary injury produces hypoxemia in a number of ways as noted in Table 11.2.

**Table 11.2.**
**Consequences of Aspiration of Fluid**

Pulmonary edema
Injury of the alveolar membrane
Direct toxicity of aspirated fluid
Surfactant washout
Fresh water inactivation of surfactant
Direct membrane injury

## Type of Aspirated Fluid

Aspiration of even small quantities of water can lead to a drastic change in $PO_2$. The usual differentiation between aspiration of salt and fresh water is often emphasized, but the toxicity of the aspirated fluid and the presence of contaminants, such as silt, mud, sewage, bacteria, and diatoms, also can influence the development of the pulmonary complications. Aspiration of stomach contents and other debris, such as sewage, sand, mud, diatoms, or algae, contributes to the membrane injury with an aspiration chemical pneumonitis.

Water containing chlorine appears to produce problems similar to those of fresh-water drowning. Water containing particulates as noted above may present problems in postresuscitation care. Bronchoscopy may be needed to remove these particulate deposits.

Theoretically, there should be a difference between fresh and salt water submersion, if a significant amount of fluid has been aspirated. Although the differences between aspiration of fresh water and sea water have been demonstrated in experimental studies and emphasized in the past, few survivors of drowning aspirate enough water to cause any life-threatening changes in blood volume or serum electrolytes. Experimental studies show that if less than 20 ml/kg of body weight is aspirated, no life-threatening electrolyte abnormalities occur, and at least 11 ml/kg is necessary to cause changes in blood volume. This means that a 20 kg child must aspirate 400 ml of solution in order to have significant electrolyte disturbances. Most adults have somewhat less than 150 ml of solution in the lungs at the time of death by drowning. The main reason for the lower volume of aspiration in human versus animal studies appears to be the previously described laryngospasm that is induced in humans by fluid in the posterior pharynx.

Clinical information on near-drowning patients indicates that there is no significant difference in serum electrolytes and hematocrit values among fresh, salt, and brackish water aspiration. Following fresh and salt water near-drowning of experimental models, the ultrastructure and light microscopy findings of the lungs are remarkably similar. The sole reported exception to this is from Israel where Dead Sea drowning victims and survivors alike are found to have marked electrolyte changes, even with aspiration of only modest amounts of fluid.[17] One might expect similar results for near-drowning victims from the Great Salt Lake, but no cases have been reported in the literature.

There are some important differences in the mechanism of pulmonary injury in fresh-versus salt-water drownings, however.

### FRESH WATER

In fresh-water drowning, when a **large** quantity of water is aspirated, hypotonic fluid passes rapidly from the lungs to the circulation. This causes a rapid washout of the surfactant and hemodilution (when large amounts of water are aspirated) due to osmotic uptake of the water.[18]

Hemodilution may rarely result in hemolysis and lowering of blood concentrations of sodium, chloride, calcium, and blood plasma proteins. The serum potassium may rise due to the hemolysis of red blood cells, but marked electrolyte shifts are rarely seen. Volume overload is occasionally seen with large aspirations of fresh water.

### SALT WATER

Aspiration of sea water is twice as lethal as fresh water per unit volume because of the impurities and bacteria it contains. Sea water contains over 20 known pathogenic bacteria including *Pseudomonas putrefactions*, *Staphylococcus aureus*, and *Vibrio parahemolyticus*.[19]

Salt water also appears to produce a larger direct insult to the lung than fresh water.[20] When a significant amount of sea water is aspirated, the salt diffuses into the blood with rapid elevation of the plasma sodium. Osmotic forces pull protein-rich fluid from the circulation into the pulmonary interstitium. The result is a fulminant pulmonary edema with direct parenchymal damage. With salt-water aspiration, hypovolemia may develop, especially if a large volume of water has been swallowed.

### Immediate Sequelae of Aspiration

As previously noted, about 15% of patients have asphyxia from the laryngospasm without significant aspiration at the time of resuscitation. These patients recover from asphyxia rapidly if they are successfully resuscitated before cardiac arrest or irreversible brain damage occurs.

Soon after the aspiration of fluid, there is an elevation of the $PaCO_2$ and a fall of the $PaO_2$ that is the combination of several mechanisms. Immediate vagal reflexes cause pulmonary vasoconstriction and a pulmonary hypertension after the aspiration of the fluid. Passage of water through the alveolar epithelium, the basement membrane, and the endothelial capillary lining causes a rapid disruption of the pulmonary ultrastructure.[21,22] Loss or inactivation of pulmonary surfactant causes an alveolar collapse with a subsequent decrease in pulmonary compliance.

This combination of mechanisms results in increased membrane permeability, exudation of proteinaceous material into the alveoli, and pulmonary edema. The other result of these mechanisms is a profound ventilation/perfusion mismatch and subsequent hypoxemia. The pulmonary blood flow and lung functions do not return to normal for days after the incident. Aspiration of as little as 1 to 3 ml of fluid per kg of body weight results in these persistently abnormal pulmonary functions.

The struggling prior to aspiration and the subsequent hypoxemia will lead to a combined metabolic and respiratory acidosis with contributions from both anaerobic metabolism and hypercapnia. The hypercapnia can be corrected with ventilation, however.

Pulmonary edema is the most common physical finding after aspiration of either salt or fresh water. Following the development of pulmonary edema, intrapulmonary shunting will contribute to the hypoxemia.

### Postmortem Findings

The findings in death by drowning in water are extremely variable and quite inconsistent. The tissues may be pinkish to frankly cyanotic. Frothy fluid from aspiration and/or pulmonary edema usually fills the lungs and airways. This froth may exude from the nose and mouth.

Examination of the lungs may reveal petechiae and seaweed, sand, mud, or other bottom debris. There is a higher incidence of such bottom particulate matter aspiration in those who have died in rapidly moving water or surf. Vomitus is also frequently present in the lungs. The upper gastrointestinal tract is often filled with ingested fluid and foreign debris.

## EMERGENCY MANAGEMENT
### Rescue and Initial Resuscitation

---

*Immediate Actions for Near-Drowning Victims*

Airway Control
  Endotracheal tube if patient is
    unconscious
  Supplemental oxygen with PEEP at
    5 mm Hg
  Consider intubation for patients with
    $PaO_2 < 90$ mm Hg
  or with $PaCO_2$ above 45 mm Hg
  Bicarbonate 1 to 2 mEq/kg guided
    by ABGs
  Arterial blood gases stat and every
    6 hours (minimum)
Laboratory Studies
  CBC and examination of serum for
    hemoglobin
  Electrolytes
  Urinalysis
  BUN, creatinine
  Coagulation studies
X-rays
  C-spine series!!!!!
  Chest x-ray (other x-rays as indicated)
ECG and Monitor for Arrhythmias
Adjunctive Therapy
*Foley catheter*
*Nasogastric tube*
*Consider placement of:*
  Swan-Ganz pulmonary artery monitoring
  Intracranial bolt pressure monitoring
  Arterial line
*If comatose, consider:*
  Diuretics
  Hypothermia
  Paralysis
  Barbiturate Coma
  Steroids
  Vasopressors
RECHECK THE PATIENT FOR ANY
  ASSOCIATED INJURIES.

---

### SUBMERSION TIMES

Time is crucial in the management of the near-drowning victim. Full neurologic recovery is not likely if the victim has been sub-merged for longer than 30 minutes in cold fresh water or longer than 15 minutes in warm fresh water. In hot springs and hot tubs, suc-cessful resuscitations are unlikely after even shorter times.[23]

Submersion time is inherently inaccurate and can serve as only a rough guide toward the decision to resuscitate. The emotional ex-citement at the time of submersion is so in-tense that few reliable observers can be found to accurately document the duration of sub-mersion. Unless a very prolonged immersion time is unquestionably documented, it is best to attempt resuscitation on all victims. The time of the call to the rescuers and the arrival of the rescuers are often known and in ex-treme cases may be used to approximate the submersion times.

### RESCUE

The attempt at a rescue of a drowning victim has claimed many a rescuer's life. Except for shallow pools and open, shallow waters with uniform bottoms, the problems faced in water rescue are likely to be too great and too dan-gerous for the poor swimmer and the un-trained person to attempt. The American Red Cross and the YMCA provide abundant courses in proper water rescue techniques for simple water rescue. This material is easily available and will not be repeated here.

The basic order of procedures for rescue are: REACH, THROW, ROW, and only as a last resort GO. The safely positioned rescuer can **reach** with a stick, ladder, article of clothing, or even a towel and pull the con-scious victim to shore. Any item that floats and may be **thrown** can provide enough buoyancy to allow for a more deliberate and leisurely approach to the conscious victim. Once the conscious patient has a floating ob-ject to hold on to, the next step is to find a way to tow or **row** him or to shore. In the cases where the victim is either already un-conscious or is too far from shore to allow for throwing and towing, the rescue must be at-tempted by going to the victim. It should be emphasized that this is the most dangerous act for the rescuer and the time when many rescuers lose their lives. It is certainly heart-ening to read of the heroics of rescue but more difficult to face the families of multiple vic-tims who lost their lives in the attempt to save another. Rescue is likelier and the danger to the rescuer reduced if a flotation device or a boat is used in the rescue.

The above principles of Reach, Throw, Row, and then Go also apply to the far more complex problem of the ice rescue. Ice rescues should never be attempted without both personal flotation devices and a safety line attached to a point on the shore. Adequate help is essential and ice rescues should not be attempted "solo." Thermal protective suits are a necessity in colder areas. A ladder may serve as a tool to push to the victim or to allow a rescuer to spread his weight over a larger area of thin ice. A small, flat-bottomed, aluminum boat is probably the best device for the ice rescue. It can be pushed stern first into the area with a rope attached to the bow end. The rescuer will remain dry and warm should the ice break. The patient can be either pulled from the water over the stern or allowed to grasp the side of the boat and be pulled to shore.

## MECHANISMS OF INJURY

All patients who are involved in boating accidents, fall into rapidly moving water, rapids, or surf, fall from a height greater than 10 feet, or are involved in head-first diving accidents should be considered to have multiple trauma and potential cervical spine injuries.[24] The easiest and quickest splint that can be used for these critical near-drowning victims is the long backboard. No time should be wasted in meticulous splinting techniques for the patient who is not breathing or who is in respiratory embarrassment from a submersion injury. Likewise, the patient should not be subjected to a movement without appropriate cervical splinting precautions, and the long backboard provides this immobilization. Once on shore, the long backboard will provide a surface suitable for CPR if needed.

In ice rescues, rapidly moving water, and falls from heights into the water, injuries are likely. Fractures to the lower extremities are more likely with ice accidents and falls from a height, but spinal injuries are common with any head-first entrance into the water. Falls into fast-moving water may have any combination of injuries as the victim may be tumbled and smashed into rocks and other debris. Victims of surfing accidents and floods may also be expected to have aspirated substantial

quantities of silt and sand. Cervical spine precautions should be taken for all of these patients. Obviously, in the difficult rescue from a raging river, heavy surf, flood, or the like, the situation may preclude any precautions.

## AIRWAY MANEUVERS

Since the primary mechanism of injury for this disease is hypoxia, maneuvers to restore ventilation are of paramount importance. If the victim is apneic, mouth-to-mouth breathing should be initiated as soon as possible. It can be started as soon as the patient can be placed on a flotation device or the rescuer can stand. If neck injury is suspected by either findings or mechanism of injury, the head-tilt method should not be used as it markedly flexes the neck. Use of the jaw-thrust method of airway management will give better protection for the cervical spine and should open the airway sufficiently.

Except for placing the victim in a relatively head-down position, most clinicians do not recommend maneuvers designed to expel water from the chest.[25,26] However, because of the higher rate of complications from sea water aspiration, some authors advocate postural maneuvers for draining sea water out of the lungs but never at the expense of expeditious CPR.

A notable exception to the policy of no "chest drainage maneuvers" is expounded by Dr. Heimlich, who advocates the use of the "Heimlich" maneuver to express water out of the lungs.[27] There are no data to support the use of a Heimlich maneuver in a near-drowning victim who does not have a particulate matter foreign body obstruction.[28] Care must be taken to prevent aspiration of gastric contents since vomiting is very common with this maneuver. Anecdotal data that support the use of the Heimlich maneuver in this arena are of little merit, since there is no way to ascertain if water "drained" from the lungs is from the lungs or actually gastric contents.

It is imperative that no time be wasted with this or other maneuvers. Since animal studies and human postmortem studies show that most victims do not aspirate significant amounts of liquid, the overall clinical significance of this or any other maneuver designed to "clear the water out of the lungs" is open to many questions.

## CARDIOPULMONARY RESUSCITATION

Immediate and adequate resuscitation is of paramount importance and is the single most important factor influencing survival. The immediate actions of the primary responder have the potential to significantly affect the outcome for the near-drowning victim.

If the patient has no pulse or is not breathing, CPR should be initiated. It is difficult to provide effective chest compressions while the patient is still in the water, but ventilations can be instituted immediately. The patient may be extricated from the water on a backboard or a Stoke's basket litter. Chest compression may be started as soon as the backboard can be supported either on a boat or in the shallows. Initial advanced cardiac life support measures do not otherwise differ from those used in other patients.

If the rescuer or subsequent field emergency medical personnel are trained and appropriately credentialed, an intravenous line should be started for medications. As with all unconscious patients, a trial of naloxone and intravenous dextrose is indicated at this point.

## SUPPLEMENTAL OXYGEN

Supplemental oxygen is a mainstay in the prehospital care of the near-drowning victim. Early efforts should include 100% oxygen, should be administered immediately by bag-valve-mask, and should be followed by rapid intubation in the unconscious patient. Field intubation must necessarily be delayed or techniques modified if spinal immobilization is required. Nasopharyngeal intubation does not usually require manipulation of the neck and is to be preferred if there is any suspicion of spinal injuries.

## SUCTION

Suction equipment must be available since many of these patients will vomit with subsequent further aspiration or may have copious secretions from the pulmonary edema. If vomiting occurs or seems imminent, the lateral decubitus position is recommended. Early intubation of the patient will protect the patient from further aspiration and allow both suctioning and administration of high-flow oxygen.

## POSTRESUSCITATION MANAGEMENT

If the patient responds to initial management, oxygen must be started at high flow with a nonrebreathing face mask. An intravenous line should be started if available and within the rescuer's ability and training. Wet clothing should be removed, if possible, and the patient covered with blankets for warmth. Constant attention should be paid to vital signs, to the potential of vomiting, and to the possibility of deterioration of the patient during transport. Potential problems include pulmonary edema and shock from associated trauma. The potential of cervical spine trauma in diving accidents cannot be overemphasized.

### Emergency Department Management

Initial management of the victim in the emergency department involves three priorities:

1. **Assessment of the ABCs**
2. **Treatment of the hypoxia**
3. **Protection of the cervical spine**

## ASSESSMENT OF THE ABCs

Airway management and restoration of ventilation and circulation are the first priority tasks. These tasks should not be delayed in an emergency department to drain the lungs of fluid. As noted above, most patients aspirate only small quantities of fluid. Better survival is found with rapid restoration of ventilation and circulation.

If the patient is not receiving 100% oxygen, this should be instituted immediately, followed by rapid intubation of the unconscious victim. The nasotracheal route is preferred, particularly with the accident victim.

Cardiac monitoring is needed for all patients, as both the acidosis and the hypoxia will decrease the fibrillation threshold. An intravenous line for medications should be started at this time if not already present. Core body temperature should be measured and measures to dry off the patient and conserve the patient's body temperature should be undertaken.

Defibrillation of the patient in ventricular fibrillation should be accomplished in the field if possible. If hypothermia is found, successful defibrillation may be possible only after core rewarming is accomplished. A cold heart is always difficult to restart, so it is important to not give up too soon. There have been reports of complete recovery after CPR times of up to 2 hours, particularly in small children. Resuscitation efforts should be continued until circulation and respiration are reestablished or cerebral death has occurred.[29] The rescuers and clinicians should be reminded that a dry environment is safer during attempts at defibrillation.

## TREATMENT OF THE HYPOXIA

Management of the pulmonary system abnormalities of near-drowning begins with airway management and continues until the discharge of the patient.

Oxygen should be administered at the highest $FiO_2$ available. Immediate and frequent arterial blood gas determinations and an initial chest x-ray are necessary. The goal of routine respiratory management is to achieve a $PaO_2$ of 70 to 100 mm Hg. Although some patients will be able to maintain this $PaO_2$ with supplemental oxygen alone, over 70% of patients will require more aggressive therapy.

Rapid intubation allows both protection of the airway and administration of higher oxygen concentrations. Positive end expiratory pressure (PEEP) or constant positive airway pressure (CPAP) with intermittent mandatory ventilation (IMV) can be easily used on the intubated patient. Ideally, PEEP should be started in the emergency department and monitored with blood gases as the patient's course progresses.

In experimental near-drowning in pigs, 5 cm of PEEP increased arterial oxygen tension, even when instituted 20 minutes after the insult.[30] The addition of PEEP will decrease the degree of intrapulmonary shunting, decrease the V/Q mismatch, and increase the functional residual capacity. The increased $PaO_2$ from the use of PEEP and CPAP will occur regardless of whether the patient has suffered fresh-water or sea water submersion. Fresh water drowning victims may require the use of either PEEP or CPAP in order to maintain the patency of the surfactant-deficient small airways.

Bronchospasm may be treated with either intravenous aminophylline or a variety of bronchodilators administered by nebulizer. The dosages of these agents do not change due to the insult of near-drowning.

Fiberoptic or rigid bronchoscopy may be indicated in patients who have aspirated particulate matter or especially contaminated fluids. Particularly noteworthy is the high percentage of patients who have had silt or sand in the trachea and lungs after falling in rapidly moving streams or in surfing accidents.

## PROTECTION OF THE CERVICAL SPINE

The cervical spine should be rapidly evaluated in all near-drowning victims. This is particularly important if there are signs of trauma or if the patient is unconscious. The cervical spine should be protected by a cervical collar and long spine board, and cervical spine x-rays should be obtained as soon as possible.

## ADJUNCTIVE IMMEDIATE THERAPY

Victims of near-drowning exhibit a combined respiratory and metabolic acidosis. The respiratory component should be corrected with prompt airway control and ventilation. Severe metabolic acidosis is common and will require correction with empiric 1 mEq/kg of sodium bicarbonate. Upon the victims' arrival at the emergency department, metabolic acidosis can be further corrected with the aid of arterial blood gas determinations.

Hypothermia and alcohol, alone or in combination, may cause hypoglycemia, and drowning victims may benefit from dextrose.

## HISTORY

After all of the immediate resuscitative efforts are underway, it is appropriate to obtain as much medical history as is available, paying particular attention to those factors that will influence the prognosis and possible complications. The physician should be able to document what kind of fluid the patient was submerged in, the temperature of the solution, a rough approximation of duration of submersion, and what resuscitative efforts were made at the scene. The patient's age should be estimated, if not readily available, and any pre-existing diseases that are known should be identified. In many cases, these data will be readily available from friends or family, but some victims are never identified. If possible, while questioning the patient or those who came with him, obtain details of the accident. The details may provide clues to fractures or intra-abdominal injuries that may go temporarily unrecognized during the excitement of the resuscitation.

If the victim is an infant or a child, the possibility of child abuse must be considered. Children may be forcibly submerged under water as a form of punishment. If other evidence of trauma or child abuse is noted that is not completely consistent with the given story, this should be carefully documented.

In the majority of child near-drownings, at least one parent is near the scene of the accident.[31] Most parents are emotionally distressed, devastated, and remorseful. The parents often relate that the child was playing, and they momentarily lost sight of the child, only to find him floating face down or submerged in the backyard pool. Another classic story is that the parent was babysitting, left the child playing in the bathtub only for a few moments, and returned to find the child face down in the tub. If the parents are not reacting appropriately or give an overly detailed or unusual story, the examiner's suspicions should be heightened.

## CRITERIA FOR ADMISSION

### Routine Ward Admission Criteria

Many patients initially appear well following an immersion incident and subsequent resuscitation, but it is not unusual for these patients to progress to respiratory distress syndrome. In one series of near-drowning victims, of 16 patients with initially normal chest roentgenograms, 7 required mechanical ventilation, 3 developed pneumonia, and 2 showed evidence of delayed pulmonary edema.[32] If the conscious near-drowning victim has an elevated $PO_2$ on supplemental oxygen, a normal $PO_2$ on room air, and a normal chest x-ray, this patient probably has a low chance of a significant aspiration. The patient should still be evaluated and observed for 24 hours because of the high incidence of delayed symptoms.

### ICU Admission Criteria

Symptomatic patients should be admitted to the ICU for at least 24 hours of observation. In one report, up to 15% of near-drowning victims who were conscious at the time of admission subsequently died as a result of pulmonary or cerebral complications. Respiratory insufficiency is common, with two thirds of the patients requiring mechanical ventilation and half of these needing PEEP.

If, after 24 hours, the patient has no signs of distress, the chest x-ray is normal, and the ABGs show a $PO_2$ of 80 mm Hg or more on room air, then the patient will probably have no problems. If the patient has any cough, the sputum should be cultured. If chest x-rays show a new infiltrate, the patient should not be discharged and should be observed.

## HOSPITAL MANAGEMENT

Once the immediately life-threatening problems have been corrected, the physician should focus on the treatment of the neurologic, pulmonary, and cardiovascular systems and any associated trauma.

## Cerebral Resuscitation

### NEUROLOGIC STATUS

One of the ultimate concerns of the physician is the status of the patient's neurologic system and the therapies that can reverse the effects of anoxia on the brain. Cerebral dysfunction is unfortunately common after near-drowning.

Neurologic classification scales for assessment of the function and prognosis of the near-drowning survivor have been developed.[33-37] These authors recommend assessment of the patient immediately after the successful resuscitation (see Table 11.3). Survivors are then classified as class A—awake; class B—blunted; or class C—comatose. They further subdivide class C into subcategories that further correlate with prognosis. The Glasgow coma scale also allows different examiners to monitor the changes in the patient's neurologic status (see Table 11.4).

After rescue and resuscitation, the extent

**Table 11.3.**
**Conn-Modell Classification of Near-Drownings**[61]

| Category | Prognosis |
|---|---|
| **Alert** | Near 100% survival with normal brain function |
| **Blunted** consciousness combative, agitated, disoriented, lethargic | 90% survival with normal brain function |
| **Comatose** | 73% survival—normal (adults) |
| | 44% survival—normal (children) |
| | 17% brain damaged— (children) |
| C-1 Flexor response to pain | |
| C-2 Decerebrate with extensor response, hyperventilation, and fixed dilated pupils | |
| C-3 Deeply comatose, flaccid, absent respirations | |

**Table 11.4.**
**Glasgow Coma Scale**

| | |
|---|---|
| *Verbal Response* | |
| None | 1 |
| Incomprehensible sounds | 2 |
| Inappropriate words | 3 |
| Confused | 4 |
| Oriented | 5 |
| *Eye Opening* | |
| None | 1 |
| To pain | 2 |
| To speech | 3 |
| Spontaneously | 4 |
| *Motor Response* | |
| None | 1 |
| Abnormal extensor | 2 |
| Abnormal flexion | 3 |
| Withdraws | 4 |
| Localizes | 5 |
| Obeys | 6 |

The CGS evaluates the patient's level of consciousness in three ways: verbal response, eye opening, and motor response. The GCS score is obtained by adding the individual scores for each of the three components. A fully oriented, alert patient would receive the maximum score of 15. A mute, flaccid patient who has no eye opening to any stimuli would receive a score of 3.

of cerebral recovery appears to be related to five factors:

1. **The response of the victim to the diving reflex**
2. **The development of hypothermia**
3. **The duration of submersion**
4. **The effectiveness of resuscitation**
5. **The methods used to support cerebral salvage**

The first three factors are discussed in detail later.

## THE EFFECTIVENESS OF RESUSCITATION

After rescue, the victim may appear to be clinically dead, either because a true cardiac arrest has occurred or because the bradycardic weak pulse is not palpable. It is emphasized that the development of immersion hypothermia prior to the anoxic insult is protective for the brain. This has been confirmed by a considerable amount of clinical experience with deliberate hypothermia in cardiovascular surgery. Therefore, all drowning victims should have a trial of resuscitation with immediate ventilation and closed chest massage. Brain death is difficult to determine at lower body temperatures, so rewarming the patient to at least 30°C is required before

abandoning CPR. CPR exceeding 2 hours has been successful, and victims have survived submersion times as long as 40 minutes.

## CEREBRAL SALVAGE TECHNIQUES

At the time of admission, the patient may appear to be "brain dead" or to show substantial evidence of brain injury. It should be assumed that all patients are potentially salvageable, and all therapeutic measures should be instituted immediately. If the brain injury is irreversible, this will be obvious by 24 hours, and therapy can be terminated.

Unfortunately, the child who is severely brain damaged may become a tragedy that is worse than death. With modern technology, this child can lie in a nursing home for 30 to 40 years, pauper his parents, and provide emotional problems for the family far beyond that ensuing from a death. As a result, cerebral resuscitation should have priority over all body systems except the respiratory and cardiovascular.

There are at least four separate effects that follow any acute brain injury, regardless of cause. The first is a loss of neuronal function, grossly manifested by a loss of consciousness. Any acute brain injury is then accompanied by a diffuse brain swelling. This swelling causes an increase in intracranial pressure. It is felt that this edema and subsequent intracranial pressure rise kills neurons that may have survived the original insult. The lethal effects of intracerebral edema are well known. In drowning, this process is predictable, controllable, and often preventable. The third and fourth effects, hyperemia and cerebral tissue acidosis, are usually corrected with the standard supportive regimens.

### HYPER Protocol

Conn's multimodality protocol uses a combination of diuretics, fluid restriction, hyperventilation with monitoring of ABGs, intracerebral pressure monitoring, barbiturates, deliberate hypothermia, and chlorpromazine designed to reduce cerebral edema and hypoxia. Modell's protocol does not use barbiturates and deliberate hypothermia and is somewhat less aggressive. A comparison of the two protocols is difficult because the two study sites deal with drownings in markedly different water temperatures. They have not been adequately studied in adult patients and the conclusions reached may not apply to the adult.

### Calcium Channel Blockers

In one reported case, verapamil was anecdotally used in resuscitation of a near-drowning victim with good effect.[38] Calcium has been implicated in the development of post-anoxic encephalopathy, and calcium channel blockers may play some future role in cerebral resuscitation. Certainly, further studies of this class of medication are needed. Until this evidence has been gathered, the effects of calcium channel blockers remain speculative.

### Evaluation of Protocols

Like all therapies, the initially reported good results and subsequent optimism found with cerebral resuscitation becomes tempered with experience. Initial investigators felt strongly that reduction of intracranial pressure (ICP) and careful respiratory monitoring were associated with good outcomes. All studies emphasize the importance of aggressive initial resuscitative measures to maintain cerebral perfusion and systemic oxygenation.

On the other hand, the value of the HYPER protocols and the intensive respiratory therapy is now thought by some to be no better than the careful personal monitoring found in an intensive care unit. Yet other investigators have noted that treatment of intracranial hypertension with hypothermia, barbiturates, and ICP monitoring apparently has no effect on the neuropsychologic outcome.[39,40] The differences of opinion and outcome seem to be partially predicated upon the water temperature, with cold water studies being optimistically guarded and warm water studies being pessimistic.[41,42]

Unfortunately, clinical trials that include both warm and cold water near-drownings with similar protocols for management do not exist. It seems illogical to compare results in a 2-month-old child who falls into an icy swimming pool in winter for 15 minutes with the results of a 40-year-old with a toxic level of alcohol who is submerged in a hot tub for 8 minutes. Even if they were both submerged for the same time, if one has intubation and respiratory support in 4 minutes and the other requires transport with a basic life support crew for 45 minutes to get to the nearest emergency facility, the results may not be entirely comparable. Are the times of submersion and rescue accurate or merely guesses? Again, unfortunately, most reports of therapy of near-drowning are retrospective, relatively small in numbers of patients, and limited in scope.

## Cardiovascular System

Stabilization of the cardiovascular system requires a careful assessment of the intravascular volume and correction of hypoxia, acidosis, and hypothermia.

Hypotension should be initially managed with fluid replacement. If the patient appears hypovolemic, occult thoracic and abdominal trauma and spinal injury should be vigorously sought. If the patient is normovolemic, inotropic agents should be used. Central venous pressure lines or, ideally, a Swan-Ganz catheter will facilitate the assessment of vascular volume. Hemolysis due to aspiration of fresh water is quite rare, but blood replacement may be needed if extensive hemolysis is found. It cannot be emphasized enough that the most common etiology of hypotension in near-drowning is occult bleeding.

Cardiac dysfunction is usually limited to rhythm disturbances, but the hypoxia may result in progression to such lethal rhythms as ventricular fibrillation and asystole. Correction of hypoxemia and acidosis is often sufficient therapy, but core rewarming of hypothermia, if present, is also necessary.

## Pulmonary System

The lethal common denominator in drownings and in rapidly fatal near-drowning is hypoxia. Profound hypoxia is found in animals that have aspirated as little as 1 ml per kg of body weight. Factors that have caused hypoxia in near-drowning include decreased lung compliance and increased intrapulmonary shunting of blood.

### SURFACTANT

As noted earlier, fresh water inactivates surfactant, and salt water draws interstitial fluid into the alveoli, which dilutes surfactant. The compliance decreases with the atelectasis due to the decreased surfactant.

### SHUNTING

Shunting will likewise occur with the atelectasis, but it is also noted with the fluid-induced bronchospasm seen with aspiration. Aspiration of debris, such as sand, mud, or sewage, may also cause the development of shunting and decrease the compliance. Noxious chemicals in the water or fluids other than water may markedly exacerbate shunting.

### CHEST RADIOGRAPHS

Three types of chest x-ray patterns may be noted:

**Normal**
**Perihilar pulmonary edema**
**Generalized pulmonary edema**

The presence of a normal chest x-ray does not mean that the patient has a normal pulmonary status. Of all initial chest x-rays, 28% are normal but become abnormal in 6 to 12 hours. Clinically obvious pulmonary prob-

lems are found with normal chest x-rays in one fourth of the patients. Chest x-ray studies should be repeated every 6 hours and ABGs measured every hour until the patient's condition stabilizes. Failure to clear the chest x-ray after 1 week or a worsening picture after 3 to 5 days should suggest a pneumonia or a possible foreign body aspiration, and the patient may need bronchoscopy.

### RESPIRATORY INSUFFICIENCY

Patients who have respiratory distress despite adequate ventilatory therapy or who require oxygen in excess of 40% in order to maintain an adequate $PO_2$ may have extensive interstitial and alveolar pulmonary edema or atelectasis and will require aggressive respiratory therapy for the resulting adult respiratory distress syndrome (ARDS).[43] ARDS can result from either water or gastric fluid aspiration and is usually seen in the first 72 hours.

For those who are submerged in brackish water or sewage, pulmonary edema, chemical pneumonitis, and pneumonia may all be found in the same patient. Sand aspiration from surf accidents may result in a "sand bronchogram" that outlines the pulmonary tree on a chest x-ray and will, likewise, require aggressive respiratory therapy.[44]

The hypoxia that develops from these pulmonary complications may cause acute tubular necrosis in the kidney, acute cerebral edema in the brain, and ischemic necrosis and arrhythmias in the heart. Treatment of any of the other organ systems requires successful treatment of the pulmonary complications.

The goal of aggressive respiratory therapy in the management of near-drowning is to keep the $PaO_2$ above 60 mm Hg without compromise of cardiac output or excessive intrapulmonary shunting. If the patient is awake and has adequate spontaneous respirations, continuous positive airway pressure by mask may be employed.

If the patient's condition is not stable, the patient should be intubated, if this has not already been done. Mechanical ventilation with a volume-limited ventilator and PEEP should be instituted. Generally, 5 to 7 cm of water is an acceptable initial PEEP. This may be increased gradually until the arterial oxygen tension is greater than 65 mm Hg. If high levels of PEEP are required, a Swan-Ganz pulmonary artery catheter will aid monitoring mixed venous pH and $PO_2$, fluid balance status and will allow measurement of cardiac output. In some cases IMV will allow use of higher airway pressure without adverse effects on cardiac output.

## Long-Term Respiratory Complications

Those patients who survive may have long-term alterations in pulmonary functions.[45] The major long-term abnormalities found have been bronchial hyperreactivity and small airway dysfunctions. These may represent important risk factors in the development of chronic obstructive pulmonary disease. Other authors have felt that the acute pulmonary abnormalities are completely reversible.[46,47]

## PNEUMOTHORAX

Oakes and associates reported pneumothorax in 6 of 21 patients, with 3 occurring iatrogenically from procedures and the other 3 occurring in patients undergoing ventilation with PEEP. Spontaneous pneumothorax did not occur.

## Miscellaneous Abnormalities

### ELECTROLYTE ABNORMALITIES

Only 15% or so of near-drowning victims aspirate enough fluid to alter the serum electrolytes significantly. Significant volume and electrolyte abnormalities are unlikely in the presence of a normal hematocrit. Electrolyte imbalance occurs primarily through GI absorption of swallowed water. Emptying the stomach of water and air with nasogastric suctioning may help to prevent this problem.

Acidosis, on the other hand, is often a major problem. About 70% of near-drowning victims have severe acidosis that requires correction with bicarbonate.[48] This correction should be done with the guidance of blood gas results, rather than empirically.

### HYPOTHERMIA

Hypothermia is a more frequent cause of death in the water than formerly realized. When the Titanic sank in 1°C water, 1500 people died within 90 minutes, yet there were ample life preservers to go around.[49] Unconsciousness occurs when the core temperature reaches about 32 to 33°C; in the water, swimming efforts cease, and the unprotected person will drown. (See Chapter 4 on hypothermia for a further discussion of these effects.)

In cold water, hypothermia will develop in a short time in unprotected adults.[50] If the water is not only cold, but moving quickly, hypothermia may develop at an incredibly rapid rate. A child's temperature drops even more quickly because of the relatively large surface-area-to-mass ratio and the lack of subcutaneous fatty insulation. Add to this the swallowing and aspiration of icy water, and the cooling rate may be enhanced.

Studies on subjects in cold water (as low as 4.5°C) demonstrate that the maximum heat loss occurs from the head, the neck, the sides of the chest, and the groin.[51] Swimming and other motion enhances this loss, increasing the risks of hypothermia. Since the cooling process is enhanced by movement, the better swimmers often die first, since they are more likely to try to tread water or swim rather than just float. Likewise "drownproofing," a technique of bobbing in the water, will markedly increase the heat loss as water circulates about the head. Based upon these studies, a heat escape lessening posture (HELP position) was devised in which the victim draws the knees up close to the chest, presses the arms to the sides, and remains as quiet as possible. For three or more persons, huddling quietly and closely together will decrease the heat loss from the groin and front (see Figs. 11.1 and 11.2).

## The Diving Reflex

The diving reflex is found in all mammals and consists of bradycardia, profound systemic vasoconstriction, and suppression of respiratory activity. It is evoked by the presence of cold water on the victim's face or nose. The inhibition of respirations apparently continues until the brain shuts down due to hypoxia. The reflex is strongest in young animals and with colder water. It is present but not particularly strong in adult humans.[6]

## Detrimental Effects

Hypothermia presents a therapeutic dilemma in the management of the near-

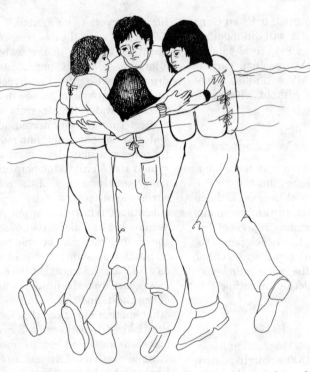

**Figure 11.1.** "Huddle" for warmth where immersed in cold water.

drowning victim. On one hand, the cardiovascular complications of hypothermia include hypotension, bradycardia, conduction deficits, and ventricular fibrillation. Electrical defibrillation of the heart is difficult at low core temperatures. Drugs, such as antiarrhythmics and insulin, may be ineffective and accumulate, reaching toxic levels due to the slowed metabolism and excretion.

### Protective Effects

On the other hand, it should be emphasized that the development of hypothermia prior to the final anoxic insult protects the brain for a considerable period following a cardiopulmonary arrest. The combination of hypothermia and the diving reflex probably plays a major role in salvage after prolonged submersion. Because of the diving reflex, which is most active in infants and small children, the heart rate drops to about 8 to 10 beats per minute, while core body temperature rapidly falls to about 28 to 30°C.

The development of hypothermia protects the brain by decreasing metabolic demands and preventing severe cerebral hypoxia. This process has been confirmed by extensive clin-

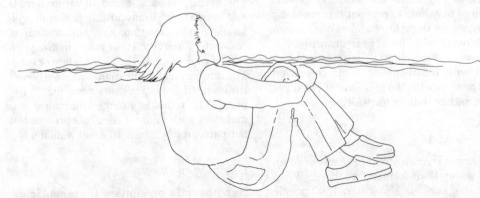

**Figure 11.2.** If alone, assume a fetal or HELP Position (Heat Escape Lessening Posture).

ical experience in cardiovascular surgery. Of course, the drowning victim is not a well-controlled, well-oxygenated preoperative patient! It should be emphasized that the simultaneous onset of anoxia with hypothermia carries a less favorable prognosis than when the hypothermia precedes the anoxia. When cardiac arrest finally occurs, there may be only an additional 10- to 15-minute period before the brain is irreversibly damaged in the anoxic hypothermic patient. Even with this understanding, the prolonged periods of submersion that have a subsequent good outcome and total recovery are not quite so miraculous as they appear.

Studies of drowning victims from warmer climates show lower survival and higher morbidity. This is probably due to the loss of protective reflexes and protective hypothermia. The difference is so marked that practitioners who see warm water near-drowning patients from the southern states have an entirely different outlook on this disease than northerners who deal with cold water near-drowning victims. Indeed, the worst outcome appears to be in victims of hot tub immersion accidents.

## Rewarming Methods

The evaluation and treatment of hypothermia whether wet or dry, on land or in the water, is essentially the same.[52] The most basic method of prevention of heat loss should be used from the very start of the resuscitation; the patient should be dried! Evaporation causes rapid heat losses and wet clothes rarely protect sufficiently from heat losses. Wet clothing should be removed as soon as possible in the resuscitation, and the patient should be covered with warmed, dry blankets.

The rewarming method of choice in the hypothermic nonbreathing near-drowning victim is probably cardiopulmonary bypass with in-line heat exchanger. This method has the very practical advantage of rewarming the core and oxygenating the brain at the same time. Water baths for rewarming are dangerous to both patient and staff if cardiovascular monitoring is employed. Other methods, such as peritoneal dialysis and hemodialysis, also allow invasive monitoring and rapid rewarming of the core simultaneously. For the conscious patient without significant respiratory embarrassment, active external

heating may suffice. Although heated moistened oxygen and warmed intravenous fluids do not contribute significant heat calories to the resuscitation, this form of adjunctive warming will often balance heat losses.

## DISSEMINATED INTRAVASCULAR COAGULATION

Coagulopathies will develop in the form of disseminated intravascular coagulation. Coagulation defects rarely may be related to the hemolyzing effects found in fresh-water drowning, to development of ARDS, or to the use of extremely warm fluids in core temperature rewarming efforts. As noted previously, very few near-drowning victims will aspirate sufficient fresh water to cause hemolysis.[53]

A decreasing hemoglobin level is more likely to be a reflection of fluid resuscitation and a continuing intrathoracic or intra-abdominal blood loss. If the clinician notes a falling hematocrit, it is wise to ensure that the patient does not have blood loss from the common sites of occult bleeding due to trauma.

## RENAL FAILURE

Acute tubular necrosis is the most common renal injury. It is a complication of one or more of the following factors: hypoxia, decreased renal blood flow from hypotension, lactic acidosis, myoglobinuria, or trauma. Renal damage is unlikely if hypoxia is prevented and renal perfusion is maintained. Acute tubular necrosis is usually found only with severe hypoxic insults.

## Adjunctive Therapies
### CATHETERS AND TUBES

Complete emergency department management should include a nasogastric tube and a Foley catheter.

### STEROIDS

Use of steroids in the management of near-drowning is controversial but is appealing on two fronts.[54] First, steroids are known to decrease brain swelling in patients with increased intracerebral pressure from a variety of causes. Secondly, steroids are also found to decrease pulmonary inflammation. They also, unfortunately, tend to blunt immune responses to infection.

Unfortunately, steroids have not been proven beneficial in any controlled, prospective, double-blinded, study of near-drowning victims. Most investigators have found no difference in outcome between patients treated with steroids and patients who have had no steroids. The studies have all been retrospective, however, and good prospective studies are needed to prove or disprove the effectiveness of steroids. Until this evidence has been gathered, steroids are not recommended.

## ANTIBIOTICS

There is little evidence for, and substantial logic against, the use of prophylactic antibiotics. In one study where 21 patients were given prophylactic antibiotics, 16 developed a pneumonia from an organism resistant to the antibiotic used.[55] Many clinicians advocate culture of a tracheal aspirate and treatment with appropriate antibiotics for that culture only if there is clinical evidence of an infection. Antibiotics should be given to those patients who exhibit signs of infection or sepsis. Less controversy exists over the use of prophylactic antibiotics when the patient aspirates grossly contaminated water, such as from sewers or septic tanks. With such contamination of the lungs, most authorities recommend antibiotics.

## Prognosis

A prognosis of the patient with near-drowning may be difficult to estimate, but current data justify guarded optimism. If the patient has made a first respiratory effort within 30 minutes of rescue, the prognosis is good.[56] The adult patient who arrives at the hospital with a beating heart has a good chance of recovery of all neurologic function. Those patients with progressive neurologic deterioration appear to have a uniform incidence of prior deterioration of pulmonary status. Survival after the near-drowning event appears to depend upon a number of interrelated factors (see Table 11.4).

In warm water submersion, a clinical picture that includes one or more of the following features will imply a severe neurologic impairment or mortality, even in children:[25,57,58]

> **Submersion for greater than 5 minutes**
> **Fixed and dilated pupils (in the ED)**
> **No CPR for 10 minutes or more**
> **pH less than 7.1 on arrival at the hospital**
> **Need for in-hospital resuscitation or ventilation**

These indicators are not absolutely reliable, and the prognostic criteria should be regarded with caution. In the absence of any unusual circumstance, such as cold water immersion or barbiturate use, a reasonable guideline is to continue resuscitation for 30 to 40 minutes. After that time, consider stopping all efforts if no effective cardiac activity has been restored (see Table 11.5).

The same prognostic factors cannot be applied to submersion in cold water. As has been noted before, there is a profound protective effect of hypothermia on cerebral survival. In very warm water, prognosis becomes guarded at best after even short periods of immersion (see Table 11.6).

## PREVENTION

Like all diseases, it is much easier to prevent a drowning or near-drowning than it is to treat one. Many of the major factors that contribute to a near-drowning are preventable, such as an inability to swim, failure to wear proper protective gear, consumption of drugs or alcohol, and stunts. Because the greatest proportion of drownings occur in nonswimmers, the protection afforded by swimming lessons is easy to support.

**Table 11.5.**
**Factors Affecting Prognosis**

1. Duration of the submersion
2. Duration and degree of hypothermia (water temperature)
3. Age of the patient
4. Water contaminants*
5. Duration of respiratory arrest*
6. Duration of cardiac arrest*
7. Rapidity and effectiveness of resuscitation*
8. ? The diving reflex*

*Without controlled studies, it is difficult to determine which of these factors have the greatest effect on the outcome of the patient after a near drowning.

Table 11.6.
**Prognostic Factors in Near-Drowning
Resuscitation**

| Good | BAD |
|---|---|
| Alert and Awake | Coma |
| | Fixed, dilated pupils |
| Cold water | Warm water |
| Short submersion | Submersion > 5 minutes |
| Older child or young adult | Extremes of age |
| On scene ACLS/BLS | No CPR for > 5 minutes |
| Healthy | Pre-existing diseases |

Children require special preventative measures. It is interesting to note that a Virginia study of toddler pool saves found that the children who had had some form of swimming lessons by 18 months of age were only half as likely to require retrieval from a pool.[59] A child with "water wings" or in a floating support, without adequate supervision immediately available, is a fatality waiting for a place to happen. Overestimation of swimming skills and trauma associated with horseplay may contribute to a child's demise.

Fencing around pools has markedly reduced the incidence of submersion injuries in those areas where it is required.[60] Because fencing requires no training or action on the part of the child, it deserves a very high priority in prevention efforts. The fencing should be at least 4 feet high and include self-locking gates.

The adult who is intoxicated not only cannot supervise a child, he or she cannot supervise personal actions. To reach the "legally drunk" 100 mg per dl level, the average 70-kg person needs to consume only four beers in the space of an hour. Any steps that reduce the rate of intoxication among swimmers will reduce the frequency of injury and death. Patients with seizure disorders or other handicaps must be properly supervised as their risk is higher.

For those who are exposed to the elements, particularly at sea in the higher latitudes, instructions in methods of conserving body heat during immersion should be mandatory. Proper protective gear should be worn at all times in these areas, including both survival suits and approved flotation devices.

## SUMMARY

An estimated 6000 to 8000 drownings will occur each year in the United States, and there is a like number of near-drownings that are reported. There is not a mandate to report near-drownings, so the figures may be far higher.

The management of near-drowning is still far from perfect. The single most important factor in recovery of the patient is the time from submersion until definitive airway care. Rapid delivery of advanced cardiac life support procedures provides this airway care and allows correction of complications of both aspiration and asphyxia. Training of lay and paramedical personnel is a priority task in reducing morbidity from this series of illnesses.

Younger victims in cold water have the best prognosis of long-term survival. Those who suffer submersion in hot tubs have the worst prognosis. Unfortunately, there is no good way to predict which person will survive intact, which will die, or which will suffer damage that leaves only vegetative functions intact. All patients deserve a full and aggressive resuscitation, with only a very few exceptions.

Finally, the best treatment for this disease is prevention. Swimming lessons, water safety, and adequate supervision should be stressed for children. Liquor and other intoxicants should be banned from swimming areas.

## References

1. Liss HP. A history of resuscitation. Ann Emerg Med 1986;15:65–72.
2. Schuman SH, Rowe JR, Glaxer HM, and Redding JS. Risk of drowning: an iceberg phenomenon. J Am Coll Emerg Physicians 1977;6:139–143.
3. Metropolitan Life Insurance Company. Statistical bulletin. May 1977;2–3.
4. Neal JM. Near-drowning. J Emerg Med 1985;3:41–51.
5. Davis S, Ledman J, Kilgore J. Drownings of children and youths in a desert state. West J Med 1985;143:196–201.
6. Smith DS. Sudden drowning syndrome. Physician Sportsmed 1980;8:76–83.
7. Orlowski JP. Prognostic factors in pediatric cases of drowning and near-drowning. J Am Coll Emerg Physicians 1979;8:176–179.
8. Seiden RH. Where are they now? A follow-up

study of suicide attempters from the Golden Gate Bridge. Suicide Life-Threat Behav 1978;Winter 8:203–216.

9. Modell JH. Drown vs near-drown: a discussion of definitions. Crit Care Med 1981;9:351–352.

10. Pratt FD, Haynes BE. Incidence of "secondary drowning" after saltwater submersion. Ann Emerg Med 1986;15:137–140.

11. Goode RC, Duffin J, Miller R. Sudden cold water immersion. Respir Physiol 1975;23:301.

12. Keating WR, Hayward MG. Sudden death in cold water and ventricular arrhythmia. J Forensic Sci 1981;26:459

13. Hermann LK. Drowning, a common tragedy. Rocky Mountain Medical J 1979;76:169–173.

14. Orlowski JP, Rothner AD, Leuders H. Submersion accidents in children with epilepsy. Am J Dis Child 1982;136:777–780.

15. Craig AB Jr. Causes of loss of consciousness during underwater swimming. J Appl Physiol 1961;16:583–586.

16. Craig AB Jr. Summary of 58 cases of loss of consciousness during underwater swimming and diving. Med Sci Sports 1976;8:171.

17. Yagil Y, Stalkikowicz R, Michaeli J, Mogle P. Near drowning in the Dead Sea: electrolyte imbalances and therapeutic implications. Arch Int Med 1985;145:50–53.

18. Pruessner HT, Zenner GO, Hansel NK. Management of the near-drowning victim. Am Fam Phys 1988;37:251–260.

19. Sims JK, Enomoto PI, Frankel RI, Wong, LM. Marine bacteria complicating seawater near-drowning and marine wounds: a hypothesis. Ann Emerg Med 1983;12:212–216.

20. Karch SB. Pathology of the lung in near-drowning. Am J Emerg Med 1986;4:4–9.

21. Pearn J. Pathophysiology of drowning. Med J Aust 1985;142:586–588.

22. Nopanitanya W, Gambill TG, Brankhous KM. Fresh water drowning: pulmonary ultrastructure and systemic fibrinolysis. Arch Pathol 1974;98:361–366.

23. Tron VA, Baldwin VJ, Pirie GE. Hot tub drownings. Pediatrics 1985;75:789–790.

24. Lukas GM, Hutton JE Jr, Lim RC, Mathewson C Jr. Injuries sustained from high velocity impact with water: an experience from the Golden Gate Bridge. J Trauma 1981;21:612–618.

25. Orlowski JP. Heimlich Maneuver for near-drowning questioned (Letter). Ann Emerg Med 1982;11:111.

26. Wilder RJ, Wedro BC. Heimlich maneuver for near-drowning questioned (Letter). Ann Emerg Med 1982;11:111.

27. Heimlich HJ. Subdiaphragmatic pressure to expel water from the lungs of drowning persons. Ann Emerg Med 1981;10:476–480.

28. Ornato JP. The resuscitation of near-drowning victims. JAMA 1986;256:75–77.

29. Orlowski JP. Drowning, near-drowning, and ice-water submersions. Pediatr Clin North Am 1987;34:75–92.

30. Lindner KH, Dick W, Lotz P. The delayed use of positive end expiratory pressure during respiratory resuscitation following near-drowning with fresh or salt water. Resuscitation 1983;10:197–211.

31. Fandel I, Bancalari E. Near-drowning in children: clinical aspects. Pediatrics 1976;58:573–579.

32. Oakes DD, Sherck JP, Maloney JR, Charters AC. Prognosis and management of victims of near-drowning. J Trauma 1982;22:544–549.

33. Conn AW, Edmonds JF, Barker GA. Cerebral resuscitation in near-drowning. Pediatric Clin North Am 1979;26:691–701.

34. Conn AW, Montes JE, Barker GA, Edmonds JF. Cerebral salvage in near-drowning following neurological classification by triage. Can Anaesth Soc J 1980;27:201–210.

35. Conn AW, Barker GA. Fresh water drowning and near-drowning: an update. Can Anaesth Soc J 1984;31:s38–s44.

36. Modell JH, Graves SA, Kuck EJ. Near-drowning: correlation of level of consciousness and survival. Can Anaesth Soc J 1980;27:201–210.

37. Cicale MJ, Block AJ. Management of near-drowning, on the scene and in the hospital. J Crit Illness 1986;1:19–32.

38. Kollar DJ. Cerebral resuscitation by use of verapamil in a victim of near-drowning. Am J Emerg Med 1984;2:148–152.

39. Allman FD, Nelson WB, Pacentine GA, et al. Outcome following cardiopulmonary resuscitation in severe pediatric near-drowning. Am J Dis Child 1986;140:571–575.

40. Bohn DJ, Biggar WD, Smith CR, et al. Influence of hypothermia, barbiturate therapy, and intracranial pressure monitoring on morbidity and mortality after near-drowning. Crit Care Med 1986;14:529–534.

41. Jacobsen WK, Mason LJ, Briggs BA, et al. Correlation of spontaneous respiration and neurologic damage in near-drowning. Crit Care Med 1983;11:487–489.

42. Frewen TC, Sumabat WO, Han VK, et al. Cerebral resuscitation in pediatric near-drowning. J Pediatr 1985;106:615–617.

43. Pfenninger J, Gerber A, Tschappler H, Zimmermann A. Adult respiratory distress syndrome in children. J Pediatr 1982;101:352–357.

44. Bonilla-Santiago J, Fill WL. Sand aspiration in drowning and near-drowning. Radiology 1978;128:301–302.

45. Laughlin JJ, Eigen H. Pulmonary function abnormalities in survivors of near-drowning. J Pediatrics 1982;100:26–30.

46. Jenkinson SG, George RB. Serial pulmonary function studies in survivors of near-drowning. Chest 1980;77:777.

47. Butt MP, Jalowayski A. Modell JH, Giam-

mona ST. Pulmonary function after resuscitation from near-drowning. Anesthesiology 1970;32:275.

48. Modell JH, Davis JH, Giammona ST, et al. Blood gas and electrolyte changes in human near-drowning victims. JAMA 1968;203:99–105.

49. Redding JS. Drowning and near-drowning. Postgrad Med 1983;74:85–97.

50. Steinman AM. Immersion hypothermia. Emerg Med Serv 1977;6:22–25.

51. Collis ML. Survival behavior in cold water immersion. In: Proceedings of the cold water symposium. Toronto, Ontario, Royal Life Saving Society of Canada: 1976.

52. Samuelson T, Doolittle W, Hayward J, et al. Hypothermia and cold water near-drowning treatment guidelines. Alaska Med 1982;24:106–111.

53. Boyson PG. Dispelling the myths and controversies of near-drowning. Emerg Med Rep 1984;5:23–28.

54. Sladen A, Zauder HL. Methylprednisolone therapy from pulmonary edema following near-drowning. JAMA 1971;215:1793–1795.

55. Oakes DD, Sherck JP, Maloney JR, et al. Prognosis and treatment of victims of near-drowning. J Trauma 1982;22:544–549.

56. Pearn J. The management of near-drowning. Br Med J 1985;291:1447–1452.

57. Danzl D. Pediatric near-drowning: aggressive CPR is best. Patient Care 1987ǧust 15:14–16.

58. Robinson MD, Seward PN. Submersion injury in children. Pediatr Emerg Care 1987;3:44–49.

59. Spyker DA. Submersion injury: epidemiology, prevention, and management. Pediatr Clin North Am 1985;32:113–125.

60. Pearn J III, Hsia EY. Swimming pool drownings and near-drownings involving children: a total population study from Hawaii. Milit Med 1980;190:15–18.

61. Modell JH, Graves SA, Kuck EJ. Near-drowning: correlation of level of consciousness and survival. Can Anaesth Soc J 1980;27:211–215.

# CHAPTER 12

# Barotrauma and Diving Emergencies

## INTRODUCTION

Once the province of the military and specially trained professionals, diving is now a family sport. It is estimated that about 3 million persons pursue recreational or sport scuba diving in the United States, with about 200,000 new divers trained each year.[1] With the influx of this great number of new divers, diving medicine has moved from the realm of military and naval physicians and an occasional occupational physician to the realm of general emergency medicine. To many emergency physicians, this is an uncomfortable change, since the treatment of diving emergencies is not taught in most residency and medical school programs, and those skills learned are often not used frequently. Most diving accidents and emergencies happen in the three prime coastal areas (Hawaii, the Pacific coast states, and Florida), but people dive in every state, on the coasts, and at altitude in mountain lakes. Nor is this trauma confined to divers. Aviators who are subjected to sudden decompression or who attempt high-altitude ascents in unpressurized aircraft are at risk for the same injuries.

As may be expected, diving accidents are more common among novice divers than trained professionals. Usually, it is during the first or second dive in open water that problems with cerebral air embolism occur. Since this dive may occur in the "open water" of a quarry or lake or in an inland area where the hospital staff is unfamiliar in the management of diving emergencies, this serious problem may be compounded by inexperience on the part of the physician.

## EFFECTS OF PRESSURE

At sea level, the atmosphere exerts a continuous, inescapable pressure of about 760 mm Hg. This is the standard atmospheric pressure or 1 atmosphere absolute (1 ATA). The human body is accustomed to this ubiquitous pressure and must compensate when it increases or decreases. Effects of the generalized decrease of atmospheric pressure are discussed in Chapter 6.

## Definitions

### PRESSURE

In diving, atmospheric pressure is often used as a reference, and dives are given as excursions from this reference. The pressure of the atmosphere will support a column of liquid under a Torricellian vacuum. Measurement of pressure in units of millimeters of mercury or inches of water dates back to the first barometric pressure measurements with glass tubes filled with columns of mercury or water.

**1 atmosphere absolute =**
33 feet of salt water (fsw) (density 1.027)
34 feet of fresh water (ffw) (density 1.000)
760 mm Hg
10 meters of sea water (density 1.010)

# Depth vs Pressure

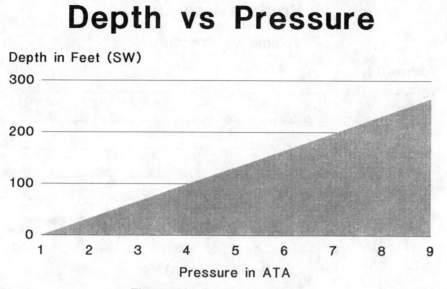

Depth in Feet (SW)

**Figure 12.1.** Depth versus Pressure.

Pressure may also be measured in terms of force per area in a number of standard units.

**1 atmosphere absolute =** 14.7 pounds/square inch (PSI)
 1 bar
 1.033 kg/cm²
 0 Atmosphere gauge

As the diver submerges, the pressure will increase because of the weight of the water over the diver. As the climber ascends, the pressure decreases as the weight of the air overhead is lessened. Since air is much less dense than water, large changes in pressure are noted as the diver descends only a short distance. Climbers must climb thousands of feet in order to effect only modest pressure changes, however. As shown in Figure 12.1, at a depth of 33 feet in salt water, the pressure surrounding the diver will be 2 ATA (two atmospheres absolute). As the diver descends, at 132 feet below the surface, the pressure will be 5 ATA.

A gas will be compressed by this increase in pressure. The majority of the tissues are composed of water and are not compressible.

## THE GAS LAWS

There are two major consequences of increased pressure on the human body that are

of concern. One is the direct mechanical effects of the pressure on body cavities, such as lungs or bowels and the soft tissues that bound these cavities. The medical consequences of compression or subsequent release of pressure on the gas-filled organs comprise the barotrauma disorders. The other consequence, decompression sickness, is a result of the change in solubility of gases in the tissues. The overall effects of both of these disorders are predictable by basic physical laws.

### BOYLE'S LAW

"At a constant temperature, the volume of a gas is inversely proportion to its absolute pressure." This means that if the absolute pressure acting on a volume of gas is doubled, the volume that the gas occupies is cut in half (see Fig. 12.2).

The equation

$$P_1 V_1 = P_2 V_2$$

is a useful expression of Boyle's law that allows the calculation of any variable if the other three variables are known.

Combining Dalton's law with Boyle's law allows the calculation of the partial pressure of a known percentage of a gas as the pressure changes.

# Boyle's Law

## Volume vs Pressure

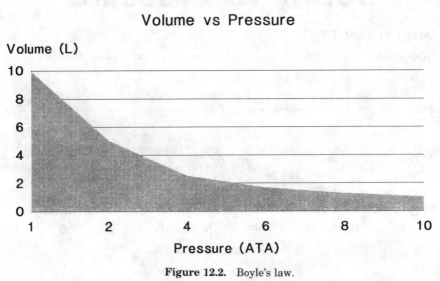

**Figure 12.2.** Boyle's law.

## DALTON'S LAW

"In a mixture of gases, the total pressure exerted is equal to the sum of the pressures exerted by each separate gas." Because the space between the molecules of a gas is very large in relation to the size of the molecule when the gases are mixed, the space is thought to be available to all of the particles of the gas (i.e., the separate gases will each occupy the entire volume). The molecules of each gas will exert force on the inner surface area of the container, and each gas will, therefore, be responsible for a portion of the pressure—the "partial pressure of the gas."

## HENRY'S LAW

A liquid's (or tissue's) capacity for holding gas is described by Henry's law, which states that the amount of gas in solution in a tissue or liquid is proportional to the external pressure of that gas surrounding the liquid (after equilibrium is achieved) (see Fig. 12.3). Henry's law can be roughly expressed as:

$$\% \, Y = (P_Y / P_T) * 100$$
Where %Y is the amount of gas dissolved
$P_Y$ is the partial pressure of gas Y
$P_T$ is the total pressure

Obviously, if the pressure is reduced, the liquid will hold less gas in solution. Henry's law explains why carbonated beverages fizz when the cap is removed and, more importantly for this discussion, why decompression sickness develops.

## BAROTRAUMA

Barotrauma is the term used for clinical manifestations of Boyle's law as a pressure disequilibrium forms between a captive gas pocket and the outside environment. These clinical manifestations may be seen either on ascent or descent and are the most common pressure-related injuries suffered by both professional and sport divers. Injuries on descent are normally squeeze injuries, such as ruptured eardrums and mask, goggle, or suit squeezes (see Table 12.1). Problems on ascent are normally air expansion injuries and are the most serious. Despite all training in ascent techniques, there are times and circumstances when divers ignore all safety procedures and suffer serious injury (see Table 12.2).

### External Ear Squeeze

External ear squeeze is found on descent and is caused by impacted cerumen or growths

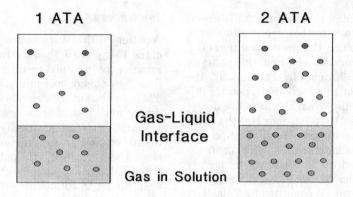

**1 ATA**　　　　　　　**2 ATA**

Gas-Liquid
Interface

Gas in Solution

$$\% \; Y = ( \; Py \; / \; Pt) \; * \; 100$$

# Henry's Law

**Figure 12.3.**　Henry's law.

that block the outer canal. The diver may cause the problem with earplugs or a tightly fitting wetsuit hood. This condition has been noted in children who dive to the bottom of a 6 to 10 foot pool while wearing earplugs.

## CLINICAL PRESENTATION

As the diver descends, the increasing pressure pushes the obstruction or growth further into the canal. The tympanic membrane (TM) bulges outward and may rupture as nature attempts to equalize the pressure. Edema and hemorrhage may also develop in the walls of the external canal. Physical findings include erythema and blood-filled blebs in the walls of the canal. The tympanic membrane may have petechiae or bloody blebs.

## TREATMENT

Treatment of external ear squeeze includes analgesics as needed for the pain, otic antibiotic solutions, and systemic antibiotics if the patient was diving in contaminated water or has a ruptured tympanic membrane. The patient should refrain from both swimming and diving until the canal is healed.

### Barotitis Media

The most frequent type of barotrauma in aviators and divers is middle ear squeeze or barotitis media. This condition results when the pressure in the middle ear cannot be equalized with that of the outside environment, due to an obstructed eustachian tube or inappropriate or ineffectual attempts at equalization of the pressure.

**Table 12.1.**
**Diving Emergencies of Descent**

Otologic Barotrauma
　External ear squeeze
　Barotitis media
　Rupture of round or oval window
Sinus squeeze (barosinusitis)
Lung squeeze
Surface area squeezes

**Table 12.2.**
**Diving Emergencies of Ascent**

Aerogastralgia
Alternobaric vertigo
Pulmonary overpressure accidents
　Dysbaric air embolism
　Pneumothorax
　Interstitial emphysema

The eustachian tube is a normally closed soft tissue structure that opens and allows equalization when the pressure differential between the middle ear and the pharynx reaches about 20 mm Hg. Fortunately, the earliest sign of this increased pressure differential is pain. When the pressure differential reaches about 100 mm Hg, the diver will experience ear pain from the stress on the tympanic membrane.[2] This pain increases as the diver descends and frequently prevents further descent. The pain is abated when the pressure is equalized by Valsalva's maneuver, chewing motions, or pressure against closed glottis with nostrils pinched (Frenzel's maneuver). Equalization through the eustachian tube is far easier when the diver is in a head-up position.

## RUPTURED TYMPANIC MEMBRANE

If the diver continues to descend despite the pain, the pressure gradient continues to increase and the tympanic membrane will eventually rupture. Nausea, vertigo, and disorientation will follow the rupture. Before rupture, the tympanic membrane may become engorged and edematous and may bleed into the canal. A tear in the middle layers of the tympanic membrane may cause the patient to develop an edematous tympanic membrane or even a hemotympanum.

Teed developed a grading for the severity of this middle-ear squeeze on a scale of 0 to 5 with 0 having no symptoms and 5 being a rupture of the tympanic membrane.[3] Most injuries to sport divers are grades 2 and 3 with erythema or hemorrhage in the eardrum (see Table 12.3).

**Table 12.3.**
**Teed Barotitis Media Categories[1]**

| Category | Description |
| --- | --- |
| Teed 0 | Normal |
| Teed 1 | Erythema of pars flaccida, umbo, and anulus |
| Teed 2 | Erythema of entire tympanum |
| Teed 3 | Hemorrhage within tympanum |
| Teed 4 | Hemorrhage into middle ear with or without TM rupture |
| Teed 5 | Hemorrhage fills middle ear |

Teed RW. Factors producing obstruction of the auditory tube in submarine personnel. US Nav Med Bull 1944;44:293–306.

## Treatment

A patient with a suspected or proven rupture of the TM (grade 5) should refrain from swimming or diving until healing has been confirmed by otoscopic examination. A ruptured TM is an absolute contraindication to further diving until healed because of the danger of infection and the possibility of caloric-induced vestibular dysfunction. Antibiotics should be prescribed if the patient has a ruptured TM, has a tympanic hematoma, or has been diving in contaminated water. Generally, a grade 2 or 3 injury should make a full recovery within a week to 10 days. Divers that are symptomatic should refrain from diving, because continued diving will worsen the condition. Prevention is simple; the diver needs to heed the warning of pain in the ears and should not dive when unable to equalize the pressure in the ears.

## SEROUS OTITIS MEDIA

Serous otitis media is common among sport divers and is caused by a relative vacuum formed in the middle ear upon ascent. Fluid is exuded by the cells of the middle ear to equalize the pressure, and this fluid fills the middle ear.

## Treatment

The condition can be treated acutely with Valsalva's maneuver. Over the longer course, the patient may use pseudoephedrine or antihistamines to open the eustachian tube.

### Round and Oval Window Rupture (Inner Ear Squeeze)

If the eustachian tube is blocked, the pressure imbalance may rupture the round window before the TM ruptures. Rarely, the rupture may occur in the oval window rather than in the round window.[4] The pressure may also push the stapes footplate into the inner ear by inward pressure on the eardrum. The diver may also perform an excessively violent Valsalva's maneuver and increase cerebrospinal fluid pressure to such a degree that the round window is exploded outward or increase middle ear pressure to such a degree that the round window implodes into the middle ear, resulting in a fistula from the round window. A combination of these factors is most likely found in many of these cases, but the basic etiology is a marked pressure difference between the inner ear and the middle ear.[2]

The resulting leakage of perilymph and development of a fistula can cause permanent cochlear damage and hearing losses. Round window rupture should be considered a medical emergency requiring prompt recognition and treatment.

## Clinical Presentation

The classic triad of signs of round window rupture includes vertigo, tinnitus, and sensorineural hearing losses. The most frequent symptom is severe vertigo. Tinnitus may be described in terms of rushing water or loud roaring sounds instead of the classic ringing. Hearing losses may be pronounced, but the patient may not note the hearing losses due to the vertigo. Audiologic testing may show complete loss of hearing. Other symptoms that have been noted with round window rupture are ataxia, nausea, and vomiting, associated with the vertigo, and a feeling of fullness in the affected ear.

As with all patients who have severe vertigo, these patients are often diaphoretic, pale, and very quiet. Frequently, signs of middle ear barotrauma described above will be noted. Nystagmus is commonly noted but may be absent in the rare case that both ears have round window ruptures.

## TREATMENT

Management of a round window rupture and the ensuing perilymph fistula is complex and controversial. Some authorities recommend immediate surgical repair of the fistula. Others feel that a trial of bed rest and antivertigo drugs will allow spontaneous closure of the fistula. Management of this condition should best be left to the otolaryngologist.

During transport of the patient, ensure that the head of the bed is elevated. Air transport in unpressurized vehicles is not recommended. The patient should not be subjected to recompression as it may worsen the leakage of perilymph.[4,5] This causes a therapeutic dilemma as many of the signs of a round window rupture mimic those of cerebral air embolism and decompression sickness of the inner ear. The latter conditions respond well to recompression. If there is very good evidence for the presence of decompression sickness or cerebral air embolism, the patient should be transported to a dive chamber and evaluated by a trained dive physician.

## Vertigo

Vertigo underwater is always serious and, frequently, life threatening. Vertigo in combination with a deep dive in dark water, a night dive, loss of air supply, entanglement, or another problem can result in tragic consequences. Nausea and subsequent vomiting due to the vertigo may foul air supplies with subsequent panic. Vertigo may be produced by an oval window rupture, TM rupture, or unequal pressure on the TM.

Alternobaric vertigo is produced by unequal pressure on both sides of the TM during ascent or descent. On ascent, the diver may feel a fullness in the ear prior to the vertigo. Nausea and vomiting frequently accompany the onset of vertigo. Dizziness may persist on the surface, but decongestants will hasten the clearing.[6,7] On descent, the onset of alternobaric vertigo usually follows a "tough" descent with many attempts at equalization of pressure followed by a sudden success.[8,9] Alternobaric vertigo of descent can be prevented by descending slowly while gently equalizing middle ear pressure. Dislocation of the stapes has been noted in this condition and is characterized by a purely conductive hearing loss.[10]

If the TM ruptures in cold water, the direct stimulus on the exposed nerve endings may cause severe vertigo, as in a caloric vestibular stimulation test.[11] In extreme cases, it may cause unconsciousness. Round window rupture also produces severe vertigo and may cause profound nausea.

Immediate treatment of the vertigo underwater is not usually possible. If the patient has not panicked, reorientation may prevent this deadly complication. A firm grip on the arm or shoulder will usually allow adequate spatial reorientation and will allow the buddy to guide the patient to the surface. Often after the guide has made certain of the problem and both are ascending, the patient may feel more comfortable with eyes closed. Surface therapy should include antivertigo agents, but efforts should be made to rapidly identify the cause of the vertigo.

## Barosinusitis

Since the sinuses are frequently afflicted with blocked passages in surface dwellers, it is no surprise that divers suffer from barotrauma to the sinuses. The most commonly affected sinuses are the maxillary and the frontal sinuses and the condition usually occurs upon descent. Predisposing conditions include the upper respiratory infections, preexisting sinusitis, nasal polyps, or prior facial trauma.

### CLINICAL FINDINGS

The patient will often describe a feeling of fullness in the affected sinus and may complain of substantial pain. In a maxillary barosinusitis, the upper canines or premolars may be exquisitely painful. Frontal headache is frequently found in frontal barosinusitis. Epistaxis is common and is usually mild in all forms of barosinusitis.

The findings of a sinusitis mimic barosinusitis in most cases. The clinician will frequently find tenderness over the affected sinus. If the injury is acute, fever will be absent, but contamination with polluted water may cause frank infectious sinusitis. Swelling and periorbital edema are usually absent.

### TREATMENT

The treatment for a barosinusitis is also the same as for a sinusitis. Immediate treatment during the dive is to ascend to a depth that affords relief and attempt to equalize the pressure with Valsalva's or Frenzel's maneuver. The mainstays of therapy are decongestants and, to a lesser degree, antihistamines. Both systemic and topical decongestants, such as Afrin, are indicated. Antibiotics are clearly indicated if the patient has a fever, purulent discharge from the nose or in the posterior pharynx, or has any other signs of infection. In most cases, ampicillin or a cephalosporin will suffice. The patient should not dive until the sinuses are clear both symptomatically and radiologically. Prevention may be afforded by a topical decongestant, such as Afrin, prior to the dive and by aborting the dive if symptoms persist.

## Miscellaneous Squeezes

As the diver descends, increasing external pressure will cause captive air spaces to shrink. The resultant loss in volume may cause damage to the diver. The most potentially serious squeezes occur about the head and face. Goggles have a captive air space that is impossible to vent and can cause ocular damage. This "goggle squeeze" can cause conjunctival hemorrhage and bleeding into the eyelids. Face masks can be vented with nasal exhalation so are less likely to cause facial damage. Professional divers with hard helmets must be careful to have the helmet pressure appropriately equalized, or they will suffer "helmet squeeze." Rarely, a diver who descends from the surface may also develop a "lung squeeze" syndrome. Wet or dry protective suits must have no folds or creases where captive air spaces can cause "suit squeeze" on deep dives. This suit squeeze can be manifested as just a reddened ridge or may cause bleeding into large folds and ridges of the skin.

## Pulmonary Overpressure

Air in the respiratory tree follows Boyle's law and expands and contracts with decreasing and increasing pressures. Normally, the pulmonary system is vented well to the outside pressure and no problems are encountered. Unfortunately, when this venting is overridden by accident or design, the lung is ill equipped to cope with the increased pressures generated. The elastic limit of the lung tissue is exceeded at about 80 to 100 mm Hg pressure differential. Constant exhalation upon ascent from a pressurized vessel or with scuba apparatus is required in order to prevent these overpressure accidents. If the diver or aviator fails to do so, the alveoli will rupture and one or more of three events will occur, producing either interstitial emphysema, pneumothorax, or an arterial gas embolization. It is impossible to predict the pathway that the air will take. Clinical symptoms depend upon the location and amount of escaped gas.

The most common cause of a pulmonary overpressure accident is inadvertent breath holding during an emergency ascent. An aviator or passenger in a plane that suffers a sudden depressurization will also suffer pulmonary overpressure phenomenon if they attempt to hold their breath at the time of the accident. Local air trapping due to bronchospasm or mucous plugs will likewise increase risks of a pulmonary overpressure accident (POP).

**SCUBA**

Danger of
Pulmonary Barotrauma

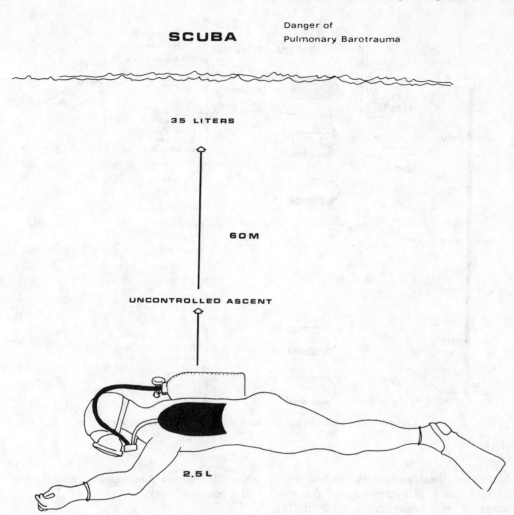

35 LITERS

60 M

UNCONTROLLED ASCENT

2.5 L

**Figure 12.4.** SCUBA: High danger of pulmonary barotrauma.

Because the volume and pressure changes are largest during the last few feet of ascent, this becomes the most dangerous part of ascending. The lung does not sustain the shear pressure well and the expanding gas tends to tear lung tissue. A POP of only **80 cm of water** is needed to rupture alveoli, and this can easily be achieved in merely 4 feet of sea water[12,13] (see Figs. 12.4 and 12.5).

**Pulmonary Overpressure Accidents (Precipitating Events)**
Breath holding on ascent from depth
Breath holding on rapid decompression to altitude (aviators)
Submarine escape training
A POP is quite possible at shallow depths (4 feet of sea water)

## INTERSTITIAL EMPHYSEMA

Mediastinal and subcutaneous emphysema are the most common manifestations of pulmonary overpressure accidents. Interstitial emphysema is also noted with the other, more severe forms of pulmonary overpressure accidents. Air will dissect from the area of the alveolar rupture into the mediastinum and from there migrate to the neck as subcutaneous emphysema, into the pericardium, and possibly into the retroperitoneum.[14-16]

The diver may experience a mild substernal chest pain, a feeling of fullness about the neck, and a "brassy voice." Dyspnea is common. The examiner may note subcutaneous emphysema about the neck, a mediastinal crunch (Haman's sign) on auscultation of the

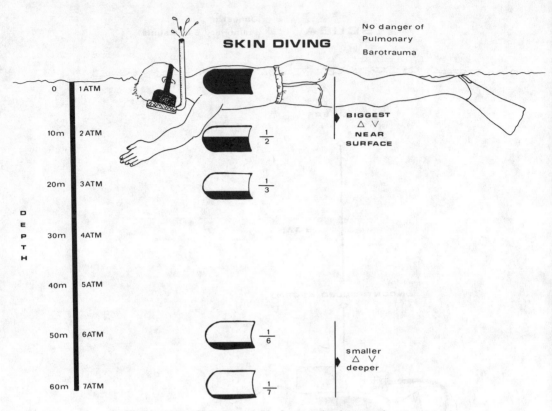

**Figure 12.5.** Skin Diving: No danger of pulmonary barotrauma.

chest or heartbeat, and possible distension of the neck veins. In extreme cases, the subcutaneous emphysema may extend into the face and about the shoulders. Radiograph findings will show obvious air about the mediastinum and neck, with possible pericardial air.

Interstitial or subcutaneous emphysema indicates the presence of escaping air from the alveoli, and the patient must be carefully monitored for other pulmonary overpressure syndromes. Unless there is compromise of circulation or breathing by the entrapped air, treatment is symptomatic. This condition should resolve in a few days without further treatment. Intubation rarely may be required with serious neck swelling. Hospitalization is indicated for these patients, due to the necessity to watch for other complications. Recompression of the patient is not associated with any significant problems, as the increased pressure will decrease bubble and pneumothorax size, but the physician should be wary as ascent in the recompression chamber will expand bubbles and increase the size of a pneumothorax.

## PNEUMOTHORAX

If the escaping air from the alveoli is free to go into the pleural space, the result is a pneumothorax. If the air migrates into the pericardium, a pneumopericardium may ensue. Rarely, the pulmonary tear may form a ball-valve effect, and a tension pneumothorax will result. This complication can be life threatening, but the pneumothorax associated with a pulmonary overpressure accident is usually not under tension.

### Clinical Presentation

A pneumothorax from a pulmonary overpressure incident is diagnosed and treated in the same manner as from all other causes. The patient who has a pneumothorax should be carefully observed for the presence of the other manifestations of a pulmonary overpressure syndrome.

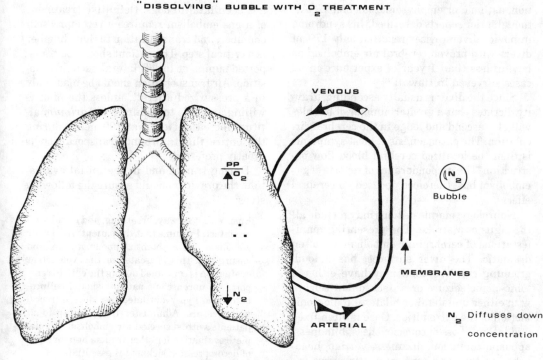

**Figure 12.6.** Alveoli rupture.

## Treatment

A small pneumothorax may be closely observed in the hospital, without further therapy. A pneumothorax greater than about 15% usually requires a chest tube. A patient with a pneumothorax is not a candidate for air transport until a chest tube has been placed. Heimlich valves or finger-cot valves are best for air transport or recompression therapy. Needle decompression may suffice for emergent air evacuation, but the provider needs to be particularly wary of reoccurrence. If the patient requires recompression therapy for another condition, a chest tube should also be inserted. Ascent in either an aircraft or recompression chamber will be associated with expansion of the pneumothorax and may cause life-threatening respiratory compromise.

## GAS EMBOLISM

When the lung tear communicates with a pulmonary vein, the result is a gas embolism that travels to the heart and then into the arterial circulation (dysbaric air embolism, DAE). Arterial gas embolism is the most serious and rapidly fatal of the pulmonary over-

pressure accidents. It is second only to drowning as a cause of death in divers.[17]

**Synonyms of Dysbaric Air Embolism**
   Aeropathy
   Aerobullosis
   Aeroembolism
   Dysbarism—pulmonary trapped gas
   Venous gas embolism
   Altitude dysbarism

## Clinical Presentation

After passing through the heart, the gas emboli are distributed randomly though the systemic circulation. Upon lodging in a small vessel, distal circulation is occluded. The clinical results will depend upon this random scattering of occlusions. If bubbles lodge in critical locations, such as the coronary arteries, the results can be rapidly fatal.

Dysbaric air embolism presents soon after the diver ascends, indeed, it is an axiom that the symptoms will be present *within 10 minutes after surfacing from a dive.*[17] A common scenario reported in the literature is the diver short on air or in a panic ascent. It may also occur during normal ascent in patients with pulmonary disease, such as airway obstruction, asthma, or emphysematous blebs.[18] Although prior reports described this syndrome in novice divers, Kizer reported only 17% of divers with proven cerebral air embolism as having less than 1 year of experience in 42 cases surveyed in Hawaii.[19]

Since the diver is usually ascending, gravity dictates that a greater number of bubbles will also ascend and lodge in the cerebral circulation. The pathogenesis of most symptoms is then the localized cerebral blood flow obstruction. The preponderance of reports of gas embolism has, therefore, focused on cerebral effects.

Neurologic manifestations may include all the signs of a stroke. The presenting manifestations of cerebral air embolism are often dramatic. The diver surfaces, has a loud, groaning cry, and then may have either a tonic-clonic seizure or a Jacksonian seizure with either unilateral or bilateral tonic-clonic motion of the extremities. Gaze is often fixed and lateral. Loss of consciousness, blindness, aphasia, confusion, dizziness, vertigo, headache, paresis, and sensory disturbances are commonly reported.[20-22] Indeed, a loss of consciousness upon ascent or shortly after surfacing should be considered an air embolism until proven otherwise. Limb and abdominal pain were infrequently seen.

Dysbaric cerebral air embolism may often be less dramatic. Diplopia, disorientation, or headache may be the original symptoms. Occasionally, ill-defined sensory losses in the facial areas or involvement of the cranial nerves may mark the presence of the emboli. Subtle changes in mental status in questionable cases may be revealed by thorough neurologic examinations.[23]

Cardiac air emboli are more frequently found in iatrogenic disease rather than due to a dysbarism. Cardiac findings may include either dysrhythmias, or pump failure.[24,25] Hemoptysis was often described as a common finding but appears much less frequently than originally thought.[19,26]

Since the diver is frequently ascending in panic or very short on air, decompression stops are often omitted. This means that a significant differential diagnosis is neurologic decompression sickness.

## Treatment

DAE is a medical emergency. As little as 0.5 ml of air injected into the cerebral circulation has been fatal to dogs. Definitive treatment of a gas embolism requires a recompression chamber, and transportation to that chamber is a critical step. The patient should be transported supine or in left lateral decubitus position. Air transportation should be made only in a pressurized aircraft, unless the pilot is willing and able to maintain a *maximum* altitude increase of less than 100 meters during the entire flight. Ground transportation is greatly preferred.

During transit and in the initial evaluation, the provider should ensure the following steps:

Ensure that airway, breathing, and circulation are intact. Presume that the patient with an air embolism has a potential pneumothorax and ensure that this is treated or that competent evaluation is continued during the entire transport. All unconscious patients should be intubated and hyperventilated to reduce intracranial pressure. Administer 100% oxygen to all patients with suspected air embolism. A complete evaluation for other trauma and for signs of decompression sickness is essential.

A large-bore intravenous line should be started on all patients. Hypotension may best be treated with pressor agents, such as dopamine, rather than boluses of fluid.[24]

Dysrhythmias should be treated as appropriate. Dysrhythmias evoked by gas emboli tend to be refractory to therapy until the bubble is reabsorbed or reduced in size by recompression.[17]

Foley catheters and endotracheal tubes should be filled with saline or water. Volume changes during recompression therapy may make air-filled catheters and tubes impractical.

Since many recompression chambers are not located in hospitals, it may be useful to get initial laboratory data, chest x-ray, and electrocardiogram while awaiting transport for the patient. Laboratory data should include CBC, electrolytes, glucose, BUN, prothrombin times, and PTT. The transport should not be unduly delayed by this evaluation.

Although past therapies have included Trendelenberg positioning or head down positioning to decrease the possibility of further distribution of emboli, this position will increase intracerebral pressure. The best position for transport of the patient with a suspected gas embolism is probably either the supine or left lateral decubitus position.[27] In both of these positions, the gas may be distributed to both the cerebral and the coronary circulations. In the head up position, air will preferentially

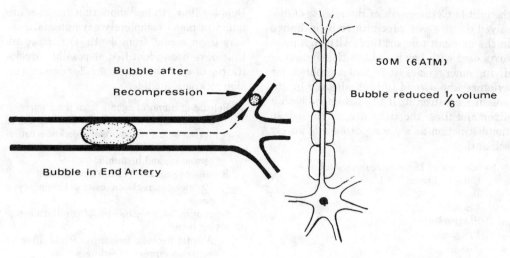

Bubble after
Recompression →

Bubble in End Artery

50M (6 ATM)

Bubble reduced $\frac{1}{6}$ volume

Neural Tissue

**Figure 12.7.** Effects of hyperbaric therapy.

rise to the neck and the cerebral circulation. The head up position should not be used if at all possible.

Therapy for the gas embolism is aimed at allowing the bubbles to dissolve and to shrink the size of the bubbles. Administration of 100% oxygen will cause more rapid diffusion of the nitrogen and help to dissolve the bubbles. To maximally shrink the bubble size, recompression to 6 ATA in a multiplace chamber on U.S. Navy Table 6A is the standard therapy for air embolism. After 30 minutes at this depth, the patient is gradually returned to 60 feet and alternating supplies of oxygen and air are given in scheduled periods during the remainder of the ascent over 5 hours. The limitations of length and depth of exposure make it impossible to reproduce Table 6A in a monoplace chamber.

There are some authorities who feel that recompression at 2.8 ATA with 100% oxygen for a lesser time will suffice.[28-33] The treatment outcomes achieved in these series suggest that this therapy may be adequate, but insufficient data exist for sweeping recommendations to change a working therapy. Given the scarcity of the much more expensive multiplace chamber versus the proliferation of the less durable and cheaper monoplace chambers, this data should be forthcoming rapidly.

### Therapeutic Adjuncts

The utility of steroids and mannitol in the treatment of arterial gas embolism is anec-

dotal, and there are no good studies that validate or refute use of these therapies. There is anecdotal evidence that steroids may be of some use in treatment of arterial gas embolism, however.[34]

### Delayed Therapy

Divers or aviators may be far removed from an appropriate treatment facility when the accident happens. Civilians may be inadequately trained in recognition of this potentially lethal syndrome and seek aid only when home remedies fail. Recompression may be attempted in-water by cognizant divers. Whatever the reason for the delay, recompression seems to help even the patient who has been delayed for days in seeking appropriate help.[34] Extensions of U.S. Navy treatment Table 6A may be helpful in many cases.

### DECOMPRESSION SICKNESS

Decompression sickness is the syndrome of problems that develop following a relatively rapid reduction in environmental pressure. It is an illness that simply did not exist until modern mechanization gave man the ability to work at higher than ambient environmental pressures. Decompression sickness has been known since the mid-1800s when construction workers in caissons and underwater tunnelers developed joint pain upon emerging from their work. Decompression sickness (also called caisson disease or the bends) is now thought to be the result of the release of dis-solved tissue gases, precipitated by a change in the ambient temperature. Although most texts deal with bends only in the context of diving emergencies, it is also a problem for aviators who ascend to high altitude in un-pressurized aircraft. If the patient is both a diver and flies, the risks are magnified, so the distinction as a diving disease is purely semantic.

### Synonyms of Decompression Sickness
Caisson disease
Bends
Chokes
Staggers
Prickles
Fits
Dysbarism
Diver's bends
Diver's palsy
Diver's itch
Diver's paralysis
High-altitude diver's disease
High-altitude caisson disease

Just like a can of ginger ale, the blood stream contains dissolved gases held in solution by the ambient pressure. Henry's law describes the amount of gas that the solution can con-tain as a function of the partial pressure of the gas. In the can of soda, the gas is carbon dioxide, while in a human the greatest pro-portion of dissolved gas is usually nitrogen. Oxygen might be in sufficient concentration to play a part but is rapidly removed from the circulation by tissue metabolism and the uptake of hemoglobin. To carry the analogy further, if the diver descends and absorbs more nitrogen under the increased pressure, it is functionally equivalent to pressurizing the soda can. If the can is opened, or the diver ascends rapidly, bubbles form. When these bubbles are released into the blood stream and tissues, they can obstruct blood flow, damage tissues, or cause tissue or blood chemistry changes. Bubbles appear to pref-erentially form in areas of decreased pres-sure, such as the bifurcations of blood vessels or along fascial planes. The effects of these bubbles throughout the body has been thought to cause the syndrome of the bends or, better named, decompression sickness.

Although this relatively simplistic expla-nation implicates bubbles as the cause of de-compression sickness, bubble formation alone does not result in decompression sickness.

Doppler flow studies show that bubbles are found in many completely asymptomatic di-vers upon ascent from depth. Other factors that have been identified as possible precip-itating or contributing factors for decompres-sion sickness include:

Release of humoral agents from the tissues
Smooth muscle activating factor released during severe decompression sickness causes elaboration of bioactive amines, bradykinin, serotonin, and histamine
Blood sludging and red cell aggregation
Platelet aggregation causes thrombocyto-penia
Disruption of endothelium of capillaries sup-plying bone
Aseptic necrosis frequently found after se-vere decompression sickness
Stasis and sludging of the epivertebral venous plexus
May cause cord damage

It should be emphasized that although the literature notes that decompression sickness is rare, this rarity is probably due to underre-porting, not scarcity of cases. The best avail-able statistics, those of the U. S. Navy, have an incidence of about 5 to 6 cases per 1000 dives, overall with a range from less than 1% in operational training dives to about 30% in experimental dives.[35] It is unlikely that the casual civilian sport diver, who is far less extensively trained or carefully monitored during dives, would have a lesser rate of de-compression sickness than the U.S. Navy's overall rate of 5 to 6%. Indeed, compiled sta-tistics from popular diving areas indicate that 50 to 60% of treated cases of decompression sickness among sport divers were neurologic in nature rather than the expected 10 to 20%.[36] One implication of this is that many of the joint-pain-only cases occurring in sport divers may not be reported to medical authorities.

### Etiology

The factors that influence the accumulation of a dissolved gas in tissue due to a change in the external pressure are:

Depth of dive
Duration of dive
Partial pressure of the gases
Tissue metabolism

Henry's law, as noted above, dictates the maximum amount of dissolved gases in tissues as related to the partial pressure of the gas. The most important variable factor in Henry's law is the depth of the dive. Since solution of a gas in tissue or liquid is not instantaneous, the time spent at that dive is also critical. Tissue and respiratory metabolism will remove oxygen and carbon dioxide.

Not every tissue will absorb nitrogen equally well. Gases become dissolved in different tissues at different characteristic rates known as "tissue half times."[37] This term describes the time it takes for a tissue to reach 50% of its total soluble gas capacity. The time required for a tissue to become saturated with a gas at a given depth depends not only on the solubility of the gas but on the tissue perfusion.[38] Nitrogen and other gases are rapidly dissolved in muscle, and exercise increases this uptake. Bone, on the other hand, takes up a gas slowly.

Nitrogen gas is slowly dissolved in fat, but it is five times more soluble in fat than in water.[39] Adipose tissue, with this high solubility for nitrogen and relatively poor perfusion, is an example of a "slow" tissue in terms of reaching saturation. It is equally slow in releasing nitrogen upon ascent. This has practical implications for the obese, who seem to experience decompression sickness more frequently than lean divers.

Heat and, indirectly, exercise also increase the solubility of a gas in tissue or blood. Exercise not only increases perfusion but warms the tissues. When the diver stops exercising upon ascent, the tissues cool and are less well perfused. The rate of removal of nitrogen will be slower in this case than was the rate of uptake.

It appears that a small amount of supersaturation can be tolerated before evidence of decompression sickness occurs. Haldane, in a study of compressed air illness in 1908, predicted the degree of tolerated supersaturation as about a 2:1 ratio, that is, the ambient pressure can be reduced to about half the original pressure and the ascent would be symptom free.[40] This is the basis for allowing an unlimited bottom time at depths less than 2 ATA pressure (33 feet). At this level, any duration of dive will be tolerated and not exceed the 2:1 ratio for supersaturation.

When the diver remains under pressure, the saturation reaches a steady state, and no more nitrogen can be dissolved. This is the basis of saturation diving, where the diver is maintained at pressure for extended periods of time to allow more useful work at depth.

As the diver starts to ascend, the ambient pressure decreases and the gas starts to diffuse out of tissues. The "slow" tissues will require more time for desaturation. If the diver ascends before the tissues are saturated, gas elimination will occur gradually and without formation of bubbles. If the ascent is made more rapidly than the nitrogen can be removed by perfusion and respiration, then the tissues become supersaturated with nitrogen. At this point, the diver is in a situation similar to the uncapped can of soda and bubbles evolve (see Fig. 12.6).

In this case, the diver must stop at an intermediate depth and allow the gas to equilibrate with the intermediate pressure. This decompression stop allows gradual off-gasing to bring the gas concentration in the tissues to a lower level and allows the diver to continue the ascent without bubble formation. Deeper dives or dives with extended stays at a depth may require more than one such decompression stop in order to safely ascend to the next higher level.

Since some tissues, such as fat, require more than 12 hours to return to normal nitrogen levels (steady state), the diver is at increased risk for this entire time. A subsequent descent within this time does not start from surface base levels of the gas. There is a residual amount of nitrogen remaining within the body. Because of this residual dissolved gas from the previous dive, the time until saturation occurs is decreased. Practically, this means that when a diver then reenters the water, he must act as if he has already experienced some "bottom" time and adjust (lengthen) the decompression accordingly. Time spent in decompression stops must be increased even more if the diver enters the water for a third or fourth dive on the same day. A partial solution to this marked increase in decompresion time encountered with these multiple dives is to maintain the diver in saturation, at either the working depth or at an intermediate depth, as discussed earlier. Note that this problem also exists when the diver flies after a dive.

Decompression tables are based upon experimental and theoretical data to allow calculation of the time that a person can spend at a depth for a given duration and return safely. The number and duration of decompression stops depends upon the duration and the depth of the dive. The tables are checked with healthy, physically fit naval divers, and may not be completely applicable for sedentary and casual sport divers. Navy diving tables have no safety margin built in and must be strictly followed for safety. Indeed, for some less fit divers, bends may occur even when they strictly follow the naval diving tables.

Susceptibility factors that increase the likelihood of decompression sickness include:

---

*Susceptibility Factors for Decompression Sickness*

Rate of ascent
Fat
Prior recent injuries
Exercise
Sex (females have greater risk)
Smoking
Dehydration
Hypothermia
Febrile illnesses
Higher than normal $CO_2$ content of gas mixture
Age greater than 40
Lack of sleep
"Adaptation"

---

## Clinical Manifestations

The general term *decompression sickness* is used to describe all signs and symptoms that result when the supersaturated solution gives up the nitrogen into the tissues and bloodstream. These signs and symptoms are roughly grouped into either mild (joint pain and itching ) or serious (neurologic or other serious illness) classifications. These classifications are also called type I and type II, respectively.

---

*Decompression Sickness Groups*

Type I (Pain Only)
    Malaise
    Skin manifestations
    Lymphatic
    Bends
Type II (Serious)
    Chokes
    Neurological
    Vasomotor (rare)
Caveat: These categories can overlap and 10–15% of Type I may progress to Type II.

---

Decompression sickness pains normally appear within minutes to hours after the dive, in contrast to the almost instantaneous symptoms of the air embolism. Because decompression sickness is caused by the effects of bubbles in the vessels and different types of tissues, it has a very complex range of symptoms and signs. The effects may range from the common vascular occlusion to pulmonic infarction, lymphedema, immune reactions, or damage to the vascular epithelium. In rare cases, symptoms or damage may be noted days after the dive.[41]

The mechanical effects of the bubbles are thought to be more influential in brain, pulmonary, periarticular, and spinal decompression sickness. In spinal cord decompression sickness, the bubbles are thought to obstruct the venous return in Batson's plexus with a subsequent venous infarction. After the flow is stopped, the bubbles may act as foreign bodies causing platelet and red cell clumping and activation of the clotting syndrome as described below.

The indirect effects of intravascular bubbles are thought to be more important in patients with delayed treatment of decompression sickness. Intravascular bubbles may act as a center for platelet aggregation after decompression. The bubbles also accelerate clotting, presumably by activation of Hageman factor, with subsequent alterations in PTT and factors V and VII.[42,43] The syndrome then becomes progressive and irreversible. Fibrin-split products are elevated and may serve as a screening test for serious decompression sickness.[44] The fibrinogen consumption increases, even in asymptomatic divers.

### TYPE I (PAIN ONLY)
#### Malaise/Fatigue

Fatigue is a common, normal response to the stresses of diving. It is also a mild and first symptom of decompression sickness that may accompany more serious symptoms. More debilitating fatigue or malaise should heighten the physician's suspicions of possible decompression sickness.

#### Joint Pain (The Bends)

The most common symptoms of decompression sickness are pains confined to the limbs

(50 to 75% of cases). Strictly speaking, the term bends should be used only to mean this joint pain. Unfortunately, it is often used generically as a synonym for decompression sickness. The term is derived from the tunnelers and caisson workers who would walk with hips bent and the upper body thrown forward.

In the typical diver who has the bends, acute pains develop in the shoulder, elbow, or, most commonly, in a knee shortly after surfacing. Aviators, on the other hand, develop pains in the upper extremities more frequently. Usually, the pain occurs within 4 hours after the episode but, occasionally, may show up as long as 12 hours later. The joints are usually involved, and the pain may vary from deep aching, toothache like, throbbing pains to a dull, vague, grating sensation. The pain is often exacerbated by movement or exercise.

There is usually no visible abnormality and little tenderness to palpation. Occasionally, erythema, edema, and decreased range of motion may be noted. Inflation of a blood pressure cuff over the site of the pain may decrease or abolish the pain. There may be some numbness or paresthesias about the affected joint, but this will not be in a cutaneous nerve distribution.

## Cutaneous Decompression Sickness

Skin bends are associated with both serious and mild forms of decompression sickness. Skin bends present as the diver's complaint of itching, formication, or burning of the skin. The examiner may note mottling, scarlatiniform, or erysipeloid rashes, or marbleization of the skin. Rarely, subcutaneous emphysema will be noted.

Most commonly, these rashes are scarlatiniform or punctate in nature and found about the chest, shoulders, back, upper abdomen, and thighs. The onset of these rashes is within 3 to 6 hours, and they may last only minutes to hours. It is thought that scarlatiniform rashes are due to a piloerector response and a histamine release.

More serious involvement is noted when the rash is erysipeloid. The distribution is the same as in the scarlatiniform rash. In this manifestation, there is interference of the venous drainage system by the gas bubbles. The lesions are a collection of papules that may merge to form plaques with firm, flat borders. Coughing or a Valsalva's maneuver accentuates the lesions (Mellinghof's sign).

Marbleization or cutis marmorata is the most serious manifestation of skin bends and is thought to be associated with the more serious forms of decompression sickness. It consists of a small, pale area with cyanotic mottling that spreads peripherally. The skin may be erythematous with extension of the cyanosis and mottling, warmer than the surrounding skin, and and some swelling and edema. Marbleization connotes gas in the tissues and blood vessels and is an ominous sign of decompression sickness.

If subcutaneous emphysema is noted about the head and neck, it should be presumed to be from a pulmonary overpressure accident, however. Crepitance about localized areas and tendon sheaths may be noted.

## Lymphatic Manifestations

Localized swelling or peu d'orange may result from lymphatic obstruction by off-gased bubbles. It is common over the trunk and occasionally found about the head and neck.

## TYPE II

Manifestations of decompression sickness other than central nervous system lesions and joint pain are less common. A number of symptoms and syndromes have been recognized.

## Neurologic Decompression Sickness

Neurologic decompression sickness may affect any part of the central nervous system and comprises between 8 and 35% of cases of DCS. Among divers, spinal cord involvement is the classic picture, while among aviators who sustain an explosive decompression, cerebral involvement is more common. About 75% of divers with spinal cord involvement will have a lower thoracic, lumbar, or sacral deficit. (Lesions in the middle one third of the cord are most often seen.) A common first symptom among divers is back pain followed by numbness or paresthesias in the legs.[45] Complaints of pins and needles or "gone to sleep" are most frequently seen in these cases. The distribution of this numbness may be along classic dermatomes, or may be patchy or even in the hysterical pattern of stocking and glove.[46] These symptoms may progress to urinary retention, paraplegia, or even quadraplegia or death.[17,47–49] Urinary retention is such a common symptom that professional divers once carried urinary catheters in their equipment.[50]

Cerebral decompression sickness commonly presents with visual symptoms, such as scotoma, diplopia, or tunnel vision. Aviators commonly have a migraine-like headache as a first manifestation. More ominous symptoms include seizures, hemiplegia, and coma, which, fortunately, are rare. Fatigue of uncertain etiology or a sense of detachment may sometimes be noted, both with or without associated symptoms. Personality changes are also found and may present as a psychotic break.

## Pulmonary Decompression Syndrome

Pulmonary decompression syndrome or the "chokes," results from diffuse off-gasing that becomes trapped in the pulmonary circulation. It becomes symptomatic when about 10% of the pulmonary vascular tree is obstructed. Clinical findings include substernal, burning chest pain, tachypnea, cough, dyspnea, and signs of circulatory compromise. The cough is described as being easily initiated by cigarettes and progresses to an uncontrollable paroxysm. These patients often have an inexorable and rapid downhill course. It should be noted that the signs of the chokes are similar to those of a pulmonary overpressure accident. Since many divers with pulmonary overpressure accidents have made a panic ascent, it is quite likely that both entities coexist.

## Vestibular Decompression Sickness

Vestibular decompression sickness or the staggers is noted by hearing loss, vertigo, nystagmus, vomiting, or tinnitus.[51] It is normally associated only with helium-oxygen diving mixtures. It is an extremely serious manifestation of DCS and, if not treated promptly, will lead to permanent damage to the vestibular mechanism. The differential diagnosis includes middle ear barotrauma and round window rupture. A history of difficulty clearing the eustachian tube should prompt the physician to consider the latter diagnosis.

## Decompression Shock

Rarely, patients may have a generalized liberation of gas bubbles in the circulation. These patients will develop decompression shock and have a fulminant picture with high mortality. A synonym for this is vasomotor decompression sickness. It is thought that hypovolemia due to hemoconcentration and increased vascular permeability is the etiology. Since this disease is rare, there is little clinical experience to validate this theory.

## Diagnosis

The diagnosis of any diving injury is most often made by history associated with a high index of suspicion. Any complaint of pain, neurologic symptoms, difficulty breathing, or unconsciousness coupled with a history of diving with compressed air or other gases or a history of an explosive decompressive event in an aviator should warrant an intensive search for pulmonary barotrauma or decompression sickness. If possible, obtain an accurate history of the dive including duration and depth of all dives done that day. Include surface times between dives and calculate the safe limits for dives with the U.S. Navy tables to get a better indication of the possibility of decompression sickness. For aviators, determine the altitude, protective gear, and steps taken after the decompression.

As has been noted, dysbaric air embolism and decompression sickness may coexist in the same patient who has made a panic ascent. Although symptoms of a dysbaric air embolism start more quickly than those of decompression sickness, it is difficult to accurately differentiate the two illnesses in the field. All patients should be treated as if they have both until accurate lab and x-ray data is available.

## Treatment

Both dysbaric air embolism and decompression sickness are emergencies that need recompression therapy in a hyperbaric chamber as soon as possible. It is important for the emergency provider to consider all symptoms that begin after a dive with compressed gases or a decompressive flight accident as being due to decompression sickness or dysbaric air embolism until proven otherwise.

---

*Important Questions to Ask*

1. How deep was the diver?
2. How long was he at that depth?
3. What kind of gases was he breathing?
4. Was this a repetitive dive?
5. Was this a multilevel dive?
6. Was this a multialtitude dive?
7. Was the diver's weight belt still on?
8. How long after surfacing did the symptoms start?
9. What symptoms are present now?
10. Has the diver ever had decompression sickness?
11. What treatment has the diver had already?
12. What tables were used to decompress?
13. Has the diver been flying?

---

## PREHOSPITAL

Cardiopulmonary rescusitation and management of the ABCs should take the usual priority. Hypothermia should be corrected, and the patient protected from further heat loss. Associated injuries should be sought and treated appropriately. It is poor form to allow the patient to expire of entirely correctable causes, with a relatively minor dysbaric injury. It is equally inelegant to underestimate the severity of the dysbaric injury. *The most common error in medical care of dysbaric injuries is failure to recognize the seriousness of the patient's condition.*

Supplemental high-flow oxygen with a nonrebreathing face mask should be given to all suspected diving injuries as soon as possible. This high-flow oxygen is best given using an aviator's tight-fitting, double-seal mask, if available. High-flow oxygen will improve clearance of nitrogen from the blood stream by increasing the diffusion gradient. Improved oxygenation of tissues will be an added benefit.

Positioning of the patient with a suspected decompression injury is controversial. As indicated previously, head down positioning has disadvantages, particularly in the longer transport. Left lateral decubitus and supine positions are both recommended and are probably of equal value. There are no good data supporting either position.

Generally, the patient with suspected dysbaric air embolism or decompression sickness should be taken directly to a hyperbaric chamber. If possible, the provider should opt for a multiplace chamber. If there is a monoplace chamber with appropriately trained staff nearby, this would be better than no recompression or hours delay. Transport should be at 100 meters net altitude gain or less. Greater net altitude gains have been associated with worsening of the injury. Do not refer the patient to a recompression chamber that is at higher altitude than the patient.

Two large-bore intravenous lines should be started with normal saline or Ringer's lactate. Fluid replacement in patients not in shock should be about 250 ml to 500 ml per hour. Fluid overload should be avoided. If blood pressure falls, fluid administration should be increased proportionally. Urine output should be maintained at 0.5 to 1 ml per kg per hour.

Two aspririn tablets (625 mg) should be given to the alert patient. This dose will provide platelet antiaggregation effects. Ibuprofen may be substituted if ASA is not available. No oral medications should be given to patients who have compromised levels of consciousness or nausea. If CNS signs are present, steroids may be given in the field by intravenous routes, if competent medical providers are available.

If the EMT or physician is unsure about the need for recompression, appropriate therapy, or the location of the nearest hyperbaric treatment facility, the National **Diving Alert Network** (DAN) maintains a listing and advice **24 hours per day at 919–684–8111**. Information of a noncritical nature may be obtained by calling **919–684–2948**, Monday through Friday from 9 to 5 Eastern Standard Time.[52]

Field recompression by a repeat dive has been advocated occasionally. Field recompression is generally discouraged because it wastes time and increases the nitrogen load of the tissues. It is virtually impossible to provide adequate patient support to a compromised patient in the water. A sole viable exception to this policy might be where an undersea habitat exists that can provide adequate medical care for the diver.

## EMERGENT RECOMPRESSION

The mainstay of therapy for decompression sickness is recompression therapy. Nothing should be done in an emergency department that will delay that therapy, unless it is to secure an airway, support breathing, ensure circulation, or staunch external bleeding. Even

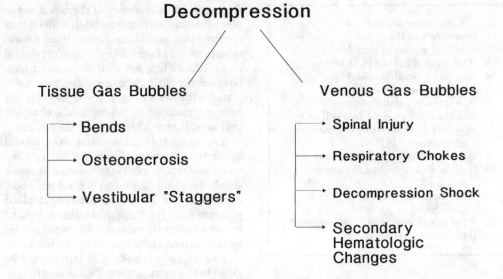

**Figure 12.8.** Decompression.

these therapies should be managed en route to the chamber if possible. Patients who have been delayed, for whatever reason, should still be transported for prompt recompression therapy (see Figs. 12.6–12.9).

As noted in the section of dysbaric air embolism, laboratory and x-ray evalution for other trauma should be accomplished while awaiting transport, if possible. CBC, serum electrolytes, blood urea nitrogen, and clotting studies can be drawn in any event and the results called to the treatment facility.

Those patients with minor decompression sickness will need only oral fluids, pain medication, and transport to a chamber. Those patients with signs of a serious decompression sickness should be transported expedi-

tiously, with a physician in attendance, to the nearest appropriate chamber. En route, advanced life support medications may be used as appropriate. The aircraft should be pressurized to 1 ATA or should stay below 100 meters net altitude gain. Physicians should realize that a pressurized aircraft is often better for the patient than an unpressurized helicopter.

**Aircraft Known to Pressurize to Sea Level**
C–130 Hercules (Military)
C–9 (Military aeromedical evacuation)
C5A
Boeing 707
Boeing 727
Boeing 737
Boeing 747

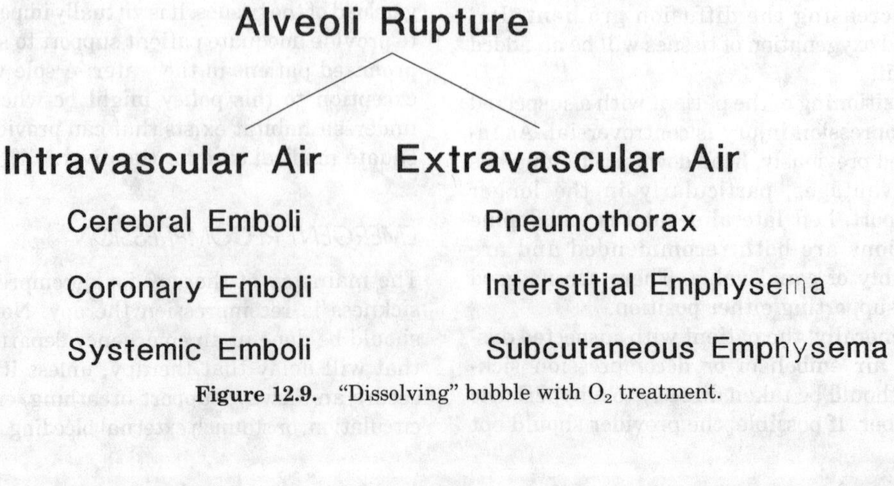

# Alveoli Rupture

## Intravascular Air

Cerebral Emboli

Coronary Emboli

Systemic Emboli

## Extravascular Air

Pneumothorax

Interstitial Emphysema

Subcutaneous Emphysema

**Figure 12.9.** "Dissolving" bubble with $O_2$ treatment.

Douglas DC–8
Douglas DC–10
BAC –111
Cessna Citation
Learjet (preferred for speed and pressurization system)
Lockheed Supersabre

Pilots should be consulted to ascertain if a specific aircraft can be pressurized for the duration and at the altitudes required for the evacuation. Other aircraft may also be pressurized to sea level while at operational altitude.

The objectives in recompression are three-fold: reduce the size and number of the evolved bubbles, prevent further formation of bubbles, and increase diffusion (off-gasing) of the nitrogen. The increase in pressure to 6 ATA will rapidly decrease the size of the bubbles, allowing more distal migration of the bubbles. This will decrease the size of the ischemic area and allow better perfusion of the tissues. Absorption of bubbles is aided by the increased pressure, thus increasing the solubility of the gas in the tissues. The increased pressure also eliminates supersaturation of the tissues and new bubble formation. Diffusion off-gasing is then promoted by having the patient breathe pure oxygen at steps in the recompression therapy.

Details of recompression therapy are normally handled by a specially trained team at the chamber. The details for treatments are spelled out in Navy Treatment Table 5, 6, or 6A.[53] The choice of table is best handled by a militarily trained dive physician or by a graduate of the Undersea Medical Society's 3-week dive medicine course.

Generally, Table 5 is used for pain only, type I, or bends. The patient response is frequently complete in 10 minutes. Table 6 is used for type II cases, type I cases that do not respond to therapy, or bends that occur under pressure. Table 6 is normally 285 minutes, but additional extensions may be added if symptoms persist.

## Adjunctive Therapy

The most important adjunctive therapy is rapid administration of fluids. About 1 liter should be given in the first hour after the accident. Oral fluids can be given to the alert patient, while intravenous fluids are gener-

ally preferred. Various investigators have used different fluids, but all agree that any saline solution, such as normal saline or Ringer's lactate with or without dextrose, is adequate. Dextrose in water, alone, should not be used as it tends to worsen pulmonary edema. Several authors have reported relief of symptoms with oral fluids alone in relatively minor cases of decompression sickness.[54]

Dopamine has been used successfully to maintain pressure in cases refractory to fluids administration. It should be remembered that loss of the spinally mediated vascular tone may cause a marked hypotension. MAST trousers seem logical, but have not been reported, for these cases. MAST trousers should generally not be used inside a chamber, because the pressure changes will cause wide fluctuations in MAST inflation. Epinephrine, neosynephrine, and levophed have been described but would all be expected to increase myocardial oxygen consumption and decrease distal tissue perfusion, perhaps to the patient's detriment.

Seizures may be managed with diazepam, but the patient needs to be carefully monitored, since diazepam can cause significant respiratory depression.[55] Respiratory depression may be increased by diazepam, so administration should be carefully monitored. Diazepam may also be of use with nausea, vomiting, and vertigo but may also mask inner ear decompression sickness.[56] As the patient is recompressed and then slowly decompressed with oxygen, diazepam may also mask CNS oxygen toxicity.

Steroids are recommended by some authors to decrease the edema and to activate the prostaglandin system.[57] The exact mechanism of the action of steroids in the patient with decompression sickness is unclear. Steroids are, as usual, controversial, and the real utility awaits controlled studies. If steroids are used, a recommended therapy schedule includes 125 mg of methylprednisolone intravenously along with 4 mg of dexamethasone.[58] The dexamethasone is continued 4 times per day for 3 days and then discontinued. Steroids will exacerbate oxygen toxicity. Some authors advocate use of steroids as a preventative measure following the recompression therapy.

Various measures to decrease the sludging of blood, platelet aggregation, and microthrombus formation have been advocated.

Aspirin is thought to decrease platelet aggregation and to reduce the incidence of microthrombus formation. Aspirin may be given to alert patients in a dose of two adult (625 mg) tablets every 3 days. Dextran and plasmanate have been proposed to decrease the sludging of blood and subsequent microthrombus formation. Controlled studies are lacking for the use of these two drugs. Heparin has also been proposed, more for clearing of lipemia than for anticoagulant effects. Doses recommended include 7500 units intravenously with 5000 units every 4 hours. Data for heparin appears to be anecdotal, and no controlled studies are available.

## Potential Problems

The most common potential problems associated with recompression therapy are probably related to the condition of the diver or aviator undergoing therapy. Appropriate life support and monitoring should be available at all times. Generally speaking, monoplace chambers are unsuitable for critically ill patients as they afford no access to the patient without abrupt decompression. If at all possible, the patient with a serious dysbarism should be treated at a multiplace chamber where drugs, equipment, and additional help may be "locked into" the chamber, while the dive is in progress.

Oxygen toxicity may be noted in any patient who is given oxygen at high pressures. Oxygen toxicity has been noted in patients breathing 100% oxygen at all pressures greater than 1 ATA. A wide range of symptoms and signs have been described, the most dramatic of which is tonic-clonic convulsions. Unfortunately, the first manifestation of oxygen toxicity may be seizures, and there is no consistent premonitory signs. Facial twitching is often noted prior to the seizures but is not a consistent finding. Nausea and vomiting are particularly common at pressures between 1 and 2 ATA. Hallucinations, lightheadedness, anxiety, muscular twitches, amnesia, and confusion are all found, both alone and in combination. Dives are thought to be a greater risk than recompression or "dry" oxygen therapy.

Treatment of oxygen toxicity is to remove the 100% oxygen source. Normally, even seizures will promptly resolve when the mask is removed and the patient is allowed to breathe room air. Anticonvulsants may be used in exceptional cases. It is safe to resume oxygen 15 minutes after the reaction has completely subsided, but the provider must be aware that reactions occur again.

## Outcome

The outcome of recompression therapy following a decompression accident will depend upon the nature of the decompression sickness and the amount of delay in starting recompression therapy. Between 80 and 90% of those who have a decompression sickness will improve or become symptom free. Dramatic recoveries have been made even after long treatment delays, but early therapy is associated with better outcomes.[59-61]

## Postrecompression

After the dive, the patient should be kept at the area of the chamber for a minimum of 6 hours to facilitate retreatment. Intensive care observation is recommended for all but minor dysbaric injuries. The patient should be advised not to fly (including airlines) for a minimum of 3 days following recompression therapy. Exceptions may be made on an individual basis for patients with access to aircraft that can be pressurized to sea level. Aircrew members, particularly of unpressurized aircraft, and altitude chamber crew should not fly for a minimum of 7 days.

## Repeated Diving After Decompression Sickness

Patients should generally not dive for 1 to 2 months after a minor decompression sickness. Patients with multiple minor decompression sicknesses should be carefully evaluated, particularly for training, ability to interpret decompression tables, and comprehension of risks involved. Multiple minor decompression sicknesses do not medically preclude resumption of diving, however. Serious decompression sickness should "ground" the diver from further diving for 4 to 6 months. Repeated type II episodes should warrant cessation of diving. A CNS "hit" should remove an aviator from flying status.

## MISCELLANEOUS DIVING EMERGENCIES

### Barodentalgia

Barodentalgia occurs when a diver or aviator has an enclosed pocket of air beneath a crown, filling, or cavity. This problem may develop on either ascent or descent and is a trapped gas syndrome. As the diver descends, negative pressure develops and the nerve is "sucked" into the pocket causing marked pain. If the pressure equalizes, there will be no pain. As the aviator or diver ascends, the expansion of the trapped gas pocket in the filling may cause pressure on the nerve, again causing extreme pain. As the pressure slowly equalizes, the pain recedes. Definitive treatment is proper dental care. Although painful teeth may be relatively common, a rare form of the problem has been described where the tooth is cracked or explodes by the pressure gradient.

### Diving Trauma

Diving trauma should be treated as any other trauma. The basics of airway, breathing, circulation, protection of the cervical spine, and prevention of exsanguinating blood loss should not be neglected. If a near-drowning or sudden ascent is caused by the trauma, then the diver needs to be appropriately resuscitated and evaluated for these potentially lethal problems. The diver who is diving in contaminated water may require prophylactic antibiotics. Wound cultures should be obtained.

A specific problem to military and commercial divers is underwater blast injury. A diver who experiences a nearby underwater blast may sustain more trauma than that caused by a similar blast in air. Since water is incompressible, the blast is transmitted with less attenuation than in the air. The resulting pressure wave tends to cause damage in the tissues that are adjacent to gas spaces, such as intestine and lungs. Lesser damage may be sustained about the brain, ear, and sinuses.

### Hypothermia

Hypothermia is frequently associated with divers and with diving injuries. Despite adequate protective gear, divers may develop hypothermia rapidly due to the markedly increased heat losses associated with immersion in cold water. Respiratory heat losses are also increased due to the increased density of the inspired gases. Professional divers breathing noble gas mixtures are at particular risk from respiratory heat losses. Since hypothermia is associated with decreased judgment and impaired mentation, accidents may result.

Treatment of the hypothermia is unchanged from immersion hypothermia due to any other cause. The patient should be carefully evaluated for trauma and for the presence of decompression sickness.

### Nitrogen Narcosis

Clinically, nitrogen narcosis resembles ethanol intoxication or the effects of nitrous oxide anesthesia. In compressed air dives, most divers experience some impairment in cognitive abilities at about 100 feet. Popular texts use "martini's rule" that, in terms of effect, each 33 feet of depth is equivalent to one martini. At 200 feet, most divers experience such deterioration in cognitive and performance abilities that no useful work is possible (200/ 33 = about 6 martinis).

### Carbon Monoxide Poisoning

Carbon monoxide poisoning from improper tank filling procedures is a particular problem when divers fill their own tanks from portable compressors. Another source of contaminated air is improperly positioned surface-supplied diving equipment. The subsequent contaminated air supply causes the classic confusion, short attention span, and nausea of early carbon monoxide poisoning, Unfortunately, confusion in a scuba diver may be rapidly lethal. Intentional or accidental tampering has been implicated in some accidents involving carbon monoxide poisoning in diving.

Other contaminants may be noted in the divers' gases, including carbon dioxide and oil. Rarely, uninformed divers will attempt to dive on pure oxygen or use an oxygen-augmented mixture of gases to dive. The resultant oxygen toxicity may be rapidly fatal for the diver in the water.

### Shallow Water Blackout

The problem of hyperventilation, carbon dioxide washout, and subsequent anoxic blackout is covered in Chapter 11, Near-Drowning Emergencies. It is a problem associated with the skin or free diver who attempts to lengthen his stay under water by hyperventilation or using a "hit" of oxygen.

### High Pressure Nervous Syndrome

This refers to the effects seen after a rapid compression, breathing helium-oxygen mixture, to greater than 400 feet. In the simplest form, the patient has a shaking of the hands, but on deeper dives, the patient may develop nausea, dizziness, and vomiting. There is some evidence that judgment is impaired concomitantly with this complication. The problem can be treated with slower compression rates or the addition of a small amount of nitrogen in the air mixture.

### Compression Arthralgia

Divers who descend greater than 500 feet generally report a sensation of dry and painful joints. It is thought to be due to a reduction in joint fluid and does not require treatment.

### SUMMARY

Sport diving is a rapidly growing hobby with an enthusiastic following. With the looser controls in civilian sports, divers may fly and develop DCS far from the place where they played. As such, medical personnel must be familiar with the problems associated with diving and the use of compressed gases. Problems that occur on descent are usually associated with a trapped gas phenomenon, while those on ascent are due to either expansion of trapped gases or release of dissolved gases. Simple equalization of pressures is the key to solving most of the problems of descent. The problems of ascent are more dangerous, complex, and time critical. For most ascent-related emergencies, the key to successful therapy is rapid recompression. Proven adjunctive therapy includes 100% oxygen and intravenous fluids.

### References

1. Strauss RH. Diving medicine. Am Rev Respir Dis 1979;119:1001–1023.
2. Kizer KW. Diving medicine. Emerg Med Clin North Am 1984;2:513–530.
3. Edmonds C, Lowry C, Pennefather J, eds. Otologic aspects of diving. Glebe, New South Wales, Australia: Australasian Medical Publishing Company, Ltd., 1973.
4. Money KE, Buckingham IP, Calder IM, et al. Damage to the middle ear and the inner ear in underwater divers. Undersea Biomed Res 1985;12:77–84.
5. Freeman P. Rupture of the round window membrane in inner ear barotrauma. Arch Otolaryngol 1974;99:437–443.
6. Parell GJ, Becker GD. Conservative management of inner ear trauma resulting from scuba diving. Otolaryngol Head Neck Surg 1985; 93:393–397.
7. Ingelstedt S, Ivarsson A, Tjernstrom O. Vertigo due to relative overpressure in the middle ear. Acta Otolaryngol 1974;78:1–74.
8. Vorosmarti J, Bradley ME. Alternobaric vertigo in military divers. Milit Med 1970;135:182–185.
9. Tjernstrom O. Middle ear mechanics and alternobaric vertigo. Acta Otolaryngol 1974; 78:376–384.
10. Lundgren CEG. Alternobaric vertigo—a diving hazard. Br Med J 1965;2:511–513.
11. Lundgren CEG. On alternobaric vertigo—epidemiologic aspects. In: Hesser CM, Linarrson D, eds.: Proceedings of the First Annual Scientific Meeting of the European Undersea Biomedical Society. Forsvarsmedicin 1974; 9:406–409.
12. Bruch FR Jr. Pulmonary barotrauma [Letter]. Ann Emerg Med 1986;15;1373–1374.
13. Boettger ML. Scuba diving emergencies: pulmonary overpressure accidents and decompression sickness. Ann Emerg Med 1983;12:563–567.
14. Schaefer KE, McNulty WP, Carey C, et al. Mechanisms in development of interstitial emphysema and air embolism on decompression from depth. J Appl Physiol 1958;13:15–29.
15. Malhotra MS, Wright HC. The effect of a raised intrapulmonary pressure on the lungs of fresh chilled bound and unbound cadavers. Med Res Council (RN PRC) Rep 1960;189.
16. Evans DE, Hardenbergh E, Kobrine AI, et al. Effects of cerebral air embolism on cardiovascular function. Undersea Biomed Res 1978; 5:33,A–42.
17. Arthur CD, Margulies RA. A short course in diving medicine. Ann Emerg Med 1987;16:689–701.
18. Liebow AA, Stark JE, Vogel J, et al. Intra-

pulmonary air trapping in submarine escape training casualties. US Armed Forces Med J 1959;10:265–289.

19. Kizer KW. Dysbaric cerebral air embolism in Hawaii. Ann Emerg Med 1987;16:535–541.

20. Pierce EC. Cerebral gas embolism (arterial) with special reference to iatrogenic accidents. HBO Review 1980;1:161–184.

21. Menkin M, Schwartzman RJ. Cerebral air embolism. Arch Neurol 1977;34:168–170.

22. Gillen HW. Symptomatology of cerebral gas embolism. Neurology 1968;18:507–512.

23. Neumann TS, Hallenbeck JM. Barotraumatic cerebral air embolism and the mental status examination: a report of four cases. Ann Emerg Med 1987;16:220–223.

24. Cales RH, Humphreys N, Pilmanis AA, et al. Cardiac arrest from gas embolism in scuba diving. Ann Emerg Med 1981;10:589–592.

25. Eguchi S, Bosher LS. Myocardial dysfunction resulting from coronary air embolism. Surgery 1962;51;103–111.

26. Brooks GJ, Green, RD, Leitch DR. Pulmonary barotrauma in submarine escape trainees and the treatment of cerebral arterial air embolism. Aviat Space Environ Med 1986;57:1201–1207.

27. Toole JF. Effect of changes of head, limb, and body position on the cephalic circulation. N Engl J Med 1968;279:307–311.

28. Bove AA, Clark JM, Simon AJ, et al. Successful therapy of cerebral air embolism at 2.8 ATA. Undersea Biomed Res 1982;9:75–80.

29. Leitch DR, Greenbaum LJ, Hallenbeck, JM. Cerebral arterial air embolism. I. Is there benefit in beginning HBO treatment at 6 bar. Undersea Biomed Res 1984;11:221–235.

30. Leitch DR, Greenbaum LJ, Hallenbeck, JM. Cerebral arterial air embolism. II. Effect of pressure and time on cortical evoked potential recovery. Undersea Biomed Res 1984;11:237–248.

31. Leitch DR, Greenbaum LJ, Hallenbeck, JM. Cerebral arterial air embolism. III. Cerebral blood flow after decompression from various pressure treatments. Undersea Biomed Res 1984;11:249–263.

32. Kizer KW. Monoplace chamber treatment of dysbaric diving diseases. J Hyperbar Med 1986;1:137–138.

33. Hart GB, Strauss MB, Lennon PA. The treatment of decompression sickness and air embolism in a monoplace chamber. J Hyperbar Med 1986;1:1–7.

34. Kizer KW. Delayed treatment of dysbarism: a retrospective review of 50 cases. JAMA 1982; 247:2555–2558.

35. Diving Statistics, Diving Accidents, and Injuries Analysis. Norfolk, VA: Naval Safety Center, 1981:1–3.

36. Kizer KW. Disorders of the deep. Emergency Med 1984;*:18–58.

37. Elliot DH, Hallenbeck JM. The pathophysiology of decompression sickness. In: Bennett PB, Elliot DH, eds. The physiology and medicine of diving and compressed air work. Baltimore: Williams & Wilkins, 1975:76–92.

38. Tobias CA, Jones HB, Lawrence JH, et al. The uptake and elimination of krypton and other inert gases by the human body. J Clin Invest 1949;28:1375–1385.

39. Hills BA. Biophysical basis of prevention and treatment. Decompression sickness, Vol 1. New York: J Wiley & Sons, 1977:76–91.

40. Boycott AE, Damant GC, Haldane JS. The prevention of compressed air illness. J Hyg (London) 1908;8:342–443.

41. Myers RAM, Bray P. Delayed treatment of serious decompression sickness. Ann Emerg Med 1985;14:254–257.

42. Philp RB, Inwood MJ, Ackles KN, et al. Effects of decompression on platelets and hemostasis in men and the influence of antiplatelet drugs (RA233 and VK744). Aerospace Med 1974; 45:231–240.

43. Philp RB. A review of blood changes associated with compression-decompression: relationship to decompression sickness. Undersea Biomed Res 1974;1:117–150.

44. Hart GB. Screening test for decompression sickness. Aviat Space Environ Med 1976; 47:993–994.

45. Strauss RH, Prockop LD. Decompression sickness among scuba divers. JAMA 1973;223:637–640.

46. Boettger ML. Scuba diving emergencies: pulmonary overpressure accidents and decompression sickness. 1983;12:563–567.

47. Frankel HL. Paraplegia due to decompression sickness. Paraplegia 1977;14:306–311.

48. Reviera JC. Decompression sickness among divers: an analysis of 935 cases. Milit Med 1964;129:314–334.

49. Dick AP, Massey EW. Neurologic presentation of decompression sickness and air embolism in sport scuba divers. Neurology 1985;35:667–671.

50. Blick G. Notes on diver's paralysis. Br Med J 1909;4:1796–1798.

51. Farmer JC, Thomas WG, Youngblood DG, et al. Inner ear decompression sickness. Laryngoscope 1976;86:1315–1327.

52. DAN Diving Accident Network [Letter]. J Emerg Med 1987;2:223–224.

53. Strauss RH. Decompression sickness. In: Straus RH, ed. Diving medicine. New York: Grune & Stratton, 1976:63–82.

54. Treatment of serious decompression sickness and arterial gas embolism. In: Davis JC, ed. The Twentieth Undersea Medical Society

Workshop. Bethesda MD: Undersea Medical Society, Inc., 1979.

55. Catron PW, Flynn ET. Adjuvant drug therapy for decompression sickness: a review. Undersea Biomed Res 1982;9:161–173.

56. Farmer JC, Thomas WG, Youngblood DG, et al. Inner ear decompression sickness. Laryngoscope 1976;86:1315–1327.

57. Bove AA. The basis for drug therapy in decompression sickness. Undersea Biomed Res 1982;9:91–111.

58. Kizer KW. Corticosteroids in the treatment of serious decompression sickness. Ann Emerg Med 1981;10:485–488.

59. Kizer KW. Delayed treatment of dysbarism: a retrospective review of 50 cases. JAMA 1982; 247:2555–2558.

60. Butler FK, Pinto CV. Progressive ulnar palsy as a late complication of decompression sickness. Ann Emerg Med 1986;15:738–741.

61. Myers RAM, Bray P. Delayed treatment of serious decompression sickness. Ann Emerg Med 1985;14:254–257.

62. Teed RW. Factors producing obstruction of the auditory tube in submarine personnel. US Nav Med Bull 1944;44:293–306.

# CHAPTER 13

# Field Treatment of Water

## INTRODUCTION

Not long ago, or at least that is how the rumor goes, most wilderness trekkers would drink from streams at will, without giving much thought to the possible contamination of the water while in "civilized countries." Whether this happy state was due to the hardiness of the trekker or the pristine state of the wilderness is open to some question. Now that there are more folks using those clear mountain streams, more of those folks are acquiring *Giardia* and other waterborne diseases. Since there are few studies that have measured the level of contamination of streams that few folks frequent, the cause and effect relationship is not really that clear.

It is certain that some of the travelers in the wilderness have been less than completely careful in disposal of their personal wastes. It is likewise certain that *Giardia* and other intestinal invaders have been found recently in places where few souls have ventured, yet. These invaders are also carried and transmitted by mammals other than humans (see Figs. 13.1 and 13.2). The nickname of one of these diseases, "beaver fever," reflects the potential for transmission by another common mammal.

The situation was, of course, different in less-developed countries. There tales of "don't drink the water" and "don't eat the salads" and the consequences of failure to heed the warnings abound. The trekker to a far off wilderness expected to be exposed to water and foodborne illness and was not often dis-

appointed. Indeed, the variety of waterborne parasites and pathogens found in the tropics are still incompletely cataloged. In more populated areas, indiscriminant spread of sewage and wastes in public watersheds and use of untreated nightsoil for fertilization has led to intriguing patterns of disease transmission.

Will the wilds of the United States and Canada follow as places that we "don't drink the water"? Is this trend for infection due to

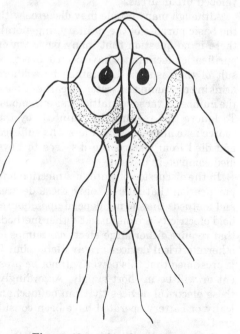

**Figure 13.1.** *Giardia* organism.

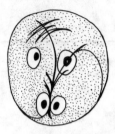

**Figure 13.2.** *Giardia* cystic form.

better reporting, more people in the wilderness areas, poor waste disposal practices, or a combination of all three? Should the traveler purify his water. If so, how? Where?

## FIELD WATER DISINFECTION

It should be made clear that field water disinfection principles are not just applicable to mountain climbers, backpackers, and trekkers. Disasters, such as floods and earthquakes, may render city water systems unusable or contaminated for long periods of time. Contamination of public water supplies has occurred even in quite civilized countries under the best of circumstances. Travelers to third world or underdeveloped countries should be routinely advised to disinfect their water supplies when traveling outside of well-developed urban areas.

Although many people may disagree with the basic purpose of the military in general, there is no question that many basic water purification techniques have been a direct result of the casualties sustained by soldiers drinking contaminated water. In earlier times, the number of these casualties was enormous. To ignore this research as "tainted" by the source is to allow those soldiers who suffered and died from waterborne diseases to have died completely in vain.

In the discussion of water disinfection and purification that follows, only those devices and methods that do not depend upon household electricity are discussed. Other methods that require either large electrical pumps or other electrical devices are available, but it is presumed that this power will not be present or will be in short supply. Accordingly, those electrical devices that can be mechanically or battery operated have been considered.

Devices, such as distillation units, will not only destroy bacteria and other infective organisms but will remove inorganic minerals. Unfortunately, these devices use considerable energy, and have a low output and are, thus, recommended only for specific laboratory or medical applications and not for routine water purification.

In addition, many of these units provide enough water only for drinking and cooking. In some areas of the world, water sources are so contaminated that they are unfit for bathing or shaving. These waters may contain cercariae or other parasites of animal, bird, or even human origin. Provision of enough disinfected water for laundry and bathing is not generally within the scope of this chapter although some devices discussed may be capable of purification of quantities sufficient for small parties.

## Definitions
### STERILIZATION

Sterilization is the process of inactivation of ALL disease-causing agents. Water treated for sterilization may be safely drunk or used for internal surgical procedures. Sterilization does not remove minerals or debris, however.

### DISINFECTION

Disinfection is the inactivation of all infective agents. Not all organisms need to be killed or destroyed for disinfection, but all disease-causing agents must be killed or destroyed. Needless to say, sterilized water is always disinfected. Most city water supplies in the United States are disinfected, not sterilized.

### CLARIFICATION

Clarification is the removal of debris from the water. Literally, it is clearing the water of particulate matter. Bacteria, virons, and parasites may or may not be removed by clarification, depending upon the process. Dissolved minerals may also be left in the water by clarification processes.

### POTABLE

Potable water is safe (but not necessarily pleasant) to drink. All waterborne, disease-causing organisms have been removed or destroyed. Some minerals may be removed by procedures like desalination, but substantial quantities of taste-changing minerals or particulate matter may remain. Potability is only determined by chemical and microbiologic examination.

## PALATABLE

Palatable water is pleasant to taste and appearance (but not necessarily safe). Unfortunately, there is no significant relationship between potability and palatability.

## HARDNESS

Water containing certain compounds of calcium and magnesium is termed "hard" water. Water can be "softened" by exchanging water soluble sodium ions for the hardness ions. Water softeners are not purifiers nor do they remove other chemical contaminants. Their intended function is to extract calcium and magnesium ions from the water, making it more desirable for bathing, laundering, and other cleaning chores. Modest amounts of iron and hydrogen sulfides may incidentally be removed in the softening process.

---

*Effective Water Treatment Methods*
**Heat**
  Boiling
  Pasteurization
  Distillation
**Physical Removal**
  Filtration
**Halogens**
  Chlorine
  Iodine

---

## Heat

### STANDARD BOILING

The standard recommendations to boil all water for 10 to 30 minutes will completely sterilize it. Boiling for this length of time will kill not only all waterborne bacteria, parasites, and virons but will also kill the organisms most resistant to heat, such as clostridial spores. Water boiled in this manner is suitable for surgical procedures and dressing wounds. It is also suitable for drinking, of course. Unfortunately, boiling water for 30 minutes will be expensive in both time and fuel consumption. For many trekkers and backpackers, the fuel necessary to boil water

for 30 minutes may be a prohibitive weight. This process does nothing to improve palatability or remove minerals from the water. When cooled, the boiled water must be kept in a covered, uncontaminated container since boiling does not impart any residual disinfectant.

## SHORTENED BOILING TIMES

Acceptable water for drinking may be obtained by bringing the water to a rolling boil and then cooling. Please note that water treated in this manner is not suitable for surgical scrubs and treatment of wounds, as the spores present may not be killed. Fortunately, spores, which are the most heat-resistant organisms, do not cause any waterborne diseases. This water is technically not sterilized but disinfected. The technique was first proposed in the 1800s by Pasteur as a treatment for milk and is successfully used to this day (pasteurization).

The reason that the technique is so successful is that time and temperature are inversely related for heat disinfection: the higher the temperature, the less time is required. For much of the time used to heat the water to a boil, the water is above the disinfection temperature, so by the time it reaches the boiling point, it is safe to drink.

As altitude increases, atmospheric pressure decreases, and the ability to vaporize water is enhanced, leading to a decrease in the boiling point of water. No matter what terrestial altitude is reached, the temperature at which water boils is sufficiently high for proper disinfection (see Table 13.1). When

**Table 13.1.**
**Boiling Point Depression with Altitude**

| Elevation | Baro Press | Boiling Point |
|---|---|---|
| 2 ATA | 1520 mm Hg | 121°C (pressure cooker) |
| Sea Level | 760 mm Hg | 100°C |
| 5000 feet | 632 mm Hg | 95°C |
| 10000 feet | 522 mm Hg | 90°C |
| 14000 feet | 446 mm Hg | 86°C |
| 19000 feet | 364 mm Hg | 81°C |
| 22000 feet | 321 mm Hg | 77°C |

Adapted from Keenan JH, Keyes FG. Thermodynamics of Steam. New York: John Wiley and Sons, Inc., 1936.

**Table 13.2.**
**Thermal Death Points (Typical)**

| | | |
|---|---|---|
| *Giardia* | 131°F (55°C) | 5 minutes |
| Amoeba[17] | 131°F (55°C) | 5 minutes |
| Enteric | 150°F (65°C) | 1 minute |
| Bacteria[17] | 131°F (55°C) | 30 minutes |
| Virus[13,19] | 135°F (58°C) | 20–30 minutes |
| | 158°F (70°C) | 1 minute |
| | 194°F (90°C) | Seconds |

the atmospheric pressure is increased, the boiling point will also increase, therefore, when boiling water in a pressure cooker, the time needed for either disinfection or sterilization is decreased (see Table 13.2). This is the principle behind the steam autoclave commonly used in medicine.

## Filtration

Larger infective agents and particulate matter may be effectively removed by filtration, but many filters suitable for field use are not small enough to remove all infective viruses. Generally speaking, filters are graded by measurement in microns of the largest particle that will pass through the filter. For routine disinfection of water by filtration alone, a filter size of no greater than 0.4 microns is recommended (see Table 13.3 and 13.4).

**Table 13.3.**
**Least Diameters of Potentially Infective Agents**

| Organism | Least Diameter |
|---|---|
| Parasite eggs | 20 μm |
| *Schistosomiasis* ect | |
| *Giardia* (cyst form) | 5 μm |
| *Entomeba histolytica* | 5 μm |
| *Clostridium perfringens* | 1.0 μm |
| Anthrax | 1.0 μm |
| *Salmonella typhosa* | 0.6 μm |
| *Salmonella* (various sp) | 0.5 μm |
| *E. coli* | 0.5 μm |
| *Shigella* | 0.4 μm |
| *Salmonella hirshfeldii* (enteric fever) | 0.3 μm |
| *Mycoplasma pneumonia* (smallest free-living organism) | 0.3 μm |
| Viruses | 0.01 μm |

**Table 13.4.**
**Comparative Sizes of Common Filters**

| | |
|---|---|
| Filter paper (lab grade) | 10 μm |
| Pocket purifier | 10 μm |
| Timberline filter | 2.0 μm |
| First Need filter | 0.4 μm |
| Katadyne "pocket" filter | 0.2 μm |

As the size of the particle that a filter allows to pass through decreases, more pressure will be required to push the water through the filter. For relatively large filters, gravity pressure alone will suffice, but, unfortunately, these filters are not suitable for routine disinfection of water. Fine filters (often termed ultrafilters) that will remove ALL infective material require pressures that are not easily achievable in the field and are not practical .

### KATADYN

The best physical filter on the market is also the most expensive: the Katadyn (see Fig. 13.3). This company manufactures several sizes ranging from a 1.5 pound "pocket" filter to large expedition filters with hundreds of liters per day capacity. The two smallest models filter .75 liters per minute and 8 liters per minute respectively. The surface of the clay filter—the candle—must be cleaned regularly, and each cleaning removes a small amount of the surface. Eventually, the filter is worn away and must be replaced (after years of use and cleaning). Having no disposable parts, it is conceivable that the Katadyn will outlast its owner. The candle is fragile and may be broken by rough handling.

The Katadyn will effectively and rapidly clean water of all particulate matter, parasites, protozoans, and bacteria.[1] It should be noted that the filter size is far larger than the viruses, so they pass through freely.

The company asserts that viruses are bound to the clay candle and that the silver impregnation of the clay then kills them. The U. S. Environmental Protection Agency (EPA) does not recognize this assertion, but foreign advertising for these Swiss-made filters commonly has this claim. If in a hepatitis-A endemic area, postfiltration treatment with a modest amount of halogen is recommended. It should be noted that postfiltration treat-

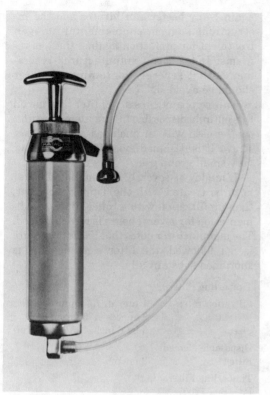

**Figure 13.3.**  Katadyn filter.

ment of stored water with modest amounts of halogen is a wise idea in any case, since it will decrease the effects of inadvertent contamination.

**Katadyn Filter Products**

| | |
|---|---|
| Katadyn pocket filter | $170 (occasional sale $140) |
| Pocket filter "candle" | $ 90 |

Hand pump model in zipper case
Brush and candle wear measuring device included
28-inch intake hose and particulate strainer included

| | |
|---|---|
| Filtration rate: | 0.75 liters per minute |
| Weight: | 23 oz (650 grams) |
| Size: | 10 inches by 2 inches (25 × 5 cm) |

No disposable components

| | |
|---|---|
| Filtration size: | 0.2 microns |

**Group Model KFT**

Although the Katadyn pocket filter can easily support the drinking water needs of several people, hand pumping three fourths of a liter per minute may get tiresome for the larger quantities needed for laundry and hygiene. The group model with 8 liters per minute capacity will solve this problem for small groups.

| | |
|---|---|
| Filtration rate: | 8.0 liters per minute |
| Weight: | 4.9 kilograms (10 lbs) |
| Size: | 58 cm length (23 inches) |

No disposable components

| | |
|---|---|
| Filtration size: | 0.2 microns |

Katadyn USA Inc
6907 East McDowell Road
Scottsdale, AZ 85257
602-990-3131

Katadyn Products, Ltd.
P.O. Box 154
CH-8304 Wallisellen
Switzerland

## FIRST NEED PURIFIER

This disposable element filter produced by General Ecology, Inc. is substantially less expensive than the Katadyn filter. It also has a silver impregnated filter, with a charcoal matrix and 0.4 micron filter size. The flow rate is one half liter per minute. It is small, weighing less than 12 ounces. The charcoal filter will remove some chemical pollutants. Each hand-pumped filter is rated for 400 liters (800 pints) of water and comes with an intake strainer (see Fig. 13.4).

It should be noted that this unit is also substantially less fragile than the Katadyn pocket filter unit. If inexperienced hands are involved in water preparation, this unit certainly would be the first choice. Its only major disadvantage is the need to carry replacements for the disposable cartridge. For an extended trek this may be a considerable disadvantage, depending upon the turbidity of the water and amount of use.

To the filtration of the water is added the

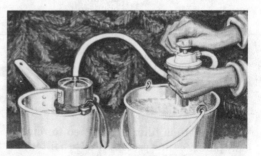

**Figure 13.4.**  First-Need filter.

advantage of charcoal adsorption of other contaminants so that the water from the General Ecology filters often actually tastes better than the original source.

The same company produces the Seagull IV Pres-sure-pure electrically pumped filter. This larger system requires a 12 volt, 1 amp power supply and will produce 1 gallon per minute. This unit has an 8000 liter lifetime per filter.

The same caveat about viral contamination noted with the Katadyn filter also applies to this filter. Testing of the First Need and Seagull IV shows that *E. coli*, and amoebic and *Giardia* cysts are completely removed by these products. The charcoal filter may improve the taste of the water somewhat, but it does not remove all dissolved minerals or salts. Prefiltration treatment of water with halogen should allow for adequate contact time, since the charcoal will remove the halogen. With prefiltration and a charcoal filter device, there is no halogen taste. A **POST**-filtration treatment allows for safer storage of water if the water must stand for any period of time but the water has a distinctive halogen taste.

**General Ecology Filter Products**

First Need purifier                    $39.95
  Replacement cannister       24.95
Filtration rate:                       0.5 liters per minute
Size:                                  6 by 6" cylinder
                                       (15 × 15 cm)
Weight:                                12 ounces (340 grams)

Disposable cannister element
0.4 micron filter size (absolute)

Seagull IV                             $785.00
  Replacement cannister       80.00

Disposable core canister element
0.4 micron filter size

Filtration rate:                       4 liters per minute
Size:                                  20 by 14 inches (50 × 35 cm)
Weight:                                20 lbs (9 kg)
Requires 12 volts DC at 1 amp

General Ecology, Inc
151 Sheree Boulevard
Lionville, PA 19353

## Timberline Filter

The Timberline filter is designed to remove only parasites and protozoa due to a filter size of 2 microns. This filter will not be effective against any bacteria or viruses and the instructions suggest supplemental halogen treatment for protection against these organisms. Indeed, the manufacturer recommends that severely contaminated water should be avoided.

This company cites a 400 liter lifetime on this entirely disposable filter system. The unit can be used with an included pump or as a straw. It is designed more for individual or very small group use.

If muddy or severely contaminated water is to be treated with the Timberline filter, then prefiltration with a coffee filter or sedimentation for several hours is recommended. The manufacturer notes that if this procedure is not followed, the filter element's life is shortened substantially.

Timberline Filter

Filtration rate:       1 liter in 1.5 minutes
Weight:                6 ounces (170 grams)
Size:                  3 by 6 inches (7.5 × 15 cm)

Disposable element
Filter size:           2 micron

Timberline Filters, Inc.
P.O. Box 12007
Boulder, CO 80303

Note that filters do not remove chemicals and minerals. They do remove all but the very finest particulate matter. Unless a lab-grade ultrafilter is used, viral elements are not removed. Water may require further treatment for chemical or viral contamination. Professionals dependent upon water supplies for life and livelihood use a dual system, such as preboiling followed by microfiltration or microfiltration followed by halogen treatment to ensure safe water supplies.[2]

## Halogenation

The halogens include chlorine and iodine. These are both effective disinfectants for viruses, enteric bacteria, and protozoan cystic forms, such as amoebas and *Giardia*. The ability of the halogens to destroy an organism depends upon the resistance of the organism, the concentration of the halogen, the temperature of the water, and the length of time that the organisms are exposed to the halogen (contact time). The concentration of the halogens is measured in parts per million (ppm) or the equivalent milligrams per liter.

The effective concentration of the halogen is dependent not only upon the amount of the halogen but upon the other contaminants in the water and the pH of the water. Organic material will absorb some of the halogen, so more will be required for cloudy or heavily polluted water. A residual halogen concentration will mean that the potential of contamination of stored water will be decreased.

Viruses are somewhat more resistant to halogenation than bacteria. Virucidal residuals of iodine and chlorine are 5 to 70 times higher than bactericidal residuals.[3] Resistance of the organism to chlorine and iodine appear to be similar (see Table 13.5).

It should also be noted that many parasites and their eggs and encysted forms are quite resistant to all of the halogens.[4] Since all of the eggs and parasites capable of infesting humans are greater than 10 microns in size, quite inexpensive filters will remove them from the water. Infestation with para-

**Table 13.5.**
**Experimental Effective Disinfection Data (for 99.9% Kill of Organisms)[13,20–22]**

| Time | Conc | pH | Water Temp |
|------|------|------|------|
| *Giardia* | *Chlorine* | [Clear Water] | |
| 6+ hr | 0.5 ppm | 6–8 | 3–5°C |
| 120 min | 2.0 | 6–8 | 3–5°C |
| 60 min | 4.0 | 6–8 | 3–5°C |
| 30 min | 8.0 | 6–8 | 3–5°C |
| 15 min | 3.0 | 6–8 | 20°C |
| 15 min | 10.0 | 6–8 | 3–5°C |
| 10 min | 3.0 | 6–8 | 15°C |
| 10 min | 1.5 | 6–8 | 25°C |
| | | | |
| *E. Coli* | *Chlorine* | [Clear Water] | |
| 5 min | 0.03 | 6–8 | 2–5°C |
| | | | |
| *Enteric Viruses* | *Chlorine* | [Clear Water] | |
| 40 min | 0.5 ppm | 7.8 | 2°C |
| 30 min | 0.3 | 7.8 | 25°C |
| | | | |
| *Giardia* | *Iodine* | [Clear Water] | |
| 15 min | 3.0 | 6–8 | 20°C |
| 30 min | 7.0 | 6–8 | 3–5°C |
| 15 min | 7.0 | 6–8 | 3–5°C |
| | | | (96.5% kill) |
| | | | |
| *Salmonella* | *Iodine* | [Clear Water] | |
| 2 min | 0.5 | 6–8 | 20°C |
| | | | |
| *E. Coli* | *Iodine* | [Clear Water] | |
| 1 min | 1.0 | 6–8 | 2–5°C |

sites is not usually a problem in major municipal water supplies, since filtration is an essential step in commercial water preparation. In the field, however, filtration should be an essential step in purification of water in areas where parasitic infestations have been reported. This filtration will also remove large organic particulates and thereby decrease contact time needed for the halogens.

For a given set of conditions of pH, temperature, and organic pollutants, the contact time multiplied by the concentration is equal to a constant factor. This means that doubling the contact time will allow the use of half as much halogen. This becomes important with cold and cloudy water where the halogen concentration for an effective dose may become distasteful.

Contact time and dose calculations recommended are very conservative under the philosophy that a single infective organism is more dangerous than a minimal change in water taste. In cases of commercial products, if the manufacturer's recommendations were followed, there was a 100% kill of *Giardia* cysts in studies reviewed. If the relative risk of infection in an area is small, then downward modifications of dose or contact time recommendations may be made at the user's risk. If there is any question, remember that increased contact time will result in increased disinfection.

## CHLORINE

Chlorine is used throughout the United States for treatment of public water supplies in residual (unbound) concentrations of less than 1 ppm. Effective chlorine concentrations are strongly affected by temperature, pH, organic material, and nitrogenous pollutants. This means that amount of chlorine routinely employed as a disinfectant may not be sufficient to consistently kill such resistant species as *Giardia*. This data has been confirmed in the laboratory under experimental conditions.[5,6]

This does not mean that chlorine does not work, it only means that the conditions must be optimal for chlorine to be consistently effective. Urban *Giardia* epidemics appear to be the result of inadequate contact time, breaks in the water delivery system, or inadequate concentration of free chlorine. Maintenance problems in municipal water systems may not be detected until an outbreak surfaces.

## pH effect

When chlorine is added to water, it dissociates to hydrochloric and hypochlorous acids. The hypochlorous acid appears to be the active ingredient and is unstable, rapidly dissociating into hydrogen ion and hypochlorite ions at pHs above 7. With acidic pH, the hypochlorous acid will predominate, at a pH of 8.5, nearly all of the acid has dissociated. Hypochlorous acid will kill *E. coli* nearly 70 times as fast as hypochlorite ion, so acid pH is essential for proper disinfection by chlorine.

## Organic Compounds

Chlorine also reacts with nitrogen compounds, including organic compounds, in the water. The reaction produces chloramines, also called "combined available chlorine." The chloramines are much less effective than hypochlorous acid in disinfection of water, so sufficient chlorine must be added to produce free chlorine and overcome the chlorine demand. While cloudy water is one indication of a high chlorine demand, many compounds that react with chlorine are dissolved and found in clear water.

## Disadvantages

Disadvantages of chlorine include an unpleasant taste in concentrations of greater than 4 to 5 ppm. Unfortunately, unless accurate measurements are readily available, the 1 ppm free chlorine concentration used in municipal water supplies is an unobtainable bottom limit. When using chlorine in the field, one should always use enough so that there is at least some slight odor or taste to ensure that enough chemical remains after combination with organic matter to deal with the pathogenic organisms. After an appropriate contact time, the water can be filtered through a charcoal filter to remove the objectionable taste or a flavoring agent can be added.

Chlorine may also combine with halogenated hydrocarbons in the water to produce teratogenic, mutagenic, and carcinogenic chlorine compounds. The potential of chlorine combination exists, but the effects and actual quantities of these compounds is a speculation, and there have been no studies to prove or disprove this effect. It is further doubtful that any problem would exist with the ex- ceedingly small quantities involved in field water supply disinfection.

## FIELD CHLORINATION PROCEDURES

Again, the basic idea is to achieve a free halogen level of greater than 1 ppm. Contact time must be increased for cold water, and either contact time, concentration, or both should be increased with cloudy water. As noted above, the effectiveness of chlorine is severely reduced by the presence of organic material, low temperature, and alkaline pH. If the water is cold, the water container can be carried inside a vest next to the body to warm the water and decrease the contact time needed.

Note that efficacy of all of these halogen products will be markedly improved by prefiltration of water to remove sediment and organic debris. THESE RECOMMENDED CONTACT TIMES ARE NOT SUFFICIENT TO KILL PARASITES AND PARASITE EGGS. Parasites and parasite eggs are easily removed by filtration, which is recommended in areas where waterborne parasites are endemic.

## Halazone

Halazone tablets have been dutifully lugged into the bush by generations of trekkers and backpackers. Unfortunately, many of these trekkers have been essentially unprotected. Halazone tablets are unstable and tend to deteriorate rapidly. There is no physical change in the tablet that will indicate potency. If exposed to air, the tablets lose 75% of their activity within 2 days. On the shelf, the tablets will deteriorate within 5 months at 32°C. When storage is at 40 to 50°C, this shelf life dwindles to 1 to 2 months. The backpacker that depends upon halazone should get a fresh bottle for each trip from a reputable supplier and should not store this bottle for longer than 2 months prior to use.

Halazone Tablets

Each tablet releases about 2.3 to 2.5 ppm chlorine

|  | Clear | Cloudy |
|---|---|---|
| Warm | 5 tabs/30 min | 5 tabs/30 min |
| Cold | 5 tabs/30 min | 5 tabs/30 min |

Manufacturer's contact/dose recommendations for each liter of water. Some studies allow one half dose for clear water. This may be effective as the lowest halogen residuals measured in one study were 7 ppm with the above doses. Please note that the studies used FRESH tablets.

## Liquid Bleach

Liquid household chlorine bleach has between 5 and 6% free chlorine. Bleach is inexpensive and readily available in large quantities. Bleaches with additives should be avoided as the additives may be toxic. Spills of bleach may be corrosive to equipment, but at household strengths, it should not be corrosive to skin after short contact. Bleach is not a stable compound; it will evaporate from open bottles or be released into the air within the bottle when some of the solution has been used. Ultraviolet light will cause deterioration if bleach is stored in the sunlight.

Current recommendations for bleach for field disinfection:

5 to 6% Liquid Sodium Hypochlorite (Household Bleach)[7]

|      | Clear          | Cloudy         |
|------|----------------|----------------|
| Warm | 2 drops/30 min | 4 drops/30 min |
| Cold | 2 drops/45 min | 4 drops/45 min |

Added to 1 liter of water. Commercial bleach, such as those products found in commercial laundries, have concentrations ranging up to 17% and are not recommended due to their causticity.

## Calcium Hypochlorite

The military has used 0.5 gm calcium hypochlorite ampules for a chlorine source in field water treatment for many years.[8] The military recommends using enough calcium hypochlorite until 5 ppm residual chlorine has been obtained for a 30-minute contact time. No changes in dose or contact time are made for cold water, but the dose is titrated at 10 minutes with a N,N-diethyl-p-phenylenediamine (DPD Method) color change to 5 ppm chlorine residual. The DPD method kit is included with the military calcium hypochlorite package. Cloudy water would therefore be treated with increased chlorine to provide exactly 5 ppm after 10 minutes.

The military-issued calcium hypochlorite is a powder and requires a separate premixing step to ensure complete dissolution. The recommended amounts of calcium hypochlorite to process water are:

| 33 gallon lyster bag (132 L) | 5 amps (1.5 gm)   |
|------------------------------|-------------------|
| 5 gallon can (20 L)          | 1/2 amp (.25 gm)  |

If the N,N-diethyl-p-phenylenediamine (DPD method) test does not show 5 ppm at 10 minutes, then add one third of the above dose and retest the water in 10 more minutes.

Needless to say, at the 5 ppm level, the disinfected water has a substantial "chlorine taste" and the procedure for disinfection of water is rather complex.

Recently, 4 in 1 Water Systems introduced a two-step process with calcium hypochlorite crystals to achieve a very high concentration of chlorine for disinfection. The water may be stored in this highly chlorinated form with safety from contamination. When ready for use, the chlorine is removed with "industrial strength" hydrogen peroxide. The calcium hypochlorite is converted to calcium chloride and the excess oxygen is released. The disinfected water has no chlorine taste and the oxygenation may actually improve the taste. Unfortunately, the 30% hydrogen peroxide is corrosive to both equipment and skin and precautions against spillage must be made. The disinfection process is simple and elegant.

4 in 1 Water Systems
142 Lincoln Avenue Suite 701
Santa Fe, NM 87501

## IODINE

The problems in predicting a proper dose of chlorine for water that has an unknown pH and unknown chlorine demand make chlorine a difficult disinfectant to use in the field. In extensive studies of field water disinfection for individual soldiers, the U. S. Army concluded that iodine is superior to chlorine. The basic reasons are:

1. Iodine does not react as much with organic material in the water.
2. Iodine is more effective over a wide temperature and pH range.
3. Iodine has a less objectionable taste for equipotent doses.
4. mDosage forms of iodine are more stable than similar preparations of chlorine.

This feeling has slowly percolated to the civilian world.

High germicidal activity is maintained over a wide range of pH in the presence of a variety of water contaminants. Its germicidal action is less dependent upon pH, temperature, and time of contact.

Iodine concentrations of 5 to 10 ppm have

been found effective against all types of waterborne pathogenic organisms, including the enteric bacteria, amebic cysts, cercariae, *Leptospira* and viruses, within 10 minutes at room temperature.[9] Iodination will easily destroy both cystic forms of protozoans and enteroviruses after 15 minutes in concentrations of 3 to 5 ppm in water of 25°C temperature.

Nitrogenous impurities do not impair the effectiveness of iodine. Iodine does not combine readily with amino acids, ammonia, or organic material, so it remains effective in cloudy and polluted water. Relatively pH insensitive, iodine is an effective virucide at wide pH ranges.

Possible contraindications for iodine water purification include unstable thyroid disease, pregnancy, or, of course, iodine allergy. Although drinking water systems have experimentally used iodine, there are no current commercial or municipal water systems that use iodine for purification due to the contraindications.

Iodine can be added to water in three basic ways: as a solution, as a tincture (solution in alcohol), and as tetraglycine hydroperiodide. Various halogenated resins have also been used in combination with filters to add iodine to water.

## Iodine Tablets

Tetraglycine hydroperiodide tablets have been chosen by the U. S. Army for the individual soldier's water disinfection.[10] Similar iodine tablets are sold commerically as Potable Aqua or Globaline (see Fig. 13.5). Water pH is corrected by a buffer to make the iodine content of the tablets more effective. The tablets are easily carried, the shelf life is measured in months when properly stored, and the tablet is a calibrated dose for a 1 liter canteen. The tablets do lose strength after opening or if stored in hot places but will change from gray to yellow with a decrease in potency. At room temperature and 100% humidity, iodine tablets will lose 33% of their iodine in 4 days if exposed to air.[11] Unused tablets should be discarded 3 months after opening a bottle.

> The dose recommended by the Army is 2 tablets per liter of water for cloudy water and 1 tablet per liter of water for clear water with a contact time of 30 minutes. They also note that the contact time should be increased to 1 hour if the

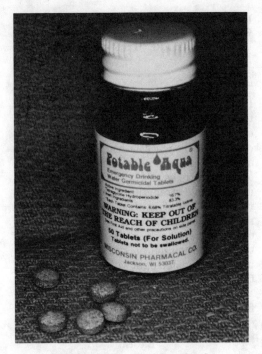

**Figure 13.5.** Aqua Pure bottle.

water is very cold. Each tablet releases about 7 to 10 ppm of iodine.

**Use iodine tablets only if they are:**
1. **Steel gray in color**
2. **Not stuck together**
3. **Not crumbling**

## Iodine Crystals

A simple method of employing a disinfecting dose of iodine has been available for years but only recently has become popular. Described in detail in 1975 by Kahn and Visscher, the original reports were published in the late 1950s by Chang.[12,13] Inmates of three Florida prisions have consumed water disinfected with 0.5 to 1.0 mg/L of iodine for 15 years. No detrimental changes were noted in the general health or thyroid function of normal inmates.[14]

Crystalline iodine is nearly insoluble in water, and a saturated solution at 25°C contains only 320 ppm. If 12.5 cc of 320 ppm iodine solution are added to 1 liter of water, an initial dose of about 4 ppm is obtained. If the iodine solution is kept at near body temperature, only 10 cc of the solution is needed for a 4 ppm disinfection dose.

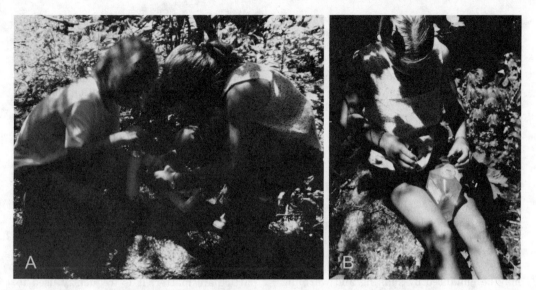

**Figure 13.6.** **A**, use of Katadyn water filter; **B**, use of Polar Pure.

A 1- or 2-ounce glass bottle with a cap that measures 2.5 cc of solution is needed. If 4 to 8 grams of iodine crystals are added to the bottle, which is filled with water, capped, and shaken vigorously for 30 to 60 seconds, a saturated solution results. If the filled bottle is kept in an inside garment pocket in cold weather, the solution will be both premixed and at skin surface temperature. This higher temperature insures that there is at least 300 ppm of iodine dissolved in the water.

A commercial version of this saturated solution of iodine is marketed as Polar Pure water disinfectant (see Fig. 13.6). The bottle containing iodine crystals also has a liquid crystal thermometer and a fine mesh filter to trap the iodine crystals.

Dangers and disadvantages of this procedure are inadvertent ingestion of iodine crystals or breakage of the bottle. Iodine crystals are toxic, but no fatalities have been reported following ingestion of less than 15 gm of iodine. Ingestion of an ounce of saturated iodine solution would be harmless. Iodine crystals are heavier than water and sink in the supernatant after only a few seconds. If the supernatant is carefully poured, no crystals will fall into the cap, and iodine toxicity should not be a problem. Glass bottles will not take on a brown stain and will allow observation of the crystals. If the bottle is broken, or the solution is spilled, staining of skin or equipment will occur.

Since 8 gm of iodine will treat about 2000 liters of water, this method is extremely cost effective, even in the commercial version. Pure iodine will not lose effectiveness with storage, if there is water in the bottle. If there is no water, the iodine will sublime and be lost.

Another solution of iodine that has been recommended by some authors is the 10% povidine-iodine solution (Betadine and other trade names) commonly used for surgical disinfection.[15] The soap should not be used for this purpose. The use of this substance as a water disinfectant is still controversial, has had no organized studies, and is not recommended for routine disinfection.[16] This solution is commonly used to cleanse wounds and may serve as a "reserve" method of disinfection should other methods be broken or unavailable.

**Povidone-Iodine Solution**

|       | Clear    | Cloudy   |
|-------|----------|----------|
| Warm  | 8 drops  | 16 drops |
| Cold  | 16 drops | 16 drops |

Add dose to 1 liter of water. Recommended contact time is 30 minutes in all cases.

**Saturated iodine solution**

| Iodine Temp   | Volume   | Capfuls | ppm  |
|---------------|----------|---------|------|
| 3°C (37°F)    | 20.0 cc  | 8       | 200  |
| 20°C (68°F)   | 13.0 cc  | 5 +     | 300  |
| 25°C (77°F)   | 12.5 cc  | 5       | 320* |
| 40°C (104°F)  | 10.0 cc  | 4       | 400  |

*Approximately skin surface temperature

This dose will result in 4 ppm in 1 liter water. In all cases, 30 minutes contact time is recommended, although 15 minutes contact time may be safe for clear and warm water.

Iodine crystals USP are available from most pharmacies.

Polar Pure Water Disinfectant: About $10.00

Polar Equipment
12881 Foothill Lane
Saratoga, CA 95070.

## Tincture of Iodine

Tincture of iodine may be commercially obtained as the 2% alcoholic solution or may be made as an 8% solution. The 8% solution is made by adding 8 gm of iodine crystals to 100 cc of 95% ethanol. The solubility of the iodine may be enhanced by shaking and warming the alcohol. The tinctures should be dispensed with an insulin or tuberculin syringe since only small amounts are required.

There are no advantages or substantial disadvantages of this method to the water solution of iodine covered above. The alcohol can evaporate or leak more readily than the water solution, leaving the traveler without a means of water purification. The alcohol-iodine solution is more concentrated, so there is often substantially more iodine taste to the treated water.

**2% Iodine Tincture**

|  | Clear | Cloudy |
|---|---|---|
| Warm | 0.25 cc | 0.5 cc |
| Cold | 0.25 cc | 0.5 cc |

In all cases, 30 minutes contact time is recommended.

**8% Iodine Tincture**

|  | Clear | Cloudy |
|---|---|---|
| Warm | 0.1 cc | 0.2 cc |
| Cold | 0.1 cc | 0.2 cc |

In all cases, 30 minutes contact time is recommended.

## Halogen-Impregnated Resin Filters

Various manufacturers tout special effects and better taste by halogenation of water, followed by charcoal filtration. In many cases, "preboosters" of sodium hypochlorite or iodine are recommended by the manufacturer. This amounts to halogenation as described earlier, with all of the disadvantages and advantages of halogenation, combined with an extra cost for the booster.

There is no convincing data that these combinations are any better or more convenient than filters and halogenation combinations already discussed. They certainly are not less expensive than iodination of water with the saturated solution method.

The "gimmick" of a special-release-halogen impregnated resin is also used. Be cautious of filters that claim that impregnation with a substance will destroy a pathogen. To destroy any pathogens, contact time is necessary, and resins do not speed up this contact time.

Charcoal filtration of water will improve taste, remove halogens, minerals, and some particulate matter. It is frequently used to clarify and purify water from public mains. If the taste of halogenated water is objectionable, and cannot be adequately masked by beverages, then charcoal filtration will provide fresher tasting water.

At least one manufacturer has an iodine-impregnated resin followed immediately by charcoal in a strawlike filter. This combination is not rational and should be avoided. The concept of charcoal filtration after halogen disinfection is rational only when the full contact time and dose recommendations for the halogen are followed completely. If the water is filtered prior to full contact time, then the charcoal adsorbs the halogen before complete disinfection has occurred, leaving the user at risk.

## Prevention

The question is still: Should the traveler purify his or her water? The author's answer is yes. The method chosen depends upon the degree of contamination expected.

While in the United States, Canada, Australia, and most European countries, tap water may be presumed to be safe unless specific instructions are given by local authorities to the contrary. Fruits and vegetables may be consumed after peeling. All other foods are only as good as the hygiene of the person preparing them. In wilderness areas, simple filtration with a good filter is probably adequate.

In areas, such as Africa, Central America,

Southeast Asia, ALL water is presumed contaminated and must be treated with both filtration and halogenation or boiling prior to use. In certain rural areas, the water is unfit for bathing and must be treated prior to personal hygiene. Likewise, all foods are presumed to be contaminated unless thoroughly cooked and freshly served. Salads and leafy vegetables are particularly dangerous because of the potential for nightsoil fertilization and the difficulty cleansing them. Although usually safe, even bottled water has been known to cause outbreaks of disease. Hot tea and coffee are probably safe due to the preparation temperature. Wine and beer that are locally bottled may or may not be safe, while imported wine and beer are probably uncontaminated. Ice cubes are considered contaminated unless made from treated water in clean trays. Carbonated beverages appear to be safe due to the bacteriostatic properties of the carbonation.

In the remainder of the world, the question remains open. Raw and uncooked seafood should be avoided. Private homes may be safest, with public stalls and vendors most dangerous. Restaurants may be rated highly for the taste of the food and elegance of service yet fail in the hygiene of preparation. Cost or independent ratings appear to not have much relation to the cleanliness of the cooking and serving staff. The authors tend to be relatively conservative in treatment and prudent in food consumption while in foreign lands. Water is filtered and food is consumed fully cooked and hot. Little trouble has resulted with this conservative approach.

The larger question is, of course, prevention of contamination. Sound field sanitation practices may prevent future contamination of wildlands sources. Latrine locations should be at least 150 feet from any water supply, trail, or campsite and downstream from the water supply. Avoid damp, moist areas and drainage into watersheds. Privies should be constructed for the length of the stay and should be at least 6 to 8 inches deep, within the biologically active upper layer of soil. For frequent use areas, such as alpine tundra or river beds, that cannot recover from such digging, wastes should be packed out and disposed of properly. Privies should be covered after use and the area returned to a natural condition.

## SUMMARY

Treatment of water is relatively simple, straightforward, and necessary. The question of potential water contamination is not answerable in the field. Multiple expedition leaders and military commanders can vouch for the consequences of poor field sanitation. The failure to treat water supplies and procure safe food can cause a trek to be a miserable experience and may necessitate evacuation for severe illness.

In the majority of cases, the disease complex is preventable by foresight and planning. Prudence and patience while awaiting for the action of filter, halogen, or fire can replace the time wasted in multiple trips to the outhouse, commode, or latrine.

## References

1. Schmidt SD, Meier PG. Evaluation of *Giardia* cyst removal via portable water filtration devices. J Freshwater Ecology 1984;2:435:439.
2. Taplin D, Meinking TL. Health and safety in the field: provision of potable water. General Ecology Water Research Updates 1986;May:1–7.
3. National Academy of Sciences, Safe Drinking Water Committee. The disinfection of drinking water. In: National Academy of Sciences. Drinking Water and Health, Vol 2. National Academy Press, 1980.
4. Department of the Army. Sanitary control and surveillance of field water supplies (TB MED 577). Washington, DC: U.S. Government Printing Office, 1986.
5. Jarrol EL, Bingham AK, Meyer EA. Effect of chlorine on *Giardia lamblia* cyst viability. Appl Environ Microbiol 1981;41:483–487.
6. Jarrol EL, Bingham AK, Meyer EA. *Giardia* cyst destruction: effectiveness of six small-quantity water disinfection methods. Am J Trop Med Hyg 1980;19:8–11.
7. Centers for Disease Control. Health Information for International Travel. HEW Publication No. (CDC) 79–8280. Atlanta: U.S. Department of Health, Education, and Welfare, 1979;90–91.
8. Department of the Army. Soldier's manual of common tasks (FM 21–2). Washington, DC: U.S. Government Printing Office, 1979.
9. Chang SL, Morris JC. Elemental iodine as a disinfectant for drinking water. Ind Eng Chem 1953;45;1009.
10. Department of the Army. Field Sanitation and Hygiene (FM 21–10). Washington, DC: U.S. Government Printing Office, 1980.

11. Morris JC, Chang SL, Fair GM, Conant GH Jr. Disinfection of drinking water under field conditions. Ind Eng Chem Ind Ed 1953;45:1013.

12. Kahn FH, Visscher BR. Water disinfection in the wilderness: a simple, effective method of iodination. West J Med 1975;122:450–453.

13. Chang SL. The use of active iodine as a water disinfectant. J Am Pharm Assoc 1958;47:417–423.

14. Thomas WC Jr, Malagodi MH, Oates TW, McCourt JP. Effects of an iodinated water supply. Trans Am Clin Clim Assoc 1978;90:153.

15. Vines T. *Giardia*: forcing 'don't drink the water' practices. Response 1985;September/October:13–21.

16. Preventative measures. In: Wilkerson JA, ed. In: Medicine for mountaineering, 3rd ed. Seattle: The Mountaineers, 1985.

17. Neumann HH. Bacteriological safety of hot tapwater in developing countries. Public Health Rep 1969;84:812.

18. Ginoza W. Mechanisms of inactivation of single stranded virus nucleic acids by heat. Nature 1964;203:606

19. Krugman S, Giles JP, Hammond J. Hepatitis virus: effect of heat on the infectivity and antigenicity of the MS–1 and MS–2 strains. J Infect Dis 1970;122:432.

20. Jarrol EL, Bingham AK, Meyer EA. Giardia cyst destruction: effectiveness of six small-quantity water disinfection methods. Am J Trop Med Hyg 1980;19:8–11.

21. Backer H. Field water disinfection. Wilderness Medical Society, Snowmass: Wilderness Medicine Symposium, August 23–28, 1987.

22. Laubusch EI: Chlorination and other disinfection processes. In: American Water Works Association. Water Quality and Treatment: A Handbook of Public Water Supplies. New York:McGraw-Hill, 1971.

# CHAPTER 14

# Environmental Emergencies in the Wilderness Context

## INTRODUCTION

### The Field of Wilderness Medicine: An Overview

If we define wilderness medicine as care without sophisticated medical facilities, then wilderness medicine is old. Before the advent of modern medical science, all medical care was wilderness medicine, and only in the past 75 years have we stepped away from this standard.[a] One now sees a resurgent interest in medical problems in (and of) the wilderness.

Our frontier forebears treated their medical problems without physicians, with success dependent on what harm the remedy might cause. Today, most consider these medical problems appropriate to bring to their family physicians or an emergency department. Pharmacists and other medical providers may be consulted for a remedy from the ever-expanding, over-the-counter (OTC) pharmacopoeia.

An outdoors enthusiast (one who isn't a physician) who experiences a medical problem in the wilderness faces three choices. First, one might leave the wilderness area and seek a physician. As a second option, the patient may attempt self-care with OTC, or prescription medications, if available. For minor surgical problems, one might attempt a simple

surgical procedure (e.g., lancing a small boil or removing a splinter). The third option is simply to suffer and hope the problem resolves before one reaches trailhead and the doctor. Certainly, a relatively minor problem in the urban environment can rapidly ruin a wilderness outing. This means that some primary or self-care must be taught to the wilderness trekker.

For some conditions, appropriate medical care on the street or in an emergency department might not be applicable in the wilderness. This "civilized" care might even be inappropriate in the wilderness. A dramatic example is CPR in the snow for a cardiac arrest at 14,000 feet. The "civilized" standard teaching of CPR "until the rescuers are exhausted" is, for both the climbing party and the victim, a sentence of death. Clearly, a reorganization of current knowledge in light of the constraints of the wilderness is needed.

The medical community also faces several other questions in teaching medical care to the outdoor public. Who may receive the training to deal with these problems? At what level do we teach:

1. No medication or therapy
2. OTC medications and therapy
3. Prescription medications and "invasive" therapy

Who teaches the classes? In this litigious society, who takes responsibility for training the public?

---

[a]For a refreshing view of modern medicine in its historic context, we suggest: Newman A. The illustrated treasury of medical curiosa. New York: McGraw-Hill, 1988.

## PROBLEMS WITH CURRENT TRAINING

Many wilderness search and rescue team members have medical or nursing education or have attended EMT or paramedic classes. However, once in the wilderness, it is hard for them to apply these teachings. Few people can carry a 40-pound survival pack and 60 pounds of medical equipment and drugs for long. A medical protocol that simply calls for emergency transport is not a useful instruction where evacuations may be measured in "yak-days." Neither the pharmacopoeia nor equipment that the experienced medical provider is accustomed to use is often available in the outback.

Providing wilderness medical training just to park and national forest law enforcement officers and members of search-and-rescue teams ignores a large population needing wilderness medical training. Those who travel the wilderness regularly as part of their jobs or for recreation are often confronted with both minor and major emergencies. For many years, highly motivated outdoors enthusiasts attended EMT classes, assuming this was the best preparation for the wilderness emergency. They, too, found that "street" EMT training is of limited use beyond the trailhead. These outdoorspeople need education on how to care for minor medical problems, those not covered by "street" EMT training. This is wilderness "primary care."

When the wilderness trip is extended from a few days to several weeks, a different set of problems emerges, and one arrives at yet another wilderness medicine topic: expedition medicine. When a group sets out to trek along the China-Tibet border, the walk out to a medical facility might take weeks, so one must plan for any malady or injury. This scope of medicine has been faced in the past by the medical providers on expeditions and ships at sea. Because of the length of time involved, expedition medical providers need training different from that required for shorter outings. Even physicians may find themselves deficient in skills and knowledge for this far-remote practice.

An excellent textbook on expedition medicine, *Medicine for Mountaineering* by James Wilkerson, is now in its third edition. The U.S. Public Health Service also publishes a medical manual for seamen that is of use to the expedition medic. Hamilton Bailey's *Emergency Surgery* is an excellent field surgical textbook for those with more advanced training (see Suggested Readings). Military-oriented texts tend to concentrate on the problems of ballistics-related injuries but also have excellent advice on sanitation and expedient field evacuation methods.

The topics of search-and-rescue medicine, wilderness primary care, and expedition medicine focus mostly on familiar emergency medicine problems in the wilderness setting. A different component of wilderness medicine looks at environmental problems that are characteristic of the wilderness. Not all environmental emergencies occur in the wilderness (radiation exposures are rare), but certain environmental problems commonly occur in wilderness travelers. Some environmental emergencies immediately conjure an image of the wilderness traveler (e.g., high-altitude pulmonary edema and the mountaineer), and others, while found in the urban setting, are more common in the wilderness-traveling populace (e.g., hypothermia and frostbite). Some of these environmental problems, such as sunburn, animal bites, envenomations, and insect stings, "fall in the cracks" between the traditional medical and surgical disciplines. Many of these "orphan problems" have been claimed by emergency medicine. A large part of this book deals with these problems.

For these environmental problems, the goal of wilderness or environmental medicine is to describe optimum medical management of the problem. However, for wilderness first aid and wilderness EMS, medical management is constrained by the environment.

### Hard Problems of Wilderness Emergency Medicine, or How Many Pounds Can You Cram into a 10-Pound Bag?

The first problem is weight. Wilderness backpackers, climbers, and, to a lesser extent, canoeists can only carry a small medical kit. (Some backpackers are known for cutting the handles off their toothbrushes and the margins off their maps to save weight. To them, a 1-pound medical kit would be exorbitantly heavy.) It is hard to select a backpacker's medical kit that is light and hardy, yet will be adequate for most common wilderness medical problems. (More on this topic may be found in Appendix A.)

In wilderness EMS, the rescue team's primary purpose is rescue and medical care of the wilderness patient. These providers are often superbly conditioned, and the sojourn is clearly defined, so the medical kit can be only a few pounds heavier than the backpacker's, but weight is still a major factor. The rescue team member must carry all personal and survival equipment, food, and water needed for the task and all predictable problems. Depending on the environment, this can range from a few to 30 or 40 pounds. Rescue and life-support equipment is heavy and can easily add 40 pounds to an already-heavy pack. Rockfall, mountains, caves, rain, and snow require specialized survival gear, adding more weight. These specialized rescuers may tote equipment in excess of 100 pounds.

In contrast to the rescue squad, search field team members may spend hours or days traveling cross-country on a search. The search team must carry equipment in case they find the victim, but weighting down with heavy rescue equipment will decrease their effectiveness and may delay finding the victim until after he or she dies. As with a backpacker's first aid kit, a search team member's medical kit must be light and compact and must provide for minor team illnesses as well as possible major illness or trauma.

The second problem is the environment. The most ubiquitous environmental problem faced by all rescue parties is hypothermia. Though we tend to think of hypothermia as a winter problem, if glycogen reserves for thermogenesis are impaired by shock, the climber will very quickly become hypothermic. Unless well insulated, even healthy volunteer victims who are immobilized in a Stokes litter during rescue practice find themselves quickly beginning to shiver on warm spring or fall days. Of course, the equipment needed to combat the hypothermia hazard obligates even more weight.

Hyperthermia should not be neglected either. It (together with dehydration) may have caused the initial victim and can affect all rescue operations. The effort and dehydration encountered in moving a patient out of a desert canyon should never be neglected in planning rescue operations. A rescuer who succumbs in the field to exhaustion or heat illness may double the number of patients.

Other environmental hazards for rescuers must not be dismissed lightly. Obvious hazards, such as avalanches, rockfall, cliffs, and whitewater, abound, but more important are the less-spectacular, but more subtle, hazards. Common problems include underestimating the time required for a rescue, consequently spending the night with an unstable patient, with no light or bivouac gear; setting out for a rescue on a sunny afternoon, unprepared for the fog, rain, and wind that come at dusk; or inability to find the patient despite several hours of searching and discovering that the team's radio has insufficient gain to contact Medical Command Base.

The third problem is time (usually too much). Wilderness EMTs (WEMT) must care for their patients over a much longer period than street EMTs. Some problems can be safely ignored by an urban EMT, because the patient will soon be whisked away to a nearby emergency department. These same problems, although not immediately threatening to life or limb, may become life- or limb-threatening during the course of a wilderness rescue, depending on the length of the rescue. In parts of the West, or in a catastrophic natural disaster, the WEMT may need to care for patients for longer than 24 hours. Courses for WEMTs in these situations may add modules with additional skills. Certainly, the WEMT must be able to evaluate common medical problems, decide which can be ignored, which can be treated in the field, and which require immediate evacuation. Fluid monitoring and balance, long-term wound care, nutrition, and dealing with bodily wastes are problems not covered in "street" EMS training. Prevention of hypothermia in immobile patients is given lip service in many parts of the United States. Thwarting hypothermia is essential management of a patient in a litter for even a few hours. Training EMTs to perform procedures such as field suturing or reduction of dislocations is controversial, although military medics have been doing it for years.

## CURRENT RESEARCH AND TRAINING ORGANIZATIONS

Currently, organizations such as the Wilderness Medical Society, the Appalachian Search and Rescue Conference, National Association for Search and Rescue, National Cave Rescue

Commission, National Ski Patrol, and Mountain Rescue Association, and independent businesses such as Wilderness Medical Associates, are researching and teaching wilderness medicine. ASTM (formerly the American Society for Testing and Materials), a national and international standards development organization, has recently (spring 1988) established a committee on search and rescue and, in concert with their committee on Emergency Medical Services, may develop national standards for wilderness search and rescue medical training. Contact information for these and other related organizations is provided in Appendix C.

One cannot discuss wilderness medical training without giving due credit to the various military medical corps. Military medics formed the model for the civilian EMT programs. The military, through necessity, has dealt with medical care in remote areas, environmental constraints, field sanitation, and water purification problems for years. Indeed, landmark articles on field medical problems have been written by military authors such as Walter Reed. Military medical corps documents are an excellent source of information for those developing wilderness medical programs. Military medics may use skills beyond the current capabilities of civilian wilderness medics (e.g., field radiology, laboratory studies, and emergency surgery). However, the military medic's field training is in part, a model for WEMT training. Though wilderness medicine is pursuing an independent path from the military, the cross-fertilization between civilian wilderness medicine and military medicine continues.

Having now mentioned a few examples of the adaptation of standard medical principles and the management of environmental problems during a long wilderness rescue, let's now look more closely at the field of wilderness EMS.

## Wilderness Emergency Medical Services

### URBAN EMS, WILDERNESS EMS, DISASTER EMS: WHAT'S THE DIFFERENCE?

"Special rescue" EMS teams, such as medically oriented wilderness search and rescue teams, often provide prehospital EMS services far away from an ambulance and in hostile environments. If one looks closely at the medical problems of wilderness search and rescue, one finds the distinction between the emergency medical services (EMS) and the search and rescue (SAR) systems blurred. Wilderness rescue includes a variety of disciplines, with many differences compared to most urban and rural rescue training (e.g., land navigation, short-term survival, wilderness travel, search, and semitechnical evacuation). Knots and rappelling are just minor parts of wilderness rescue. Indeed, many mountain rescue techniques have been adopted for urban rescue, further blurring the distinction.

Let's consider two examples:

One might think of cliff rescue as a type of wilderness rescue, but if one can drive an ambulance or rescue truck to the top or bottom of a small cliff, there's really no "wilderness" involved: Standard building rescue techniques can be employed effectively.

On the other hand, depending on the terrain, one quarter mile from the nearest navigable road represents the limit of most urban and many rural EMS systems' ability to effectively function. Beyond this point, carrying bulky rescue gear, litters, and patient is more effort than a two- or three-person paramedic crew can muster. Consider a patient a half mile from the road, at night, in wind and freezing rain, down in a deep, rugged ravine. In this case, standard stretchers and EMT techniques will be very inefficient. Untrained help will often be of no help at all in this situation and may well create multiple new victims to rescue! Using mountain rescue techniques might reduce this 10-hour operation down to a 2-hour evacuation.[b] Given the conditions described above, it might make a difference, not only to the patient's life and limb, but also to the rescuers' lives and limbs.

Figure 14.1 places some search and rescue activities along the spectrum between Search and Rescue and Emergency Medical Services.

### INTEGRATION WITH THE EXISTING SYSTEM

City or county EMS managers sometimes slight the problems of Wilderness Emergency

---

[b]Examples include careful land navigation, the Incident Command System for coordination, and standard rope team rotations for changing belayers during a semi-technical evacuation.

SAR

| | | |
|---|---|---|
| ******* | # | Downed aircraft search |
| ***** | ## | Backcountry lost person search |
| **** | ### | Rescue of victims found during a search |
| *** | #### | Cave and cliff rescue far from the road |
| ** | ##### | Rescue one fourth mile from the road |
| * | ###### | Medical care in the above situations |
| | | EMS |

**Figure 14.1.** The spectrum of EMS and SAR responsibilities.

Medical Services, because there are so few wilderness patients compared to the vast numbers being brought in by "standard" ambulances. Wilderness patients may be rare, but they arouse the intense interest of the press and public, and they are often in the public's eye for a long time. They also require many different EMS and rescue resources and bring out issues of command, control, and coordination. For EMS and other emergency service managers, wilderness patients are a potent source of suits and other legal/management problems. All these are powerful reasons why any EMS system with nearby backcountry areas should be actively involved in wilderness EMS.

Because of the unique problems of wilderness rescue, specialized organizations evolved to deal with them. In the early days, wilderness rescue teams assumed that the patient's first medical care would be at the hospital. Over the years, the prehospital EMS system blossomed, and the patient would receive some medical care from the ambulance waiting at the end of the trail or at the entrance of the cave. Special rescue teams containing EMTs, EMT-Ps, RNs, and MDs now bring medical care directly to the victim. Despite high standards and outstanding volunteer support, these special rescue teams often find it hard to integrate their services into the mainstream of prehospital EMS.

At least in the East, wilderness rescues are rare in any given county, so it is hard to justify a special rescue team for each county. Most teams have members in several counties and may even respond to other areas of the state. (For difficult operations, some organizations, such as the Appalachian Search and Rescue Conference and the National Cave Rescue Commission, draw rescuers from several states.) Since most EMS systems operate on a county or municipal level, wilderness rescue teams operating across many different jurisdictions find it hard to integrate with local EMS systems: Their services are rarely needed in the county, so it is hard to persuade the local "street" EMS services to accept them; since they routinely provide services outside the county, it is also hard for them to obtain county EMS funding. Even in states where each county has its own search and rescue team, the SAR team is often quite separated from any EMS responsibilities or capabilities.

A simple way to avoid this problem, one could suggest, would be to simply include a local medical provider when a wilderness rescue team comes into a given jurisdiction. This has been a standard policy for many years but, in practice, is only marginally satisfactory.

The first major problem with assigning local providers to SAR teams is safety: Not every EMS agency can supply an experienced field provider with the training and personal equipment for wilderness travel, land navigation, night operations in winter storms, and use of ropes. Moreover, if, once in the field, the rescue team discovers inadequacies in the provider's outdoor equipment or capabilities, it puts the provider, the rescue team, and the victim all at risk of injury or death. Even in relatively safe situations, some providers are reluctant to go into the field without the heavy ambulance or hospital-based equipment they are trained to use. In recent rescues, local prehospital providers said "I'm not going down (up) there, and neither is my equipment! You bring the patient to me."

Even if one could assure an adequately trained local provider another issue arises: Most wilderness rescues are in areas where standard EMS communications are at best marginal, so local non-MD providers will operate on prior written standing orders. Are local prehospital protocols adequate to deal with the routine problems of wilderness rescue, such as hypothermia and major infections, during an 18-hour evacuation? There are arguments for different protocols for wilderness rescues.

Even if we can establish reliable communications from the patient's side, is the local EMS command physician appropriate to manage these difficult problems, or should we consult a wilderness specialist? Some believe in specially trained wilderness command doctors and hope to establish a roster of physicians with special training in the management of specific wilderness rescue problems. Though such experienced field physicians may be few and far between, communications to a distant Wilderness Command Physician will be little problem once we can assure communications from the back of a cave or from a deep valley in a wilderness area.

Just as EMS and trauma systems extend the reach of emergency medical and surgical facilities into surrounding communities, so the WEMS System should extend their reach into the backcountry. Other components of a suitable WEMS system might include clinical training with testing and certification at all levels, continuing education programs, medical direction by experienced wilderness physicians, and a sophisticated communications network. Quality control and accountability are imperative for such a system, if it is to be accepted by the medical community.

## THE WILDERNESS EMERGENCY MEDICAL TECHNICIAN/DISASTER EMT

Back in the mid–1970s, some basic EMT courses were offered with a wilderness slant. Such courses would cover all the ambulance-related material required to meet the Department of Transportation (DOT) standards but would expand the coverage of wilderness-specific problems and include wilderness-oriented practical sessions. These were the first "Wilderness Emergency Medical Technician" courses.[c] Such wilderness-oriented EMT classes are still offered throughout the country. As Wilderness EMT training matured, variations on this original WEMT curriculum idea appeared. One approach was to offer a "Wilderness Medical Technician" class that replaced all ambulance-specific material with wilderness-specific material. This curriculum didn't meet DOT standards for an EMT class, so students were not eligible to receive EMT certification. Another popular variant was to offer a special "add-on" for those who

were already EMTs. Most current WEMT course offerings follow this model.

Though some WEMT classes offer training for the general outdoor public, the most reputable courses provide training aimed at medical and paramedical personnel working with wilderness search and rescue teams, or EMS agency personnel with wilderness rescue responsibilities. Such courses include the management of patients over extended periods, the treatment of exposure, trauma, shock, and infections, and, for advanced EMTs and EMT-Ps, the use of drugs, IVs, and other invasive procedures in the wilderness environment. Some argue that special skills that are needed for proper medical management are beyond the skills of a basic EMT, (for instance, reducing a subcoracoid dislocation of the shoulder).

The extended transports of wilderness rescue highlights the need for intravenous hydration. Adding a few simple intramuscular or intravenous medications (epinephrine, morphine sulfate) is also attractive. The EMT licensing structure in some states makes this difficult; for instance, Pennsylvania only recognizes basic EMTs and EMT-Ps and creation of an intermediate level would be politically difficult. In Virginia, where a variety of intermediate advanced EMT levels are licensed, a basic WEMT course with IV skills seems probable in the near future as part of the state EMT licensing structure.

Add-on wilderness training for EMT-Ps is also being offered. In some cases, this is the same training as for basic EMTs, since few if any advanced skills are unique to the wilderness paramedic. Skills such as nasogastric tubes, Foley urinary catheters, and central intravenous lines are all required or optional in street EMT-P training. However, EMT-Ps generally have a stronger background in basic sciences (e.g., anatomy, physiology, and pharmacology), and, on this basis, it is reasonable to offer separate classes for EMTs and EMT-Ps.

As discussed in the first part of this chapter, wilderness primary care should be considered a legitimate part of WEMT training, even though it is oriented to the WEMT and teammates. If a SAR team physician writes prescriptions for prescription medications in the WEMT's primary care kit and provides protocols, WEMTs may use prescription medications for well defined minor problems.

---

[c]The authors have participated and conducted several such classes for the Blue Ridge Mountain Rescue Group of the Appalachian Search and Rescue Conference in the early 1970's.

Think about what a WEMT should do. WEMTs must be self-sufficient, that is, they should be able to carry all their own food, water, and shelter and can stay mobile in a hostile outdoor environment. With little equipment, the WEMT should be able to care for people with medical emergencies, especially those with trauma or environmental illnesses. And the WEMT should be able to manage patients for a long time, even if on-line medical control isn't available. The WEMT should be able to provide definitive care for some minor medical and surgical problems. (Although WEMTs should do so only if the patient can't be taken to a doctor or hospital.)

These are ideal qualifications for a field medic in a war or major disaster—widespread enough to overwhelm or destroy medical and EMS systems. The recent Mexico City or Afganistan earthquakes are good examples of this mass calamity. Training wilderness search and rescue team medics for disaster response also may allow teams and WEMT programs to access funds allocated for disaster training.

## THE WILDERNESS COMMAND PHYSICIAN

Providing medical command to a wilderness medic on a 36-hour evacuation in freezing rain on the side of a mountain involves problems encountered by few physicians in their routine practice. A wilderness command physician must have a solid understanding of general emergency medicine, possess particular expertise in wilderness medical problems (hypothermia, environmental poisonings, and the like) and the problems encountered by WEMTs. To become a Wilderness Command Physician, a command physician, even an experienced outdoors enthusiast, should participate in wilderness rescue simulations to appreciate the difficulty of wilderness rescue and the severity of the environment.

## APPENDIX A: WILDERNESS FIRST AID AND MEDICAL KITS

An ideal wilderness first aid/medical kit is difficult to define. The number of people in the party, the length of the trip and distance to medical care, the area through which one is traveling, and the training of those on the trip all bear on the size and contents of the kit. The kit should be able to provide "second aid," as well as first aid, for serious medical problems that occur on the trail. The kit should also have what is needed to treat many minor medical problems on the trail without having to cut short the trip.

Any prescription for a wilderness medical kit for the general outdoor public should have a disclaimer such as:

> You should obtain prescriptions for these medications from your doctor. A reason your doctor may hesitate to write prescriptions for your medical kit is that you should NOT substitute your medical kit for a doctor's care. For example, if you start taking an antibiotic out on the trail, you may just be diminishing the signs of infection without eradicating it. Therefore, when you get back after a trip that has required more than minor use of your medical kit, CALL YOUR DOCTOR. He or she may be able to tell you that everything's fine but, on the other hand, might want you to come in for additional evaluation or treatment. Only a physician may tell you how to use prescription medications, so the doses in this article must be confirmed or modified by your private physician. Also, medications your physician prescribes for you are for you, not for others; it is neither wise nor legal for you to offer your medications to others.

### Primary Care Member's Kit

The selection of medications and other items for a wilderness medical kit often occasions lengthy debate. Here, we present a representative example, based in part, on a kit designed for members of the Mountain Rescue Association's Appalachian Search and Rescue Conference. This kit is a suggested list for individual WEMTs to carry in their field packs on searches and rescues. A large field team could leave several members' kits at base, taking only two or three for the entire team. The kit is designed to provide for individual team member's incidental problems and to provide some supplies that may be pooled to care for a rescue patient. Physicians often add a small suture kit and a few injectable drugs, e.g., morphine or meperidine, epinephrine, and Valium or Ativan.

Other good examples of personal wilderness medical kits may be found in Auerbach, Breyfogle, Darvill, Forgey's Wilderness Medicine, Lentz et al., and Wilkerson (see Suggested Readings).

## MEDICATIONS

(Prescription-only items are noted by the Rx, trade names in italics)

| Number/amount | Item and size/strength |
|---|---|
| #30: | Acetaminophen tablets, 500 mg for fever or minor pain |
| #60: | Ibuprofen tablets, (Nuprin, Advil) 200 mg for pain or inflammation (such as a sprained ankle), frostbite (400 mg Rufen or Motrin tablets are available by prescription) |
| 1: | 3 cc squeeze bottle oxymetazoline nasal spray (Afrin) for allergic or viral rhinitis, sinusitis, otitis |
| #8: | Sustained-release pseudoephedrine tablets, 120 mg (Sudafed) for allergic or viral rhinitis, sinusitis, otitis |
| #8: | Sustained-release chlorpheniramine tablets, 8 mg (Chlor-Trimeton) for allergies, colds, poison ivy |
| #20: | Diphenhydramine capsules, 25 mg. (Benadryl) for allergies, colds, poison ivy, or sedation |
| #10: | Maalox or similar antacid tablets for gastritis, ulcers, or when taking ibuprofen |
| #5: | Bisacodyl tablets, 5 mg (Dulcolax) for minor constipation from field diets (Administration of this medication for abdominal pain is not recommended by most medical authorities.) |
| Rx #6: | Transdermal scopolamine patches (Trans-Derm/Scop) for prophylaxis of motion sickness |
| Rx #10: | Acetaminophen with 30 mg codeine (Tylenol #3 tablets) for more severe pain, cough suppression, possibly for diarrhea |
| Rx #10: | Immodium capsules for diarrhea |
| Rx #10: | Prochlorperazine tablets, 10 mg (Compazine) for nausea (acceptable alternative may be Phenergan) |
| Rx #1: | 2 cc dropper bottle proparacaine HCl ophthalmic solution for painless eye exams |
| Rx #1: | 3.5 gm tube polymyxin/bacitracin ophthalmic ointment (Polysporin) for eye injuries, skin wounds, otitis externa (an |

| Number/amount | Item and size/strength |
|---|---|
| | alternative to this would be a 3.5 gm tube of gentimycin opthalmic ointment) |
| Rx #1: | Anaphylaxis kit (includes injectable epinephrine) (Anakit) for severe allergic (i.e., anaphylactic) reactions |
| Rx #1: | 15 gm tube fluocinolone acetonide cream 0.2% or similar high-strength steroid cream or lotion (Valisone, Benisone, Lidex, Kenalog, Aristocort, Uticort, Synalar) for insect bites, skin allergies, poison ivy |
| #1: | 15 gm tube miconazole nitrate cream 2% (Micatin or Rx Monistat) for athlete's foot, jock itch, ringworm, or yeast vaginitis |
| #4: | 1 gm foil packets povidone-iodine ointment for wounds |
| #1: | 30 cc bottle mild liquid surgical soap (Hibiclens, Phisohex) for general wound cleaning and for scrubbing hands |
| #1: | 15 cc bottle Sting-Eeze solution for immediate relief of stings |
| #1: | 15 gm tube of nupercaine for hemorrhoidal and chafing relief. |
| #2: | Packets Gatorade or ERG powder, each to make 1/2 liter for rehydration, heat exhaustion, heat cramps[d] |
| #1: | Bottle 18+ SPF sunburn prevention lotion. |
| #1: | 30 gm tube zinc oxide ointment (useful for prevention of sunburn and as a protection for chapped areas) |
| #1: | Pocket inhaler (such as Brethine or Ventolin) |

(The following medications are for longer trips or expeditions)

| Number/amount | Item and size/strength |
|---|---|
| Rx #40: | Erythromycin tablets, 250 mg |
| Rx #40: | Cephalexin tablets, 250 mg (Keflex, Keftabs) |
| Rx #20: | Trimethoprim-Sulfa tablets (Bactrim DS) |
| Rx #40: | Metronidazole tablets, 250 mg (Flagyl) |

These antibiotics are useful for skin and wound infections, strep throat, otitis media, and urinary

---

[d]We assume that team members will have plenty of electrolyte drink mix available in their packs for routine use and therefore only specify 1 liter for the MEDKIT.

infections. Erythromycin may be used for pneumonia, Keflex for most wound infections, and Bactrim for aquatic wounds. Flagyl is useful for treatment of Giardia infections and for some gynecologic infections.

| | |
|---|---|
| #1 oz: | Oil of cloves (Eugenol) |
| #2 | Temporary dental filling kit (Cavit) |

This equipment may be used to effect emergency dental repairs

| | |
|---|---|
| Rx #12: | Phenazopyridine tablets 250 mg (Pyridium) |

Pyridium is useful for treatment of symptomatic cystitis.

| | |
|---|---|
| Rx #1: | 2 cc dropper bottle Cyclopentolate HCl ophthalmic solution 0.5% or 1% (Cyclogyl) |

Cyclogel is useful for pain due to corneal abrasion or snowblindness.

| | |
|---|---|
| Rx #20: | acetazolamide tablets 250 mg (Diamox) |

Diamox is needed at altitudes greater than 8000 feet for prophylaxis of altitude illness in those teammembers who are not completely altitude acclimated

## DRESSINGS AND BANDAGES[e]

| | |
|---|---|
| #4: | 3″ x 4″ pieces of moleskin |
| #1: | 1″ (by at least 3 yards) waterproof adhesive tape |
| #1: | 3″ by 5 yards (stretched) elastic (Ace) bandage |
| #2: | 3″ by 5 yards (stretched) conforming roller gauze (Kling) |
| #10: | small adhesive bandages (1″ × 3″ Band-aids) |
| #8: | medium-sized (3″ × 3″ or 4″ × 4″) gauze pads |
| #5: | medium-sized butterfly strips or suture strips (Steristrips) |
| #3: | triangular bandage with two safety pins |
| #1: | wire mesh splint or SamSplint |
| #2: | eyepads |

## MISCELLANEOUS

| | |
|---|---|
| #1: | 15 cc bottle povadone-iodine solution (Betadine) |
| #6: | Alcohol prep pads, in foil |
| #6: | sterile cotton applicators (Q-tips) |
| #3: | #11 scalpel blades, sterile (with handle) |
| #1: | paper clip, medium size |

| | |
|---|---|
| #1: | dental tamping instrument—for longer trips |
| #1: | pair small sharp scissors |
| #1: | pair fine-point splinter forceps |
| #1: | low-reading clinical thermometer |
| #1: | nylon zipper bag for MEDKIT |
| #1: | plastic-laminated contents/instructions |
| #5: | freezer-style zip lock plastic bags (if not available elsewhere in SAR pack) |

Oral and nasal airways
Water purification system (recommended is either the First Need or Katadyn filter, with iodine post-filtration treatment). This water is suitable for irrigation of wounds and for consumption.

## APPENDIX B: WILDERNESS EMERGENCY MEDICAL SERVICES EQUIPMENT

### A "Wilderness Ambulance"

Let's make an analogy between an ambulance and a wilderness rescue team. The litter team members' booted feet are its "tires." Blistered feet or slippery shoes on a rescue team may be just as hazardous as bald tires on an ambulance. Training in good foot care and proper personal equipment are essential parts of the "wilderness ambulance[f]."

The rescuers' headlamps and flashlights are the "wilderness ambulance's" headlights. Night wilderness rescuers trying to carry (and care for) a patient using hand-held flashlights are probably worse off than EMTs in an ambulance with no headlights and no interior lighting.

These analogies can, of course be carried to extremes, but are a useful starting place for examining the equipment needs of a wilderness rescue team. Just as ambulances must have a full complement of required equipment, state EMS agencies might require every wilderness EMS agency to have the minimum equipment and personnel to successfully build a "wilderness ambulance."

The Appalachian Search and Rescue Conference made a proposal for modifications to one state's EMS regulations that would es-

---

[e]The standard ASRC kit contains only 1 roll of roller gauze and one triangular bandage. This is done to save weight, since with any significant injury during an operation, several members will soon be present, each able to contribute his or her own roller gauze and triangular bandages.

[f]One might argue that the rescue team's equipment can be all team equipment, with no need for personal equipment, but a quick thought about boots will belie this. A 5-mile hike in "team" boots would turn any rescuer into a casualty.

tablish standards for such a "wilderness ambulance" for every wilderness EMS agency.[2] Personal gear, including proper boots, clothing, survival gear, and headlamps are part of the proposal. Other sections of the proposal specify the use of proper evacuation gear (i.e., Stokes litter, ropes, semitechnical evacuation equipment), patient immobilization and packaging equipment, radios, field-portable extrication gear, medical equipment and supplies, and a minimum of nine evacuation team members who are certified to the state's search and rescue Field Team Member standards.

## Drugs and Equipment for Wilderness EMS

This is merely a list to provide a broad general idea of the type of equipment recommended for wilderness EMS agencies. Actual equipment needs vary depending on terrain, resources, training, and patient population. Certain materials should be available from team member's own packs, such as food, water, water purification tablets or filters, and fire-starting materials. Two-way radios are essential to the rescue party, and, at a minimum, two identical units need to be carried by the party (three units with 6 spare batteries is better)[g].

Oxygen bottles, masks, valves, and tubing are not included in this equipment due to the weight considerations. If there is opportunity to air-resupply, then these could be added to the resupply package.

## PREPACKAGED KITS

Airway and endotracheal intubation kit (a single handle with lithium dry cells for laryngoscope and for otoscope/ophthalmoscope is recommended): At least two endotracheal tubes of each of the the common sizes should be carried to allow for damage to the tubes. Extra oral and nasal airways in various sizes should be carried as well.

Catheterization kit with Texas catheters and various sizes of Foley catheters.

Chest tubes, tubing, and valves for tube thoracostomy—if there is a qualified medical attendant in the party. Although a simple suture set and scalpel will allow insertion of a chest tube, a large, curved clamp will improve technique and rapidity. Although trochar tubes are available, use of the trochar is considered risky.

IV Kit (see below)

Suture Kit[h]—Disposable suture kits are now readily available, with excellent quality instruments. These may be discarded after use or may be sterilized and reused. Sutures in a variety of sizes in both absorbable and nonabsorbable materials may be easily carried. Surgical staples may offer an alternative with less training and anesthesia required. (Originally developed by the Soviets, these staples are available in small, disposable, preloaded packages by Ethicon, 3M and others.) Steri-strips and other adhesive closures also provide good wound approximation for areas without substantial tissue tension.

Splints (SamSplints, wire mesh splints, or other light but easily adapted splinting materials; fiberglass casting material is an excellent material for splinting.) Inflatable leg and arm splints are light and provide good immobilization, but must be monitored frequently for pressure changes during both ascent and descent.

Tubes, bottles, and and an irrigation syringe for nasogastric intubation should be carried.

## BANDAGES AND DRESSINGS

Litter Packaging (Ensolite or other pad, sleeping bag, tarps, tie-ins)

Spinal immobilization (a full-body vacuum splint in a Stokes Litter with duct tape provides excellent immobilization as well as insulation and protection[i]). Standard backboards are servicable, but uncomfortable for extended evacuations. Additional insulation will be required for these devices.

Additional sterile gauze pads, to include abdominal dressing pads for management of larger wounds.

Additional eye pads

Additional triangular bandages

Additional elastic bandages

Additional moleskin

---

[g]Murphy, A noted exponent of critical component failure philosophy would have us take 4 radios and 10 battery packs to expect 2 working radios at the end of a three day sojourn.

[h]Wound irrigation may use any source of clean water. Water brought to a boil for 10 minutes, or that from a backcountry micropore water filter, is ideal. A small bit of salt (i.e., adding a standard fast-food restaurant salt packet to a liter of water) will bring the irrigation solution nearer to isotonic and minimize wound edema from irrigation.

[i]Such devices may be purchased through Med-Tech, 9833 Belmont, Bellflower, CA 90706 and numerous other suppliers of gear for emergency medical services.

Additional adhesive tape
Electronic rectal thermometer Kit (a remote-eading indoor-outdoor thermometer with a rectal temperature probe[j])
Device for providing warm, humidified air or oxygen
Heat adding device[k]
Sterile gloves
Sterile lubricant jelly
Plastic sheeting to protect dressings from rain or mud

## MISCELLANEOUS EQUIPMENT

Stethoscope
Otoscope/ophthalmoscope kit (both Propper and Welch/Allyn make excellent small kits that work on AA or AAA batteries)
Flashlight (headlamp preferred) with extra batteries
Sphygmomanometer
Tongue blades
Hot water bottle
Ring cutter
Strong wire cutters
"EMT" scissors
Duct tape (Military "100 MPH tape")

## IV EQUIPMENT[l]

Ringer's Lactate (4 Liters)
Normal Saline (4 Liters) (50% dextrose from the drug pack may be added to make up $D_5NS$ for patients who need the dextrose, i.e., those 18 to 36 hours or more after severe trauma.)

---

[j]Inexpensive indoor-outdoor thermometers are available from suppliers such as Radio Shack but must be treated with care, must be calibrated against a known standard thermometer, and the readout box must be kept from extremes of temperature. However, at $15 and 2 ounces per unit, they fit most wilderness search and rescue teams' financial and weight budgets admirably.
[k]Multiple devices designed to rewarm or ward off hypothermia have been proposed from sarong-like garments to plumbed garments with circulating hot water. None of these garments or devices are without substantial weight and safety considerations. Use of a hot charcoal heater in a dry forest area, for example, may change a "simple" rescue into a fire rescue. Increased weight of plumbing and heating devices may be prohibitive. Choice of which heat adding device to use is left to the discretion of the rescue squad.
[l]One hears of military and NASA attempts to provide filter systems so that water may be purified of both pathogenic organisms and pyrogenic materials. This would allow wilderness rescue teams to carry several bags, empty of all but a pinch of salt or sugar, and fill them with water purified at the scene, eliminating the weight of IV solutions. Alas, such systems are not yet available to wilderness search and rescue teams.

$D_5W$ 500 cc
Plasma or plasma expanders
IV catheters e.g.,
#4—18 gauge short
2—18 gauge long
4—14 gauge short
4—16 gauge short
Accessory supplies (e.g., tape, silk sutures for securing lines, tourniquets, dressings, infusion sets, blood warming tubing, and heat packs and small strips of closed-cell foam for warming)

Depending upon the skill and expertise of the medical attendants, equipment for insertion of central lines may be carried. For field insertion of central lines, external jugular and groin lines are preferred due to the lessened complication rates (in the short term).

## DRUGS

The choice of drugs depends on the patient population, the medications carried in members' personal MEDKITs, and the preference of the operational medical director. This list is, therefore, designed to complement the member's personal MEDKIT. Some items may be kept on standby for airlift as needed or added to the kit based on knowledge of a specific victim's medical problems. Examples include insulin, antivenin, and specific anticonvulsants. Quantity of each medication provided depends greatly upon the situation and is, therefore, entirely at the discretion of the team and medical advisors. A physician should be consulted when determining the quantities and dosages of the items to be included.

Albuterol or terbutaline inhaler
Aminophylline (IV and PO)
Atropine (IV)
Bretylium tosylate (IV) (This is the only antiarrhythmic thought to be effective in hypothermic patients.)
Cephalosporin antibiotic (IV or IM) (Ceftriaxone is an excellent choice.)
Dexamethasone (IV and PO)
Dextrose solution 50% (IV)
Diazepam or lorazepam (IV and PO)
Diphenhydramine (IV and PO)
Dopamine or dobutamine (IV)
Epinephrine (IV or SQ) (for weight reasons, only carry 1:1000)
Furosemide (IV and PO)
Glucagon (IV)
Haloperidol (IM and PO)

Lidocaine (IV, can be used as local anesthetic)
Mannitol (IV)
Metronidazole (IV and PO)
Morphine sulfate or other potent narcotic (PO, IV and SQ)
Naloxone (IV)
Nitroglycerine tablets or spray
Oxytocin (IV)
Phenobarbital (IV and PO)
Phenytoin (IV and PO)
Propanolol (IV)
Sodium bicarbonate (IV and PO)
Sunburn screen (18+ SPF minimum)

The following items are appropriate only in certain areas and should generally be obtained just before the mission.

Antimalarials (specific for area)
Antiparasitic agents (specific for area)
Snake antivenom (specific for area snakes)

## SURVIVAL AND RESCUE GEAR

Survival and rescue gear is not listed. Since each area and rescue presents individual problems and requires specific gear, it was felt that local agencies should best describe the gear needed for the survival and rescue efforts. If air resupply is available, extra survival gear may be obtained as needed.

## APPENDIX C: WILDERNESS EMS CONTACTS

Appalachian Search and Rescue Conference (ASRC)
P.O. Box 440 Newcomb Station
Charlottesville, VA 22904
1-804-674-2400 (Emergency Only)

ASTM
(Committee F-30 on Emergency Medical Services)
(Committee F-32 on Search and Rescue)
1916 Race Street
Philadelphia, PA 19103
1-215-299-5400

Mountain Rescue Association
P.O. Box 2513
Yakima, WA 98907-2513

National Association for Search and Rescue
P.O. Box 3709
Fairfax, VA 22038
1-703-352-1349

National Cave Rescue Commission
Don Pacquette, National Coordinator,
835 Hickory Drive
Bloomington, IN 47401

National Cave Rescue Commission
Noel Sloane, National Medical Advisor,
5243 Luzzone #609
Indianapolis, IN 46220

National Ski Patrol System
Warren Bowman, M.D.
National Medical Advisor
Box 35100
Billings, MT 59107-5100

Wilderness Medical Associates
RFD 2 Box 890
Bryant Pond, ME 04219
1-207-665-2707

Wilderness Medical Society
P.O. Box 397
Point Reyes Station, CA 94956

Acknowledgments

Portions of this Chapter were adapted from publications of the ASRC-CEM Wilderness Emergency Medicine Curriculum Development Project and from published materials of the Groups of the Appalachian Search and Rescue Conference, with permission.

## Suggested Readings

Appalachian Search and Rescue Conference. Training Guide, 3rd ed. Charlottesville, VA: Appalachian Search and Rescue Conference, 1980.

Auerbach PS, Geehr EC. Management of wilderness and environmental emergencies, 2nd ed. New York: MacMillan, 1988.

Auerbach PS. Medicine for the outdoors: a guide to emergency medical procedures and first aid. Boston: Little, Brown, 1986.

Breyfogle ND. The common sense medical guide and outdoor reference. New York: McGraw-Hill, 1981.

Burton AC, Edholm OC. Man in a cold environment: physiological and pathological effects of exposure to low temperatures. London: Edward Arnold, 1955. Reprint, New York: Hafner Publishing Co., 1969.

Cooper D. It's about time: the fundamental SAR skills course. Response 1985;4(Nov/Dec):19–25.

Darvill FT. Mountaineering medicine—a wilderness medical guide, 9th ed. Mount Vernon, WA: Skagit Mountain Rescue Unit, 1980.

Department of Emergency Services, Commonwealth of Virginia. Search and rescue training and certification program. Part 1. Ground search and rescue. Richmond, VA: Commonwealth of Virginia, 1986.

Forgey WW. Hypothermia: death by exposure. Merrillville, IN: Indiana Camp Supply Books, 1985.

Forgey WW. Wilderness medicine. Merrillville, IN: Indiana Camp Supply Books, 1979.

Goldsmith MF. Physicians enamored of the adventurous life make the great outdoors safer for all. JAMA 256(23):3197- 3199, 1986.

Goodman PH, Kurtz KJ, Carmichael J. Medical recommendations for wilderness travel. 1. Health maintenance in the great outdoors. Postgrad Med 1985; 77(June):173–184.

Goth P. Wilderness EMT: Evaluation of a new curriculum. Response 1985; 4(Sep/Oct):21–29.

Green WG. Search and rescue for EMTs. Newport News, VA: VASI, 1986.

Hackett PH. Mountain sickness: prevention, recognition, and treatment. New York: American Alpine Club, 1980. (American Alpine Club Climber's Guide).

Hunt TK. Epidemiology of rockclimbing injuries in yosemite. Wilderness Medicine 1986; 3(Oct): 6–7

Johnson TS, Rock PB, Fulco CS, et al. Prevention of acute mountain sickness by dexamethasone. N Engl J Med, 1984; 310:683–686.

Kaufman TI; Knopp R; Webster T. The Parkmedic program: pre-hospital care in the national parks. Ann Emerg Med 1981;10:156–160.

Larson EB, Roach RC, Schoene RB, Hornbein TF. Acute mountain sickness and acetazolamide: Clinical Efficacy and Effect on Ventilation. JAMA 1982; 248:328–332.

Lathrop TG. Hypothermia: killer of the unprepared (revised edition). Portland: Mazamas, 1975.

LeBlanc J. Man in the cold. Springfield, IL: Charles C. Thomas, 1975.

Lentz JM, Macdonald SC; Carline JD. Mountaineering first aid: a guide to accident Response and First Aid Care, 3rd ed. Seattle: The Mountaineers, 1985.

Lloyd EL. Hypothermia and cold stress. Rockville, MD: Aspen Systems Corporation, 1986.

Maclean D, Emslie-Smith D. Accidental hypothermia. Oxford: Blackwell Scientific Publications, 1977.

National Association of Diver Medical Technicians. Field guide for the diver medical technician. Bay City, TX: National Association of DiverMedics, 1983.

National Cave Rescue Commission. Manual of U.S. cave rescue techniques. Huntsville, AL: National Cave Rescue Commission, National Speleological Society, 1981.

Popovic V, Popovic P. Hypothermia in biology and medicine. New York, Grune & Stratton, 1974.

Pozos RS, Wittmers LE. The nature and treatment of hypothermia. Minneapolis: University of Minnesota Press, 1983.

Safety and Techniques Committee, National Speleological Society. American caving accidents. Huntsville, AL: National Speleological Society (annual).

Safety Committees, The American Alpine Club and The Alpine Club of Canada. Accidents in North American mountaineering. New York: The American Alpine Club (annual).

Stewart CE. Perspectives in rational management: eelected environmental emergencies. Eden Prairie, MN: Cardinal Health Systems, 1987.

U.S. Army Institute for Military Assistance. U.S. Army Special Forces medical handbook, USA Manual ST 31–91B. Boulder, CO: Paladin Press, 1982.

U.S. Public Health Service. The ship's medicine chest and medical aid at Sea, HEW Publication No. (HSA) 78–2024. Washington, DC: U.S. Government Printing Office, 1978.

Virginia Division of Emergency Medical Services. Rules and regulations of the board of health, Commonwealth of Virginia: emergency medical dervices. Richmond, VA: State Department of Health, 1980.

Wilderness Medical Society. Backcountry first aid workshop, Yosemite Park, November, 1984. (position paper). Point Reyes Station, CA: Wilderness Medical Society, (no date).

Wilkerson JA, Bangs CC, Hayward JS. Hypothermia, frostbite, and other cold injuries: prevention, recognition, and prehospital treatment. Seattle: The Mountaineers, 1986.

Wilkerson JA. Medicine for mountaineering, 3rd ed. Seattle: The Mountaineers, 1985.

## References

1. Conover K. Wilderness emergency medicine curriculum development project: prospectus. Pittsburgh, PA: Appalachian Search and Rescue Conference, and Center for Emergency Medicine of Western PA, 1987.

2. Conover K, and members of the Appalachian Search and Rescue Conference, Inc. Changes to the Virginia emergency medical services regulations regarding wilderness emergency medical services: a draft proposal. Charlottesville, VA: ASRC, 1987.

# Prevention of Arthropod Envenomation

## INTRODUCTION

There are but three ways by which we can protect ourselves from arthropod bites or envenomation: kill the insect, spoil the insect's meal, or deny the insect entry into our skin. These three methods correspond, roughly, to insecticides, insect repellents, and barrier protection.

## Insecticides

Insecticides such as DDT or malathion are more useful in agriculture and area protection. It is unlikely that the wilderness traveler in small groups will employ these area insecticide agents as a protection from arthropods. Permathrin, a derivative of the pyrethrum flower, may be a useful insecticide for application to the individual's clothing and is discussed below.

## Repellents

An insect repellent is a chemical that causes the insects to redirect their path away from the subject. They should not be confused with insecticides, which kill the insect. Insect repellents merely discourage the animals from biting. The ideal repellent should be chemically stable over long periods of time, effective against multiple arthropods, nondamaging to applied surfaces (including both skin and clothes), nontoxic to humans, and esthetically pleasing in taste, smell, and color. This ideal repellent does not exist.[1]

---

### Self-protection From Bites and Stings

Remain indoors during late afternoon, early evening, and night, if possible. Plan outside activities during these times to take place in screened-in areas.

Do not wear brightly colored clothing. Bright, floral prints are attractive to stinging insects.

Avoid flowers and flowering or fruiting trees and shrubs. Although this will not protect from mosquitoes, it will decrease the possibility of bee or wasp stings.

Cover skin with clothing if possible. Lightweight and tight-fitting garments may present little or no obstacle to some mosquitoes, so application of repellent to clothing is recommended.

Keep sweet foods and drinks covered. Stay away from garbage bins or pits, and keep all garbage securely wrapped in plastic.

Apply insect repellents to skin surfaces and clothing. (When venturing into tick-infested areas, treat cuffs, socks, and shoe tops as well as clothing.)

Use of small, open containers of beer or soda some distance away from the picnic area or campsite may give the insects their feast and allow them to avoid you.

Current insect repellents are useful in prevention of mosquito, flea, tick, and fly bites. They are not effective in prevention of stings such as from bees, wasps, and yellow jackets.

The two major repellents available are N,N-diethyl-*m*-toluamide (DEET or *m*-DET) and ethyl hexanediol (Rutgers 612). Both repellents are effective against the common biting insects in the United States. DEET has a longer duration of action than ethyl hexanediol, but both can be washed away by water or sweat. Ounce for ounce, DEET is longer lasting and repels a broader spectrum of pests.[2]

The action, site, or mode of known insect repellents in repelling or redirection of insects is unknown.[3,4] DEET may interfere with the initial absorption of lactic acid to the mosquito's sensory organs, but the mechanism is still speculative. Lactic acid is known to be a "host attractant" molecule evaporating from all warm-blooded animals. Since lactic acid is thought to be an attractant for chiggers, ticks, fleas, some flies, and mosquitoes, insect repellents are somewhat effective against all of these species.

Despite this cross-reactivity, compounds useful for repelling mosquitoes are not necessarily the most effective for other species. Other compounds recently have been found to be more effective as tick repellents than DEET.[5,6] It is hoped that these more effective agents will soon be available commercially.

Theoretically, the more DEET in the formula, the longer lasting the protection. Solutions of DEET stronger than 50 or 55% probably have little greater effectiveness than 50% DEET. One study involving troops felt that repellents with 75% DEET were sufficient to adequately protect against disease-carrying mosquitoes.[7] The more concentrated solutions are also more likely to feel uncomfortably oily.

Repellents are available in a variety of forms from aerosols to wipe-on tissues. Clothing impregnated with DEET (e.g., "Shoo Bug") is also available. Be certain to cover all exposed areas with repellent. Mosquitoes need only an area about 2 cm square—the size of a dime—in order to feed. Cream or lotion repellents that are directly applied are probably the best. Sprays are more popular, but only about 60% of the solution makes it to your skin, and this must then be spread around.

DEET and other insect repellents are washed off skin surfaces by swimming, sweating, and rain. Application of the repellent to clothing will increase the duration of action. Heat and activity will decrease the protection time by increasing the evaporation of the repellent.[8] When the insect repellent wears off, insects will gradually become bolder. Finally, they will land for short times and then will start to bite. Without rain or sweat this will occur in 3 to 14 hours with 75% solutions of DEET. This is time to apply a new coating.

## REPELLENT ADDITIVES

Some manufacturers add dimethyl phthalate (DMP), which theoretically protects more against chiggers and ticks. DEET is fairly effective against both pests, so it is dubious whether DMP adds anything to the solution.

Permathrin, an extract of the pyrethrum flower, is a good adjunct to DEET, particularly in areas where ticks abound.[9,10] Permathrin is an odorless insecticide, rather than a repellent. It is available as Permanone Tick Repellent and should be sprayed on clothing. It is thought to be a valuable adjunct to DEET since it will kill mosquitoes and other insects, rather than merely annoying them. Permathrin may be more effective against crawling insects than DEET. Impregnation of clothing with permathrim will also enhance the effectiveness of DEET against mosquitoes, since the local mosquito count is reduced.[11]

### Untested Repellents

Some authors advocate oral B-complex vitamins as insect repellents.[12] Oral administration of 75 to 150 mg of thiamine daily is thought to produce a body odor offensive to insects. The thiamine is excreted in sweat with variable results. There are no controlled studies, and evidence appears entirely anecdotal. If insects are noted to be biting despite the thiamine, perhaps another method should be considered.

Electronic devices that purport to repel mosquitoes by emitting an irritating buzzing sound are not effective. The sound waves are completely outside the hearing range of the mosquito. Electronic blacklight "zappers" are more effective against harmless moths and beetles than against pests. For this reason, the zappers are most effective in an enclosed area.

Finally, several insecticides such as Raid and Black Flag, Skin-So-Soft (a mineral oil product by Avon), and dog or cat flea collars have been used by some for their insect repellent features. Use of these untested and undocumented agents may be fraught with hazard and should be avoided.[13] Schreck and Kline have reported that Skin-So-Soft is effective in prevention of biting midges by entrapment in the mineral oil base.[14] It is difficult to logically advocate the use of full-strength application of a product designed to be added by the capful to a bathtub of water, without further testing. Sunscreens and lanolin-based creams and lotions may provide a similar mode of barrier protection from midges with well-tested products.

---

**Concentration of DEET in Some Insect Repellents***

| | |
|---|---|
| 6/12 Plus spray | 5 (25% ethyl hexanediol) |
| 6/12 Plus stick | 9 (56% ethyl hexanediol) |
| 6/12 Plus liquid | 10 (80% ethyl hexanediol) |
| OFF regular spray | 14 |
| Cutter's regular spray | 17 |
| Cutter's evergreen spray | 17 |
| OFF Deep Woods Spray | 20 |
| Muskol Spray | 25 |
| Cutter's liquid | 22 |
| OFF Deep Woods lotion | 30 |
| OFF disposable towels | 25 |
| Cutter's stick | 33 |
| Cutter's cream | 35 |
| Repel spray | 40 |
| Repel lotion | 55 |
| Sportsmate II Premium | 55 |
| Skram | 74.5 |
| Space-Shield II | 75 |
| Military Insect Repellent | 75 |
| Muskol | 95 |
| Ben's 100 Lotion | 100 |
| Cutter Formula 100 | 100 |
| Deep Woods Off (maximum) | 100 |
| Skeeter Stop 100 | 100 |
| Repel 100 | 100 |
| Muskol Maximum Strength | 100 |
| Tecnu 10-Hour Repellent | 100 |

---

*Compiled from multiple sources and manufacturers.

---

## COMPLICATIONS

Local and systemic toxic effects of insect repellents are reported only rarely in humans. Most reports are about DEET, probably since it is the active ingredient in virtually all insect repellents on the market. As use of alternative and newer agents increase, one may expect more reports of complications found with these repellents.

DEET is absorbed through intact skin and as much as 9% of the dose applied may be absorbed.[15] Absorption is rapid; 48% of the topical dose is absorbed within 6 hours, and the highest plasma levels occur within 1 hour. When concentrated solutions are applied, there is a distinct possibility of systemic toxicity. Preparations containing less than 50% DEET appear to have fewer side effects in adults.[16]

Prior studies have emphasized that DEET causes little skin irritation or reaction. A growing body of literature now notes that the application of DEET may be associated with a number of potentially serious rashes and irritations. Many of these studies were performed with solutions of less than 50% concentration.

### Dermatitis

In both children and adults, localized dermatitis and urticaria have been noted with use of lower concentrations of DEET.[17,18] Papular urticaria is often thought to be due to the biting arthropods but, in fact, may be due to the application of DEET.[19] More concentrated solutions have caused erythema, bullous skin necrosis, and scarring in up to 40% of adults who apply DEET to sensitive areas such as the antecubital fossa.[18,20]

### Encephalopathy

Repeated and extensive application of 20% or greater solutions of DEET to children (and more rarely to adults) has been purported to cause encephalopathy. This encephalopathy was manifested by altered behavior, staggering gait, agitation, tremors, restlessness, and seizures, and has been fatal in isolated cases.[21–24] In these cases, multiple applications of DEET were noted, but DEET and metabolite levels were not measured. In one of the cases, a deficiency of ornithine-carbamoyl-transferase was noted and was thought to have precipitated the reaction.[25,26] Solutions of 70% DEET applied daily for 2 weeks have been implicated in acute manic psychosis in adults.[27,28] Cutaneous applications of as little as 1 to 2 ml of 50% concentration have caused paresthesias in humans.[19]

A toxic reaction should be considered when a patient, particularly a child, presents with bizzare neurologic symptoms and has a history of exposure to DEET. Since insect repellents are generally not noted in medical histories, the examiner must be careful to elicit this data. Treatment is entirely supportive, and only symptomatic care is advised. There is no specific therapy for the complications caused by DEET.

## Ingestion

Ingestion of DEET can cause convulsions, coma, hypotension, and respiratory depression.[16] The case fatality rate of ingestions may be as high as 40%. Anaphylaxis has been noted with cutaneous application of DEET but is quite uncommon.[29]

## PRECAUTIONS

Frequent application to large exposed surfaces for days or weeks should be avoided. DEET solutions greater than 50% should not be used in children and infants because of the increased potential for absorption. Unless traveling to an area where disease-carrying pests abound, solutions greater than 75% concentration are not useful. Outer clothes impregnated with DEET will provide similar protection without significant skin contact.[30–33]

A final note: DEET is safe on cotton, wool, and nylon. Synthetics like spandex, rayon, and acetate can be destroyed both by DEET and by many of the solvents it is mixed in. DEET and solvents may also destroy watch crystals, plastic eyeglasses, and some polyester fabrics.

## Barrier Protection

Long-sleeve clothing, trousers, and hats will reduce the surface area available for mosquitoes to bite. Pants tightly tucked into boots and sleeves rolled down and buttoned will likewise decrease the available area for ticks to bite. Although ticks are not able to bite through clothing, mosquitoes are able to penetrate tight-fitting and loose-weave clothes. As noted above, impregnation of clothing with repellents will markedly increase the protection afforded by garments. Desert dwellers become accustomed to shaking out clothes and boots prior to donning them, thus preventing scorpion bites.

Bed nets or mosquito nets provide substantial protection from nocturnal insect bites. In one study, use of bed nets in a malaria-endemic area decreased the incidence of parasitemia by 50%.[34] Impregnation of the insect netting with permathrim or other repellent/insecticide would logically increase the protection of the netting.[35–37]

## Area Protection From Insect Stings and Bites

These devices and strategies are useful only in fixed camps or homesites. It usually is not possible to use area protections while in the wilderness.

The first line of control of mosquitoes is to eliminate the standing water that becomes a breeding area. Eliminate water-containing receptacles near homes and play areas.

Treat breeding sites with appropriate insecticides. Failing that, the areas may be covered with oily substances that prevent the larvae's siphon from obtaining oxygen. In urban areas, birdbaths, swimming pools, gutters, and tree stumps are common breeding areas. Stagnant ponds and marshes are classic outback breeding areas, but even small surface water puddles may harbor larvae.

Use insect repellents such as citronella candles or mosquito coils.[38] These ancient devices work by burning a joss or incense stick-like base with mosquito repellent or insecticide contained in the base. The active substances are then slowly released in the smoke.[39,40] The insecticide is distributed through a spatial volume to deter the offending arthropods. These coils and candles do show substantial effectiveness within closed spaces, such as houses or tents, but are ineffective in open spaces.

## References

1. Reifenrath WG, Rutledge LC. Evaluation of mosquito repellent formulations. J Pharm Sci 1983;72:169–173.
2. Robbins PJ, Cherniack MG. Review of the biodistribution and toxicity of the insect repellent N,N-Diethyl-m-toluamide (DEET). J Toxicol Environ Health 1986;18:503–525.
3. Weiss R. The sound of no mosquitoes biting. Science News 1988;134(3):37.
4. Davis EE. Insect repellents: concepts of their mode of action relative to potential sensory mechanisms in mosquitoes (Diptera:culicidae). J Med Entomol 1985;22:237–243.
5. Skinner WA, Rosentreter U, Elward T. Tick repellents. I. Ethylene glycol acetamides. J Pharm Sci 1983;71:837–839.
6. Skinner WA, Rosentreter U, Elward T. Tick repellents. II. N-substituted azacyclopentanones and azacylopentanones. J Pharm Sci 1983;72:1354–1356.
7. Hooper RL, Wirtz RA. Insect repellent used by troops in the field: results of a questionaire. Milit Med 1983;148:34–38.
8. Reifenrath WG, Robinson PB. In vitro skin evaporation and penetration characteristics of mosquito repellents. J Pharm Sci 1983;71:1014–1018.
9. Schreck CD, Snoddy EL, Spielman A. Pressurized sprays of Permethrin or DEET on military clothing for personal protection against *Ioxodes dammini* (Acari:Ixodidae). J Med Entomol 1986;23:396–399.
10. Mehr ZA, Rutledge LC, Morales EL, Inase JL. Laboratory evaluation of commercial and experimental repellents against *Ornithodoros parkeri* (Acari:Argasidae) J Med Entomol 1986;23:136–140.
11. Schreck CE, Haile DG, Kline DL. The effectiveness of permethrin and DEET, alone or in combination, for protection against *Aedes aeniorhynchus*. J Trop Med Hyg 1984;33:725–730.
12. Honig PJ. Arthopod bites, stings, and infestations: their prevention and treatment. Pediatr Dermatol 1986;3:189–197.
13. Sundlof SF, Mayhew IG. A neuroparalytic syndrome assocated with an oral flea repellent containing diethanolamine. Vet Hum Toxicol 1983;25:247.
14. Schreck CE. Kline DL. Repellency determinations of four commercial products against six species of ceratopogonid biting midges. Mosq News 1981;41:7–10.
15. Feldman RJ, Maibach HI. Absorption of some organic compounds through the skin in man. J Invest Dermatol 1970;54:399–404.
16. Are insect repellents safe? [Editorial] Lancet 1988;2:610–611.
17. Maibach HI, Johnson HL. Contact urticaria to diethyltoluamide. Arch Dermatol 1975;111:726–730.
18. Rueveni H, Yagupsky P. Diethyltoluamide-containing insect repellent: adverse effects in worldwide use. Arch Dermatol 1982;118:852–854.
19. Mack RB. Lord of the flies, fleas and mosquitos—DEET (Diethyltoluamide intoxication) NC Med J 1986;47:353–354.
20. Lamberg SI, Mulrennan JA. Bullous reaction to diethyl toluamide (DEET). Arch Dermatol 1969;100:582–586.
21. Edwards DL, Johnson CE. Insect-repellent-induced toxic encephalopathy in a child. Clin Pharm 1987;6:494–498
22. Gryboski J, Weinstein D, Ordway NK. Toxic encephalopathy apparently related to the use of an insect repellent. N Engl J Med 1961;264:289–291.
23. Roland EH, Jan JE, Rigg JM. Toxic encephalopathy in a child after brief exposure to insect repellents. Can Med Assoc J 1985;132:155–156.
24. de Garbino JP, Laborde A. Toxicity of an insect repellent; N-N-diethyltoluamide. Vet Hum Toxicol 1983;25:422–423.
25. Heick HMC, Shipman RT, Chir B, et al. Rey-like syndrome associated with use of insect repellent in a presumed hetercygote for ornithine carbamoyl transferase deficiency. J Pediatr 1980;97:471–472.
26. Heick HMC, Peterson RG, Dalpe-Scott M, et al. Insect repellent, N,N-diethyl-*m*-toluamide, effect on ammonia metabolism. Pediatrics 1988;82:373–376.
27. Snyder JW, Poe RO, Stubbins, Garrettson LK. Acute manic psychosis following the dermal application of N, N-diethyl-*m*-toluamide (DEET) in an adult. Clin Toxicol 1986;24:429–439.
28. Poe RO, Snyder JW, Stubbins JF, Garretson LK. Letters to the editor: psychotic reaction to an insect repellent. Am J Psychiatry 1987;144:1103–1104.
29. Miller JD. Anaphylaxis associated with insect repellent [Letter]. N Engl J Med 1982;307:1341–1342.
30. Harlan HJ, Schreck CE, Kline DL. Insect repellent jacket tests against biting midges (Diptera: culicoides) in Panama. Am J Trop Med Hyg 1983;115:185–188.
31. Grothaus RH, Haskins JR, Schreck CE, Gouck

HK. Insect repellent jacket: status, value and potential. Mosq News 1976;36:11–18.

32. Curtis CF. Letters to the editor: making insect repellents safe. Lancet 1988;2:1020.

33. Curtis CF, Lines JD, Ijumba J, et al. The relative efficacy of repellents against mosquito vectors of disease. Med Vet Entomol 1987;1:109–119.

34. Bradley AK, Greenwood AM, Byass P, et al. Bed-nets (mosquito-nets) and morbidity from malaria. Lancet 1986;:204–207.

35. Ranque P, Toure Y, Soula G, et al. Use of mosquito nets impregnated with deltamethrin in malaria control. Abstract of a paper presented at the Xth Conference of Tropical Medicine and Malaria, Calgary, 1984.

36. Lines JD, Myamba J, Curtis CF. Experimental hut trials of permethrin-impregnated mos-quito nets and eave curtains against malaria vectors in Tanzania. Med Vet Entomol 1987;1:37–51.

37. Snow RW, Rowan KM, Greenwood BM. A trial of permethrin-treated bed nets in the prevention of malaria in Gambian children. Trans R Soc Trop Med Hyg 1987;81:563–567.

38. Charlwood JD, Jolley D. The coil works (against mosquitoes in Papua New Guinea). Trans R Soc Trop Med Hyg 1984;78:678.

39. Liu K, Wong MH, Mui YL. Toxic effects of mosquito coil (a mosquito repellent smoke on rats). I. Properties of the mosquito coil and its smoke. Toxicol Lett 1987;39:223–230.

40. Liu K, Wong MH, Mui YL. Toxic effects of mosquito coil (a mosquito repellent smoke on rats). II. Morphological changes of the respiratory system. Toxicol Lett 1987;39:231–239.

# Index

Page numbers in *italics* denote figures; those followed by "t" denote tables.